Current Medical Therapy

Current Medical Therapy

Editor

Robert W. Schrier, M.D.
Professor and Chairman
Department of Medicine
University of Colorado School of Medicine
Denver, Colorado

Raven Press ■ New York

Raven Press, 1140 Avenue of the Americas, New York, New York 10036

Made in the United States of America

Library of Congress Cataloging in Publication Data
Main entry under title:

Current medical therapy.

"Written entirely by faculty of the University of
Colorado School of Medicine"—Pref.
Includes bibliographical references and index.
1. Therapeutics. I. Schrier, Robert W. II. University of Colorado at Denver. School of Medicine.
[DNLM: 1. Therapeutics—Handbooks. WB 39 M489]
RM121.M47   1984   615.5   84-6800
ISBN 0-89004-548-8

The material contained in this volume was submitted as previously unpublished material, except in the instances in which credit has been given to the source from which some of the illustrative material was derived.

Great care has been taken to maintain the accuracy of the information contained in the volume. However, Raven Press cannot be held responsible for errors or for any consequences arising from the use of the information contained herein.

Preface

The handbook *Current Medical Therapy* was written entirely by faculty of the University of Colorado School of Medicine. These faculty members have substantial clinical experience and expertise and are dedicated and effective teachers. The commitment of the authors and the editor was to provide a high quality handbook of medical therapeutics for medical students, houseofficers, primary care physicians, and other medical professionals.

A practical clinical approach to medical therapeutics (including the major areas of internal medicine) is emphasized by the authors. The handbook also addresses areas of medical therapeutics that are frequently neglected by primary care internists including dermatological and neuropsychiatric disorders and preventive medicine. Tables are used where conciseness is advantageous and important general references are listed at the end of each chapter. Primary and alternative treatments are discussed including their side effects. When various therapies are commonly used but their efficacy has not been well documented, the authors have so stated. When appropriate, differences in the therapeutic costs are presented. The handbook includes information on both inpatient and outpatient therapeutics. Mechanisms of disease have been emphasized when such knowledge is an important basis for judicious therapy. Lastly, it should be stressed that this therapeutics handbook provides only guidelines which must be individualized for each patient; it cannot replace expert consultation when necessary. In this context, we expect that *Current Medical Therapy* will provide a unique vehicle to assist the physician in the implementation of the most timely, efficacious, safe and cost effective therapy once a specific diagnosis has been made.

Robert W. Schrier

Contents

Contributors

University of Colorado School of Medicine
4200 East 9th Avenue
Denver, Colorado 80262

Martin J. Blaser, M.D.
Assistant Professor of Medicine
Division of Infectious Diseases;
and
Denver Veterans Administration
Medical Center

Thomas J. Braun, M.D.
Assistant Professor of Medicine
Division of Medical Oncology; and
Denver Veterans Administration
Medical Center

Boris Draznin, M.D.
Assistant Professor of Medicine
Division of Endocrinology; and
Denver Veterans Administration
Medical Center

Steven L. Dubovsky, M.D.
Associate Professor of Psychiatry
and Medicine

Richard T. Ellison III, M.D.
Instructor of Medicine
Division of Infectious Diseases;
and
Denver Veterans Administration
Medical Center

Gregory T. Everson, M.D.
Assistant Professor of Medicine
Division of Gastroenterology

Lawrence E. Feinberg, M.D.
Associate Professor of Medicine
Division of Internal Medicine

John Goff, M.D.
Assistant Professor of Medicine
Division of Gastroenterology

Ute Hasiba, M.D.
Associate Professor of Medicine
Division of Hematology

Kenneth Hossack, M.D.
Associate Professor of Medicine
Division of Cardiology; and
Attending Physician
Denver General Hospital

J. Clark Huff, M.D.
Associate Professor of
Dermatology and Medicine

Martin P. Hutt, M.D.
Professor of Medicine
Division of Renal Diseases

William D. Kaehny, M.D.
Associate Professor of Medicine
Division of Renal Diseases; and
Denver Veterans Administration
    Medical Center

Talmadge E. King, Jr., M.D.
Assistant Professor of Medicine
Division of Cardiology; and
Denver Veterans Administration
    Medical Center

Brian L. Kotzin, M.D.
Assistant Professor of Medicine
Division of Rheumatology; and
Denver Veterans Administration
    Medical Center

Stuart L. Linas, M.D.
Associate Professor of Medicine
Division of Renal Diseases; and
Attending Physician
Denver General Hospital

Thomas J. Meyer, M.D.
Assistant Professor of Medicine
Division of Internal Medicine; and
Denver Veterans Administration
    Medical Center

Michael J. Reiter, M.D.
Assistant Professor of Medicine
Division of Cardiology

Richard Robbins, M.D.
Assistant Professor of Medicine
Division of Endocrinology

Neil L. Rosenberg, M.D.
Assistant Professor of Neurology;
    and
Attending Physician
Denver General Hospital

Craig N. Sadur, M.D.
Assistant Professor of Medicine
Division of Endocrinology; and
Attending Physician
Denver General Hospital

Alan L. Schocket, M.D.
Assistant Professor of Medicine
Division of Clinical Immunology;
    and
Associate Director of Internal
    Medicine
Presbyterian/St. Luke's Medical
    Center

Robert W. Schrier, M.D.
Professor and Chairman
Department of Medicine

Allen J. Sedman, M.D.
Assistant Professor of Medicine
Division of Internal Medicine

James C. Steigerwald, M.D.
Associate Professor of Medicine
Division of Rheumatology

Current Medical Therapy

1.

General Care of the Medical Patient

Lawrence E. Feinberg

1.

General Care of the Medical Patient

I. HOSPITAL ORDERS

A. Routine Orders

1. Admitting diagnoses and medical condition.

2. Allergies.

3. **Vital signs.** Observe standard monitoring of temperature, pulse, respiration, and blood pressure (BP). Consider measurements of orthostatic pulse and BP changes, checks of neurologic signs, and reasons to contact a physician—i.e., specify allowable variations in vital signs or maximum doses of p.r.n. medications. Avoid unnecessarily frequent monitoring that might disturb the patient's rest and sleep.

4. **Diet.** Specify consistency (liquid versus solid); specific restrictions such as sodium, protein, or lactose; need for snacks or supplements; or other specific modifications (i.e., high-fiber, kosher, vegetarian, etc.). Ideally, hospital meals should conform to the patient's long-term nutritional program (see Chapter 21).

5. **Activity.** Mobilize the patient as much as possible. Deep breathing, regular turning, range-of-motion exercises, sitting in a chair, and assisted walking promote well-being and serve to lower the incidence of decubiti, venous thrombosis, atelectasis, and pneumonia.

6. **Specific nursing instructions.** Intake and output, serial weights, skin or wound care, respiratory measures, checking stools for occult blood, urine testing, blood glucose monitoring, abdominal girth measurements, seizure precautions, and isolation.

7. **Intravenous fluids.** Composition of fluids, rate of administration, and dosage of constituents (i.e., potassium chloride, multivitamins).

8. **Medications.** Dosage, frequency, and route of administration (see II. A.).

9. **Admission laboratory tests.** There is no routine admission test battery; testing must be individualized. A complete blood count, urinalysis, biochemical survey, electrocardiogram, and chest radiograph are obtained in most patients. The overall yield of admission **screening** tests in terms of important new diagnoses is very small; the physician must guard against overinterpretation and pursuit of possibly false-positive screening tests. No daily or standing orders for laboratory test should be written.

3

10. Consultations. Consider input from physical and occupational therapists, social worker, substance-abuse counselor, nutritionist, visiting nurse coordinator, etc.

11. Medical orders should be reevaluated frequently.

B. **Common Medication Orders**

1. Prevent constipation and fecal impaction.

   a. Maintain maximum tolerable level of in-hospital activity.

   b. Provide a high-fiber diet (cereals, raw fruits, and vegetables).

   c. If necessary, prescribe a psyllium hydrophilic bulk-forming preparation (Metamucil®, Modane®, Effersyllium®) initially 1 to 2 teaspoons in water or juice, ingested immediately after the largest meal.

   d. Routine use of docusate (Colace®, DDS®, etc.) is not justified; it is less physiologic, less effective, and less compatible with the longer-term benefits of fiber.

2. **Bedtime sedation.** The unfamiliar hospital environment and the anxiety related to illness may necessitate hypnotic medication. Nonetheless, one should always explore the nature of the in-hospital sleep disturbance.

   a. Avoid unnecessary nighttime measurements of vital signs.

   b. Improve the analgesic program for patients experiencing pain at night or made anxious by inconsistent pain relief.

   c. Avoid sedative hypnotics in patients with dementia or confusion (see III.).

   d. Drugs of choice are the short-acting benzodiazepines:

   (1) Temazepam (Restoril®); dose: 15 to 30 mg h.s.; $t\frac{1}{2} = 5$ to 15 hr.

   (2) Oxazepam; dose: 10 mg h.s.; $t\frac{1}{2} = 5$ to 20 hr.

   e. For elderly patients use temazepam, initially 15 mg 1 hr before bedtime. Triazolam 0.125 mg may be used if the problem is solely in falling asleep and not one of restless or discontinuous sleep. Chloral hydrate 250 to 500 mg is an alternative, but its metabolites may displace drugs such as warfarin and phenytoin from plasma-binding sites and cause extreme hypoprothrombinemia or phenytoin toxicity. **Avoid antihistamines.** They are associated with a higher risk of delirium than are the benzodiazepines.

3. **Heparin prophylaxis.** In order to reduce the incidence of deep vein thrombosis and pulmonary thromboembolism, low-dose heparin prophylaxis is a consideration for all immobilized medical patients who are not at increased risk of bleeding.

   a. The standard dose, initiated on admission, is 5,000 U sodium heparin, s.c., every 12 hr.

   b. **Exclusions:** active bleeding, history of bleeding tendency, ongoing anticoagulant therapy, recent gastrointestinal hemorrhage, active peptic ulcer disease, chronic renal failure, chronic liver disease, severe hypertension (DBP > 120 mm Hg), acute stroke, or pericardial effusion.

   c. Discontinue subcutaneous heparin at the time the patient is fully mobilized or when there is occurrence of side effects possibly related to heparin, appearance of contraindications to heparin, or at the time of hospital discharge.

C. "Do Not Resuscitate" Orders

1. Establish and record when the patient is not a candidate for cardiopulmonary resuscitation (CPR). Otherwise, in the event of cardiac or respiratory arrest, full resuscitative measures would be likely to be undertaken.

2. A decision not to resuscitate is considered for many reasons: the previously stated or current wishes of the patient or family; advanced age of the patient; poor prognosis; severe brain damage; extreme suffering or disability in a chronically or terminally ill patient. The decision-making also must be guided by the input of the patient's ongoing physician. Persons whose underlying condition has steadily progressed to cardiac or respiratory arrest (death) should not necessarily be resuscitated when that event finally occurs.

3. Consider the lack of efficacy of traumatic and time-consuming CPR maneuvers in certain groups of patients; i.e., patients with metastatic cancer have virtually no chance of responding to resuscitative measures and eventually leaving the hospital.

II. PREVENTION OF IN-HOSPITAL COMPLICATIONS

A. Drug Therapy

1. **General comments.** Pharmacotherapy provides remarkable benefits to sick people but often produces adverse effects. At least 15% to 20% of hospitalized patients experience one or more adverse drug reactions during their in-patient stay. These drug reactions may be life-threatening.

2. **Have a clear-cut indication for the administration of any drug.** If the diagnosis is uncertain, a course of watchful waiting is generally preferred to a therapeutic trial. Reserve therapeutic trials for patients who are seriously ill or show a threat to essential organ function. Once such treatment is undertaken, it should be maintained long enough to test its effectiveness conclusively.

3. **Know the action and adverse effects of drugs.** Almost all effective drugs can cause serious adverse effects in some patients. These risks are generally acceptable with serious illnesses. The use of a potentially toxic drug for a minor illness or symptom is generally unacceptable.

4. **Drug dosage must be individualized.** Take into account the patient's age, size, general health, possible hepatic, cardiac, or renal disease, and the expected or observed clinical response. If there is any question about dosage, start with smaller doses and gradually increase, constantly monitoring for efficacy and adverse effects. At the time the drug is started, **explicitly decide how you will measure the effectiveness of drug therapy and monitor for possible toxicity.**

5. **For drugs eliminated predominantly by the kidney,** use formulas to approximate renal function and adjust doses accordingly.

$$\text{Creatinine clearance (Cl}_{Cr}) = \frac{(140 - \text{age}) \times \text{weight (kg)}}{70 \times \text{serum creatinine}}$$

For women multiply the derived Cl_{Cr} by 0.85.

6. **Check the nurses' medication record the day after admission and review this drug record daily.** Any nonessential drug should be eliminated.

7. **Always consider that ongoing or new signs, symptoms, or laboratory abnormalities could be drug-induced. Ask yourself: Could a drug be causing or aggravating this patient's condition?**

8. **Most common types of adverse reactions** and side effects include abnormal mental status, nausea and vomiting, abdominal distress, diarrhea, constipation, rash, or fever.

9. **Drugs most commonly implicated** as a cause of serious adverse effects include

Digoxin	Beta-adrenergic blockers
All antiarrhythmic drugs	Other antihypertensive drugs
Theophylline	Penicillin
Heparin	Benzodiazepines
Warfarin	

10. **Measurement of serum drug concentrations** can help monitor therapy with potentially toxic drugs such as aminoglycosides or theophylline. However, **clinical monitoring and sound judgment remain of utmost importance.** One selects a proper dose and dosing interval, carefully follows the patient for signs of drug efficacy, and observes for adverse drug effects. The most common mistakes involve disregarding signs and symptoms of toxicity because the serum concentration is in the "therapeutic range," or failing to increase the dose in a patient who remains without clinical benefit and without side effects but has a drug level in the middle of the "therapeutic" range. **The goal of drug therapy is to treat the individual patient, not a serum concentration.**

11. **Drug interactions increase with the number of drugs prescribed.** The effect of one drug can be increased or decreased by the previous or concurrent administration of another drug. Drugs such as warfarin, digoxin, theophylline, and sulfonylureas may be involved in life-threatening drug-drug interactions. These are predictable and can be avoided by addressing the possibility of drug interaction every time a new drug is added to an existing drug regimen. One should refer frequently to an accessible reference source on drug-drug interactions.

12. **Newly released drugs** are indicated if an established drug has failed to produce the desired results in a given patient. Be aware that as experience with a new drug accumulates, various kinds of toxicity become manifest, particularly adverse effects that are influenced by disease, drug interactions, or age. These are not likely to be uncovered during preliminary drug trials. **If a new drug is to do no more than an old medication, use the older preparations,** which are likely to be safer and cheaper.

13. **Prescription writing and discharge planning.** Prescriptions should be carefully written. The name of the drug, dosage, amount dispensed, instructions for administration, and legible signature are all important. Label medications according to the indication such as "Clonidine, 0.1 mg, 1 tab p.o., b.i.d. **for high blood pressure.**" At discharge **outline the treatment program and**

explain about potentially significant side effects. If necessary, prepare a sheet or card with individual tablets or capsules taped to the surface with names, indications, and directions for use next to the medication. Involve relatives or friends to help dispense medications to the elderly or disabled. Consider use of a multicompartment container (7 × 4) to allow for a week's dispensing and display of drugs.

B. Catheter Management

1. **General comments.** Medical devices such as intravenous and urinary catheters are a necessary part of high-quality medical care. Unfortunately, these and other intravascular devices are major causes of hospital-acquired infection. They facilitate infection by damaging or invading epithelial and mucosal barriers.

2. **Intravenous catheters**

   a. **Replace plastic catheters after 48 hr.** When percutaneously inserted plastic catheters are left in for longer than 48 hr, the associated septicemia rate ranges between 2% and 5%.

   b. **Insert in aseptic fashion,** with skin cleansed by 1% iodine solution after vigorous scrubbing of the skin. Iodine or iodophores should be allowed to dry for 30 sec, then washed off with 30% alcohol to reduce chance of skin burns (70% alcohol is an acceptable alternative disinfectant). Use sterile gloves and drapes when feasible.

   c. **The catheter should be firmly anchored** after insertion to prevent to-and-fro motion that may facilitate entry of organisms.

   d. **Record the time and date** of catheter insertion on the dressing and in the medical record.

   e. **Reassess the indications for continued i.v. catheterization daily.**

   f. Be mindful that neither topical antibacterial ointments nor systemic antimicrobial therapy protects against catheter-related infection.

   g. **Inspect the insertion site every 24 to 48 hr.** Remove and culture the catheter in the event of local pain or inflammation or clinical signs of sepsis without an obvious source. Removing the catheter is the single most therapeutic maneuver in the management of catheter-related septicemia. Patients who are clinically septic, with purulence that can be expressed from the wound, or those who have positive blood cultures, should receive antibiotic therapy; i.e. an antistaphylococcal drug and an aminoglycoside.

3. **Indwelling urinary bladder catheter**

   a. Short-term catheterization is often necessary in monitoring acutely ill patients who are incontinent or unable to void and whose management demands that urine output be measured. **The catheter should be removed as soon as possible.** Do not use such catheters simply for the convenience of the nursing staff or physician. Long-term catheterization is associated with a high, almost inevitable risk of bacteriuria and possible sepsis.

   b. In order to decrease or minimize the risk of infection, two or three single straight catheterizations over a 48- to 72-hr period may be preferable to insertion of an indwelling catheter. (Avoid this practice in persons with prostate disease or urethral stricture.)

c. When an indwelling catheter is indicated, aseptic insertion and a sterile closed drainage system must be employed. The junction of the catheter and the drainage tube should not be disconnected unless irrigation of an obstructed catheter is necessary. Do not change the catheter unless it malfunctions, leaks, or becomes contaminated or obstructed.

d. Maintain a urine flow exceeding 100 ml/hr if at all possible. Maintain downhill drainage at all times with frequent emptying of the collection bag.

e. Meatal care with povidone-iodine or soap and water solutions does not reduce the incidence of catheter-related infection.

f. Do not treat catheter-associated asymptomatic bacteriuria while the catheter is still in place. Do not use antibiotic irrigants nor antibiotic suppressive therapy during an anticipated short-term catheterization. Continuous antibiotic irrigation has not been shown to be more effective in delaying onset of infection than the careful maintenance of a closed drainage system. Antimicrobial therapy of catheter associated infection generally leads to colonization with resistant organisms.

g. Condom catheters may work well for males who are cooperative or at least are unable to manipulate the drainage system.

C. Prevention and Management of Bed Sores

1. General comments. Pressure sores can lead to debility, deep indolent infections, and polymicrobial sepsis. Pressure, shearing forces, friction, and moisture contribute to the development of these lesions. Most are located in the sacral and coccygeal area, ischial tuberosites, and greater trochanters.

2. Prevention depends on meticulous nursing care. Relief of pressure on bony prominences is the main objective. The patient must be rotated from side to side, back to front, ideally every 2 hr. Bridging with soft pillows relieves pressure at strategic sites. Avoid having the patient dragged or slipping on the bed sheets and prevent or promptly attend to incontinence. If necessary, rocking beds or special fluid-support or air-support systems may be used to prevent or assist healing of ulcers. In summary, **keep the skin clean and dry, and relieve pressure on bony prominences.**

3. Management of established decubiti includes optimal nutrition and general medical care, particularly improved glycemic control in diabetic patients. Pressure is relieved and wound debridement with wet to dry dressings and packing with saline-soaked gauze is accomplished every 4 hr. Fibrinolysin ointment (Elase®) may assist in wound debridement. Surgical intervention may be necessary for deeper or more complex pressure sores.

D. Prevention of Falls

1. General comments. Impairment of postural control and injurious falls are problems for debilitated and elderly hospitalized patients. Changes in baroreceptor sensitivity, proprioception, coordination, and gait, as well as dementia, lack of fitness, and drug side effects may contribute to this problem.

2. **Exercise caution in prescribing CNS-active drugs** to patients who have had prolonged bed rest, postural falls in blood pressure, or complaints of unsteadiness or dizziness, or who have a history of falls or severe musculoskeletal or neurologic disease.

3. Such patients should be referred to physical therapists for training and balance exercises. Walking aids such as canes and walkers should be encouraged where appropriate.

III. ANALGESIC THERAPY

A. **General Comments** The goal of analgesic therapy is to allow patients to tolerate the time and testing needed to assess the nature of their pain or to allow time for other therapies to alleviate it. Pain may be the only clue toward diagnosis and the only symptom that can be followed to determine whether the patient's condition is getting better or worse. The physician must always reassess the underlying mechanism of pain. What is the diagnosis? Is there a better way to ease the patient's discomfort? What are the emotional determinants and/or consequences? The choice of a specific drug approach is based on the cause, severity, and duration of pain as well as the patient's age, personality, cultural background, and other factors that influence the perception of pain. In general, the physician does best to believe the patient's report of pain. **Non-narcotic preparations are the initial choice for treatment of mild to moderately severe pain.**

B. **Salicylates** These analgesic and anti-inflammatory agents are effective in treating many types of pain. All of the salicylate preparations have comparable analgesic potency. Avoid using aspirin as an analgesic when the presence of **fever** is an important diagnostic issue or when the response of an established fever must be monitored.

1. **Adverse effects.** Gastrointestinal distress and occult blood loss are common; erosive gastritis with pain, vomiting, and hemorrhage may occur. Enteric-coated aspirin and the non-aspirin salicylates appear to be less irritative to the gastric mucosa. Low doses of aspirin inhibit platelet aggregation and prolong bleeding time. Patients with bleeding tendencies, including those receiving warfarin or heparin, should not receive aspirin. Because this effect lasts up to 1 week, it is advisable to omit aspirin during the week prior to a scheduled biopsy or surgical procedure. Nonaspirin salicylate preparations do not exert this effect on bleeding time. Aspirin, but not the other salicylates, may provoke idiosyncratic reactions (urticaria, wheezing, laryngeal edema, hypotension), particularly in persons with asthma or nasal polyps. Dose-related side effects include tinnitus, dizziness, and hearing loss.

2. **Dosage and preparations.** Aspirin is given orally, 0.3 to 1.0 g every 4 hr. The dosage of other salicylate preparations is listed in Chapter 16. Diflunisal (Dolobid®) is a newer and more potent salicylate preparation. An initial dose of 500 to 1,000 mg followed by 250 to 500 mg every 8 to 12 hr is recommended for most patients.

C. **Acetaminophen** This drug has analgesic effects comparable to aspirin but lacks anti-inflammatory activity.

Adverse effects. Acetaminophen does not injure the stomach, nor does it inhibit platelet aggregation. Chronic heavy ingestion or acute overdosage may cause toxic hepatitis and may rarely promote hemolysis in patients with glucose-6-phosphate dehydrogenase deficiency. Approximately 6% of patients with aspirin intolerance (e.g., wheezing) may experience a similar response to acetaminophen.

D. Other Nonsteroidal Anti-Inflammatory Agents   These drugs are effective analgesics and may be tried when aspirin or acetaminophen are ineffective or poorly tolerated. Naproxen, fenoprofen, mefenamic acid, and ibuprofen have specific approval for use as analgesics. These agents may promote less gastric distress and do have more convenient dosage schedules. They are much more expensive, however (see Chapter 16).

E. Narcotic Analgesics

1. **These drugs should be used only when other drugs and maneuvers will not provide adequate pain relief.**

2. **Opiates are relatively contraindicated** in acute disease states in which the pattern and course of pain may have diagnostic significance or in situations such as cerebral hemorrhage or acute head trauma where the state of the sensorium or pupillary responses must remain unaltered by drugs.

3. **Opiates must be used cautiously** in conditions associated with extreme sensitivity to their sedative effects, such as in patients with hypothyroidism, anemia, hypovolemia, liver disease or concurrent use of other CNS depressant drugs.

4. For moderate to severe pain employ codeine or oxycodone (see Table 1). For severe pain morphine or meperidine are drugs of choice.

5. **Start with a low dose,** particularly for conditions listed in section 3 above.

TABLE 1.   *Narcotic-type analgesics used orally for moderate to severe pain*

Name	Equianalgesic dose (mg)[a]	Duration (hr)	Comments/precautions
Codeine	32–65	4–6	Adverse effects are qualitatively similar but less than morphine
Oxycodone	2.5	3–4	Like codeine
+aspirin (Percodan®) +acetaminophen (Percocet®) (Tylox®)			Available only in combination forms Preparations listed contain 5 mg oxycodone
Pentazocine (Talwin®)	30	4–6	Mixed agonist-antagonist Less respiratory depression Slower development of tolerance or dependence May precipitate withdrawal in narcotic-dependent patients
Propoxyphene hydrochloride	65–130	4–6	Long half-life; may accumulate with repetitive dosing Overdose may be complicated by convulsions and require continuous naloxone infusion

[a]Compared to aspirin (650 mg).

If the initial dose proves ineffective and does not produce limiting adverse effects, then increase the dose and monitor closely.

6. **Provide an adequate trial before switching to an alternative agent.** An adequate trial includes regular administration of a sufficiently high dose at frequent intervals. Regular administration provides superior pain relief, allows reduction of the total amount taken in a 24-hr period, and reduces abnormal pain behavior—i.e., administration on an as-needed basis may be associated with increased anxiety, increased perception of pain, and reinforcement of pain behavior more prone to lead to psychological dependence. Patient-controlled analgesia via a programmable infusion offers promise as an effective and rational method for delivery. However, more experience is needed using this technique.

7. **Anticipate tolerance.** Increasing doses are required to maintain the same analgesic effect. This may occur several days after starting drug therapy. Increase the amount of dose or frequency of drug administration or consider adding a nonnarcotic drug.

8. **Consider combinations of drugs**

   a. Narcotic + non-narcotic (aspirin, acetaminophen).

   b. Narcotic + antihistamine (hydroxyzine 25 to 50 mg i.m.). This potentiates the analgesic effect and adds antiemetic action with minimal increase in sedation.

   c. Narcotic + tricyclic antidepressant for chronic pain.

9. **Know the equianalgesic doses** when switching from one chronically used narcotic analgesic to another. Halving the equianalgesic dose of the new drug often provides effective pain control. Be aware that substitution of mixed agonist-antagonist drugs may induce withdrawal symptoms in chronic users of other narcotic analgesics (Table 2).

10. Physical dependence may occur, but usually requires at least 2 weeks of continuous use. In fact, the medical use of narcotic analgesics in a general hospital population rarely is associated with the development of addiction.

11. **Adverse effects** are common to equianalgesic doses of all the narcotic preparations. However, substitution of one drug for another may be associated with amelioration of the unwanted signs or symptoms. Naloxone reverses major signs of toxicity (see Chapter 24). Regarding sedation, a reduced dose of a narcotic analgesic given more frequently improves this symptom. Other sedative drugs should be discontinued, if possible. Other medical problems or a superimposed encephalopathy should be suspected if **excess sedation** develops on a stable narcotic regimen for pain. **Nausea and vomiting** may be avoided or controlled by keeping the patient down in bed, switching to another narcotic, or adding an antiemetic agent. **Constipation** should be handled in a prophylactic manner with liberal oral fluids, dietary and medicinal fiber, and stool softeners. **Urinary retention,** particularly in elderly patients, must be anticipated by close monitoring of voiding habits and urine output, attention to complaints of suprapubic pain or fullness, and assessment of bladder size.

12. **Do not use placebos.** Occasionally, patients who receive or demand narcotic

TABLE 2. *Narcotic-type analgesics commonly used for severe pain*

Name	Route	Equianalgesic dose (mg)[a]	Duration (hr)[b]	Comments/precautions
Morphine	i.m.	10	4–6	Prototype opiate analgesic
	p.o.	60	4–7	May cause sedation, respiratory depression, hypotension, nausea and vomiting, constipation, urinary retention
				Avoid in settings of diagnostic uncertainty
Meperidine	i.m.	75	4–5	Poor choice for oral analgesic
(Demerol®)	p.o.	300	4–6	With repetitive i.m. administration, CNS hyperirritability, mood changes, tremors, myoclonus, occasionally seizures
				Caution in renal insufficiency
Methadone	i.m.	10	c	Reliable oral potency
	p.o.	20	c	May accumulate with repetitive dosing
Hydromorphone	i.m.	1.5	4–5	Potency is advantage for patients
(Dilaudid®)	p.o.	7.5	c	requiring large i.m. doses
Oxymorphone	i.m.	1	c	
(Numorphan®)	p.o.	6	c	
Pentazocine	i.m.	60	c	Mixed agonist-antagonist
(Talwin®)	p.o.	180	c	Less respiratory depression
				Slower development of tolerance or dependence
				May precipitate withdrawal in narcotic-dependent patients
Nalbuphine (Nubain®)	i.m.	10	c	Like pentazocine
Butorphanol (Stadol®)	i.m.	2	c	Like pentazocine

[a]These doses are recommended starting doses from which the optimal dose for each patient is determined by titration and the maximal dose limited by adverse effects.
[b]Duration of analgesia is based on mean values and refers to the stated equianalgesic doses.
[c]Comparable to equianalgesic dose of morphine.

analgesics are perceived as manipulative problem patients and are thought to be exaggerating their symptoms. It is inappropriate and imprecise to use placebo injections in order to prove the patient "wrong" or to differentiate whether the pain is organic or psychogenic. In fact, 30% to 40% of patients with pain, such as postoperative pain, are placebo-responsive. Placebos are less likely to promote pain relief among demanding or manipulative patients, the usual recipients of placebos.

IV. MANAGEMENT OF FEVER

A. General Comments   The **temperature curve** is an important diagnostic sign. First, determine the cause of the fever. Second, allow the response of the fever to serve as an important clue to the efficacy of treatment. If a patient is tolerating fever well, there is no reason to suppress it. Fever does not impair and may actually enhance host immune defenses.

B. Reasons To Treat Fever

   1. To diminish tachycardia and the potential for heart failure in patients with organic heart disease.

   2. To decrease adverse effects on cerebral function.

   3. To diminish catabolism and associated hyperventilation and fluid losses.

   4. To relieve patient discomfort.

C. Antipyretic Measures

   1. Aspirin or acetaminophen

      a. Give either of these drugs 325 to 650 mg every 3 to 4 hr orally or via rectal suppository if needed.

      b. Avoid p.r.n. administration.

      c. Choose acetaminophen for patients allergic to or intolerant of aspirin or in those with active bleeding, bleeding tendency, or active ulcer disease.

      d. Discontinue aspirin or acetaminophen 24 to 72 hr after initiation in order to observe response of the temperature curve to the passage of time or to antimicrobial or other therapeutic measures.

      e. Avoid salicylates in the treatment of adolescents and children with viral illnesses (particularly chicken pox and influenza) because salicylates have been associated with Reye's syndrome.

   2. Mechanical measures to lower temperature

      a. Sponging with tepid water or rubbing skin with a towel soaked in tepid water to facilitate heat vaporization.

      b. Cooling blankets. **Precaution:** Turn off blanket when body temperature reaches 37.7° to 38.3°C in order to avoid overshooting.

V. MANAGEMENT OF EMOTIONAL REACTIONS TO ACUTE MEDICAL ILLNESS

A. Caring, Supportive Relationship Establish a caring, supportive relationship with the ill person. **Communicate regularly.** Attempt to visit the patient for a second or third time each day, however briefly. Take the opportunity to learn more about the patient's family, career, interests, hobbies, etc. Explore the patient's emotional response to prior illness. Consider asking the patient, "How are your spirits?", "Is there anything else I can do for you?", or "Do you have any questions?" Don't hesitate to say, "I'm sorry you are ill." Update the patient and family regularly about progress, tests being contemplated, or changes in therapy.

B. Depressive Illness Expect to find depressive illness in every chronically ill patient admitted to the hospital. Decide whether the depression is mild and manageable by psychological support and attention to the primary illness, or whether the depression is severe and deserving of psychiatric consultation and/or a trial of antidepressant medication.

C. Recognize and Manage the Emotional Reactions to Acute Medical Illness

Adjustment to be made by patient	Common maladaptive response	Management
Acknowledgment of illness	Denial	Attempt to reassure; decrease anxiety. In general, the patient's denial need not be challenged unless it in some way interferes with medical management
The patient must depend on others for care	Noncompliance Signing out against advice (Note: medical patients have the right to leave the hospital at any time provided they are competent and the situation is not a life-threatening emergency.)	**Must explore major fear of patient.** Compromise if necessary. **Allow patient to air grievances.** Convey respect for patient's position. Determine specifically what patient fears. Give patient more autonomy. Give staff opportunity to voice their complaints and anger
	Overdemanding behavior	**Acknowledge anger-provoking nature of patient.** Understand basis for behavior. Explain to the patient the counterproductive effect of his or her demanding behavior. Work out arrangements, setting reasonable limits; e.g., regular visits by nurse rather than "on-demand" service

D. New or Decompensated Organic Mental Syndromes   Be prepared to deal with new or decompensated organic mental syndromes. Anxiety and disorientation may be fostered by the unfamiliar hospital environment, the stress of illness and pain, sleep deprivation, drug side effects, and the threatening aspects of monitoring apparatus, catheters, and tubes. Elderly patients and those with mild or subclinical dementia are most likely to experience increased confusion and agitation in this setting, particularly at night ("sundowning"). **The following guidelines serve to minimize these problems.**

1. Maintain frequent nursing and physician contact; provide frequent orienting cues and reassurance.

2. Provide calendar, radio, television, newspaper, clock, and photographs of loved ones.

3. Avoid single, isolated room.

4. Involve family and friends, extending visiting hours around the clock if nec-

essary. Arrange a nightly phone call by a family member or friend to coincide with bedtime.

5. At night employ a night light, lower the bed, and avoid bed rails if at all possible. Have urinal, eyeglasses, hearing aid within easy reach.

6. In general, avoid sedative-hypnotics for sleep. If necessary, use temazepam 15 mg or thioridazine (Mellaril®) 25 mg given 1 hr prior to bedtime; or use chloral hydrate 250 to 500 mg h.s. (not in patients receiving warfarin or phenytoin).

7. In the event of severe agitation use haloperidol, initially 1 to 10 mg parenterally, with adjusted doses every 30 min until tranquilization is achieved. Fifty percent of this tranquilizing dose could be employed at bedtime on subsequent nights to prevent recurrence.

8. Avoid restraints.

VI. CARE OF THE DYING PATIENT/TERMINAL CARE

A. **General Comments** Terminal care refers to the management of patients in whom the advent of death is felt to be certain and not too far off, and for whom medical effort is focused on the relief of symptoms and the support of the patient and family. The goal is to provide the fullest potential for physical ease and personal relationships until death.

B. **Physical Needs** One must continue to meet the basic physical needs of the dying patient, such as attention to minor infections or fecal impaction.

C. **Provide Emotional Support** Provide emotional support to the patient and family. Seek to minimize the universal feelings of the dying patient—fear of suffering and fear of abandonment. Words and frequent attention are reassuring.

D. **Depression and Poor Well-Being** These may be responsive to agents such as methylphenidate or high-dose corticosteroids. Prednisone may also improve appetite.

E. **Aggressive Control of Pain** Use regular doses of narcotic analgesics if necessary.

1. Pain usually can be controlled with regular doses of **oral analgesics,** including morphine elixir (10 mg/5 ml) or hydromorphone (Dilaudid®).

2. **Aspirin or other nonsteroidal agents** may help relieve visceral or bone pain.

3. Consider **corticosteroids** or **nerve blocks** to help combat pain.

4. For patients requiring large and frequent doses of parenteral narcotic analgesics, consider **continuous subcutaneous or intravenous infusion of morphine.** This approach offers the advantage of substantially reducing patient discomfort and apprehension often accompanying frequent intramuscular or subcutaneous injections. In addition, a constant level of morphine provides better pain relief with a lower total daily dose when compared to intermittent parenteral administration. Continuous infusion via portable automated syringe or infusion pump, such as the type used for insulin administration, may allow the patient the opportunity to move freely, and even return home.

5. Consider opiates to relieve the sensation of **dyspnea** in patients with refractory pleural effusions, pneumonia, or other terminal pulmonary complications. The subjective improvement is superior to that observed with oxygen therapy.

6. Condom or indwelling catheters can minimize the distressing results of urinary incontinence.

7. Haloperidol 1 to 10 mg may be given for agitation or restlessness.

VII. PREVENTIVE HEALTH CARE

A. **General Comments** Although prevention and early detection of disease are priorities for the outpatient setting, such considerations are a legitimate part of the comprehensive inpatient evaluation. General recommendations for health maintenance appear below. At minimum, these guidelines serve to direct patients toward a more regular program of health care subsequent to discharge. Preventive care involves identification of cardiovascular risk factors, detection of preclinical cancer, immunizations, and screening for asymptomatic infection as well as general and psychological counseling. The optimal frequency of periodic evaluation and screening procedures varies with the patient's age, family history, known risk factors, and established medical problems.

B. **Immunizations**

Vaccine	Recommendations	Adverse effects
Influenza	Persons over age 65. Persons with chronic disease potentially worsened by lower respiratory tract infection: Heart disease with potential for CHF, all chronic pulmonary diseases; renal insufficiency or nephrotic syndrome; diabetes mellitus; severe chronic anemia; neoplastic disease; patients on immunosuppressive therapy	Fever, malaise, myalgia; duration 1–2 days. Immediate-type sensitivity reactions (rare). **Contraindication:** anaphylactic hypersensitivity to eggs
Pneumococcal	Same as for influenza vaccine. Candidates for splenectomy and splenectomized individuals.	Local reactions. Rare anaphylactic reactions. Do not administer more often than every 5 yr
Meningococcal	Sickle-cell disease. Candidates for splenectomy and splenectomized individuals. Household contacts of meningococcal disease cases (sero-groups A and C)	Local erythema for 1–2 days
Tetanus toxoid (Td = tetanus, diphtheria, adult type)	Every 10 yr. **Priority:** Older patients, particularly those with diabetes mellitus, ischemic ulcers, or pressure sores.	

Hepatitis B	Chronic renal failure/ hemodialysis patients. Homosexually active males. Parenteral illicit drug users. Household and regular sexual contacts of hepatitis B carriers. Patients with clotting disorders who receive pooled blood products. Patients who happen to be: Health care workers or hospital staff who have contact with blood or blood products; clients or staff of institutions for the mentally retarded	Soreness and redness at injection site

C. Cancer Screening and Prevention

1. Counseling

a. Discourage cigarette and heavy alcohol use.

b. Teach breast self-examination and encourage monthly exams by all women, beginning at age 25 to 30.

c. Advise caution about excess sun exposure, particularly for light-complexioned persons. Use of sunscreens and reduced outdoor exposure between 11:00 a.m. and 1:00 p.m. prevent most of the daily carcinogenic UV light exposure from reaching the skin.

d. Reinforce "healthy" diet; i.e., low total fat and increased fiber. Emerging evidence implicates high-fat diet as a contributor to cancer of the colon, breast, and prostate.

2. Early cancer detection

Procedure	Onset and frequency of screening	High-risk status
MD exam: specific attention to skin, oral cavity, lymph nodes, thyroid, testicles	Yearly for high-risk persons; otherwise every 2–3 yr	Skin: light complexion; ↑ sun. Oral cavity: ethanol, cigarettes. Thyroid: childhood neck irradiation. Testicle: undescended testis.
Breast self-examination	Monthly, begin age 20–30	Prior breast cancer. Mother or sibling with breast cancer. Complicated fibrocystic disease
Breast exam by physician	Every 2–3 yr, age 20–40; over 40, every year	As above

Mammography	Baseline between age 35–40; regular screening starting between ages 40–50 and every 1–3 yr thereafter depending on ease of physical exam and risk status	As for breast self-examination
Pap smear	Age 20–65; at least every 3 yr after 2 negative exams 1 yr apart; under 20 and over 65 if sexually active	Multiple sexual partners
Pelvic examination	Age 20–40; every 3 yr; after age 40, every 1–2 yr	Personal history of breast, uterine cancer. Nulligravida
Endometrial tissue sampling	At menopause for women starting on exogenous estrogens	History of infertility; anovulation; obesity; estrogen therapy
Rectal exam	Every 1–2 yr over age 50	Risk for colorectal cancer increased by: personal history of polyps or previous colorectal cancer; family history of colorectal cancer or polyps; personal history of breast, uterine cancer; chronic ulcerative colitis
Stool testing for occult blood	Yearly after age 50	Same as above
Sigmoidoscopy	Every 5 yr after age 50	Same as above

D. Cardiovascular Risk Factors

Procedure	Onset and frequency of screening	High-risk status
Blood pressure	Every 1–3 yr after age 20	Cigarette smoking, elevated serum cholesterol, diabetes mellitus. Family history of hypertension and/or premature vascular disease
Cholesterol	Presence of atherosclerotic disease or other risk factors. Family history of hyperlipoproteinemia or premature vascular disease. Screen at age 20–25; again at age 35–40.	Same as above

E. Miscellaneous

Procedure	Onset and frequency of screening	High-risk status
PPD	If status unknown, perform	Positive family history

	at least once and document result in medical record	
VDRL, gonococcal culture	Consider yearly in sexually active individuals with multiple partners	
Hearing assessment	Based on clinical judgment	
Ocular tonometry	Every 1–3 yr after age 40	Family history of glaucoma
Serum thyroxine	Consider screening for hypothyroidism in postmenopausal women every 5 yr	Postmenopausal women; diabetes mellitus; other "autoimmune" disorders

F. Health Counseling

1. **Encourage aerobic exercise** such as vigorous walking, jogging, swimming, cycling, racquet sports, etc.

2. **Healthy diet.** Advise low saturated fat, low cholesterol; caloric intake compatible with maintenance of ideal body weight; increased dietary fiber (whole grains, cereals, raw fruits, and vegetables). Advocate decrease in meats and dairy products; instead, poultry, fish, smaller lean meat portions, low-fat dairy products; limitation of obviously fatty and fried foods, butter, margarine, dressings, etc.

3. Educate about and promote **cessation of cigarette smoking.** Discourage **excess alcohol intake** and proscribe use of alcohol and a motor vehicle. Advise the use of seat belts. Develop management skills or knowledge of **professional resources** to handle family dysfunction, marital and sexual problems, contraception and family planning, retirement distress, and grief reactions.

VIII. CIGARETTE SMOKING

A. **General Comments** Cigarette smoking is the major preventable cause of ill health and death. Coronary heart disease, lung cancer, and obstructive lung disease (bronchitis, emphysema) contribute to the 25% to 70% excess mortality in smoking men and women. Most smokers show evidence of small airway dysfunction within 5 to 10 years of regular smoking. In addition to lung cancer, neoplasms of the oral cavity, larynx, esophagus, pancreas, urinary bladder, and kidney are more commonly observed in smokers, as are all forms of atherosclerotic cardiovascular disease.

B. **Exposure to Cigarette Smoke** Involuntary or passive exposure to cigarette smoke may cause eye irritation, bronchospasm, and lowered angina threshold in nonsmokers. Children of smoking parents experience more respiratory infections, and wives of male smokers reportedly have a higher incidence of lung cancer.

C. **Cessation of Cigarette Smoking** Cessation is associated with improved health and a more favorable long-term prognosis.

1. The risk of fatal coronary heart disease, particularly sudden death, is reduced to the level of the nonsmoker within 1 to 3 years.

2. There is rapid improvement of reactive airways disease and a decreased incidence of bronchitis and pneumonia.

3. The rate of decline of FEV_1 becomes less steep and the chance of subsequent chronic bronchitis or emphysema is markedly reduced.

4. The risk of lung cancer slowly decreases to be approximately twice that of a lifelong nonsmoker after 15 years of abstinence.

5. The patient demonstrates increased concern for the health and comfort of others and experiences enhanced self-esteem.

D. **Most Ex-Smokers Quit on Their Own**   Thirty-three million Americans have given up cigarette smoking since the 1964 Surgeon General's report on smoking hazards; 95% of these persons did this on their own. Pessimism and passive acceptance of the patient's smoking behavior is not justified.

E. **Current Smokers**   Three quarters of current smokers state that they wish not to smoke.

F. **Physician Intervention**   The physician must intervene to educate, discourage smoking, and offer opportunities for cessation.

1. **Deliver a strong antismoking message** outlining the effects of smoking on the cardiovascular, respiratory, and other systems.

2. Try to relate smoking to any signs or symptoms currently experienced by the patient. One has the potentially greatest impact when smoking can be related to current symptoms or medical illness such as bronchitis or pneumonia, ulcer disease, even sinus or upper respiratory symptoms. It is less easy for patients to dissociate themselves from the adverse effects of smoking when they have symptoms. The first few days of disease and forced abstinence may facilitate breaking the habit.

3. Provide reinforcing pamphlets, films, and videotapes, many of which are provided free by the American Cancer Society and the American Lung Association.

4. **Consider referral to a structured program for quitting.** Know the resources available in your community. Formal programs emphasize self-help, behavior modification, or hypnosis-meditative approaches.

a. **Self-help programs** emphasize substitute activities (e.g., chewing gum or mints); guidelines for gradual reduction in the amount of each cigarette smoked, the degree of inhalation, and the number smoked, and simple aversive therapy such as the painful snapping of a rubber band worn around the wrist when a strong urge to smoke is experienced. This approach is for those who pride themselves in being independent, not for patients who lack self-reliance.

b. **Behavior modification strategies** focus on the stimuli in daily life that act as learned cues to trigger smoking. One attempts to break the automatic smoking responses to certain cues such as awakening, coffee drinking, or TV watching by making cigarettes less accessible or having only a certain isolated place or certain times in which to smoke.

c. **Hypnosis-meditative programs** make use of heightened suggestibility associated with hypnotic trance and learning of autosuggestive techniques. Periodic meditation (time-outs) are used to relieve tension.

5. **Successful stop-smoking programs** incorporate some or all of the following practices.

   a. **Positive orientation.** Stopping smoking is viewed as an act of gaining control of one's life, not simply an act of deprivation.

   b. Personal relationship with a trained therapist or counselor.

   c. Small group sessions providing encouragement from others who are also trying to quit.

   d. Involvement of spouses.

   e. Quitting is achieved within a 2-week period. If a more gradual reduction is planned, a quit date is set well in advance.

   f. A regular aerobic exercise program is initiated.

   g. Deep-breathing and relaxation techniques are employed.

   h. A buddy system is established whereby ex-smokers can provide individual support to those seeking to stop smoking.

   i. Monitoring of blood thiocyanate levels may be employed in order to detect covert smoking.

   j. The treatment program should continue for 6 to 12 months or indefinitely. Ninety percent of recidivism occurs within the first 3 months.

6. Abstinence or reduction of cigarettes smoked is the preferred goal rather than a switch to so-called low-tar and low-nicotine cigarettes.

7. The physician should support and enforce all hospital nonsmoking policies.

IX. ALCOHOLISM

A. **General Comments**   Alcoholism is present in 10% to 25% of patients admitted to general hospital medical services. Alcoholism is any degree of alcohol use that results in physical, emotional, or vocational dysfunction. Abuse may be difficult to recognize among those who minimize or deny ethanol intake or who present to the hospital with subtle or less specific complications, such as pneumonia or dementia. In order to confirm a suspicion of alcoholism the physician must attend to the more subtle presenting features.

B. **Patient's Reaction**   Pay attention to the patient's reaction to inquiry regarding drinking habits: hesitation, irritation, or inappropriate amusement may be significant responses.

C. **Abbreviated MAST**   Consider using the abbreviated 10-question MAST questionnaire as a screening tool to support a diagnosis of alcoholism (Table 3).

D. **Subtle Stigmata**   Be alert to the more subtle stigmata of chronic alcoholism, such as the puffy, flushed appearance of the face, hoarse voice, conjunctival infection, and scattered ecchymoses. Evaluate target organs (liver, nervous system) and review basic laboratory tests such as the mean corpuscular volume, SGOT, and alkaline phosphatase.

E. **Type and Frequency of Intake**   Assess the type of alcohol intake and frequency

TABLE 3. *The brief MAST*

Questions	Circle correct answers	
1. Do you feel you are a normal drinker?	Yes (0)	No (2)
2. Do friends or relatives think you are a normal drinker?	Yes (0)	No (2)
3. Have you ever attended a meeting of Alcoholics Anonymous (AA)?	Yes (5)	No (0)
4. Have you ever lost friends or girlfriends/boyfriends because of drinking?	Yes (2)	No (0)
5. Have you ever gotten into trouble at work because of drinking?	Yes (2)	No (0)
6. Have you ever neglected your obligations, your family, or your work for two or more days in a row because you were drinking?	Yes (2)	No (0)
7. Have you ever had delirium tremens (DTs), severe shaking, heard voices or seen things that weren't there after heavy drinking?	Yes (2)	No (0)
8. Have you ever gone to anyone for help about your drinking?	Yes (5)	No (0)
9. Have you ever been in a hospital because of drinking?	Yes (5)	No (0)
10. Have you ever been arrested for drunk driving or driving after drinking?	Yes (2)	No (0)

Score ≤ 5 = Very low likelihood of alcoholism.
Score 6–17 = Indeterminate.
Score ≥ 18 = Very high likelihood of alcoholism.

of use in order to estimate the daily consumption in grams of ethanol (half pint beer = 1 oz spirits (whiskey, gin) = 1 glass wine $\cong$ 10 g ethanol). Daily intake exceeding 80 g ethanol (>40 g/day for women) places an individual at risk for major physical, psychological, and social problems. At least 10% of such persons will experience an alcohol-withdrawal syndrome on cessation of drinking.

F. Objective Advice   Advise the patient objectively in a nonpunitive manner of your assessment of the severity of his or her alcohol problem.

G. Alcoholism as a Symptom   Consider that alcoholism may be a symptom of an underlying and treatable psychiatric disorder such as depression, anxiety neurosis, phobia or panic disorder, or schizophrenia. Seek appropriate consultation.

H. Alcohol Withdrawal   During hospitalization, manage the patient's alcohol withdrawal and attempt to motivate the individual toward the general goal of abstinence. Set firm rules for dosage and time of administration of drugs. Avoid orders for analgesics or tranquilizers on an as-needed basis. Such orders encourage bargaining by the patient and foster drug taking for the relief of pain or tension.

I. Alcoholism Treatment Programs   Alcoholism treatment programs and personal effort by the patient do work. In most patients **early** in the course of problem drinking, alcohol treatment is not frustrating or useless. Rehabilitative efforts promote improved psychosocial status and job performance. Socially stable individuals, specifically those with a steady job, stable residence, or stable relationship with a spouse predictably can have a better chance of achieving sustained abstinence.

J. Appropriate Referral   Recommend treatment and seek appropriate referral to counselors, social workers, clinics, professional or volunteer agencies, or physicians who specialize in the treatment of alcohol-dependent patients. Know the resources available in your hospital and community. Rehabilitation is best accomplished in the setting of psychological peer group support. Intensive group or individual therapy, behavior modification, and assertiveness training may be involved.

BIBLIOGRAPHY

Annsten, A. G. (1979): Strategic withdrawal from cigarette smoking. *CA,* 29:96–107.
Beaver, W. T. (1981): Management of cancer pain with parenteral medication. *JAMA,* 244:2653–2657.
Bedell, S. E., Delbanco, T. L., Cook, E. F., and Epstein, F. H. (1983): Survival after cardiopulmonary resuscitation in the hospital. *N. Engl. J. Med.,* 309:569–576.
Foley, K. M. (1982): The practical use of narcotic analgesics. *Med. Clin. North Am.,* 66:1091–1104.
Goldman, D. A., Maki, D. G., Rhame, F. S., Kaiser, A. B., Tenney, J. H., and Bennett, J. V. (1973): Guidelines for infection control in intravenous therapy. *Ann. Intern. Med.,* 79:848–850.
Halkin, H., Goldberg, J., Modan, M., and Modan, B. (1982): Reduction of mortality in general medical inpatients by low-dose heparin prophylaxis. *Ann. Intern. Med.,* 96:561–565.
Hausten, P. D. (1979): *Drug Interactions.* Lea & Febiger, Philadelphia.
Immunization Practices Advisory Committee (1983): General recommendations on immunization. *Ann. Intern. Med.,* 98(Part 1):615–622.
McLellan, A. T., Luborsky, L., O'Brien, C. P., Woody, G. F., and Druley, K. A. (1982): Is treatment for substance abuse effective? *JAMA,* 247:1423–1428.
Medical Practice Committee, American College of Physicians (1981): Periodic health examination: A guide for designing individualized preventive health care in the asymptomatic patient. *Ann. Intern. Med.* 95:729–732.
Miles, S. H., Cranford, R., and Schultz, A. L. (1982): The do-not-resuscitate order in a teaching hospital. *Ann. Intern. Med.,* 96:660–664.
Perry, S., and Viederman, M. (1981): Management of emotional reactions to acute medical illness. *Med. Clin. North Am.,* 65:3–14.
Pokorny, A. D., Miller, B. A., and Kaplan, H. B. (1972): The Brief MAST: a shortened version of the Michigan Alcoholism Screening Test. *Am. J. Psychiatry,* 129:342–345.
President's Commission for the Study of Ethical Problems in Medicine and Biomedical and Behavioral Research (1983): *Deciding to Forego Life-Sustaining Treatment.* US Government Printing Office.
Reuler, J. B., and Cooney, T. G. (1981): The pressure sore: Pathophysiology and principles of management. *Ann. Intern. Med.,* 94:661–666.
Stamm, W. E. (1975): Guidelines for the prevention of catheter-associated urinary tract infections. *Ann. Intern. Med.,* 82:386–390.
Steel, K., Gertman, P. M., Crescenzi, C., and Anderson, J. (1981): Iatrogenic illness on a general medical service at a university hospital. *N. Engl. J. Med.,* 304:638–642.
Thompson, T. L., Moran, M. G., and Nies, A. S. (1983): Psychotropic drug use in the elderly. *N. Engl. J. Med.,* 308:134–138, 194–199.
Vestal, R. E. (1978): Drug use in the elderly: A review of problems and special considerations. *Drugs,* 16:358–382.

2.

Fluid and Electrolyte Disorders

William D. Kaehny

2.

Fluid and Electrolyte Disorders

Successful management of a fluid and electrolyte problem is one of the most immediately satisfying achievements in medicine, both to clinician and patient. Treatment as always is based on sound knowledge of pathophysiology. **Critical to proper management is treatment of the underlying disorder that has generated the fluid and electrolyte disturbance.**

I. **MAINTENANCE OF BODY FLUID AND ELECTROLYTE STORES** If patients cannot ingest solids or liquids, nutrients, fluid and electrolytes are provided preferably by enteral feeding (Chapter 21). However, when the gastrointestinal tract is not functional or enteral feeding is too risky because of potential aspiration of gastric contents, intravenous administration of fluid and electrolytes is necessary.

A. **Maintenance Fluids Without Abnormal Losses**

1. **Normal Losses.** The goal is to replace normal external losses and maintain extracellular fluid (ECF) volume at a normal range that allows a buffer against unexpected external losses. **Insensible** skin and respiratory system water **losses** average 12 ml/kg/day. **Obligatory urine excretion** is about 500 ml/day to allow excretion of about 600 mOsm of solute. **Metabolism** produces about 4.25 ml/kg/day of free water. Thus a 70-kg individual needs a minimum of 1,050 ml of water daily to maintain balance. However, in the absence of protein intake the kidneys are unable to concentrate the urine maximally and thus more water must be supplied.

2. **Supplementation**

   a. Although the kidneys can maintain **sodium** balance after about 5 days of no intake, the initial losses (e.g., 150 to 250 mmol) reduce ECF volume to the lower limit of normal. Thus, sodium should be provided.

   b. The kidneys are less efficient in preserving **potassium**, and therefore potassium supplementation also is necessary.

   c. Magnesium and phosphorus supplementation is not required unless more than 5 to 7 days of maintenance are anticipated.

3. For longer maintenance periods **parenteral alimentation** should be considered early to provide calories, nutrients, and minerals (Chapter 21).

4. For short-term maintenance, provision of 100 g glucose monohydrate will retard protein losses and provide about 340 calories daily.

5. One prescription filling the needs for daily maintenance fluids includes 1,000 ml of 5% dextrose and 0.45% sodium chloride (77 mM) and 1,000 ml of 5% dextrose, both with 20 mmol of potassium chloride added (total 40 mmol).

B. **Maintenance Fluids with Abnormal Losses** Abnormal losses require **addition of water and electrolytes** to the basic prescription for daily maintenance fluids. Obviously, the best course is to treat the underlying disorder in order to mitigate the need for additional replacement therapy. If renal function is reasonable, the kidneys usually will come to the rescue and adjust urinary excretion to meet most needs. General guidelines for maintenance fluids for the more common problems are listed in Table 1. These fluids should be added to the usual maintenance prescription.

Special cases of abnormal fluid losses are so-called **"third-spacing" situations** such as peritonitis, pancreatitis, and extensive burns. The problem is usually one of intravascular volume depletion. Both colloid (protein-containing) and electrolyte solutions are needed to normalize hemodynamics.

II. **TREATMENT OF VOLUME DEPLETION**

A. **Pathogenesis and Hemodynamic Effects** The pathogenesis and hemodynamic effects of volume depletion determine the type and rate of fluid and electrolyte replacement. Volume deficits may be largely **intravascular** (acute blood loss), largely **extracellular** (gastrointestinal, renal, third-spacing losses), or **total body water** (true dehydration as with increased insensible losses). Often all compartments are affected to some degree.

   1. The degree of vascular or ECF volume depletion is estimated by the effects on systemic hemodynamics.

      a. In the absence of heart failure or sepsis, supine hypotension and signs of hypoperfusion of brain, kidneys, and skin indicate **very severe** intravascular volume depletion (shock, about **30%** intravascular volume depletion).

      b. **Moderately severe** intravascular volume depletion (about **20%** intravascular volume depletion) is manifested by a fall of greater than 15 to 20 mm Hg in systolic blood pressure on assuming an orthostatic position.

      c. **Less severe** intravascular volume depletion may be manifested by decreased skin turgor, absence of axillary and groin sweat, normal or slightly increased serum creatinine with disproportionate increase in urea nitrogen (BUN) and low urine sodium concentration.

   2. **Interpretation** of systemic hemodynamics in seriously ill patients using these clinical findings **is accurate less than 50% of the time**; therefore, use of **right heart monitoring** (i.e., Swan-Ganz catheter) is a valuable tool in directing treatment.

TABLE 1. *Additional fluid replacement needs*

Disorder	Treatment[a]
Fever	2 ml/kg/day of D5/0.2% NaCl per degree C over 37°
Nasogastric suction	ml/ml lost of 0.45% NaCl with 10 mmol KCl/liter
Ileostomy losses	ml/ml lost of 0.45% NaCl with 10 mmol KCl/liter and 44.5 mmol NaHCO$_3$/liter
Diarrhea	ml/ml lost D5/0.2% NaCl with 30 mmol KCl/liter and 44.5 mmol NaHCO$_3$/liter
Postobstructive diuresis	0.5 ml/ml urine 0.45% NaCl

[a]All treatments need adjustment for the individual patient.

3. In the absence of cardiac and pulmonary disease, monitoring central venous pressure is a reasonable guide to the state of vascular volume.

B. **Treatment of Acute Intravascular Volume Depletion**   Commonly, acute intravascular volume depletion occurs due to gastrointestinal hemorrhage or external or internal vascular disruption.

1. Several large-caliber venous catheters should be placed, and **whole blood** or **packed red blood cells** and a **plasma volume expander** infused to normalize hemodynamics as rapidly as possible.

2. While waiting for blood, plasma volume expanders should be infused rapidly. The types of volume expanders are listed in Table 2.

Occasionally, rapid shifts of fluid can cause acute reductions in intravascular volume as with burns, peritonitis, pancreatitis, or external loss of ascites (umbilical hernia rupture or excessive paracentesis). Plasma volume expanders should be infused to normalize hemodynamics as rapidly as possible. Of course, **continuing losses must be replaced**.

C. **Treatment of Extracellular Volume Depletion**   The basic rule of treatment is to **normalize hemodynamics with the rapid infusion of 0.9% NaCl** (normal saline) and then worry about correcting electrolyte disorders unless life-threatening potassium, acid-base, or calcium disorders are present. Infusion rates of 500 to 1,000 ml/hr (or more) are used to restore volume, and then maintenance rates are determined. Lactated Ringer's solution may be used, and at times plasma expanders may be needed.

D. **Treatment of Total Body Water Deficits**   Situations in which water deficits exceed electrolyte losses result in **hypernatremia** (see IV. B.).

1. Initial treatment consists of infusing sufficient 0.9% NaCl to normalize hemodynamics.

2. Then oral fluids or intravenous D5W or 0.45% NaCl are given as discussed below.

TABLE 2. *Common fluids for infusion*

Solutions[a]	Volume (ml)	Na (mmol/volume)	Relative cost per unit
Blood and plasma expanders			
Whole blood	500	64 ±	34
Packed red blood cells	300	Same	34
Plasma protein fraction	500	70 ±	53
Albumin 5%	500	70 ±	53
Albumin 25%	50	7 ±	26
Hetastarch 6%	500	77	26
Extracellular fluid expanders			
Sodium chloride 0.9% (NS)	1,000	154	1.0
Lactated Ringer's solution	1,000	130	1.2
Total body water expanders			
Dextrose 5% in water (D5W)	1,000	0	1.1
Dextrose 10% in water (D10W)	1,000	0	1.3
Sodium chloride 0.45% (1/2NS)	1,000	77	1.1

[a]Other volumes and many combinations of solutions are available for maintenance or replacement needs; see text.

E. Comments on Volume-Expanding Solutions

1. **Hazards.** **Whole blood** and **red blood cell transfusions** carry the risk of transmitting hepatitis, but the urgent need for oxygen-carrying capacity outweighs this hazard. Other hazards such as alkalosis, hypocalcemia, hyperkalemia, hypokalemia, hypothermia, coagulation factor depletion, and certainly transfusion reaction should not be overlooked. **Plasma should not be used as a volume expander** because of the risk of hepatitis and the availability and efficacy of **5% albumin, plasma protein fraction** (Plasmanate®, Plasmatein®, Plasma-Plex®, and Protenate®), and **hetastarch** (hydroxyethyl starch). **Albumin 25%** causes interstitial fluid to move into the vascular space and may be used to expand intravascular volume in subjects with excess interstitial fluid and important intravascular volume depletion. Albumin has a half-life of about 3 weeks. **Dextrans** may cause anaphylaxis, acute renal failure, and bleeding and are not recommended solely for volume expansion. The relative costs are listed in Table 2.

2. **Sodium chloride solutions. Sodium chloride 0.9%** (normal saline, isotonic saline, 154 mM NaCl) distributes throughout the functional ECF, about 20% of the body weight, and is the basic ECF volume expander. About 20% remains in the intravascular space and thus serves as a reasonable expander in the absence of critical hemodynamic problems. **Ringer's lactate** contains Na 130 mM; K 4 mM; Ca 1.5 mM; and lactate 28 mM.

   Sodium chloride is available in a variety of concentrations (0.9%, 154 mM; 0.45%, 77 mM; 0.2%, 34 mM) in 5% or 10% dextrose. **More concentrated solutions such as 3%** (513 mM NaCl) **or 5%** (855 mM NaCl) **are not used for volume expansion** but rather for treatment of highly selected patients with serious hyponatremia (see IV. A.).

3. **Dextrose solutions** contain glucose monohydrate, 3.4 kcal/g, in two commonly used concentrations: 50 g/liter, 5%, and 100 g/liter, 10%. More concentrated solutions are used for parenteral nutrition solutions. These solutions distribute in total body water, 45% to 55% of adult body weight, and thus less than 10% remains in the intravascular space.

III. **TREATMENT OF EDEMATOUS STATES**

A. **General Measures**   The common disorders that cause salt and water retention sufficient to expand the interstitial fluid space by more than 4 liters with resultant edema include congestive heart failure, cirrhosis of the liver, nephrotic syndrome, and chronic renal failure. The primary diseases require treatment if possible. General measures such as **bedrest** and **severe dietary sodium** restriction, 20 mmol NaCl (500 mg sodium) or 10 mmol NaCl (250 mg sodium), may result in a diuresis but are not practical for treatment of outpatients. If edema persists after treatment of the underlying disease and moderation of sodium intake, **diuretics** are indicated to improve respiratory or cardiac function, to allow increased physical activity or intake of a palatable diet, to prevent skin breakdown, and, in few patients only, to improve physical appearance.

1. **Treatment of acute pulmonary edema** may require parenteral administration of the loop diuretics, furosemide, bumetanide, or ethacrynic acid. Occasionally, a patient with severe chronic congestive heart failure resulting in anasarca

may have a diuresis in response to parenteral, but not oral, diuretics, perhaps because of reduced gastrointestinal absorption of medications due to bowel edema. Gradual reduction in edema to the extent of 0.5- to 1.0-kg weight loss per day is preferable in the chronic edematous states. After achievement of the indicated goals of treatment, the dose of diuretic should be reduced to maintain sodium balance at the desired weight. Although achievement of so-called "dry weight" sounds ideal, a maintenance dose of diuretic that allows a trace of pedal edema at the end of the day (provided treatment goals are met) may be safer in preventing intravascular volume depletion. Available diuretic agents are listed in Table 3.

2. **Dietary salt restriction** needs to be practical and inexpensive. Thus, avoidance of foods with high salt content and removal of salt from the table should achieve a salt intake of less than 200 mmol (4.6 g sodium)/day, a level most patients can tolerate. The need for potassium supplements is discussed later (see VI. A.)

3. **The common causes of apparent resistance to diuretics** include failure of the patient to take the diuretic as prescribed, excessive dietary sodium intake, intravascular volume depletion, concomitant use of nonsteroidal anti-inflammatory drugs, and worsening of the primary disease state.

Patients with severe primary disease may require the stepwise addition of diuretics acting in different ways on different portions of the nephron. For example, a patient with severe cardiomyopathy may require a distal tubule blocker (e.g., thiazide, chlorthalidone, metolazone), a potassium-sparing diuretic (e.g., spironolactone, triamterene, amiloride), a loop diuretic (furosemide, bumetanide, ethacrynic acid) and even a proximal tubule blocker (e.g., acetazolamide). Of course, the use of multiple agents amplifies the chances of an adverse drug reaction. Ethacrynic acid may be used for patients with allergic reactions to sulfur-containing compounds such as thiazides, chlorthalidone, metolazone, furosemide, and bumetanide.

IV. **DISORDERS OF WATER METABOLISM**   Disorders of water metabolism usually are manifested by abnormalities in the serum sodium concentration. The causative disorder determines the state of total body sodium and fluid space volumes, which are critical variables in determining the direction of treatment. Treatment directed at normalizing the serum sodium concentration is undertaken in two circumstances:

1. Rapid measures are indicated if the abnormal serum osmolality is affecting brain function.

2. Chronic measures are indicated if the underlying disorder is not correctable, and normalization of serum osmolality (sodium concentration) is desirable to provide a buffer against symptomatic worsening of the osmolar disturbance.

A. **Treatment of Hyponatremia**   A general approach to treatment is displayed in Fig. 1.

1. The patient with **decreased ECF volume** has had net loss of more salt than water. Treatment of volume depletion will correct hemodynamic problems, suppress increased vasopressin (ADH) secretion and allow the kidneys to correct the hyponatremia. (See II. for details.)

TABLE 3. *Diuretic agents*

Agent	Size (mg)	Common dose	Onset (hr)	Peak (hr)	Duration (hr)	Relative cost[a]	Side-effects or reactions	Potency[a]
Proximal tubule								
Acetazolamide	125,250	250 mg b.i.d.	1	2–4	8–12	2.8–5.8	Low [K], acidosis	0.3
Loop of Henle								
Furosemide[b]	20,40,80	40 mg q.d., b.i.d.	1	1–2	6	3.3–9.4	Volume depletion, low [K], alkalosis	3–5
Ethacrynic acid[b]	25,50	50 mg q.d., b.i.d.	0.5	2	6	11.6	Same as furosemide plus more ototoxicity	
Bumetanide[b]	0.5,1.0	1 mg q.d., b.i.d.	0.5	2	4–6	10.2	Same as furosemide	
Distal tubule								
Thiazides								
Hydrochlorothiazide	25,50,100	50 mg q.d., b.i.d.	2	4	12	3.1–59.6	All thiazides same: low [K], alkalosis, high uric acid, hyperglycemia, hyperlipidemia, low [Na]	1–2
Chlorothiazide	250,500	500 mg q.d., b.i.d.	1	4	6–12	2.9–5.5		
Bendroflumethiazide	2.5,5,10	5 mg q.d., b.i.d.	2	4	6–12	16.7		
Benzthiazide	25,50	50 mg q.d., b.i.d.	2	4	6–12	3.0–7.0		
Cyclothiazide	2	2 mg q.d., b.i.d.	2	4	6–12	10.4		
Hydroflumethiazide	50	50 mg q.d., b.i.d.	2	4	6–12	5.3–11.0		
Methyclothiazide	2.5,5.0	5 mg q.d.	2	6	24	4.0–11.2		
Polythiazide	1,2,4	2 mg q.d.	2	6	24	13.2		
Trichlormethiazide	2,4	2–4 mg q.d.	2	6	24	1–13.5		
Chlorthalidone	25,50,100	50 mg q.d.	2	6	24–48	3.2–13	Same as thiazides	1–2
Metolazone	2.5,5,10	5 mg q.d.	1	2	12–24	10.1–11.0	Same as thiazides	1–2
Quinethazone	50	50 mg q.d.	1	2	12–24	19.9	Same as thiazides	1–2
Potassium-sparing								
Spironolactone[c]	25,50,100	25–50 b.i.d.	2	48–72	48–72	2.6–15.0	High [K], gynecomastia, menstrual disorders, acidosis	0.5–1
Triamterene[c]	50,100	50–100 b.i.d.	2	6–8	12–16	6.9	High [K]	
Amiloride[c]	5	5 mg q.d.	2	6–10	24	12.8	High [K]	

[a]Costs are expressed as a ratio assigning 1 to the least expensive generic trichlormethazide (average wholesale cost per 100 tablets = $1.45 in 1983). The cost refers to the underlined dosage size. Potency also relative.

[b]Available in parenteral form (onset 5–15 min, peak 30–60 min, duration 2–3 hr).

[c]Available in combinations with various thiazides.

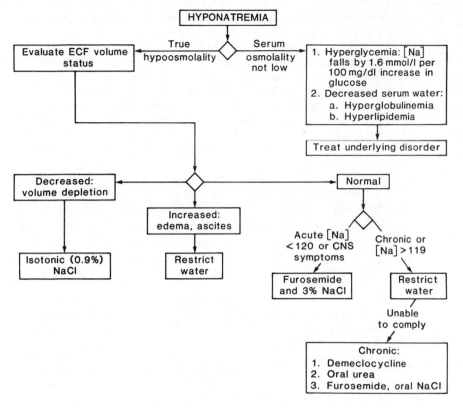

FIG. 1. Treatment of patients with hyponatremia.

2. The patient with **excess total body salt and water** (edematous states) often has increased ADH secretion in response to a perceived deficit in intravascular volume. If treatment of the underlying disorder is not successful, water intake may be restricted initially to about 500 ml less than daily maintenance needs. With normalization of the serum sodium concentration, restriction of fluid intake to equal maintenance needs should suffice (see I. A).

Diuretics may induce hyponatremia by three mechanisms:

a. Decreased intravascular volume causing increased ADH levls, decreased glomerular filtration rate, increased reabsorption of fluid in the renal proximal tubule.

b. Deficits of potassium and magnesium causing shift of sodium into cells.

c. Direct effects of the diuretic on the renal tubular diluting segment.

Thus, temporary cessation of the diuretic, administration of potassium and magnesium supplements and water restriction will allow correction of the hyponatremia in patients on a normal sodium intake. Thereafter, smaller doses or intermittent administration of the diuretic and potassium supplementation may be used to prevent recurrence of the hyponatremia.

3. The patient with relatively **normal total body salt but increased total body water** has increased ADH secretion (syndrome of inappropriate ADH secretion, drugs, hypothyroidism, stress), intake of drugs that mimic or amplify ADH effect (e.g., chlorpropamide, cyclosphosphamide, vincristine) or massive water intake. If sodium concentration falls to less than 120 mmol/liter rapidly, or is associated with altered mental status, abnormal respiratory pattern, abnormal neurological findings or seizures, measures to raise the sodium concentration to about 130 mmol/liter during an 8- to 12-hr period should be undertaken.

The amount of net water excretion necessary to raise the sodium concentration to 130 mmol/liter is calculated from the observed serum sodium concentration and the estimated total body water (60% of the weight) as follows:

Excess water $= 0.6$ weight $-$ (observed [Na]/130) $\times 0.6$ weight.

One method is to increase water excretion with **furosemide** and to replace urinary salt losses with **3% NaCl** and KCl supplements. Furosemide 1 mg/kg is administered intravenously (or p.o. if tolerated) and urine volume monitored hourly. Estimate the urine sodium concentration at 75 mmol/liter (about 70 to 100 mmol/liter). After 1 hr an infusion of 500 ml 3% NaCl with 20 mmol KCl is begun, to replace the urinary losses of the previous hour during the subsequent hour. About 150 ml of this solution replaces 1 liter of urine. Serum sodium and potassium should be monitored at 2- to 3-hr intervals. Monitoring urine electrolytes allows more precise replacement but is not usually necessary. Furosemide may be given at 3- to 4-hr intervals to maintain the diuresis. Controversial findings suggest that rapid or overcorrection of hyponatremia may cause central pontine myelinolysis. Thus, this treatment is reserved for patients with life-threatening CNS symptoms of hyponatremia.

4. If the hyponatremia is **mild or chronic and not associated with neurological abnormalities**, water restriction alone is safe and effective even with very low serum sodium concentrations. If the underlying causative disorder cannot be corrected, other measures can be used to allow the patient a less restricted fluid intake:

   a. **Demeclocycline** 13 to 15 mg/kg is effective in chronically increasing water excretion by inhibiting the action of ADH.

   b. **Urea** 30 to 60 g once daily by mouth in 100 to 200 ml of water with antacid and syrup flavoring, or *furosemide* 40 mg with 100 mmol NaCl once daily (17 mmol/1,000-mg tablet), are also reportedly effective.

B. Treatment of Hypernatremia

1. **A general approach** to the treatment of hypernatremia is outlined in Fig. 2. The net amount of free water needed to restore serum sodium concentration to 140 mmol/liter can be calculated as follows:

   Water deficit $=$ (observed [Na]/140) $\times 0.6$ weight $- 0.6$ weight.

   Deficits should be replaced over about 48 hr in order to avoid cerebral edema. Normal saline is infused to correct volume depletion, and then D5W or 0.45%

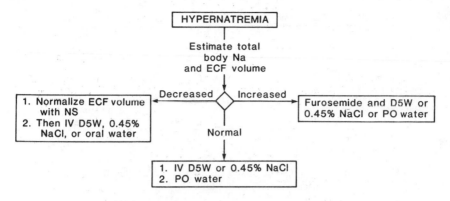

FIG. 2.   Treatment of patients with hypernatremia.

NS is infused at a rate calculated to reduce serum sodium by about 0.5 to 1.0 mmol/hr. For example, a patient with a serum sodium of 170 mmol/liter and a 9-liter water deficit is given 6.0 liters of fluid per 24 hr (5.0 liter D5W, 1.0 liter ½ NS), which provides 1,000 ml insensible loss replacement, 500 ml to match urine output, and 4,500 ml free water. Serum sodium concentration should be monitored at 4- to 8-hr intervals to insure that the prescription is achieving the predicted response. Oral water replacement is preferable for patients with serum sodium concentrations less than 160 mmol/liter.

2. Treatment of patients with **central diabetes insipidus** requires use of ADH replacement. The preferred treatment is intranasal application of dDAVP (*l*-desamino-8-D arginine vasopressin), 5 to 20 µg at 6- to 20-hr intervals. This can be blown into the nose of a comatose patient and can be used in the acute postoperative setting. Addition of a thiazide diuretic allows reduction of the dose and smoother control in chronic central diabetes insipidus.

3. In patients with **nephrogenic diabetes insipidus**, congenital or severe acquired, urine output may be reduced by thiazide diuretics and salt restriction. Nonsteroidal anti-inflammatory agents (prostaglandin inhibitors) and chlorpropamide reportedly reduce urine volumes in some patients.

V. **TREATMENT OF ACID-BASE DISORDERS**   Treatment depends on correct identification of the type of acid-base disorder, the nature of the underlying disorder, and the effect of the pH change on organ function. The following is one sequence of steps to reach a treatment decision.

1. An acid-base disorder is suspected from the patient's clinical state (e.g., hyperventilation, hypotension) and serum total CO_2 content (tCO_2) and potassium concentration.

2. The major acid-base disorder is determined from blood pH, Pco_2, $[HCO_3]$. Arterial blood sampling is necessary if any concern for adequate oxygenation exists. Venous blood obtained without tourniquet-induced stasis, or even better, following 15 min of hot pad heating (45°) of the forearm also provides values sufficient for acid-base diagnosis.

TABLE 4. *Compensation in simple acid-base disorders*

	pH	Pco$_2$	[HCO$_3^-$]
Sea-level normal	7.40	40 mm Hg	24 mmol/liter
Metabolic acidosis	↓	↓ 1.0 to 1.5 × Δ [HCO$_3^-$]	↓
Respiratory acidosis, acute	↓	↑	↑ 0.1 × ΔPco$_2$ (±3)[a]
Respiratory acidosis, chronic	↓	↑	↑ 0.4 × ΔPco$_2$ (±4)[a]
Metabolic alkalosis	↑	↑ 0.25 to 1.0 × Δ [HCO$_3^-$]	↑
Respiratory alkalosis, acute	↑	↓	↓ 0.1 to 0.3 × ΔPco$_2$
Respiratory alkalosis, chronic	↑	↓	↓ 0.2 to 0.5 × ΔPco$_2$

Δ, change in value from sea-level normal.
[a]Range about the calculated value.

3. The presence of a simple or mixed disorder is determined by judging if compensation is empirically appropriate (Table 4).

4. The underlying cause of the acid-base disorder is determined.

5. Volume depletion, electrolyte disorders, and the underlying cause are treated. If the pH is affecting organ function importantly, measures to alter pH directly are instituted.

Flow diagrams starting from abnormal serum tCO$_2$ (HCO$_3$) and leading to treatment are displayed in Figs. 3 and 4.

A. Treatment of Metabolic Acidosis

1. Treatment of **acute metabolic acidosis** may require alkali therapy if the pH is less than about 7.15 or if hemodynamic instability is present or likely. This occurs most often with the organic acidoses and toxin ingestions. Two 50-ml ampuls of 7.5% NaHCO$_3$ (44.6 mmol/50 ml, 1,784 mOsm/kg) given by slow i.v. push provide 89 mmol of bicarbonate. This will raise the plasma bicarbonate rapidly by about 2.5 mmol/liter with a resultant sharp increase in pH of 0.15 to 0.40 units, depending on the Pco$_2$ of course.[1] If large volumes of fluid are needed to replace volume deficits, the NaHCO$_3$ can be added to D5W or 0.45% NS.

The rate of administration then depends on the patient's tolerance of the volume and solute load and the need to maintain the pH above 7.20. If the generation of acid continues unabated, as with some cases of fulminant lactic acidosis or toxin ingestion, the solute and volume load with continuing NaHCO$_3$ administration may become excessive, resulting in hyperosmolarity, hypokalemia, and pulmonary edema. If this appears likely, early institution of hemodialysis using bicarbonate dialysate is indicated.

---

[1]The expected acute change in pH can be estimated using the Henderson equation, assuming no change in Pco$_2$ and a 2.5 mmol/liter increase in bicarbonate concentration following administration of 89 mmol of NaHCO$_3$:

$$\text{New } [H] = 24 \times \text{ observed Pco}_2/(\text{observed } [HCO_3] + 2.5).$$

The [H] can be estimated in nmol/liter by interpolating values between the following intervals: 6.80 = 159, 6.90 = 126, 7.00 = 100, 7.10 = 79, 7.20 = 63, 7.30 = 50. Decrements of 0.10 pH units below pH 7.00 yield [H] about 125% of the next higher pH level, whereas increments of 0.10 in pH above 7.00 yield [H +] about 80% of the next lower pH level. Between pH 7.28 and 7.45 [H] equals 80 minus the decimal of the pH—e.g., pH 7.32 = 80 − 32 = 48.

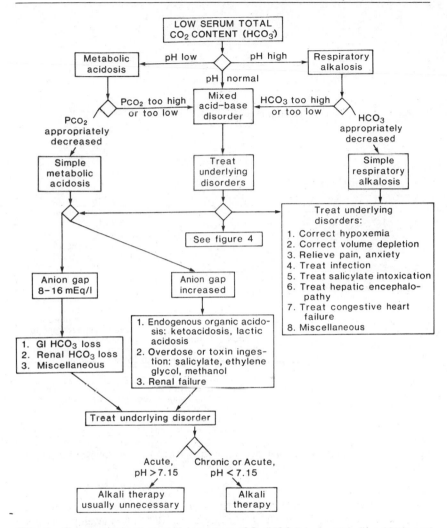

FIG. 3. Treatment of patients with low serum tCO_2 (HCO_3), i.e., metabolic acidosis and respiratory alkalosis. Anion gap is calculated as serum $[Na] - [Cl] - [tCO_2]$. The rules of compensation to determine if P_{CO_2} or $[HCO_3]$ are too high or too low are listed in Table 4.

The complications of alkali therapy thus include hyperosmolarity, volume overload, severe hypokalemia owing to shift into cells, and late "overshoot" alkalosis when the organic acid anions are metabolized to produce bicarbonate. These can be minimized by careful hemodynamic monitoring, raising pH to a safe range above 7.20 but not to normal; early, sufficient potassium administration; and use of hemodialysis.

The need for subsequent doses of $NaHCO_3$ is best determined by monitoring the acid-base variables; no formula can account for the rate of continuing acid

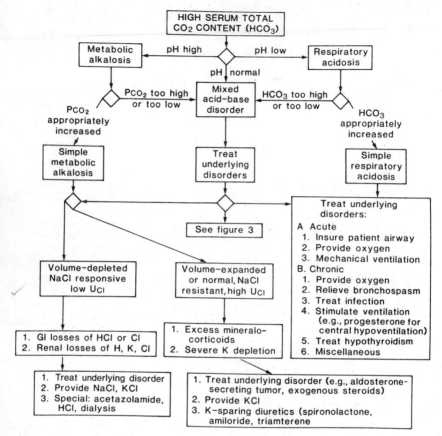

FIG. 4.   Treatment of patients with high serum tCO_2 (HCO_3), i.e., metabolic alkalosis and respiratory acidosis. The rules of compensation are listed in Table 4.

generation. However, if acid production or external HCO_3 loss has ceased, the approximate dose of $NaHCO_3$ to raise plasma [HCO_3] to a given value can be estimated using an HCO_3 distribution space of 50% to 80%, the latter applying to pH levels around 7.00 or lower, as follows:

$$mmol\,NaHCO_3\,needed = (desired - observed\,[HCO_3]) \times (.50\,to\,.80 \times kg\,wt).$$

This formula can be used to calculate the alkali repletion dose in chronic metabolic acidosis.

2. Treatment of **chronic metabolic acidosis** is necessary to prevent the lethargy, anorexia, nausea, and disturbances in mineral metabolism that may occur with serum tCO_2 levels chronically less than 15 to 18 mmol/liter. Chronic renal failure, renal tubular acidosis, ileostomy, ureterosigmoidostomy, and chronic diarrheal states constitute the group of usual causes of chronic metabolic acidosis. Alkali may be provided as **$NaHCO_3$ tablets**, 600 mg (7 mmol), or

Shohl's sodium or potassium citrate solution, 1 mmol/ml of alkali. One approach is to calculate the amount of alkali needed to raise the serum tCO_2 to about 24 mmol/liter and provide this over 3 days. Then maintenance dose is established starting at 2 mmol/kg/day and increasing by 1 to 2 mmol/kg/day as needed to maintain serum tCO_2 at the desired level.

Caution is necessary in treating patients with chronic renal failure to **prevent sodium and volume overload**. Usually 1 mmol/kg/day of alkali is a sufficient maintenance dose in these patients. Rarely, alkali may precipitate tetany by reducing ionized calcium concentration in patients with hypocalcemia as in chronic renal failure. In these subjects hypocalcemia should be corrected before giving large amounts of alkali.

B. **Treatment of Metabolic Alkalosis** Occasionally, a patient with **metabolic alkalosis** may not tolerate the volume, sodium, or potassium load needed to correct the alkalosis or may have loss of renal function to excrete the excess bicarbonate. In this instance certain special maneuvers may be used to corrrect the hyperbicarbonatemia.

1. In the patient with adequate renal function the carbonic anhydrase inhibitor **acetazolamide** may be given in 250- or 500-mg doses, i.v. or by mouth, every 6 hr as needed. This agent is very kaliuretic, and potassium replacement usually is required.

2. In special circumstances when alkalemia is hazardous (arrhythmias) and NaCl is not tolerated or ineffective, **hydrochloric acid** (HCl) may be given via a superior vena cava (not right heart) catheter as a 150 mM solution at 100 to 150 ml/hr. HCl can be infused through a peripheral venous catheter at a 150- to 250-mM concentration in an amino-acid solution without causing phlebitis or hemolysis. **Ammonium chloride** may cause ammonia intoxication, nausea, or vomiting and thus is not recommended.

3. **Hemodialysis** with a low acetate or bicarbonate dialysate is preferred for correction of metabolic alkalosis in the patient with severe or end-stage renal failure.

Prevention of metabolic alkalosis is preferable to treatment. **Cimetidine** will prevent or ameliorate metabolic alkalosis in most patients with nasogastric suction (see Chapter 11 for dosage and contraindications). Intermittent **acetazolamide** therapy is useful in patients on large doses of diuretics.

C. **Treatment of Respiratory Acid-Base Disorders** Correction of the underlying cause is optimal. Direct treatment of the simple disorders rarely is necessary. In **acute respiratory acidosis**, hypoxemia is the critical problem and should be managed as discussed in Chapter 8. In **chronic respiratory acidosis**, pH remains above 7.20, and alkali treatment is not advised. Rarely, if **acute or chronic respiratory alkalosis** causes severe alkalemia (pH over 7.55, which precipitates cardiac arrhythmias), **diazepam or morphine sulfate** may be used to reduce the hyperventilation or suppress ventilation, provided measures for respiratory support are immediately available and no contraindications exist. Certainly ventilator adjustments should be made if the level of oxygenation permits them.

D. **Treatment of Mixed Acid-Base Disorders** Frequently, the underlying disease states act to alter both the [HCO_3] and the P_{CO_2} directly, resulting in a mixed acid-base disorder. If these two variables change in the same direction, the pH tends toward normal, as in **mixed metabolic acidosis and respiratory alkalosis** or **metabolic alkalosis and respiratory acidosis**. Treatment of the underlying disorders usually suffices. However, the frequent concurrence of chronic respiratory acidosis owing to chronic obstructive pulmonary disease (COPD) and metabolic alkalosis owing to diuretic treatment of the accompanying cor pulmonale cause deleterious alkalemia. Patients with COPD have better respiratory drive and oxygenation if pH is acid. In these cases **acetazolamide** is a useful diuretic to treat the alkalemia.

If [HCO_3] and P_{CO_2} deviate from normal in opposite directions, profound **acidemia** (metabolic and respiratory acidosis) or **alkalemia** (metabolic and respiratory alkalosis) may result. If the resultant pH is life-threatening, vigorous correction of the P_{CO_2} should be undertaken at once, utilizing mechanical ventilation with respiratory suppression with morphine and muscle paralyzers if necessary. Then correction of the metabolic problem is pursued.

Occasionally, in a mixed acid-base disorder serum tCO_2 may be normal but pH and P_{CO_2} abnormal. The treatment for mixed disorders should follow the guidelines outlined in Figs. 3 and 4 and discussed earlier.

VI. DISORDERS OF POTASSIUM METABOLISM

A. Treatment of Hypokalemia   The general approach to the treatment of hypokalemia is outlined in Fig. 5.

1. **Oral repletion** of deficits is preferable. The degree of deficit can be estimated roughly in the absence of acidemia, which variably raises serum [K], and alkalemia, which lowers serum [K], without directly altering body potassium content, using the following guidelines: Serum [K] of 3.0 mmol/liter represents about a 150 mmol deficit; 2.0 to 3.0 mmol/liter, a 350- to 500-mmol deficit; less than 2.0, a 500- to 1,000-mmol deficit. Potassium chloride should be used unless chronic metabolic acidosis is present; then an organic potassium salt (citrate, acetate, gluconate) or potassium bicarbonate provides the preferred treatment of both potassium depletion and acidosis. Provision of about 100 to 160 mmol/day in divided doses for 2 to 3 days generally will replete the deficit.

   At least 20 different KCl products are available as either liquids, effervescent tablets or powder to be dissolved in liquid, or wax-matrix tablets. In addition, commercial salt substitutes contain KCl, 10 to 13 mmol per teaspoon. Wax-matrix tablets rarely cause small-bowel ulcers in contrast to the formerly used solid tablets. All products provide KCl; thus, the choice depends solely on patient tolerance and cost. Wax-matrix tablets provide 6.7 to 10 mmol KCl per tablet. Most liquids provide 10% KCl with 20 mmol per 15 ml. Effervescent tablets or powders contain 20 mmol KCl per dose. The pharmacy should be consulted for specific product contents and cost.

2. The indications for intravenous **potassium repletion** are displayed in Fig. 5. Rapid infusion rates of 8 to 20 mmol/hr of KCl as a 60- to 120-mmol/250 ml

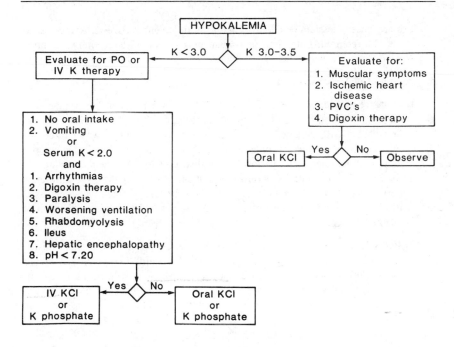

FIG. 5. Treatment of patients with hypokalemia.

D5W or saline solution may be administered through a central line with an infusion pump. This is reserved for severely ill patients in an intensive care unit with electrocardiac monitoring. In critical situations, such as respiratory paralysis or malignant ventricular arrhythmias due to hypokalemia, 10 mmol KCl in 50 ml of solution may be infused over 15 min with continuous observation. Unmonitored patients should receive no more than 200 mmol/day of KCl in a maximum concentration of 40 mM, with frequent serum [K] measurements at intervals depending on infusion rates when more than maintenance amounts are infused intravenously. Peripheral vein infusion solutions containing more than 30 mmol/liter often cause pain in the vein.

3. Chronic oral potassium supplements may be necessary in those individuals taking diuretics who develop hypokalemia as outlined in Fig. 5. The **potassium-sparing diuretics**—amiloride, triamterene and spironolactone—may be used to prevent excess potassium losses. Amiloride appears to be more potent than triamterene. Both of these agents block non-aldosterone-mediated potassium secretion, whereas spironolactone is a competitive aldosterone inhibitor. If KCl is used, 30 to 60 mmol/day is usually sufficient to maintain a normal serum [K]. All of these measures should be avoided in patients with advanced renal failure or hypoaldosteronism except in very rare circumstances. Depletion of the other major intracellular ions, magnesium and phosphate, usually ac-

companies potassium depletion. Therefore, treatment of these deficiencies also may be required. Potassium phosphate may be administered orally or intravenously as discussed below.

B. Treatment of Hyperkalemia

1. **General measures.** The basic approach to the treatment of hyperkalemia is outlined in Fig. 6. If the ECG shows a prolonged PR interval, absent P waves, or widened QRS complexes, or if the patient has paralysis, two or three 10-ml ampuls of 10% **calcium gluconate** (2 mmol or 4 mEq of calcium per ampul) should be given by slow i.v. push over 3 to 5 min while monitoring the ECG. Calcium decreases threshold potential and normalizes the difference between the threshold and resting potentials; the resting potential is decreased by hyperkalemia. The onset of effect occurs in 1 to 5 min with a duration of 30 min.

2. **Potassium shift.** The next step is to shift potassium into cells, thus raising the ratio of intra- to extracellular potassium. Fifty milliliters of 50% **dextrose** (25 g glucose) should be given by slow i.v. push along with **regular insulin**, 0.1 u/kg body weight, and two 50-ml ampuls of $NaHCO_3$ given by slow i.v. push. The hypokalemic effect occurs within 30 min and lasts 2 to 4 hr. An

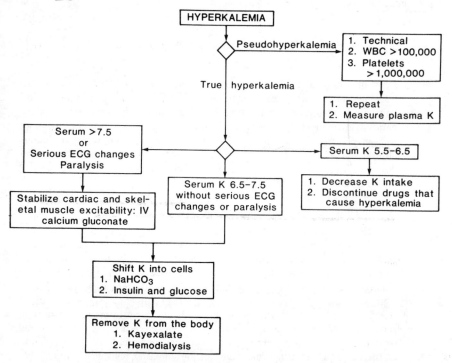

FIG. 6.   Treatment of patients with hyperkalemia.

infusion of D10W containing 20 units of regular insulin at 250 ml/hr should be started. Patients with diabetes mellitus may require more insulin.

3. **Potassium binding.** The definitive step is to remove potassium from the body either by **binding to sodium polystyrene sulfonate (Kayexalate®)** or by **hemodialysis.** The administration of 15 to 30 g Kayexalate® with 50 to 100 ml 20% sorbitol (a nonabsorbed sugar that acts as an osmotic cathartic) should be given every 6 to 12 hr. One gram of Kayexalate® binds 1 mmol of potassium in exchange for 1.5 mmol of sodium. If the patient has an ileus or is vomiting, 50 g Kayexalate® in 200 ml 20% sorbitol can be administered as a retention enema using a mushroom-balloon-tipped rectal catheter to obtain 30- to 60-min retention. Prior cleansing enemas may make this approach more effective. If the sodium load is not tolerable or other indications for dialysis exist, hemodialysis should be instituted. Peritoneal dialysis is less efficient than Kayexalate® in removing potassium. Serum potassium should be measured before each Kayexalate® or dialysis treatment.

4. **Drugs or remedies containing potassium** that may cause hyperkalemia, particularly in the presence of renal failure should be discontinued. These include **salt substitutes, amiloride, spironolactone, triamterene, nonsteroidal anti-inflammatory agents** (Chapter 16), **beta blockers,** and rarely, **heparin.**

5. Patients with chronic renal failure or hypoaldosteronism (Chapter 20) may have **chronic hyperkalemia.** Generally, cessation of the above medications and avoidance of high-potassium foods suffices to keep potassium concentration less than 6.5 mmol/liter. Occasionally, chronic intermittent Kayexalate® therapy may be necessary. Treatment of hypoaldosteronism with **fludrocortisone** is discussed in Chapter 20.

VII. DISORDERS OF PHOSPHORUS METABOLISM

A. Treatment of Hypophosphatemia

1. **Severe hypophosphatemia**—serum inorganic phosphorus less than 1.0 mg/dl—occurs most commonly with alcohol withdrawal, total parenteral nutrition (TPN), treated diabetic ketoacidosis, burns, pronounced chronic respiratory alkalosis, and use of aluminum-containing antacids. Consequences of severe hypophosphatemia include congestive heart failure, respiratory failure, rhabdomyolysis, altered mental status, hemolysis, and leukocyte dysfunction. If these manifestations are present, 0.2 mmol/kg (6.2 mg/kg) of phosphorus i.v. over 6 hr should be administered and the serum phosphorus level then measured. This dose should be repeated until the level approaches 2.0 mg/dl, and then the patient should be switched to oral phosphorus or the dose halved until the level exceeds 2.5 mg/dl. The underlying causes should have been corrected by then, with the exception of continuous TPN administration and burns. Provision of 0.25 to 0.5 mmol/kg (7.75 to 15.5 mg/kg) per day of phosphorus should be adequate maintenance for ongoing TPN.

One commercially available sodium phosphate solution for addition to infusions contains 3 mmol phosphorus and 4 mmol sodium per milliliter (Abbott). Potassium phosphate contains 3 mmol phosphorus and 4.4 mmol potassium per milliliter. The preparations in the specific hospital pharmacy should be checked for exact content. The additives to D5W or saline solutions should be ordered as both ml of solution and mmol phosphorus, e.g., add 4 ml containing 3 mM phosphate (sodium) to 500 ml NS and infuse over 6 hr.

2. **The major complications of intravenous phosphorus administration** are metastatic calcification of vessels, lung, etc.; hypocalcemia; and hypotension. Marked caution is needed in treating patients with hypercalcemia or renal failure.

3. **Moderate hypophosphatemia**—serum phosphorus 1.0 to 2.5 mg/dl—is caused by many disorders. In this setting oral repletion is preferable. About 16 mmol (500 mg) of phosphorus should be provided daily in addition to dietary phosphorus intake. Two or three times this amount may be given if serum phosphorus is less than 1.5 mg/dl, food intake is low, and renal function is normal. One quart of **skim milk** contains 30 to 35 mmol of phosphorus. **Neutra-Phos**® (Willen) contains about 0.11 mmol (3.3 mg) phosphorus and 0.1 mmol sodium and 0.1 mmol potassium per milliliter (also available as no sodium, 0.2 mmol potassium per milliliter) after reconstitution of either powder or capsules. This should be given as 150 to 300 ml in two to four divided doses daily. **Phospho-Soda**® (Fleet) contains 4.15 mmol (129 mg) phosphorus and 4.8 mmol sodium per milliliter; it should be administered as 5 ml two or three times a day. Diarrhea develops occasionally with these doses of oral phosphates.

B. **Treatment of Hyperphosphatemia**   Hyperphosphatemia generally develops only in patients with acute or chronic renal failure. Avoidance of high-phosphate foods (dairy products) and use of **aluminum-containing antacids** will control serum phosphorus concentration in most patients.

VIII. DISORDERS OF MAGNESIUM METABOLISM

A. **Treatment of Hypomagnesemia**

1. **Severe hypomagnesemia** (less than 1.2 mg/dl or 0.5 mmol/liter or 1.0 mEq/liter) may occur in patients with malabsorption, treated ketoacidosis, alcoholism, TPN, and cisplatinum or aminoglycoside therapy. If seizures, tetany, or malignant arrhythmias occur, intravenous magnesium should be given as 4 ml of **50% MgSO₄** (162 mg, 8 mmol, 16 mEq) in 100 ml D5W over 10 to 15 min. This should be followed with a 4-hr infusion of 8 ml of 50% MgSO₄ (16 mmol) in 500 to 1,000 ml D5W. During the subsequent 20 hr an additional 0.5 mmol/kg of magnesium should be provided, followed by 0.25 mmol/kg/day during the next 2 to 4 days. Serum magnesium levels should be monitored carefully.

2. For patients with **chronic moderate hypomagnesemia** due to malabsorption, or in those unable to take oral supplements, repletion with 50% MgSO₄, 4 ml (8 mmol), i.m., q6hr for 2 days followed by 2 ml q6hr for 2 to 3 days should correct the deficit. Then 2 ml (4 mmol) daily or 4 ml every other day should suffice to maintain a normal level. However, these injections are painful.

Oral magnesium supplements to prevent depletion may be provided as **magnesium oxide** tablets (240 mg = 10 mmol, variable-size tablets); usually 20 to 40 mmol per day suffice. More than 60 mmol of magnesium per day frequently causes diarrhea.

Caution is required in parenteral repletion of magnesium, especially in patients with decreased renal function. Disappearance or depression of deep tendon reflexes is a sign of hypermagnesemia that occurs at a serum concentration around 4.9 mg/dl (2 mmol/liter). Therefore, the reflexes should be checked before each dose of parenteral magnesium when acutely correcting severe depletion, especially when serum magnesium measurements (a good guide to level of depletion) are delayed or not available.

B. Treatment of Hypermagnesemia Severe hypermagnesemia occurs almost exclusively in patients with advanced renal failure who take magnesium-containing preparations or receive magnesium-containing enemas. Occasionally, a subject who ingests **Epsom salts** may develop serious hypermagnesemia.

1. Serum magnesium concentrations above 4.9 mg/dl (2 mmol or 4 mEq/liter) cause depressed tendon reflexes and GI distress.

2. Levels above 9.7 mg/dl (4 mmol or 8 mEq/liter) may ablate these reflexes and cause paralysis.

3. Levels above 14.6 mg/dl (6 mmol or 12 mEq/liter) may cause coma and respiratory arrest.

4. Heart block or cardiac arrest may occur in these latter two stages.

The immediate antidote is 10% calcium gluconate, three 10-ml ampuls (2 mmol/ampul) given by i.v. push over 5 min. Patients with moderately advanced renal failure may respond to a **furosemide-saline-calcium diuresis regimen** consisting of furosemide 40 mg i.v., 1,000 ml NS with one or two 10-ml ampuls of 10% $CaCl_2$ (7 mmol or 280 mg calcium per ampul) at 500 ml/hr. Caution must be exercised when planning to infuse calcium containing solutions in hyperphosphatemic patients because of the risk of precipitating metastatic calcification. In patients with advanced renal failure *hemodialysis* should be instituted as rapidly as possible. For subjects with mild or moderate hypomagnesemia without symptoms, discontinuing exogenous magnesium loads may be sufficient treatment.

BIBLIOGRAPHY

Berl, T., Anderson, R. J., McDonald, K. M., and Schrier, R. W. (1976): Clinical disorders of water metabolism. *Kidney Int.*, 10:117–132.

Cobb, W. E., Spare, S., and Reichlin, S. (1978): Neurogenic diabetes insipidus: Management with dDAVP(1-desamino-8-D-arginine vasopressin). *Ann. Intern. Med.*, 88:183–188.

Conners, A. F., Jr., McCaffree, D. R., and Gray, B. A. (1983): Evaluation of right-heart catheterization in the critically ill patient without acute myocardial infarction. *N. Engl. J. Med.*, 308:263–267.

Hantman, D., Rossier, B., Zohlman, R., and Schrier, R. W. (1973): Rapid correction of hyponatremia in the syndrome of inappropriate secretion of antidiuretic hormone: An alternative treatment to hypertonic saline. *Ann. Intern. Med.*, 78:870–875.

Knutson, O. H. (1983): New method for administration of hydrochloric acid in metabolic acidosis. *Lancet*, 1:953–955.

Kurtzman, N. A., and Batlle, D. C., eds. (1983): Symposium on acid-base disorders. *Med. Clin. North Am.*, 67:751–932.

Lentz, R. D., Brown, D. M., and Kjellstrand, C. M. (1978): Treatment of severe hypophosphatemia. *Ann. Intern. Med.*, 89:941–944.

Maxwell, M. H., and Kleeman, C. R., eds. (1980): *Clinical Disorders of Fluid and Electrolyte Metabolism*, 3rd ed. McGraw-Hill Book Co., New York.[2]

Schrier, R. W., ed. (1985): *Renal and Electrolyte Disorders* (3d ed.). Little, Brown and Co., Boston.[2]

---

[2]These textbooks contain detained discussions of the pathogenesis, pathophysiology, differential diagnosis, and treatment of all fluid and electrolyte disorders, with extensive bibliographies.

3.

Renal Parenchymal Diseases

Martin P. Hutt and Robert W. Schrier

3.

Renal Parenchymal Diseases

The presence of renal parenchymal disease (**RPD**) usually is recognized from **azotemia** [i.e., increased blood urea nitrogen (BUN)] or an **abnormal urine analysis** examined in routine screening tests or as part of an investigation of symptoms or signs of uremia. Therapy for RPD when directed by diagnosis (either etiologic, histologic or pathophysiologic diagnosis) is likely to be more effective than when directed empirically toward symptoms or signs.

I. THERAPY DETERMINED BY ETIOLOGY

A. Urinary Tract Infections (See also Chapter 10.) Urinary tract infections are treated as determined by the in vitro sensitivity to antibiotics of the causative bacterium. Part of prevention of recurrence consists of **eliminating predisposing factors** such as stones or stasis (e.g., prostatic hypertrophy), which are more likely to be found in males. These are usually absent in females, but other **preventive measures** are of importance in females, including postcoital voiding, wiping front to back, and frequent bladder emptying. In certain circumstances of symptomatic recurrent infections in females, prophylactic trimethoprim-sulfamethoxazole, 1 tablet nightly or before intercourse, may be used.

B. Renal Calculi Medical therapy for **stones** in the urinary tract is directed to **relief of episodes of acute pain with analgesics**—often meperidine. After the stone has passed or been removed by the urologist, it should be analyzed, because treatment to prevent recurrence of stones of differing chemical composition varies.

1. **Cystine stones** are radio-opaque and should be suspected when hexagonal crystals are seen in the urine. Therapy consists of avoiding precipitation by ensuring a high urine flow rate of at least 100 ml/hr during both day and night and rendering the urine alkaline with sodium bicarbonate (4.0 to 8.0 g daily) to increase cystine solubility.

2. **Uric acid stones** are radiolucent and may occur in the absence of hyperuricosuria (>800 mg/day). Acid urine, however, is very frequent. Therapy should include alkalinization to increase solubility of uric acid, as well as allopurinol 100 to 300 mg daily, to decrease uric acid excretion. Maintenance of a high urine flow rate (>150 ml/hr) is especially important when transient acute increases in uric acid excretion occur, such as during induction therapy for acute leukemia or lymphoma (especially Burkitt's lymphoma).

3. **Magnesium-ammonium phosphate (struvite) stones** occur in the presence of infection. Prevention of recurrence requires surgical removal of stones and clearing of infection at the time of surgery. Irrigation of the renal pelvis with a mixture of acids (renacidin) after removal of the stones may be of value to prevent recurrence.

4. Although **calcium-containing stones** occur more frequently (75% of all stones) than the stones discussed earlier, hypercalcemia and hypercalciuria are identified as causative factors in only a minority of calcium stone formers.

   a. Renal calculi associated with persistent hypercalcemia in the absence of sarcoidosis, neoplasm, or excessive vitamin D ingestion, is the hallmark of **primary hyperparathyroidism**. Hypophosphatemia, hyperchloremia, and an increased plasma concentration of parathyroid hormone confirm the diagnosis of primary hyperparathyroidism. Surgical removal of a parathyroid adenoma or partial parathyroidectomy for parathyroid hyperplasia is the treatment of choice in this setting. Adenomas may be localized with ultrasound.

   b. **Idiopathic hypercalciuria** without hypercalcemia may occur in patients with **distal renal tubular acidosis** who are unable to lower their urine pH below 5.3 when challenged with an acid load. Those patients with the complete form of renal tubular acidosis should be treated with sodium and/or potassium bicarbonate to correct the metabolic acidosis and prevent recurrence of nephrolithiasis or nephrocalcinosis. Patients with the incomplete form of distal renal tubular acidosis (absence of metabolic acidosis), in which the renal acidification defect is observed only after an exogenous acid load, may have recurrent calcium stones without hypercalciuria.

   Hypercalciuria without hypercalcemia also is encountered in some patients who are gastrointestinal **hyperabsorbers** of calcium. Following an oral load of 1.0 g of calcium, a 4-hr urine collection demonstrates urinary calcium concentration higher than 0.2 mg per mg creatinine. **Restriction of dietary calcium** by avoidance of milk and milk products is appropriate treatment in these patients.

   c. Although calcium **oxalate** is the major constituent of most renal calculi, hyperoxaluria, either primary or secondary to inflammatory small-bowel disease or intestinal bypass surgery, is uncommon. Patients with hyperoxaluria should avoid foods high in oxalate—such as nuts, spinach, rhubarb, chocolate, strawberries, and tea.

   d. Most patients with calcium-containing renal stones do not have a clear cause for stone formation. Prevention of recurrence of stones in patients with idiopathic hypercalciuria is based on **limiting stasis** within the urinary tract and maintaining low concentrations of urinary calcium and oxalate. Uric acid is thought sometimes to form a small but significant nidus in stones whose main constitutent is calcium, and therefore the **urinary concentration of uric acid is reduced** with allopurinol. To avoid stasis any mechanical obstruction is relieved and **complete bladder emptying** (sometimes with double voiding) at regular (about 3-hour) intervals is advised. To keep the concentration of potential precipitants low, a **high urine flow rate** (approximately 3 liters per day) is prescribed. Dietary calcium and oxalate are restricted. A thiazide-type diuretic, usually hydrochlorothiazide 50 mg twice daily, is given to decrease urinary calcium excretion. Modest sodium restriction is necessary to insure efficacy of thiazide diuretics in causing hypocalciuria.

II. THERAPY DETERMINED BY PATHOPHYSIOLOGY

A. Acute Renal Failure   Acute renal failure is a diagnosis of exclusion. Before an acute and profound decrease in glomerular filtration rate (GFR) to levels below 10 ml/min can be attributed to renal parenchymal disease, prerenal and postrenal disorders must be excluded.

Postrenal obstruction as a cause of azotemia may be associated with anuria, oliguria (less than 400 ml/24 hr) or polyuria (>3 liter/24 hr). Possible upper urinary tract obstruction usually is investigated with ultrasound, and rarely antegrade or retrograde pyelography is necessary. Bladder neck obstruction is best evaluated by estimation of the postvoid residual by catheterization. If urinary tract obstruction is present, it must be promptly relieved.

The presence of **prerenal factors** contributing to a reduced GFR generally is associated with extrarenal causes of renal hypoperfusion, including **intravascular volume depletion** and cardiac or liver failure. Impaired cardiac function is manifest by clinical evidence of left ventricular failure, a decreased ejection fraction, and increased pulmonary capillary wedge pressure. Therapy in that situation should be designed to improve cardiac function. Patients with **overt intravascular volume depletion and shock**, as from acute hemorrhage, obviously, should receive therapy aimed at restoring intravascular volume.

Lesser degrees of plasma volume depletion may present only as tachycardia and orthostatic hypotension. These findings also may be present in patients with a decreased cardiac output caused by myocardial (e.g., cardiomyopathy, acute myocardial infarction) or pericardial disease. It may be difficult at the bedside to be certain that mild hypovolemia is not present, and sometimes a Swan-Ganz catheter placement is necessary to measure pulmonary capillary wedge pressure.

The presence of **prerenal** factors also may be documented by evaluation of **urinary indices** (Table 1). Renal tubules capable of conserving water and salt in response to a decreased effective arterial blood volume will excrete urine with a high osmolality and creatinine and low sodium and chloride. A fractional excretion of sodium or a renal failure index (urinary sodium/urine-to-plasma creatinine) of less than 1 indicate intact tubular function in the azotemic patient, and therefore diagnose prerenal failure. Impaired tubular function in a azotemic patient with high urinary sodium, fractional excretion of sodium, and renal failure index is compatible with chronic renal disease, urinary tract obstruction, or acute tubular necrosis (ATN).

TABLE 1. *Laboratory features characteristic of the presence of prerenal factors in acute renal failure[a]*

Uosm (mOsm/kg/H_2O)	>500	U/P creatinine	>40
UNa (mEq/L)	<20	Fractional excretion Na	<1%
U/P urea N	>10	Renal failure index	<1

[a]Values outside these ranges in the azotemia patient suggest prior diuretic administration, urinary tract obstruction, chronic renal failure, or acute tubular necrosis (ATN). Patients with acute glomerulonephritis or vasculitis may have prerenal azotemia, but the sediment with hematuria, RBC casts, and proteinuria differentiates these patients from volume depletion causing prerenal azotemia.

Uosm, urinary osmolality; UNa, urinary sodium; U/P, urine-to-plasma.

If there is any question about whether intravascular volume depletion is contributing to the **azotemia**, then judicious and careful plasma volume expansion may be undertaken. For example, in a patient with chronic renal disease who becomes volume-depleted, the urinary indices may not be diagnostic of prerenal azotemia. If volume depletion is present, then volume expansion will result in an increase in GFR and cause a decrease in BUN and serum creatinine. Urinary indices also will not be diagnostic of prerenal azotemia if the patient has just received a diuretic or mannitol.

Another form of prerenal acute renal failure and **azotemia** is that **secondary to hepatic insufficiency** (hepatorenal syndrome). The low fractional excretion of sodium present in this setting indicates that tubular function is intact. The severe reduction in GFR is caused by vasoconstriction of renal resistance vessels. The **poor prognosis** results from the fact that hepatorenal syndrome is seen only in the most severe forms of hepatic disease. Efforts at plasma volume expansion to increase GFR are usually futile or achieve a transient improvement in renal function. Such efforts also may be associated with increased portal hypertension and precipitate bleeding from esophageal varices. Some patients with hepatorenal syndrome may respond to a **peritoneojugular (LeVeen) shunt**. The complications of the LeVeen shunt include the risk of infection and disseminated intravascular coagulation.

After both postrenal obstruction and prerenal factors have been excluded, the presence of intrarenal factors is established as the cause for the acute renal failure.

Different types of renal parenchymal disease may cause acute renal failure. The probability of complete recovery of renal function is greatest in nonoliguric acute tubular necrosis caused by nephrotoxic antibiotics, and treatment primarily involves cessation of antibiotics. Acute renal failure in adults owing to intrarenal factors also include ATN, which may be oliguric or nonoliguric; the former has a 50% mortality and the latter a 20% mortality. **Acute interstitial nephritis, glomerulonephritis, and cortical necrosis** are other causes of acute renal failure that are not reversible by altering either prerenal or postrenal factors. Therapy prescribed to increase recovery of renal function will vary for each condition, whereas supportive therapy to sustain the patient with acute renal failure until recovery of function is similar for each condition.

1. Therapy to increase recovery of acute renal failure

a. ATN. Since the patient mortality and morbidity with **oliguric** ATN is greater than with **nonoliguric** ATN, some investigators have recommended that the oliguric patient with ATN should receive furosemide in graded doses up to 1,000 mg/day in an effort to convert the oliguric to a nonoliguric state. Whether such an approach will decrease morbidity and mortality in these patients has yet to be shown in a prospective, double-blind study.

Therapy with **total parenteral nutrition** with essential amino acids has been shown to have a beneficial effect in one well-controlled study done in patients who developed ATN after surgery. However, the efficacy of this form of costly therapy has not been confirmed. Nevertheless, since the mortality may exceed 50% in catabolic patients, total parenteral nutrition in ATN is advocated, using preparations such as nephramine, which contains the essential amino acid equivalent of 40 g of protein per liter.

b. **Acute interstitial nephritis** is diagnosed with certainty only with a **kidney biopsy**. It may occur in association with various drugs (Table 2) or viral infections, or it may occur as an idiopathic entity. Rash, fever, eosinophilia, and eosinophiluria are clinical clues to the presence of acute interstitial nephritis but are frequently absent. Once the diagnosis is made, any drugs known to cause acute interstitial nephritis should be discontinued. In the absence of improvement in renal function within a few days after stopping the offending agent, a 2-week course of **prednisone** 1.5 mg/kg/day should be instituted. Although some workers claim that such therapy enhances recovery, a controlled study needs to be performed.

c. **Acute glomerulonephritis** may lead to acute renal failure, and the treatment depends on the cause of the glomerulonephritis. The treatment of bacterial endocarditis, or "shunt" nephritis, with antibiotics is generally sufficient for the resolution of the associated glomerulonephritis. **Multiple myeloma** also may be associated with acute renal failure. Dialysis, volume repletion, and treatment of any hypercalcemia and/or hyperuricemia, are indicated, as well as chemotherapy for the myeloma (see Chapter 15). There is no successful treatment of acute poststreptococcal glomerulonephritis causing acute renal failure, but most patients with that condition generally recover renal function with control of hypertension and heart failure, and a period of dialysis. Acute renal failure secondary to systemic lupus erythematosus or **idiopathic rapidly progressive glomerulonephritis (RPGN)** may be treated with bolus therapy (1 g methylprednisolone, i.v., during EKG monitoring for 3 consecutive days) and plasmapheresis (3 units/day for 4 days then every other day for 2 weeks). Early diagnosis of **antiglomerular basement membrane** (antiGBM) disease causing RPGN by renal biopsy with immunofluorescence demonstrating linear GBM staining and crescents would support the use of **plasmapheresis**. Non-antiGBM disease causing RPGN may be treated with steroids and immunosuppressive therapy without plasmapheresis. The efficacy of these treatments has not, however, been proved in controlled studies. Plasmapheresis should always be associated with steroid and immunosuppressive therapy (e.g., 2 to 3 mg/kg cyclophosphamide) to prevent the immunologic "rebound."

2. **Therapy** to sustain the patient until recovery of renal function is as follows:

a. Treatment of **extrarenal conditions** whether causative or coincidental is

TABLE 2. *Drugs that may cause acute interstitial nephritis*

Antibiotics	Nonsteroidal anti-inflammatory
Methicillin and other penicillins	agents
Cephalosporins	Miscellaneous
Sulfonamides	Phenytoin
Rifampin	Allopurinol
Erythromycin	Phenindione
Analgesics, especially phenacetin	Cimetidine
Diuretics, including furosemide	
and thiazides	

important and may include antibiotics to treat the bacteremia that provoked septic shock and the subsequent ATN, or careful regulation of insulin dose in a patient with diabetes mellitus.

b. **General measures.** When possible, **ambulation** should be encouraged to prevent problems associated with total bed rest, such as respiratory infections and bed sores. A **diet** of at least 2,000 calories with no more than 40 g protein (mainly as meat, eggs, milk, and fish of high biologic value) should be administered to minimize endogenous protein catabolism, negative nitrogen balance, and the generation of organic acids. Restriction of dietary potassium should be instituted. Restriction of dietary sodium chloride (<4 gm/day) if the patient is oliguric (urine <400 ml/day) will prevent the positive balance of sodium chloride. This tolerable level of about 50 mEq/day of sodium chloride avoids the decrease in palatability of more severely restricted diets. A somewhat more liberal diet is possible in the nonoliguric patient with ATN.

c. Careful attention to **water balance** also is essential to minimize positive balance and hyponatremia. The goal of fluid therapy should be to achieve a weight loss of no greater than 0.5 kg/day and no weight gain.

d. **Hypertension** may be prevented by avoiding a positive salt and water balance but antihypertensive medications (see Chapter 4) may be necessary to control hypertension and prevent encephalopathy.

e. Although **infection** is the main cause of death in acute renal failure, prophylactic antibiotics should not be used. The use of all types of catheters and intravenous lines should be avoided. Infections should be sought and when found treated promptly. Dosages of many antibiotics must be reduced in the presence of renal failure (see Chapter 10).

f. **Anemia** is frequent, but transfusion should be avoided unless for specific indications such as cardiac symptoms (e.g., angina, high-output failure).

g. **Hyperphosphatemia** should be prevented by using non-magnesium-containing phosphate binders such as Basaljel® or Amphojel®, 30 ml, at least three times daily 1 hr after meals.

h. **Hypocalcemia** and **hyperuricemia** usually occur but rarely cause symptoms and do not require therapy.

i. **Acidosis** and **hyperkalemia** are likely to occur; their therapy is discussed in Chapter 2. Failure to correct these abnormalities with appropriate medication (e.g., hyperkalemia not controlled with Kayexalate®) is an indication for dialysis.

j. **Dialysis.** Absolute indications for dialysis include pulmonary edema, pericarditis, and uremic encephalopathy. Still a matter of some controversy is the level of BUN or serum creatinine which should be an indication for dialysis even in the absence of uremic symptoms. Most nephrologists, however, would dialyze to prevent the BUN from exceeding 100 mg/dl and the serum creatinine from exceeding 8 to 10 mg/dl. The presence of **uremic symptoms,** such as pruritus, insomnia, irritability, anorexia, nausea, and vomiting also would be considered indications for dialysis. In most hospitals where hemodialysis is available this form of dialysis will be used rather than peritoneal dialysis for the treatment of acute renal failure. Access to the circulation is provided through catheters placed in the central veins. These may be left in place for several weeks although they are potential sites of infection. In the absence of systemic complications, evidence of hypercatabolism, and intra-abdominal processes, **peritoneal dialysis** may be used to treat acute renal failure.

To prevent symptoms of dysequilibrium syndrome, shorter hemodialysis (3 hr) will usually be performed daily for 3 days at initiation. Then dialysis (5 to 6 hr) will be used at least three times weekly until a lower serum creatinine pre-dialysis than post-dialysis indicates that glomerular filtration has increased. In the catabolic patient daily dialysis may be necessary to prevent uremic symptoms and maintain BUN below 100 mg/dl.

B. **Glomerular Diseases** While glomerular disease sometimes presents as acute renal failure, more often it appears as hematuria, hypertension, edema, proteinuria, or mild to moderate azotemia. Proteinuria in excess of about 3.0 g/24 hr or 3.0 mg per mg creatinine in the absence of severe hypertension or heart failure support the diagnosis of glomerulonephritis. Confirmation and a histologic diagnosis require renal biopsy.

1. Treatment of systemic events that may delay progression of renal failure include the following: **Hypertension** is a frequent complication of almost all glomerular disease, and control (by methods described in Chapter 4) will remove a factor that can accelerate decline in renal function. In diabetic patients **control of hyperglycemia** (by methods described in Chapter 19) may have a protective effect on the rate of deterioration of renal function; however, this remains to be proved. **Early treatment of urinary tract infection** and any **volume depletion** also will be important to avoid progression of renal disease.

2. Evidence of **glomerular disease as an integral part of systemic disease** involves evaluation by history and physical examination for multisystem abnormalities and serology in systemic lupus erythematosus; lung or upper airway biopsy in Wegener's granulomatosis, or skin biopsy in vasculitis. Therapy for Wegener's granulomatosis with renal impairment involves **cyclophosphamide** 2 mg/kg/day, and at least 80% of patients respond to this treatment. After 3 1/2 months of cyclophosphamide treatment, azathioprine 2 mg/kg may be substituted to avoid complications of long-term cyclophosphamide treatment. An exacerbation during azathoprine treatment should then be treated by reinstitution of cyclophosphamide treatment. After 12 months of total remission on therapy, a considerable number of patients may have all therapy discontinued without exacerbations during considerable follow-up periods.

Renal involvement with systemic lupus erythematosus also should be treated with **prednisone** at a daily dose of 1.5 mg/kg. The addition of azothioprine 1.5 mg/kg may also be used for its steroid-sparing effect. Prednisone 1.5 mg/kg can be used to treat the renal involvement of vasculitis; however, recent results suggest that many patients also may need to be treated with cyclophosphamide (1 to 2 mg/kg). White blood cell count will be expected to decrease with this therapy but must not be allowed to decrease below 3,000 cells/mm^3. **Mixed essential cryoglobulemia** associated with vasculitis may respond to plasmapheresis to lower plasma concentration of cryoglobulins; prednisone, or perhaps more preferably cyclophosphamide, is then indicated to maintain suppressed plasma levels of cryoglobulins.

3. **Primary glomerular diseases** can be reliably distinguished from one another only by renal **biopsy**.

   a. **Minimal change disease (lipoid nephrosis)** has the sole abnormality on biopsy of foot process effacement and is almost always **steroid-sensitive** (proteinuria decreases to normal: below 100 mg/day or below 0.1 mg per mg creatinine). **Prednisone** in a dose of 1.5/kg/day usually will cause a complete remission within 14 days. Within 1 week after a remission occurs the dose of prednisone should be halved to an alternate-day regimen. The prednisone is then tapered slowly in decrements of 5 mg/week. The sooner the remission has occurred, the more rapidly the dose of prednisone may be reduced.

   About half of the patients who have a complete remission will **relapse**. The relapse should be treated by recycling therapy. Specifically, the dose that causes a remission is maintained for twice as long as previously and then tapered at a slower rate. Similarly, a second relapse should be treated by doubling the duration of therapy used in the first relapse. A third relapse should be treated using the same regimen as during the second but adding a cytotoxic agent; e.g., cyclophosphamide 2 mg/kg/day or chlorambucil 0.3 mg/kg/day. This latter approach usually will result in a longer duration of remission. The dose of cytotoxic agent should be tapered and discontinued within 2 to 3 months.

   In those **steroid-resistant patients** in whom a complete remission has not occurred after 4 weeks, the prednisone dose should be decreased and discontinued. After a month off prednisone, a second attempt should be made to induce a remission with prednisone, and treatment should be continued for 6 weeks. If no remission occurs, it is likely that the patient has **focal segmental glomerulosclerosis** that was missed on the renal biopsy, and treatment should be for symptoms as described below.

   b. **Membranous nephropathy** was originally described based on light microscopy but now requires electron microscopy for an accurate diagnosis. A course of prednisone—120 mg in a single daily dose given every other day for 2 months—has been associated with a remission of proteinuria in some cases. In this well-controlled study the regimen also seems to have prevented some patients from having a rapid decline in GFR over the ensuing 2 years. However, because of the rapid and increased rate of decline in renal function in the control group, some nephrologists believe that membranous nephropathy should not be treated. The incidence of renal vein thrombosis associated with membranous nephropathy is also controversial and has varied from 5% to 33%. If renal vein thrombosis is demonstrated by renal venography, chronic anticoagulation therapy should be instituted with warfarin to prevent thromboembolic events; it is not known whether such treatment alters the natural history of membranous nephropathy.

c. In the absence of systemic disease, **focal segmental glomerulosclerosis, membranoproliferative glomerulonephritis, proliferative glomerulonephritis, and mesangial proliferative glomerulonephritis** have not been shown to benefit from treatment with prednisone, cytotoxic agents, or plasmapheresis in any controlled study. However, when faced with such patients whose GFR is declining, a therapeutic trial may sometimes be undertaken with these measures. This is particularly true when the renal biopsy demonstrates superimposition of RPGN with crescents. The younger the patient and the more rapid the rate of decline of renal function, the more tempting it is to attempt such a trial.

The judgment that renal function is deteriorating rapidly is reliable in proportion to the number of observations of **serum creatinine** available and the length of time covered by these observations. **Trends** are more easily observed by **graphic display** of the data on either a linear, logarithmic, or reciprocal scale. Two main criteria are used to judge whether the therapy has been beneficial: a change in the slope of the graph of the serum creatinine indicating stability or improvement in GFR; and, a decrease in the quantity of proteinuria. For all types of glomerular disease, patients with proteinuria of less than 2 g/24 hr or 2 mg per mg creatinine have a better prognosis than those with larger amounts of proteinuria.

4. **Nephrotic syndrome.** All glomerular disease may be associated with a nephrotic phase when **proteinuria** is greater than 3.5 g/day or 3.5 mg per mg creatinine and is associated with **hypoalbuminemia** and **edema**. In addition to treating the primary disease, supportive therapy is important.

   a. **Nutrition** is important in minimizing the degree of hypoalbuminemia. Thus, an effort should be made to have the patient ingest a daily diet of at least 100 g protein. Salt should be restricted to as low a level as possible (usually about 4.0 g/day), while still allowing a palatable diet.

   b. When **edema** is present and causing the patient discomfort, **diuretics** may be used to alleviate the discomfort. However, attempts to remove all excess extracellular fluid should not be undertaken because of the danger of volume depletion and associated complications. About half the patients with the nephrotic syndrome have hypovolemia, and vigorous diuresis may reduce renal perfusion and GFR. Therapy with diuretics should begin with a **thiazide** diuretic with gradual increases in dose. A **potassium-sparing** diuretic should be added if hypokalemia appears or the thiazide diuretic is not effective. The combination of potassium supplements and a potassium-sparing diuretic is contraindicated because of the complication of severe hyperkalemia. In resistant patients **furosemide** may be added with gradually increasing doses 40 mg b.i.d. to 320 mg b.i.d.. **Metolazone** may be added for those patients in whom large doses of furosemide (i.e., 640 mg/day) have not been effective.

   A rare patient with the nephrotic syndrome will be resistant to all these diuretics. In these patients a transient diuresis may occur when **intravenous albumin** is given in an amount sufficient to increase serum albumin and thus mobilize fluid from the extravascular interstitial compartment into the vascular space. A diuresis is best achieved if the albumin infusion is accompanied by the use of furosemide. Because glomerular capillary permeability to albumin is greatly increased in nephrotic syndrome, the exogenous albumin is rapidly excreted in the urine. Because this form of therapy is so expensive and relatively ineffective, it should be reserved for patients in whom all other measures to mobilize very discomforting edema have failed.

   c. Although the nephrotic syndrome is a hypercoagulable state, prophylactic **anticoagulation** is not recommended. If there is evidence of peripheral vein or renal vein thrombosis, long-term anticoagulation with coumadin should be undertaken (see above).

  5. The natural history of chronic glomerular disease in most patients is progression to renal insufficiency. However, the rate of progression is highly variable and may be rapid (weeks or months) or so indolent (decades) as to appear to have long periods (years) in which there is stabilization of an elevated serum creatinine. The course of the disease is best followed as described above. The cause of the progression is unknown, but recent studies in experimental animals have led to two suggestions of therapy to retard the decline in renal function.

   a. Restriction of **dietary protein** may exert a salutary effect by causing a decrease in albumin filtered by inducing a decrease in plasma albumin or GFR. The glomerular hyperfiltration and the amount of albumin filtered per nephron have been suggested as inducing glomerular sclerosis as the final common pathway for many varieties of chronic renal parenchymal disease. However, this hypothesis remains to be conclusively substantiated.

   b. Administration of **phosphate binders** has been advocated in order to prevent the hyperphosphatemia that usually occurs once the GFR decreases below 25% of normal. The rationale for this therapy is to prevent the development of a high calcium-phosphate product that could lead to precipitation of calcium-phosphate in various tissues, including the kidney. Phosphate restriction with moderate protein restriction in experimental animals has been shown to prevent progression of chronic renal failure.

   c. The same rationale could be applied to support therapy with dietary protein restriction and phosphate binders in all patients with chronic renal parenchymal disease, but beneficial effects of such therapy remain hypothetical at present.

III. THERAPY DETERMINED BY SYMPTOMS AND SIGNS During most of the course of **chronic renal parenchymal disease** the patient is asymptomatic, and there are no signs of renal insufficiency on physical examination. Azotemia occurs as GFR is reduced in relation to a diminished number of functioning nephrons. Gradually, various other laboratory abnormalities appear, and initially vague and nonspecific symptoms worsen and become disabling as the clinical syndrome of **uremia** occurs.

Some of the symptoms and signs of uremia may be treated as discussed below. Many of these symptoms and signs can be prevented or relieved by substituting the function of diseased kidneys with a transplanted kidney or dialysis. An important consideration in the management of patients with chronic renal parenchymal disease is the choice between transplantation and dialysis and the timing of beginning either of these modes of **therapy for end-stage renal disease (ESRD).**

A. Choices

1. **Transplantation or dialysis.** A successful kidney transplant from either a living related donor who is a good histocompatibility match or a cadaver donor provides the patient with end-stage renal disease with a better approximation of a normal life style than chronic dialysis. However, the increased morbidity and mortality with age above 60 years or the presence of incidental cardiopulmonary disease may make transplantation surgery too great a risk.

2. **Peritoneal or hemodialysis.** Patients on chronic dialysis may alternately use both forms of therapy. Hemodialysis at home or in a center and one or more of the variants of peritoneal dialysis—intermittent, overnight, or continuous ambulatory peritoneal dialysis (CAPD)—may be attempted until patients find the mode of dialysis best suited to personal needs and life style.

B. **Preparation and Time of Initiation**   The goal of the timing of therapy for ESRD is to minimize the duration of the symptomatic phase of renal insufficiency without subjecting the patient to the discomfort of transplantation or dialysis before it is needed. In short, the **first dialysis should be initiated before severe symptoms** of renal insufficiency begin to affect the patient's pattern of living. Most patients with chronic renal insufficiency begin to develop symptoms before the serum creatinine has risen to 10.0 mg/dl; graphic analysis projects when this level of serum creatinine will occur. The capability for hemodialysis is important whether transplantation or peritoneal dialysis is the major mode of therapy chosen. Thus, **vascular access** is an important aspect of therapy.

Establishment of vascular access should be planned to take place 2 to 3 months before it is anticipated that serum creatinine will reach 10 mg/dl. Discussing the need to establish vascular access with an ateriovenous (AV) fistula or prosthetic graft and the vascular access surgery often serve as tangible evidence to the patient that the ESRD treatment is imminent. During the phase of establishing vascular access it is often worthwhile to have the patient meet others who have had kidney transplants and experienced dialysis. Social workers and nurses who work with such patients also should establish a relationship with the patient.

C. **Symptomatic Therapy**   Treating patients with renal insufficiency from chronic renal parenchymal disease:

1. **General Measures**

a. **Diet. Protein** should be restricted to 40 g/day so that the degree of elevation of BUN at any level of GFR is minimized. The protein should be of high quality.

Sodium chloride should not be restricted unless edema and hypertension are present. This is because a negative sodium balance can cause volume depletion and lead to worsening of kidney function.

Fluid should not be restricted unless hyponatremia, indicating relative water excess, occurs. Sufficient fluid intake to achieve a urine flow rate of at least 2 liters/day also will minimize the degree of elevation of BUN at any GFR.

b. Activity should not be restricted. Patients should be encouraged to continue to work and maintain their usual life style (except that patients whose occupation involves heavy manual labor should be encouraged to learn a sedentary occupation.)

Note ⟶ **2.** Symptoms or signs that indicate dialysis should be started include pericarditis; generalized pruritus; nausea and anorexia; and, anemia if no other cause is found.

Abnormalities whose therapy is described in chapters 2, 4, and 6 include fluid and electrolyte disorders, hypertension, and heart failure.

3. Some symptoms, signs, and abnormalities persist or recur after chronic dialysis has been instituted. The management of these problems is a special area of interest in nephrology.

BIBLIOGRAPHY

Acute Renal Failure

Conger, J. D., Anderson, R. J. (1983): Acute renal failure including cortical necrosis. In: *Textbook of Nephrology*, edited by S. G. Massry and R. J. Glassock, Williams and Wilkins, Baltimore/London, pp. 215–228.

Schrier, R. W. and Conger, J. D. C. (1980): Acute renal failure: Pathogenesis, diagnosis and management. In: *Renal and Electrolyte Disorders*, 2nd ed., edited by R. W. Schrier, Little Brown and Company, Boston, pp. 375–408.

Wesson, D. E., Mitch, W. E., and Wilmore, D. W. (1983): Nutritional considerations in the treatment of acute renal failure. In: *Acute Renal Failure*, edited by B. M. Brenner and J. M. Lazarus, W. B. Saunders, Philadelphia, pp. 618–642.

Dialysis

Maher, J. H. (1983): Dialysis, hemofiltration and hemoperfusion. In: *Contemporary Nephrology*, Vol. 2, edited by S. Klahr and S. G. Massry, Plenum, New York and London, pp. 649–698.

Glomerular Diseases

Glassock, R. J., Cohen, A. H., Bennett, C. M., and Martinez-Maldanado, M. (1981): Primary glomerular diseases. In: *The Kidney*, edited by B. M. Brenner and F. C. Rector, Jr. W. B. Saunders, Philadelphia, pp. 1351–1366.

Renal Calculi

Coe, F. L. (1978): *Nephrolithiasis: Pathogenesis and Treatment*. Year Book Medical Publishers, Inc., Chicago.

Paks, C. Y. C. (1978): *Calcium Urolithiasis: Pathogenesis, Diagnosis and Management*. Plenum Medical Book Co., New York.

Transplantation

Strom, T. B. (1983): Renal transplantation. In: *Contemporary Nephrology*, Vol. 2, edited by S. Klahr and S. G. Massry, Plenum, New York and London, pp. 699–726.

Urinary Tract Infections

Komaroff, A. L. (1984): Acute dysuria in women. *N. Engl. J. Med.*, 310:368–375.

4.

Hypertension

Stuart L. Linas

4.

Hypertension

Hypertension, as defined by a diastolic blood pressure (BP) of greater than 90 mm Hg, affects some 60 million people in the United States. At least 40 million of these individuals have mild hypertension with diastolic BP between 90 and 99 mm Hg. Hypertension is a major risk factor for the development of heart failure, renal failure, stroke, and coronary artery disease. While secondary hypertension is often caused by diseases that are amenable to curative therapy, the vast majority of hypertensive individuals (> 90%) have primary or essential hypertension and must be treated medically. The diagnosis of hypertension is confirmed when the **mean diastolic BP on 3 separate days is greater than 90 mm Hg**. Diastolic pressure is measured at the point at which sound disappears (Korotkoff 5) rather than at the point at which there is a change in sound quality (Korotkoff 4).

I. **DIAGNOSTIC EVALUATION** In view of the small percentage of patients with secondary hypertension, it is not cost-effective to perform the large number of laboratory tests that would be required to exclude secondary causes of hypertension. Instead the **initial diagnostic evaluation** should include a complete history and physical examination with special emphasis on: **(a)** level of BP, **(b)** end-organ damage from hypertension, and **(c)** possibility of secondary hypertension (e.g., pulse lag between upper and lower extremities as in aortic coarctation, or abdominal bruits as in renovascular hypertension). **Initial laboratory data** should be confined to tests that determine **(a)** risks of hypertension, **(b)** end-organ damage from hypertension, and **(c)** possibility of secondary hypertension. These tests include urinalysis, creatinine, potassium, glucose, uric acid, cholesterol, triglycerides, chest X-ray, and EKG.

Only certain patients should have more complete studies to exclude the possibility of **secondary hypertension: (a)** hypertension with end-organ damage; **(b)** moderate to severe hypertension without end-organ damage but with resistant hypertension; and **(c)** initial screening tests that are positive (e.g., hypokalemia in the absence of diuretics).

II. **GENERAL THERAPEUTIC DECISIONS** Hypertension is associated with increased cardiovascular morbidity and mortality. Whereas large scale epidemiological studies have shown that BP reduction reduces morbidity and mortality in patients with moderate or severe hypertension, the benefits of early and aggressive therapy in patients with mild hypertension is not as certain. The initial decision in the evaluation of the hypertensive patient (Fig. 1) is the urgency of reducing BP.

Hypertensive emergency is defined as severe elevation of arterial pressure that represents an immediate threat to life or to function of vital organs. Although diastolic pressure is usually greater than 120 mm Hg, hypertension should be considered emergent in the presence of advancing end-organ disease and a diastolic pressure

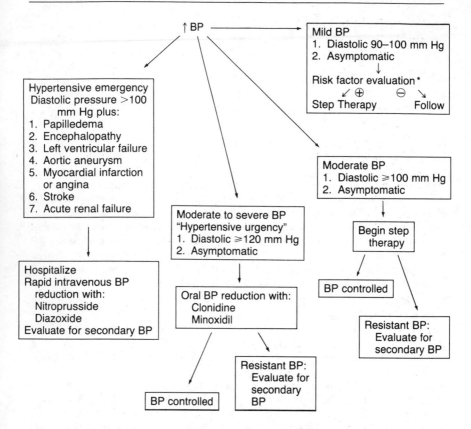

FIG. 1.   Hypertension syndromes. BP, blood pressure. *Risk factor evaluation (see text).

greater than 100 mm Hg. Immediate BP reduction should be achieved by the administration of rapidly acting, intravenously administered antihypertensive drugs such as sodium nitroprusside or diazoxide.

Hypertensive urgency is defined as moderate to severe hypertension in which there is no end-organ damage but in which end-organ damage may ensue if the hypertension is not brought under control. BP reduction can be achieved by the administration of rapidly acting, orally administered antihypertension drugs such as clonidine or minoxidil.

In the absence of end-organ damage in patients with **mild** (diastolic pressure 90 to 100 mm Hg) to **moderate** (diastolic pressure 100 to 120 mm Hg) **hypertension**, drug therapy need not be initiated immediately, pending a diagnostic evaluation and a short trial (3 to 6 months) of nonpharmacological modalities such as weight loss, salt restriction, and an exercise program. In patients whose diastolic BP remains greater than 100 mm Hg, **drug therapy** should be instituted.

In patients whose diastolic BP is between 90 and 100 mm Hg, the decision to begin drug therapy should be based on assessment of other **cardiovascular risk factors**. These include (**a**) cigarette smoking, (**b**) diabetes, (**c**) high serum cholesterol, (**d**) systolic BP over 165 mm Hg, **(e)** diastolic BP over 95 mm Hg, **(f)** target organ disease, **(g)** age less than 45 years, and **(h)** family history of severe hypertension. Drug therapy should be initiated if there is any evidence of end-organ disease or if any three risk factors are present. It should also be stated, however, that treatment of persistent diastolic BP greater than 90 mm Hg has been recommended by the results of some studies, particularly in patients older than 45 to 50 years of age.

III. SPECIFIC RECOMMENDATIONS

A. Hypertensive Emergency   (See Table 1) Patients should be treated aggressively with intravenous antihypertensive agents. The major goal of therapy is to **decrease diastolic pressure** to 100 mm Hg within 30 to 60 min, since prompt lowering of BP increases survival and reduces morbidity. Once BP control is obtained, oral agents should be initiated and intravenous medications tapered and discontinued.

1. Initial medications

a. Sodium nitroprusside (Nipride®). This is the **drug of choice** in patients with hypertensive emergency. It is an arteriolar- and venodilator (thus cardiac output rarely increases) and is effective in lowering BP in more than 90% of patients with severe hypertension. A dose of 0.5 µg/kg/min is initiated (the tubing and i.v. bottle should be wrapped in foil as the solution deteriorates in light). Every 2 to 3 min the dosage is increased by 0.5 to 1 µg/kg/min until diastolic pressure is 100 mm Hg. The average dose is 3 to 5 µg/kg/min. Dosage exceeding 10 µg/kg/min is occasionally required. Because of the rapid action of the drug, BP monitoring in the intensive care unit is crucial. If indirect measurements of pressure are not felt to be accurate, continuous direct intraarterial BP monitoring is necessary.

Nitroprusside is metabolized to cyanide, which is metabolized by the liver to thiocyanate prior to renal excretion. Thus, the drug should be used with caution in patients with liver or kidney disease. Plasma thiocyanate levels should be kept under 10 mg/dl. Cyanide toxicity is treated by reducing the dose of nitroprusside and by infusions of thiosulfate (to provide a sulfur donor to form thiocyanate), sodium nitrate (to induce methemoglobin, which combines with cyanide to form cyanmethemoglobin), and hydroxocobalamin (which combines with cyanide to form cyanocobalamin).

b. Diazoxide (Hyperstat®). An arteriolar, but not venous, vasodilator that results in a reflex increase in cardiac output. The initial dose in patients on no other antihypertensives is 100 mg given over 10 sec (it is highly protein-bound so cannot be given slowly). The maximum hypotensive effect occurs within 5 min. The duration of action of diazoxide is variable between 3 and 12 hours. The same dose or as much as 300 mg can then be repeated. In patients on other antihypertensives, excessive hypotension can occur. Thus, an initial dose of 25 mg is administered and repeated at 10- to 15-minute intervals until BP control is obtained.

Aside from hypotension, the **major side effects of** diazoxide **are sodium retention and hyperglycemia.** Diazoxide should not be utilized in patients in whom reflex activation of the sympathetic nervous system is of concern (pheochromocytoma, dissecting aortic aneurysm, angina, myocardial infarction) or in patients with intracranial bleeding.

TABLE 1. *Treatment of hypertensive emergency*

Name	Pharmacologic effect	Dosage (i.v.)	Time course of action onset/max./duration	Side effects
Sodium nitroprusside	Direct arteriolar- and venodilator	Initial 0.5 µg/kg/min Usual maintenance 3–5 µg/kg/min Upper limit 10 µg/kg/min	<1 min/1–2 min/2–5 min	Thiocyanate toxicity
Diazoxide	Direct arteriolar-vasodilator	Initial No other medications: 300 mg Other antihypertensives: 25–100 mg Maintenance Initial dose every 3–12 hr	1 min/2–4 min/4–12 hr	Hyperglycemia
Trimethaphan camsylate	Indirect ganglionic blocker	Initial 1 mg/min Maintenance 2–5 mg/min	<1 min/1–2 min/<5 min	Parasympathetic blockade (e.g. urinary retention) Tachyphylaxis

c. **Trimethaphan camsylate (Arfonad®).** A **ganglionic blocking drug** that has proved of particular use in the treatment of **aortic dissection.** Its primary effect is on upright BP, and patients should be treated in the sitting position. The initial dose is 1 mg/min. Because of the rapidity of action, the dose is increased every 5 min until diastolic pressure reaches 100 mm Hg. The toxicity of trimethaphan is related to parasympathetic blockade such as urinary retention, constipation, ileus, and pupillary dilatation. Rapid tachyphylaxis can be a major problem.

2. **Maintenance medications.** Following the initial control of BP with intravenous medication, the patient should be switched to **oral therapy.** Because of the importance of BP control, we recommend three-drug therapy during the transition phase of the treatment of hypertensive emergency. The cornerstone of therapy is a direct **arteriolar vasodilator** such as hydralazine (or minoxidil). Since these agents activate the sympathetic nervous system and cause renal sodium retention, a beta blocker and diuretic are added. This is accomplished as follows: After BP has been controlled with nitroprusside, **hydralazine** 50 mg and **propranolol** 40 mg (or the equivalent dose of other beta blockers) are administered. As BP decreases, nitroprusside is tapered. If diastolic pressure remains over 100 mm Hg, hydralazine 100 mg is administered after 8 to 12 hr. The dose of propranolol is increased (usually 80 to 120 mg b.i.d.) to maintain beta blockade. If BP is not controlled with hydralazine (200 mg/day), minoxidil is substituted for hydralazine beginning at 2.5 mg and increasing the dose of minoxidil by 2.5 to 5 mg every 8 to 12 hr until BP is controlled (usually 5 to 10 mg b.i.d.). Beta blockade is maintained, and a diuretic (e.g., furosemide 40 mg b.i.d.) is added to either hydralazine or minoxidil therapy. Table 4 lists the potential side effects of this three-drug regimen.

3. **Special syndromes of hypertensive emergency**

   a. **Aortic dissection.** Medical therapy forms the basis for the **initial** therapy of all patients with aortic dissection. Therapy is directed at halting the progression of the dissecting hematoma. The goals of pharmacological therapy are to reduce systolic BP, and to diminish the velocity of left ventricular ejection (dv/dt). For rapid reduction of arterial pressure **nitroprusside** is the agent of choice. Since nitroprusside can increase dv/dt, adequate beta blockade is essential. Propranolol is administered as a test dose of 0.5 mg i.v. If heart rate does not decrease precipitously, 1 mg is administered intravenously every 5 min until heart rate is 60 to 70 beats/min or until a total dose of 0.15 mg/kg is administered. Additional propranolol (2 to 6 mg i.v.) is given every 4 to 6 hr to maintain beta blockade. If nitroprusside is ineffective or poorly tolerated, **trimethaphan** is utilized. Since trimethaphan decreases dv/dt, beta blockade is not required. Although theoretically a better drug than nitroprusside, trimethaphan is a second choice because of side effects and tachyphylaxis.

   After BP is stabilized the patient should undergo angiography. In general, surgical therapy is recommended for a **proximal dissection** (which includes the ascending aorta and aortic arch), and medical therapy is recommended for a **distal dissection**.

   b. **Pheochromocytoma.** In patients with pheochromocytoma, hypertensive emergency is treated by the administration of the alpha-adrenergic blocking agent **phentolamine** (Regitine®), 2 to 5 mg every 5 to 10 min until BP is controlled. Only after adequate alpha blockade is obtained is beta blockade with propranolol instituted to control tachycardia.

B. **Hypertensive Urgency**   (Diastolic blood pressure >120 mm Hg in an asymptomatic patient.) Patients should be treated aggressively with **oral antihypertensive agents**. The goal of therapy is to decrease diastolic pressure to 110 mm Hg within 6 hr. If this goal is not reached, the patient should be treated with parenteral antihypertensive drugs as described in the Hypertensive Emergency section.

1. **Specific recommendations**

   a. **Clonidine (Catapres®).** Administer 0.2 mg orally followed by 0.1 mg every hour until the diastolic BP is less than 110 mm Hg or until a dose of 0.7 mg has been obtained. Maintenance therapy consists of dividing the dose of clonidine into a twice-a-day regimen. Hydrochlorothiazide is added to prevent sodium retention, and a vasodilator such as hydralazine is added if necessary.

   b. **Minoxidil (Loniten®).** Administer propranolol 40 mg and furosemide 40 mg. If diastolic BP remains greater than 120 mm Hg after 2 hr, administer minoxidil 20 mg orally. If diastolic pressure remains greater than 110 mm Hg 4 hr after the initial dose of minoxidil, administer a booster dose (5 to 20 mg depending on the initial decrease in pressure; a 20-mg dose would be expected to produce the same percentage reduction as did the 20-mg loading dose, whereas a 5-mg dose would produce 25% of the percentage reduction).

   Maintenance therapy is calculated by administering half the sum of the loading dose and a 4-hr booster dose on a twice-a-day basis. Propranolol is adjusted to maintain heart rate, and furosemide is adjusted to prevent sodium retention.

C. **Mild to Moderate Hypertension**   (Diastolic blood pressure <120 mm Hg, Tables 2, 3, and 4.) The **stepped-care approach** is utilized in mild to moderate hypertension. The general goals of therapy are to minimize the risk of hypertensive cardiovascular complications by maintaining the lowest BP (usually 80 to 90 mm Hg diastolic) in the absence of drug-induced side effects.

1. **Step-1 therapy of hypertension** (Table 2). A **thiazide** or thiazide-like diuretic is the first-line drug. These diuretics are the cornerstone of the stepped-care approach to hypertension because they are safe, inexpensive, and efficacious as monotherapy in the treatment of most patients with hypertension. In addition, since most other antihypertensive agents result in sodium retention, diuretics need to be continued when other agents are utilized for hypertensive therapy.

   Other thiazide-like agents include chlorthalidone (Hygroton®) and metolazone (Zaroxolyn®), both of which are longer-acting than thiazide diuretics. Although these agents are as efficacious as thiazides, they are rarely utilized in place of thiazides because of the higher incidence of potassium (K) depletion (chlorthalidone) and the greater expense (metolazone).

TABLE 2. *Step-1 drugs in the treatment of hypertension*

Name	Dosage	Side Effects
K-wasting diuretics		
Hydrochlorothiazide (and other thiazides)	25–50 mg b.i.d. ⎫	Hypokalemia Hyperglycemia Hyperuricemia and gout
Chlorthalidone	50 mg q.d. ⎬	Hyperlipidemia Hypercalcemia
Metolazone	25–50 mg q.d. ⎭	Hyponatremia
K-sparing diuretics		
Spironolactone	25–50 mg b.i.d.	Gynecomastia; nausea ⎫
Triamterene	100 mg b.i.d.	Nausea ⎬ Hyperkalemia
Amiloride	5–10 mg q.d.	Nausea ⎭

Mild K depletion (serum K between 3 and 3.5 mEq/liter) occurs in a small percentage of patients on thiazide therapy; this may be as high as 25% in patients on unrestricted sodium intake and doses of 50 to 100 mg of hydrochlorothiazide. Although severe K depletion may cause severe ventricular arrhythmias, serum K >3 mEq/liter does **not** appear to pose a risk to patients, and K should not be replaced unless: serum K is less than 3 mEq/liter; there is a history of ischemic heart disease, arrhythmias, or the patient is on digitalis.

Other **side effects** of K-losing diuretics include: hyperglycemia, especially in patients with underlying glucose intolerance; hyperuricemia and gout; hyperlipidemia; hypercalcemia, by both enhanced renal calcium reabsorption and by enhanced bone calcium reabsorption; and, hyponatremia.

K-sparing diuretics should not be utilized as monotherapy of hypertension but may prove useful in patients requiring K supplementation. **Amiloride** is particularly useful in this situation. Combination drugs such as Aldactazide®, Dyazide®, and Moduretic® (thiazide and spironolactone, thiazide and triamterene, thiazide and amiloride, respectively) should also not be utilized in the initial therapy of hypertension because: K supplementation is rarely required in patients with mild to moderate essential hypertension, and they are more expensive than the thiazides. K-sparing diuretics and K supplements should **never** be used together.

2. **Step-2 therapy of hypertension** (Table 3). There are a large number of agents available for step-2 therapy of hypertension. These agents interfere with the adrenergic nervous system but at different sites, and they tend to cause sodium retention and are most efficacious in the presence of a diuretic.

   a. **Predominantly central agonists**

   (1) **Methyldopa (Aldomet®).** Methyldopa reduces central sympathetic outflow and decreases blood pressure by reducing peripheral resistance. It can be utilized twice a day and does not reduce renal blood flow or glomerular filtration rate (GFR), but dosages must be reduced in renal failure since the parent compound and metabolites are excreted by the kidney.

   Side effects include sedation, depression, orthostatic hypotension, impotence, and decreased libido. Also seen are autoimmune effects in-

TABLE 3. *Step-2 drugs in the treatment of hypertension*

Drug	Dose range (usual dose)	Chronic hemodynamic effect				Side effects
		CO	TPR	HR	RBF	
Methyldopa	250–3000 mg/d (500–1000 mg b.i.d.)	± ↓	↓	→	→	Impotence Sedation Orthostatic hypotension ⊗ ANA ⊗ Coombs Increased liver function tests
Clonidine	0.2–0.8 mg/d (0.2–0.4 mg b.i.d.)	↓	± ↓	↓	→	Dry mouth Sedation Rebound hypertension
Reserpine	0.1–0.25 mg/d (0.1–0.2 mg q.d.)	↓	↓	↓	→	Depression, peptic ulcer, nasal stuffiness
Prazosin	1–20 mg/d (2–6 mg b.i.d.)	± ↑	↓	→	→	Orthostatic symptoms First-dose hypotensive effect Headache
Beta-receptor antagonists Nonselective						
Propranolol	8–480 mg/d (80–160 mg b.i.d.)	↓	↑	↓	↓	
Timolol	20–120 mg/d (10–30 mg b.i.d.)	↓	↑	↓	↓	
Nadolol	8–230 mg/d (80–160 mg/d)	↓	± ↑	↓	→	Congestive heart failure Bronchospasm[a]
Selective						Heart block
Metoprolol	100–400 mg/d (50–100 mg b.i.d.)	↓	↑	↓	→	Depression Sedation
Atenolol	50–200 mg/d (50–100 mg/d)	↓	± ↑	↓	→	Hypoglycemia[a] Nightmares
With ISA						
Pindolol	10–60 mg/d (5–30 mg b.i.d.)	→	↓	± ↓	→	

[a]Not with low-dose selective beta blockers.
CO, cardiac output; TPR, total peripheral resistance; HR, heart rate; RBF, renal blood flow; ISA, intrinsic sympathomimetic activity.
→, no effect; ↓, decreases; ↑, increases.

cluding a positive ANA (5%), a positive Coombs test (25% of patients), and rarely hemolytic anemia (1%). Hepatic damage and fatal hepatic necrosis also have been reported, as has drug-induced fever. The drug should be discontinued in patients with hemolytic anemia and in patients with hepatic injury.

(2) Clonidine (Catapres®). Clonidine is a centrally acting alpha-2 adrenoreceptor agonist that reduces BP by reducing cardiac output and on occasion peripheral resistance. Although central sympathetic outflow is reduced, the baroreceptor reflex is left intact; thus, hypotension is rarely a problem. Clonidine can be utilized once or twice a day. Renal blood flow is not altered.

Side effects: As with methyldopa, sedation, dry mouth, impotence, and dizziness occur but with less frequency. With sudden cessation of daily doses > 1 mg a withdrawal syndrome may occur that is characterized by return of hypertension to pretreatment or higher levels, headache, agitation, tremor, and GI symptoms. Therapy consists of reinstitution of clonidine. More rapid control of BP can be accomplished with nitroprusside or phentolamine. Clonidine should be carefully withdrawn in patients receiving beta blockers, since abrupt discontinuation may result in hypertension owing to the effect of circulating catecholamines on alpha-adrenergic receptors.

(3) **Guanabenz (Wytensin®).** Guanabenz is a new centrally acting adrenergic agonist that shares most of the same features as clonidine, both therapeutically and with regard to side effects. It is more expensive than methyldopa or clonidine.

b. **Drugs that act within the neuron**

Reserpine. Reserpine depletes postganglionic adrenergic neurons of norepinephrine by inhibiting its uptake into storage vesicles, thereby exposing it to degradation by monoamine oxidase. This occurs both peripherally and centrally. Peripheral vascular resistance and cardiac output are decreased. Reserpine rarely alters renal function.

The **major side effect is depression**, especially in the elderly and in patients with a prior history of depression. Other side effects include sedation, dry mouth, nasal congestion, peptic ulcer, abdominal pain, and diarrhea.

While the use of this agent has progressively declined, reserpine has certain advantages. Its **long half-life** makes once-a-day administration useful in patients with compliance problems. There is little postural hypotension, and the drug is especially efficacious when combined with a diuretic.

c. **Predominantly peripheral antagonists**

(1) **Alpha-receptor antagonists. Prazosin** (Minipress®) is a selective antagonist of the postsynaptic alpha-1 adrenoreceptor; it reduces BP by reducing peripheral resistance. In some patients (especially those with congestive heart failure) this afterload reduction may result in an increase in cardiac output. Renal blood flow is not altered.

Side effects include postural hypotension and dizziness. A rare (< 1%) self-limited hypotensive syncopal reaction has been described after the first dose. This reaction may be caused by abrupt adrenergic blockade of both arterioles and venules leading to venous pooling and postural hypotension. This problem can be prevented by limiting the first dose to less than 1 mg.

(2) **Beta-receptor antagonists.** These agents reduce BP by a number of mechanisms including (a) central effects, (b) decrease in cardiac output, and (c) decrease in renin activity. Whatever the mechanism of action, there is a decrease in cardiac output. Pindolol, an agent with intrinsic beta-agonist activity, may be an exception.

The agents are grouped on the basis of whether they are **cardioselective** (beta-1 receptor only) or **nonselective** (beta-1 and beta-2 receptors) beta blockers and whether they possess **intrinsic sympathomimetic activity (ISA)**. The heart has a predominance of beta-1 receptors, whereas the peripheral circulation and the lung have a predominance of beta-2 receptors. It is important to realize that the selectivity of various agents is only relative, and dosages that block only beta-1 receptors in most patients may block both beta-1 and beta-2 receptors in others. The clinical significance of drugs with ISA (pindolol) has not been proved. Common **side effects** include:

(a) Negative inotropic effect that may precipitate or worsen congestive heart failure

(b) attenuation of recovery from insulin-induced hypoglycemia

(c) blockade of hypoglycemic symptoms

(d) hypertensive response to hypoglycemia

(e) bronchospasm; thus only low-dose selective beta-1 agents should be considered in patients with reactive airway disease

(f) atrioventricular conduction delay (thus precluding use in most patients with second- and third-degree heart block)

(g) sick sinus syndrome

(h) CNS side effects such as sedation, depression, impotence, and nightmares

(i) precipitation of angina in patients with underlying coronary artery disease who are abruptly withdrawn from these drugs for the treatment of hypertension.

While beta blockers differ with regard to lipid solubility, a property that may determine CNS penetrability (hence CNS side effects), and with regard to metabolism (hence dosing intervals), none of the beta blockers needs to be administered more than twice a day.

d. Nonselective beta blockers

(1) **Propranolol (Inderal®).** This original beta blocker available in the United States has recently been released in a long-acting once-a-day form.

(2) **Timolol (Blocadren®).** This is the first beta blocker shown to be efficacious in the prevention of death after myocardial infarction. It is minimally protein-bound. The dosage should be decreased in either liver or kidney insufficiency.

(3) **Nadolol (Corgard®).** This beta-blocker's low lipid solubility may decrease brain penetration and decrease CNS side effects; this, however, remains to be proved. It is administered once a day, and the dosing interval should be prolonged in patients with renal failure.

e. Selective beta blockers

(1) **Metoprolol (Lopressor™).** In doses less than 100 mg/day this agent is relatively selective for beta-1 receptors.

(2) **Atenolol (Tenormin®)**. In doses less than 100 mg/day this agent is relatively selective to beta-1 receptors and may be given once a day. The dosing interval should be prolonged in patients with renal insufficiency.

f. **Beta blocker with ISA**

Pindolol (Visken®). This is the initial beta blocker with ISA. It may be useful in patients with sinus bradycardia. Hepatic clearance of pindolol is the main site of metabolism.

3. **Step-3 therapy of hypertension** (Table 4). In patients whose blood pressure is not controlled with two drugs a third agent is utilized. The agent most often utilized is **hydralazine** (Apresoline®). Hydralazine decreases blood pressure by acting directly on arteriolar smooth muscle to cause vasodilation. The antihypertensive effect of hydralazine is limited by reflex activity of the adrenergic nervous system (causing tachycardia and increase in cardiac output and myocardial oxygen demand) and by sodium retention. However, when administered with a beta blocker and a diuretic, hydralazine is a very efficacious antihypertensive agent.

Side effects: Because of secondary sympathetic reflexes, hydralazine should **not be** administered alone. With a diuretic and beta blocker the secondary adrenergic reflexes and salt-retaining effects of hydralazine are minimized. The drug should not be administered to patients with unstable coronary artery disease. A lupus-like syndrome occurs in 10% to 20% of patients receiving more than 400 mg/day and in patients who are slow acetylators of the drug. The drug should be discontinued in patients with this syndrome.

4. **Step-4 therapy of hypertension.** Patients who continue to be hypertensive on three agents are considered to have resistant hypertension (see below). Three agents are currently utilized for the therapy of resistant hypertension.

a. **Minoxidil (Loniten®)**. Minoxidil is an **extremely potent arteriolar vasodilator** that reduces BP by reducing vascular resistance. It should be utilized only in the presence of a beta blocker (on occasion clonidine has proved to be an adequate substitute) and a diuretic. All other antihypertensives, except a beta blocker and a diuretic, are discontinued, and minoxidil is begun at a dose of 2.5 mg b.i.d. and titrated up to a dose of 20 mg b.i.d. Most patients are controlled with 10 to 20 mg/day. **Side effects** in general are similar to those associated with hydralazine administration; however, a lupus-like syndrome has not been reported. **Hypertrichosis** occurs in 50% to 100% of patients receiving minoxidil and may be prevented by depilatory agents. T-wave abnormalities on the EKG occur frequently but should not preclude the use of the drug, since they do not represent ischemic heart disease. Pericardial effusions have been reported, especially in patients with renal failure or systemic lupus erythematosus. Fluid retention can be profound with minoxidil and may require large doses of furosemide (300 to 500 mg/day) for control.

b. **Captopril (Capoten®)**. Captopril reduces blood pressure by preventing the formation of the potent endogenous vasoconstrictor hormone angiotensin II. It is most useful in high-renin states. To avoid hypotensive reactions

TABLE 4. *Step-3 and step-4 drugs in the therapy of hypertension*

| Drug | Dose range (usual dose) | Hemodynamic effects | | | Side effects |
		CO	TPR	HR	
Step 3					
Hydralazine	50–400 mg/d (100–150 mg b.i.d.)	Alone: ↑	↓	↑	SLE-like syndrome Tachycardia Headache Angina SLE
		With beta blocker: →	→	↑	
Step 4					
Minoxidil	5–40 mg/d (5–10 mg b.i.d.)	With beta blocker: →	→	↑	Hair growth EKG changes Pericardial effusion
Captopril	150–450 mg/d (50–100 mg t.i.d.)	± ↑	→		Skin rash Leukopenia Proteinuria Renal failure
Guanethidine	10–100 mg/d (10–50 mg/d)	↓	→	↑	Postural hypotension Impotence

CO, cardiac output; TPR, total peripheral resistance; HR, heart rate; SLE, systemic lupus erythematosus. ↑, increases; ↓, decreases; →, no effect.

all other antihypertensives should be discontinued prior to instituting captopril. The drug is titrated from 25 mg t.i.d. up to 200 mg t.i.d. If captopril alone does not normalize blood pressure, a diuretic is added. Many patients also require a beta blocker. A **triphasic response** to captopril is often seen: initial decrease in BP followed by a return of BP to pretreatment levels and then a gradual decrease in BP over 7 to 10 days.

Side effects of captopril include skin rash, pruritus, taste impairment, and, rarely, severe leukopenia (blood counts should be monitored carefully during the first month of therapy) and proteinuria. Renal failure has been reported in patients with severe bilateral renal artery stenosis or renal artery stenosis in a solitary kidney.

c. **Guanethidine (Ismelin®).** Guanethidine acts by inhibiting the release of norepinephrine at adrenergic neurons. Agents such as tricyclic antidepressants and ephedrine completely block the uptake of guanethidine into nerves and antagonize its effect. Guanethidine decreases both peripheral resistance and cardiac output. BP falls more in the upright than the supine position.

Side effects: Since guanethidine is both an **arteriolar- and venodilator**, severe postural hypotension may occur. Unlike many other antiadrenergic drugs guanethidine is not very lipid-soluble, so that CNS side effects (sedation, depression) are infrequent.

d. **Calcium channel blockers.** Although the calcium channel blockers appear to be effective arteriolar vasodilators (especially nifedipine), their role in the treatment of hypertension is not yet clear. At present **they are not approved for hypertension** by the Food and Drug Administration.

5. **Summary of step therapy of hypertension.** Although there are many regimens for the stepped-care approach to hypertension, we have found that two are particularly useful.

Approach 1

Step 1. Begin with a thiazide diuretic (e.g., hydrochlorothiazide 50 mg/day) with modest sodium restriction.

Step 2. Add a beta blocker (e.g., metoprolol 50 mg q.d. and titrate to 100 mg b.i.d.). The choice of beta blocker is related to cost only.

Step 3. Add hydralazine; begin at 25 mg b.i.d. and titrate to 100 mg b.i.d.

Step 4. Discontinue hydralazine; begin minoxidil 2.5 mg b.i.d. and titrate to 10 mg b.i.d.

Approach 2

Step 1. Begin with a thiazide diuretic (e.g., hydrochlorothiazide 50 mg/day).

Step 2. Add clonidine; begin at 0.1 mg h.s. and titrate to 0.4 mg b.i.d.

Step 3. Add hydralazine at 25 mg b.i.d. and titrate to 100 mg b.i.d.

Step 4. Stop all antihypertensives; begin captopril 25 mg t.i.d. and increase to 150 mg b.i.d.; add hydrochlorothiazide 50 mg q.d.; increase captopril to 200 mg b.i.d.; add a beta blocker such as metoprolol at 50 mg q.d. and titrate to 100 mg b.i.d.

6. **Role of non-step therapy in the treatment of hypertension.** In some patients with essential hypertension the stepped-care approach to therapy is bypassed. This includes patients with (a) essential hypertension and high cardiac output and (b) essential hypertension and high plasma renin activity.

a. **High cardiac output.** In occasional patients hypertension is primarily caused by an abnormally elevated cardiac output rather than by an elevation in peripheral resistance. Hypertension in association with a high cardiac output has been found most often in the early stages of essential hypertension. Such patients may have other evidence of excessive sympathetic nervous system function. Rather than diuretics, beta-adrenergic blocking agents are the initial treatment of choice in these patients.

b. **High plasma renin activity (PRA).** Between 5% and 10% of patients with essential hypertension have an increase in PRA as judged by relating PRA to urinary sodium excretion. The increase in PRA is often associated with evidence of **excessive sympathetic nervous system activity**. Beta-blocking agents are the initial treatment in these individuals.

IV. SPECIAL CONSIDERATIONS IN THE MANAGEMENT OF HYPERTENSION

A. **Resistant Hypertension**   Resistant hypertension is defined as the failure to control BP to a level < 150/100 mm Hg in a patient who takes medication described in step 3 of the stepped-care approach to the therapy of hypertension. There are a number of **causes of resistant hypertension**. The most important include: patient noncompliance with medication regimens; volume excess; secondary rather than essential hypertension; and inadequate drug therapy. Before concluding that drug therapy is inadequate and that step 4 therapy is indicated, the first three possibilities should be carefully considered. This may include a more complete evaluation for secondary causes of hypertension, such as plasma catecholamines for pheochromocytoma, renal arteriography for renovascular hypertension, or plasma aldosterone and renin determinations for primary hyperaldosteronism (especially in hypokalemic patients with inappropriate renal K-wasting in the absence of diuretics).

B. **Anesthesia and Surgery in Hypertensive Patients**   Hypertensive patients should be well controlled prior to anesthesia and surgery. Guanethidine should be replaced by another agent, since it potentiates the effects of circulating norepinephrine released by anesthesia. Since parenteral clonidine is unavailable, this agent also should be replaced by another agent such as propranolol. **Severe perioperative hypertension** is managed with nitroprusside. **Less severe hypertension**, when the patient is not taking anything by mouth, is managed with hydralazine, a beta blocker, and furosemide to maintain normal volume status.

C. **Hypertension in Renal Insufficiency**   Hypertension in patients with chronic renal failure is predominantly caused by **volume expansion**. Most patients can be treated with **diuretics**. Furosemide or metolazone are required when serum creatinine exceeds 2.5 to 3 mg/dl. Ten to twenty percent of patients have a more resistant form of hypertension and can be treated with a beta blocker and a vasodilator such as hydralazine or minoxidil.

BIBLIOGRAPHY

Anderson, R. J., Hart, G. R., Crumpler, C. P., Reed, W. G., and Matthews, C. A. (1981): Oral clonidine loading in hypertensive urgencies. *JAMA*, 246:848–850.

Gifford, R. W., Jr., and Tarazi, R. B. (1978): Resistant hypertension: Diagnosis and management. *Ann. Intern. Med.*, 88:661–665.

Harrington, J. T., Isner, J. M., and Kassirer, J. P. (1982): Our national obsession with potassium. *Am. J. Med.*, 3:155–159.

The Joint National Committee on Detection, Evaluation, and Treatment of High Blood Pressure (1980): The 1980 Report of the Joint National Committee on detection, evaluation, and treatment of high blood pressure. *Arch. Intern. Med.*, 140:1280–1285.

Kaplan, N. M. (1983): Mild hypertension. *Arch. Intern. Med.*, 143:255–259.

Linas, S. L., and Nies, A. S. (1981): Minoxidil. *Ann. Intern. Med.*, 94:61–65.

Vidt, D. G., Bravo, E. L., and Fouad, F. M. (1982): Drug therapy: Captopril. *N. Engl. J. Med.*, 306:214–219.

5.

Angina and Myocardial Infarction

Kenneth Hossack

5.

Angina and Myocardial Infarction

I. ANGINA

A. Pathophysiology Angina is a symptom of **transient myocardial ischemia** owing to an imbalance between myocardial oxygen supply and demand. The pathophysiological process leading to the imbalance is often a combination of factors. Supply usually is decreased because of **fixed coronary lesions**, and superimposed vasoconstriction can further decrease supply. Demand increases as a result of **increased myocardial work**. The product of heart rate and systolic blood pressure is a reliable noninvasive index of myocardial oxygen demand. It is important to remember that angina also can be a symptom of **valvular heart disease** (particularly aortic stenosis) and **hypertrophic cardiomyopathy**. Therapy is aimed at manipulating determinants of both supply and demand.

B. Chronic Stable Angina

1. **Definition.** Patients typically describe angina as central chest tightness, pressure, or squeezing sensation that usually is related to exertion. The discomfort often radiates to arms or jaw as an ache. Relief from the discomfort with rest or nitroglycerin over 1 to 5 min is a typical feature. In some patients the discomfort is located only in the arms or jaws. When all of these features are present, the pain is **typical** or **definite** angina. If one feature is not present, then the pain is **probable** angina; and if more than one feature is absent or there are atypical features, then the pain is **atypical** angina.

   A stable pain pattern in terms of frequency, severity, duration, and initiating events are features of **chronic stable angina**.

2. **Diagnosis.** The classification of pain as atypical, probable, or definite angina provides important information about the likelihood of disease. In males the prevalences of angiographically demonstrable coronary artery disease are 22%, 66%, and 88%, respectively, and in females the respective prevalences are 5%, 35%, and 58%. The Canadian Cardiovascular Society classification (Table 1) is a useful method of grading angina severity.

   Formal assessment of **exercise capacity** provides useful information to gauge subsequent response to treatment and helps identify factors associated with a poor prognosis. Such factors include short exercise duration, marked ST depression at low workloads, and hypotension or poor blood pressure response during exercise.

   Other noninvasive tests such as thallium scintigraphy or rest/exercise ejection fraction studies are not indicated in the majority of patients with definite angina but may be of help in patients with atypical chest pain. In general,

TABLE 1. *Grading of angina of effort by the Canadian Cardiovascular Society*

I. "Ordinary physical activity does not cause...angina"—such as walking and climbing stairs. Angina with strenuous or rapid or prolonged exertion at work or recreation
II. "Slight limitation of ordinary activity." Walking or climbing stairs rapidly, walking uphill, walking or stair climbing after meals, in cold, in wind, under emotional stress, or only during the few hours after awakening. Walking more than 2 blocks on the level and climbing more than 1 flight of ordinary stairs at a normal pace and in normal conditions
III. "Marked limitation of ordinary physical activity." Walking 1 to 2 blocks on the level and climbing 1 flight of stairs in normal conditions and at normal pace
IV. "Inability to carry on any physical activity without discomfort—anginal syndrome may be present at rest"

From L. Campeau (1976): Grading of angina pectoris. *Circulation,* 54:522–523.

coronary arteriography is indicated when it is felt that a patient may be a candidate for **surgery.**

3. **Treatment.** Nitrates (Table 2), **beta-blocking agents** (Table 3), and **calcium slow-channel blocking drugs** (Table 4) are all effective in preventing episodes of angina and increasing exercise capacity. Patients appear to have better tolerance to transdermal nitroglycerin than to oral nitrates. Nitrates generally are prescribed initially, but beta blockers are preferred in patients with associated hypertension or marked rise in heart rate and blood pressure during exercise. Beta blockers improve exercise performance by means of a reduction in heart rate and blood pressure, and all agents have this effect. The choice between one beta blocker and another depends on patient tolerance. Patient compliance is improved with once-a-day agents. **Combination therapy** of nitrates and beta blockers, or beta blockers and nifedipine or verapamil, may

TABLE 2. *Nitrates*

Drug and administration	Dose	Duration of action[a]	Side effects
Nitroglycerin			All nitrates have the potential to
Sublingual	0.3–0.6 mg p.r.n.	30 min	cause side effects related to
Oral (sustained	1.3–6.5 mg t.i.d.	4–8 hr	vasodilating properties, e.g.,
release, tablets,			headaches, flushing, reflex
caps.)			hypotension, tachycardia,
Ointment (2%)	½–2 in. q 4–6 hr	4–6 hr	dizziness
Transdermal			
Nitrodisc™	8–16 cm²/d	24–48 hr	
Nitro-Dur®	5–30 cm²/d		
Transderm®-Nitro	2.5–15 mg/d		
Intravenous	10–200 µg/min	5–10 min	
Isosorbide dinitrate			
Sublingual	2.5–10 mg q 3 hr	1–2 hr	Same
Oral tablets	20–60 mg q 6 hr	4–6 hr	
Sustained release	40–80 mg q 8–12 hr	8–12 hr	
Pentaerythritol tetranitrate			
Oral	10–60 mg q 6 hr	4–6 hr	Same
Erythrityl tetranitrate			
Sublingual	5–15 mg q 6 hr	3–6 hr	Same
Chewable			
Oral			

[a]Period of time that a dose has an antianginal effect.

TABLE 3. *Beta-adrenergic blocking agents*

Drug and administration	Dose	Duration of action	Side effects
Nonselective			
Propranolol			
Intravenous	1 mg increments up to 10 mg total	½–2 hr	Fatigue, lethargy Sleep disturbance Impotence
Oral tablets	20–120 mg q6hr	4–8 hr	Hypotension
Sustained release	80–320 mg/d	24 hr	Heart failure
Timolol			Bradyarrhythmias
Oral	10–20 mg b.i.d.	12 hr	Heart block
Nadolol			Raynaud's phenomenon
Oral	40–240 mg/d	24 hr	Exacerbates reactive airways disease Masks signs of hypoglycemia Accentuates insulin-induced hypoglycemia
Relative cardioselectivity			
Atenolol			
Oral	50–200 mg/d	24 hr	Same, except relatively safe at low doses in patients with reactive airways disease Has tendency to activate hypoglycemia
Metoprolol			
Oral	50–150 mg b.i.d.–t.i.d.	8–12 hr	Same
Intrinsic sympathomimetic activity			
Pindolol			
Oral	5–15 mg t.i.d.	8 hr	Same as for nonselective but less tendency to cause bradyarrhythmias

be necessary to offer symptomatic relief in some patients. **Sublingual nitroglycerin** can be used as a prophylactic (e.g., prior to an activity that causes symptoms) as well as for relief of acute episodes of pain. Comparative effects of nitrates, beta blockers, and calcium slow-channel blocking agents are shown in Table 5.

Patients with **Prinzmetal's** or **variable-threshold angina** (cold-induced angina, angina at rest and on exertion, angina at different workloads) are a subset in which an element of vasospasm contributes to symptoms. In this group of patients use of a calcium slow-channel blocking agent is favored.

Side effects (Tables 2, 3, and 4) often limit the use of a drug. This is particularly true of oral nitrates. Beta blockers with low lipid solubility (e.g., nadolol, atenolol) are claimed to have fewer CNS side effects but this remains to be proved.

Revascularization (coronary angioplasty or bypass grafting) should be considered in patients with poor response to medical treatment or those whose life style is compromised by angina. Subsets with poor prognosis (left main

TABLE 4. *Calcium slow-channel blocking agents*

Drug and administration	Dose	Duration of action	Side effects
Nifedipine			
Sublingual	10 mg	2–4 hr	Hypotension
			Tachycardia (reflex), headaches,
Oral	10–30 mg q 6–8 hr	6–8 hr	edema, dizziness
Verapamil			
Oral	80–120 mg q 6–8 hr	6 hr	Heart failure in patients with decreased ejection fraction
			Hypotension
			Edema
			Constipation
			Heart block
Diltiazem			
Oral	60–90 mg q 6–8 hr	6 hr	Edema
			Nausea
			Headaches
			Dizziness
			Heart block

coronary artery stenosis, three-vessel disease) also should be considered for surgery.

C. Unstable Angina   Crescendo angina, preinfarction angina, and intermediate syndrome.

1. **Definition.** Unstable angina is a term used to describe several different patterns of angina. These include patients with a history of chronic stable angina who enter a phase when the pain comes on at lower levels of activity, lasts longer, and requires more nitroglycerin for relief. Others have pain coming principally at rest, or pain that is so prolonged that it resembles the pain of acute myocardial infarction.

2. **Diagnosis.** These patients should be admitted to a **coronary care unit** (CCU). In those with prolonged episodes of pain, acute myocardial infarction should be excluded with serial EKGs and creatine phosphokinase (CPK) enzyme measurements. An important aspect of monitoring is to document the presence or absence of EKG changes during episodes of pain. Evidence of **ST elevation** with pain is very suggestive of a vasospastic element.

3. **Treatment.** Patients presenting with unstable angina are often receiving medical treatment that limits therapeutic options. Some studies favor **coronary vasoconstriction** as a major pathophysiologic component, and the use of nitrates and calcium-channel blocking drugs is recommended. Other reports suggest that disease progression is a common cause of vasospasm. In terms of medical treatment, a superiority of calcium-channel blockers over beta blockers or nitrates has been suggested but not documented. Patients frequently require combination treatment. Those who demonstrate **ST elevation** with pain appear to respond to **calcium-channel blockers** because they frequently have a vasospastic component.

Often the most effective way to control pain initially is with an **intravenous nitroglycerin infusion**. The initial dose is 10 μg/min and titrated every 5 to

TABLE 5. Comparative effects

Agent	Arterial dilator	Venodilator	Prevents coronary vasoconstriction	Heart rate	Systolic blood pressure	AV conduction	Tachyphylaxis
Nitrates	+ +	+ +	+ + +	+	– –	0	Yes (long-acting nitrates)
Beta blockers							
Nonselective	0	0	–	– – –	– – –	–	No
Selective	0	0	–	– – –	– – –	–	No
Intrinsic sympathomimetic activity	0	0	–	–/0	– – –	0	No
Ca^{2+} channel blockers							
Nifedipine	+ + +	0	+ + +	+ +	– – –	0	No
Verapamil	+ +	0	+ + +	–/0	– –	–	No
Diltiazem	+	0	+ + +	–	–/0	–	No

AV, atrioventricular.

+, Increase/or positive effect; –, decrease/or negative effect; 0, no effect.

10 min according to symptomatic and blood pressure response. Excessive fall in blood pressure can be treated by reducing the infusion rate, elevating legs, and giving fluids if necessary. This route of administration is preferred to other methods for administering nitroglycerin because it allows better titration of the dose. It is important to remember that nitroglycerin is absorbed to polyvinylchloride; therefore the **infusion should be mixed in a glass bottle**. A few patients will not respond to maximal medical treatment and **intra-aortic balloon pumping** may be efficacious in those patients. Most patients presenting with unstable angina should have **coronary arteriography**.

II. **CORONARY ARTERY SPASM**   The characteristics of the pain are like typical angina in terms of quality, location, and relief with nitroglycerin, but they differ in that the pain comes on **at rest** and often wakes patients from sleep during the early hours of the morning.

A. **Diagnosis**   Spasm should be suspected on the basis of history. Patients frequently note that beta blockers make symptoms worse. **Holter monitoring** documenting ST change with pain in the absence of heart rate change is helpful. Provocation of spasm with **intravenous ergonovine** is the most effective way to diagnose spasm but this should be done only during cardiac catheterization.

B. **Treatment**   Calcium slow-channel blockers are the treatment of choice in this condition (Table 4). Nitrates also are useful, but side effects limit patient compliance. Switching from one Ca^{2+} blocker to another may be helpful when patients are refractory, and in a small number of patients combination treatment (nifedipine + diltiazem, nifedipine + verapamil) may give better control. Beta-blocking agents are contraindicated in patients with coronary spasm because the alpha-adrenergic predominance in this situation may precipitate spasm.

III. **MYOCARDIAL INFARCTION**

A. **Acute Phase**   The major goals are **pain relief** and **prevention of arrhythmias**.

1. **Pain relief. Morphine** 2 to 6 mg, i.v., should be given over 5 min. Many patients require additional doses up to a total of 15 to 20 mg.

2. **Arrhythmia prevention.** Intravenous **lidocaine** bolus 75 to 100 mg followed by i.v. infusion of 2 mg/min generally provides effective prevention of malignant arrhythmias. This dose should be reduced in patients who have signs of heart failure and in very elderly patients because of decreased hepatic metabolism. Lidocaine should be discontinued 24 hr after admission if the patient is stable. Patients with an uncomplicated course can be moved from the CCU after 48 hr.

3. **General measures. Oxygen therapy** is given, 2 to 3 liter/min via nasal prongs. **Sedation** is prescribed as necessary (e.g., diazepam). Patients should have a light diet during the first 24 hr. **Anticoagulant therapy** with subcutaneous heparin, 5,000 units every 8 hr to prevent thromboembolic disease, is recommended unless there is a specific contraindication. This should be continued until the patient is fully mobilized.

4. **Rehabilitation.** Once patients have been pain-free for 24 hr at bed rest, activity should progress from passive to active exercises. Leg dangling for short periods helps prevent deconditioning.

5. **Role of intervention to limit infarct size.** This is still a controversial area, but in some patients certain interventions appear to be effective.

   a. **Streptokinase**, either given directly into the coronary artery involved or intravenously (1.5 million units over 1 hr), opens vessels in 60% to 80% of cases. This form of treatment should be limited to patients who can receive treatment within 3 to 4 hr of the onset of symptoms and who are continuing to have chest pain or who show ST elevation without Q waves in at least several leads.

   b. **Intravenous propranolol**, 1- to 2-mg bolus, up to 10 mg, is useful in controlling heart rate and blood pressure in patients with marked sympathetic overactivity. Efficacy in limiting infarct size, however, remains unproved. Other interventions, such as a glucose-insulin-potassium infusion, nitrates, and nitroprusside, have been used; but routine use of these agents is not recommended unless there are specific indications such as continued chest pain or heart failure.

B. **Complications—General**

1. **Arrhythmias.** Arrhythmias associated with myocardial infarction are listed in Table 6.

2. **Hypotension.** This can be the result of several factors, including a vagal reaction, volume depletion, impending cardiogenic shock, and right ventricular infarction. Initial treatment includes simple measures such as **raising legs**. If volume depletion is felt to be the cause, then a challenge with 250 ml of normal saline over 30 min is suggested. Failure to respond satisfactorily necessitates placing a Swan-Ganz catheter to assess filling pressures and cardiac output. **Low filling pressure** indicates the need for additional volume expansion, whereas **high filling pressure** indicates heart failure. A disproportionately elevated right atrial pressure in comparison to the wedge pressure suggests right ventricular infarction (normally the difference is > 6 mm Hg).

3. **Heart failure** (see Chapter 6).

   a. **Mild.** Diuretics are recommended.

   b. **Moderate.** Diuretics and vasodilators are recommended.

   c. **Severe.** Diuretics, vasodilators, sympathomimetic agents, and possibly intra-aortic balloon pump are recommended. If pulmonary edema is severe and oxygenation is a problem, mechanical ventilation may be necessary. Swan-Ganz catheter monitoring is required.

4. **Cardiogenic shock.** This has a very **poor prognosis**, and patients require hemodynamic monitoring, dopamine or dobutamine, and intra-aortic balloon pumping. Swan-Ganz monitoring is indicated.

C. **Early Recovery**

1. **General.** Patients should be monitored for 48 to 72 hr on telemetry after transfer from CCU.

2. **Rehabilitation.** Gradually increase activity with sitting in chair, moving around bed, and using bedside commode. Patients without complications can be walking in halls by days 3 to 5. Those with evidence of failure should be

TABLE 6. *Arrhythmias*

Arrhythmia	Frequency	Primary therapy	Secondary therapy	Supporting therapy
Ventricular fibrillation	Common	Cardioversion 200–400 Wsec	Bretylium, i.v., 5 mg/kg Lidocaine, i.v., 75–100 mg	Cardiopulmonary resuscitation (CPR) Sodium bicarbonate Epinephrine
Ventricular tachycardia	Common	Lidocaine, i.v., 75–100 mg Precordial thump	Cardioversion Procainamide, i.v., 0.5–1g loading dose	If patient is conscious, sedation should be given before cardioversion
Ventricular premature beats ($\geq$6/min, R on T, coupling, multifocal)	Very common	Lidocaine, i.v., 75–100 mg bolus then 1–3 mg/min infusion	Procainamide, i.v., 0.5–1g loading dose; 2–6 mg/ min infusion Oral quinidine	Exclude other causes, such as low K^+ or Mg^{2+}, digitalis intoxication
Ventricular asystole	Common	CPR Intracardiac epinephrine	Transthoracic or transvenous pacing	Sodium bicarbonate Calcium chloride
Accelerated idioventricular rhythm				
Symptomatic	Rare	Lidocaine, i.v., 75–100 mg		
Asymptomatic	Common	None		
Accelerated junctional rhythm	Rare	None		
Paroxysmal junctional tachycardia				
Symptomatic	Very rare	Cardioversion (synchronized)		
Asymptomatic	Very rare	None		
Sinus tachycardia	Common	None	None	Usually reflects underlying heart failure requiring treatment

Sinus bradycardia			
Symptomatic	Rare	Atropine, i.v., 0.5–1.0 mg	Temporary transvenous pacemaker
Asymptomatic	Common	None	
Atrial premature beats	Very common	None	
Paroxysmal supraventricular tachycardia	Very rare	Carotid sinus massage Digoxin, i.v., 0.25 mg	Propranolol, i.v., 0.5–2 mg Verapamil, i.v., 5–10 mg Cardioversion
Atrial fibrillation	Rare	Digoxin, i.v., 0.25 mg	Cardioversion (synchronized) Propranolol, i.v., 0.5–2 mg Verapamil, i.v., 5–10 mg
Atrial flutter	Rare	Digoxin, i.v., 0.25 mg	Cardioversion (synchronized) Propranolol, i.v., 0.5–2 mg Verapamil, i.v., 5–10 mg
First-degree heart block	Common	None	
Mobitz type-I block			
Asymptomatic	Common	None	
Symptomatic	Rare	Temporary transvenous pacing	
Mobitz type-II block			
Asymptomatic	Rare	None	
Symptomatic	Rare	Temporary transvenous pacing	
Complete heart block	Common	Temporary transvenous pacing	Atropine, i.v., 0.5–1 mg Isoproterenol, i.v., infusion 1–2 µg/min Atropine, i.v., 0.5–1 mg Isoproterenol, i.v., infusion 1–2 µg/min

mobilized more slowly. Aim to have patients fully mobile by days 7 to 10. Advice regarding smoking, diet, and blood pressure control should be given where appropriate.

3. **Complications**

a. **Infarct extension.** Return to CCU and monitor.

b. **Postinfarction angina.** Treat with nitrates, beta blockers, or calcium-channel blockers, and consider coronary arteriography.

c. **Pericarditis.** Pain relief can be obtained with aspirin or other nonsteroidal anti-inflammatory drugs.

d. **Ventricular septal defect (VSD).** Suspicion of VSD requires Swan-Ganz monitoring, measurement of pulmonary-artery and right atrial oxygen saturations, afterload reduction, catheterization, and surgical consideration.

e. **Mitral regurgitation (MIR).** MIR requires a Swan-Ganz catheter, afterload reduction, catheterization, and consideration for mitral valve replacement.

f. **Cardiac rupture.** Cardiac rupture requires sympathomimetics and **immediate cardiac surgery.**

D. **Late Recovery** Before discharge patients should be assessed with Holter monitors and arrhythmias appropriately treated. An exercise test should be performed, and patients with exercise-induced ischemia should undergo coronary arteriography.

1. **Rehabilitation.** Normal completion of the exercise test indicates that patients are capable of normal self-care activities. The cardiovascular demands during intercourse are similar to those of the exercise test. In the absence of a formal rehabilitation program, patients should be instructed in a **daily walking program.** Initially, they should walk for 30 min and use symptoms to adjust the intensity of activity. The duration of exercise should be increased to 45 to 60 min over a 3- to 4-week period. Shopping malls are convenient places to exercise during climatic extremes. Patients may resume driving a car 2 to 4 weeks after discharge; return to sedentary occupation 6 to 8 weeks after discharge; and manual work 8 to 12 weeks after discharge. Symptom-limited **maximal** exercise testing is recommended before returning to manual work.

2. **Complications. Post-myocardial infarction syndrome (Dressler's syndrome):** The treatment of Dressler's syndrome initially consists of aspirin or other nonsteroidal anti-inflammatory drugs. Recurrent episodes should be treated with prednisone 40 mg/day and tapered slowly according to symptoms.

3. **Other measures**

a. **Anticoagulation.** Long-term treatment with **warfarin** is recommended for patients who survive very large infarcts, due to the risk of systemic emboli.

b. **Permanent pacing.** Permanent pacing is a controversial area because clear benefits have not been documented. Mortality in these cases is generally related to infarct size and left ventricular damage. **Indications for permanent pacing include**

(1) Persistent complete heart block (≥ 7 days).

(2) Anterior myocardial infarction complicated by transient complete heart block.

(3) Left bundle branch block with a transient high-degree atrioventricular (AV) block.

(4) Right bundle branch block with left anterior hemiblock and transient high-degree AV block.

c. **Secondary prevention.** A number of agents have been evaluated, including beta blockers, aspirin, dypyridamole, and sulfinpyrazone, to improve mortality postinfarction. Several studies showed favorable results with beta blockers; however, the overall gain in survival was small. Identification of patients with severe arrhythmias and/or ischemia and treating them appropriately appears to be a more rational approach than subjecting all patients to beta blockers.

BIBLIOGRAPHY

Angina

Pitt, B., Kalft, V., Rabinovitch, et al. (1983): Impact of radionuclide techniques on evaluation of patients with ischemic heart disease. *JACC*, 1:63–72.

Takaro, T., Hultgren, H. N., Lipton, M. D., and Detre, K. M. (1976): The VA cooperative randomized study of surgery for coronary arterial occlusive disease II Subgroup with left main lesions. *Circulation*, (Suppl. III) 54:107–112.

Weiner, D. A., Ryan, T. J., McCabe, C. H., et al. (1979): Exercise stress testing. Correlations among history of angina, ST segment response and prevalence of coronary artery disease in the coronary artery surgery study (CASS). *N. Engl. J. Med.*, 301:230–235.

Weiner, D. A., Ryan, T. J., McCabe, C. H., et al. (1984): Prognostic importance of a clinical profile and exercise test in medically treated patients with coronary artery disease. *JACC*, 3:772–779.

Beta Blockers

Opie, L. H. (1980): Drugs and the heart. *Lancet*, 1:693–698.

Calcium Slow Channel Blockers

Krihler, D. M., and Rowland, E. (1983): Clinical value of calcium antagonists in treatment of cardiovascular disorders. *JACC*, 1:355–364.

Coronary Artery Spasm

Maseri, A. (1979): Variant angina and coronary vasospasm: clues to a broader understanding of angina pectoris. *Cardiovasc. Med.*, 4:647.

Silvermann-Bott, C., Heupler, F. A. (1983): Natural history of pure coronary artery spasm in patients treated medically. *JACC*, 2:200–205.

Myocardial Infarction

Chamberlain, D. A. (1983): Editorial. Beta adrenoceptor antagonists after myocardial infarction—where are we now? *Br. Heart J.*, 49:105–110.

Furberg, C. D. (1984): Clinical value of intracoronary streptokinase. *Am. J. Cardiol.*, 53:626–627.

Griggs, T. R., Wagner, G. S., and Gettes, L. S. (1983): Beta-adrenergic blocking agents after myocardial infarction. An undocumental need in patients at lowest risk. *JACC*, 1:1530–1533.

Gunnar, R. M. and Laeb, H. S. (1983): Shock in acute myocardial infarction; evaluation of psychologic therapy. *JACC*, 1:154–163.

Sobel, B. E. and Braunwald, E. (1980): The management of acute myocardial infarction in heart disease. Edited by E. Braunwald, pp. 1353–1386. WB Saunders, Philadelphia.

Nitrates

McGregor, M. (1982): The nitrates and myocardial ischemia. *Circulation*, 66:689–692.

Opie, L. (1980): Nitrates. *Lancet*, 1:750–753.

6.

Congestive Heart Failure with Cardiomyopathies and Valvular Heart Disease

Kenneth Hossack

6.

Congestive Heart Failure with Cardiomyopathies and Valvular Heart Disease

Heart failure is most commonly the result of **left ventricular dysfunction**, and as the disease progresses, signs of right-side failure become apparent. Patients with long-standing chronic lung disease, however, may develop isolated right heart failure. In evaluating a patient with congestive heart failure it is important to determine a specific underlying cause and to prescribe treatment for a potentially reversible process.

I. **DIFFERENTIAL DIAGNOSIS** Surgically correctable lesions such as **valvular disease** and **ventricular aneurysm** should be excluded by careful physical examination and echocardiography. Some common causes of cardiomyopathy are listed in Table 1, but heart failure on the basis of coronary artery disease is probably the most common cause of congestive heart failure.

It is important to exclude other causes for the apparent signs of heart failure. The differentiation between restrictive and constrictive cardiomyopathy may be difficult, often requiring **detailed cardiological evaluation, including catheterization**. For example, constrictive pericarditis may present as intractable right heart failure.

II. **THERAPY** The aim of therapy in patients with heart failure is to **alter the preload, afterload, and contractility** so that cardiac function is optimized and symptoms are alleviated. The treatment prescribed depends on the severity of the heart failure, and the need for additional therapy is dictated by response to initial therapy.

The New York Heart Association functional classification is useful for categorizing patients. Formal exercise testing gives more objective information on functional status.

III. **GENERAL MEASURES** Irrespective of functional class, a **no-added-salt diet** is

TABLE 1. *Common causes of cardiomyopathy*

Infective	Infiltrative
Viral	Amyloidosis
Metabolic	Hemochromatosis
Thiamine deficiency	Sarcoidosis
Acromegaly	Others
Myxedema	Endocardial fibroelastosis
Thyrotoxicosis	Sickle-cell anemia
Diabetes mellitus	Neuromuscular disorders
Uremia	Postpartum disorders
Toxic	
Alcohol	
Bleomycin	
Adriamycin	

prescribed. Patients in classes III and IV benefit from **bed rest**, and subcutaneous **heparin** is recommended until they are mobile. **Oxygen** via nasal prongs to relieve dyspnea should be administered. Patients with atrial fibrillation should receive **anticoagulation** therapy with warfarin to prevent embolic events, and the ventricular response should be slowed to 60 to 80 beats/min with **digitalization**. Paracentesis and pleural aspiration are indicated in refractory failure.

IV. **SPECIFIC TREATMENT**   A controversial issue is the value of Swan-Ganz catheter monitoring to assess response to therapy. If heart failure is mild, necessitating only diuretics, then such monitoring is unnecessary. In the setting of acute heart failure, particularly complicating an acute myocardial infarction, and when intravenous agents are being used, **monitoring** is advisable. There are limitations of therapy in that initial favorable responses may not be maintained and deterioration can be detected early by monitoring.

   A. **Diuretics**   Medical treatment for patients in class II should initially consist of **diuretics** (see Table 2) and **digoxin** (0.125 to 0.25 mg/day depending on the patients' size and renal function). Nevertheless, the value of digoxin is debated. It is clearly indicated in patients with atrial fibrillation to slow the ventricular response. Use of **potassium supplements** or K^+-sparing diuretics is important in those receiving diuretics, particularly with digoxin administration.

   1. **Thiazides.** There is a wide choice of diuretic agents for maintenance therapy. **Thiazide** diuretics are very effective. They have the advantage of a longer duration of action than furosemide.

   2. **Furosemide** is the intravenous diuretic of choice when a **rapid effect** is required.

   3. **Ethacrynic acid** also is very effective when given intravenously. For patients with more marked fluid retention furosemide is preferred.

   4. A disadvantage of diuretics is their ability to cause a contraction alkalosis and deterioration of renal function due to hypovolemia. When this occurs, the dose of diuretic should be reduced; if heart failure symptoms are still present, additional treatment with vasodilators is prescribed.

   B. **Oral Vasodilators**   Patients in functional classes III and IV frequently require additional treatment to improve symptoms. Oral vasodilators are listed in Table 3. **Arterial dilators** are preferred initially to venodilators.

   1. **Hydralazine** and **prazosin** are the first-line agents. Prazosin is preferred because the side effect profile is much less serious than with hydralazine. Prazosin has the disadvantage that tolerance develops to the drug in about 50% of patients. The addition of nitrates to hydralazine often provides additional benefit because of the predominant effect of the nitrates on the venous side of the circulation.

   When prazosin and hydralazine are ineffective, captopril is recommended. It is important to start with very low doses (6 mg t.i.d.) and increase gradually.

   2. Minoxidil and nifedipine are second-line agents.

   3. **Amrinone** is an experimental oral and intravenous agent with inotropic effects; it is neither a catecholamine nor a glycoside. The usual oral dose is 75 to 200 mg t.i.d. The drug improves symptoms of heart failure both at rest and during

TABLE 2. *Diuretics*

Drug	Dosage	Administration	Side effects	Comments
Furosemide	20–120 mg/d or b.i.d.	Oral	Hypotension Hypokalemia Hyperuricemia	Need to give potassium supplements or K⁺-sparing diuretics
	20–80 mg	i.v.	Skin rash Abnormal liver function Deafness	
Ethacrynic acid	50–100 mg/d or b.i.d.	Oral	Hypotension Hypokalemia Hyperuricemia	Need to give potassium supplements or K⁺-sparing diuretics
Chlorothiazide	50 mg 250–500 mg/d	i.v. Oral	Hypokalemia Gout	Need to give potassium supplements or K⁺-sparing diuretics
Hydrochlorothiazide	50–100 mg/d	Oral	Hyperglycemia Hypercalcemia	
Chlorthalidone	50–100 mg/d	Oral	Cholestatic jaundice	
Metolazone	20–25 mg/d	Oral		
Amiloride	5–15 mg/d	Oral	Hyperkalemia	Mild diuretic, but very effective K⁺-sparing agent; should be avoided in renal dysfunction
Triamterene	100–200 mg/d	Oral	Hyperkalemia Nausea	Avoid in patients with renal dysfunction or diabetes mellitus
Spironolactone	50–200 mg/c	Oral	Hyperkalemia Gynecomastia	Avoid in patients with renal dysfunction

TABLE 3. *Vasodilators*

Drug	Dosage	Mode of action		Side effects	Comments
		Venodilator	Arterial dilator		
Direct acting					
Isosorbide dinitrate	20–60 mg q 6 hr	+ + +	+	Hypotension Headaches	Tachyphylaxis may develop
Nitroglycerin ointment patches	½–2" q 6 hr 5–30 cm²/d	+ + +	+	Hypotension Headaches	Tachyphylaxis may develop
Hydralazine	50–200 mg q 6–8 hr	+/0	+ + +	Reflex tachycardia Systemic lupus Skin rash May provoke angina	Tachyphylaxis may develop
Minoxidil	2.5–10 mg b.i.d.	+/0	+ + +	Hypotension Fluid retention Hirsutism	Not a first-line drug
Neurohumoral antagonists					
Prazosin	1–5 mg q 8 hr	+ +	+ + +	Hypotension	Tachyphylaxis common
Captopril	6–25 mg q 6–8 hr	+	+ + +	Hypotension Proteinuria Bone marrow suppression	Use in smaller doses than for hypertension
Ca²⁺ channel blocking agent					
Nifedipine	10–30 mg t.i.d.	0	+ + +	Hypotension Peripheral edema Headaches Flushing	May also improve diastolic compliance

exercise. Side effects are worsening of ventricular arrhythmias including sudden death, fevers, thrombocytopenia, myalgia, gastrointestinal disturbances, and hepatic dysfunction.

C. Parenteral Agents Parenteral agents used to improve heart failure are listed in Table 4. When these are administered, acute **hemodynamic monitoring** is advisable.

1. When the systemic vascular resistance is high, **nitroprusside** is the drug of choice. Manipulation of preload and afterload with nitroglycerin and nitroprusside should be attempted.

2. When **additional treatment** is required, dopamine or dobutamine is used.

3. **Aminophylline** is useful in patients who have **airways obstruction** associated with pulmonary congestion.

V. VALVULAR HEART DISEASE

A. General All patients with valvular heart disease require prophylaxis for infective endocarditis irrespective of severity of valve lesion.

B. Aortic Stenosis Valve replacement is indicated when a patient develops symptoms. Long-term medical treatment for symptoms is not recommended.

C. Aortic Regurgitation Symptoms can be improved with diuretics and vasodilators, but the concern with this lesion is the development of irreversible left ventricular dysfunction. **Surgery** is therefore indicated when symptoms develop or in asymptomatic patients with a severe regurgitation in whom left ventricular function deteriorates. **Echocardiography** is a useful method to assess noninvasively changes in left ventricular function.

D. Mitral Stenosis Mildly symptomatic patients can be improved by controlling heart rate during exercise with **digoxin** or a **beta blocker**. Gentle **diuresis** also can improve symptoms. Patients in atrial fibrillation or those with moderate to severe stenosis should receive **anticoagulation** therapy with warfarin to prevent thromboembolic phenomena. **Surgery** (commissurotomy or valve replacement) is indicated when the functional state deteriorates. Most centers use **cardiopulmonary bypass** to perform commissurotomy. Replacing the mitral valve if commis-

TABLE 4. *Parenteral agents*

Drug	Dose	Comments
Vasodilators		
Nitroglycerin	10–200 μg/min	Mix in a glass bottle because nitroglycerin is absorbed by plastic
Nitroprusside	0.5–10 μg/kg/min	Light-sensitive; container should be wrapped in foil
Sympathomimetic agents		
Dopamine	≤1–10 μg/kg/min	Tends to raise blood pressure more than dobutamine does
Dobutamine	2.5–20 μg/min	Less tendency to increase heart rate than with dopamine
Aminophylline	2.0–5.6 mg/kg loading dose 0.5–0.9 mg/kg/hr infusion	Has weak inotropic effect; also may improve renal blood flow

surotomy is not feasible in this situation is therefore not a problem. In general, calcified valves, those with marked chordal fusion and shortening, and those with associated regurgitation are better replaced.

E. **Mitral Regurgitation**   The decision to recommend surgery for this lesion can be difficult. Often patients can be considerably improved with **diuretics** and **vasodilators**. The regurgitation eventually leads to left ventricular dysfunction, and the ejection fraction usually falls after valve replacement. Thus, in some patients left ventricular function is so poor that surgery is not warranted. A severe lesion with moderate symptoms is an indication for **surgery**. Patients with atrial fibrillation should receive **anticoagulation** therapy.

F. **Mitral Stenosis and Regurgitation**   These patients behave more like those with mitral stenosis. Medical treatment is less satisfactory, and **surgery** for valve replacement is indicated when symptoms develop. These patients should receive **anticoagulation** therapy.

G. **Hypertrophic Cardiomyopathy**   **Avoid strenuous physical activity.** Symptoms can be improved with beta blockers, but often large doses are required (propranolol 120 mg q.i.d.). Patients may respond to verapamil 80 mg to 120 mg q.i.d., but the drug should be administered cautiously. Patients refractory to medical treatment who have a resting systolic pressure difference between the body of the left ventricle and the left ventricular outflow tract benefit from myoectomy.

Diuretics should be avoided, and inotropic agents and vasodilators are contraindicated because the outflow obstruction may be worsened. Patients may develop atrial fibrillation; digoxin is useful to control the ventricular rate. These patients should receive anticoagulation therapy to prevent thromboembolic phenomena.

BIBLIOGRAPHY

Cardiomyopathies
Emmanuel, R. (1970): Classification of the cardiomyopathies. *Am. J. Cardiol.*, 26:438.

Valvular Heart Disease
Rahimtoola, S. H. (1983): Valvular heart disease: A perspective. *JACC*, 1:199–215.

Vasodilators
Chatterjee, K. and Parmley, W. W. (1983): Vasodilator therapy for acute myocardial infarction and chronic congestive heart failure. *JACC*, 1:133–153.
Opie, L. H. (1980): Digitalis and sympathomimetic stimulants. *Lancet*, 1:912–918.
Opie, L. H. (1980): Vasodilating drugs. *Lancet*, 1:966–972.
Packer, M. (1983): Vasodilator and inotropic therapy for severe chronic heart failure: Passion and skepticism. *JACC*, 2:841–852.

7.

Management of Cardiac Arrhythmias

Michael J. Reiter

7.

Management of Cardiac Arrhythmias

I. MECHANISMS OF CARDIAC ARRHYTHMIAS

A. **Review of Normal Cardiac Electrophysiology**   The resting cardiac cell membrane has a potential of -60 to -90 mV (inside negative) owing to the concentration gradient of K^+ and the relatively high permeability of the resting membrane to K^+. In contrast, membrane permeability to Na^+ and Ca^{2+} is low. However, changes in the electrical field within the membrane can alter the permeability characteristics of the membrane, permitting inward movement of sodium and calcium and resulting in cellular depolarization. The action potential of normal atrial, ventricular, and Purkinje fiber tissue consists of both a fast and slow inward current. The initial rapid depolarization is the result of an increase in the membrane permeability to sodium ions. The rate of rise of the initial depolarization is a determinant of conduction velocity through myocardial tissue. Immediately after initial depolarization, membrane permeability to Na^+ falls, and the membrane starts to repolarize. A second inward current develops when the membrane has been depolarized from -90 mV to approximately -40 mV by the fast inward current. In contrast to the rapid inward-current channel, this second inward-current channel is activated and inactivated much more slowly and contributes to the plateau phase of the action potential. Under normal conditions the major ionic species accounting for the slow inward current is Ca^{2+}.

Cells in the sinoatrial (SA) and atrioventricular (AV) nodes (and perhaps Purkinje fibers under pathological conditions) appear to have action potentials primarily dependent on the slow calcium current.

In addition, certain cells in the SA node, atria, AV node, and His-Purkinje system exhibit a spontaneous, gradual depolarization during electrical diastole. These cells may reach the membrane threshold potential and generate an action potential. This property is referred to as "automaticity." Under normal conditions, cells in the SA node reach threshold first. In the event of sinus slowing, subsidiary pacemaker cells may reach threshold, giving rise to a slower escape rhythm.

B. **Physiology of Sinus Rhythm**   Since cells in the SA node have the fastest inherent rate, they assume pacemaker control of the heart under normal conditions. Depolarization of cells in the SA node is not apparent on the surface electrocardiogram, but may be inferred from the spread of the depolarization wave front through atrial tissue (P wave).

The wave of depolarization enters AV nodal tissue in the region of the low interatrial septum. Normally, the atria and ventricle are electrically isolated from each other except in this region. Conduction through the AV node is slowed, in a rate-dependent manner, because of the slow upstroke of the action potential

94

characteristic of cells in the node and because of the long relative refractory period of these cells.

The His bundle emerges from the AV node and divides at the top of the muscular interventricular septum into the right and left bundle branch systems. The electrical activity of the His bundle may be recorded by an intracardiac catheter positioned near the septal leaflet of the tricuspid valve. The right bundle branch is single. The left bundle branch divides into a left posterior fascicle and a left anterior fascicle. The bundle branch system activates ventricular myocardium by means of an extensive endocardial network of terminal Purkinje fibers.

C. **Mechanisms of Tachyarrhythmias**

1. **Enhanced automaticity** can produce cardiac tachycardias when there is an **increase in the rate of diastolic depolarization** in subsidiary pacemaker cells so that these cells reach threshold before those in the sinus node. Conditions favoring enhanced automaticity include ischemia or hypoxia, hypokalemia, hypomagnesemia, digitalis toxicity, and beta agonists. Since the inherent rate of pacemaker cells tends to change gradually, automatic (ectopic) tachycardias are usually nonparoxysmal and frequently vary in rate. With depolarization, pacemaker cells are reset, and therefore these arrhythmias are uncommonly terminated by electrical cardioversion.

   The automatic tachyarrhythmias include:

   a. Sinus tachycardia.

   b. Ectopic atrial tachycardia.

   c. Multifocal atrial tachycardia.

   d. Some types of junctional tachycardias (nonparoxysmal).

   e. Some types of ventricular tachycardias.

   f. Accelerated idioventricular rhythm.

2. **Reentrant arrhythmias** are the result of a continuous circle of activation. This requires **two potential pathways** with common origin and termination. There also has to be a critical relationship between refractoriness and conduction so that a critically timed impulse will encounter **unidirectional block** in one of the pathways but travel down the other pathway with **conduction slowed** sufficiently so that the first pathway recovers to permit conduction in the opposite direction, giving rise to a continuous circuit of activation. Reentry arrhythmias are dependent on the existence of electrically excitable (nonrefractory) conducting tissue just ahead of the depolarization wave front at all times. Reentry arrhythmias are usually regular and are frequently initiated by a single premature stimulus; they usually can be terminated by an appropriately timed stimulus and can be terminated by cardioversion.

   Clinically important reentrant arrhythmias include:

   a. Most cases of paroxysmal supraventricular tachycardia (PSVT). The reentry circuit may be of four different varieties:

      (1) In approximately 50% of patients it resides completely within an AV node in which there appears to be two pathways (AV nodal reentry tachycardia).

(2) In about 40% of patients it utilizes a "concealed" accessory (Kent bundle) atrioventricular pathway (accessory pathway reentry tachycardia). The pathway is concealed because it is capable of conducting only unidirectionally from the ventricle to the atrium. Therefore, during sinus rhythm a short PR interval and delta wave are not seen.

(3) In the remaining 10% to 15% of cases the two limbs of the reentry circuit appear to reside either completely within the atria (intra-atrial reentry tachycardia) or

(4) Within the sinus node (sinus node reentry tachycardia).

b. The common paroxysmal arrhythmias associated with the Wolff-Parkinson-White (WPW) syndrome (the accessory pathway acts as part of the reentry circuit).

c. Atrial flutter and fibrillation.

d. Most cases of ventricular tachycardia (VT) (the reentry circuit resides within the ventricle).

D. Mechanisms of Bradyarrhythmias

1. Failure of impulse origination. The slowing or failure (arrest) of inherent sinus automaticity or the inability of the sinus node potential to propagate (exit block) may lead to persistent and/or inappropriate bradycardia and to prolonged, symptomatic pauses. This can produce symptoms of congestive failure, presyncope, Stokes-Adams attacks, or sudden death and are collectively referred to as the **sick sinus syndrome.** The occurrence of significant bradycardia or prolonged pauses requires the concomitant failure of distal escape pacemaker cells. This suggests that the pathological process is more widespread.

2. Failure of impulse propagation

a. Conduction delay and block **within the AV node** at higher rates are both physiologic and under the influence of autonomic tone. In the normal AV node progressive delay prior to conduction block is normal at paced rates at or above about 120 beats/min (bpm). Abnormal delay (first-degree AV block), intermittent conduction block (Mobitz I), or high-grade AV block are usually well tolerated, because the block occurs nonparoxysmally and there are dependable subsidiary pacemaker cells with a sufficient escape rate located within the junction or in the His-Purkinje system.

b. Conduction block **below the AV node** may involve the common His bundle, all three fascicles (complete heart block), or complete failure of two fascicles and intermittent failure of the third (Mobitz II), and more frequently occurs abruptly. The emergence of an adequate and dependable escape rhythm is less likely.

II. CHARACTERISTICS OF ANTIARRHYTHMIC AGENTS

A. General   Antiarrhythmic agents available for clinical use are sometimes classified on the basis of their electrophysiologic effects in normal, isolated cardiac tissue preparations. However, at present our understanding of their antiarrhythmic action is insufficient to present definitive guidelines for the clinical selection of a particular agent. Thus, for the present, therapy for arrhythmias remains primarily empiric.

B. Quinidine

1. **Actions.** Quinidine, by **decreasing membrane permeability to sodium** ions during the rapid initial depolarization of the action potential, decreases the maximum rate of depolarization, slows conduction, and prolongs refractoriness of atrial, Purkinje, and ventricular tissue. Quinidine also **depresses spontaneous diastolic depolarization** (i.e., reduces automaticity). These effects appear to be lessened by hypokalemia. Quinidine also has an **anticholinergic** (vagolytic) action that tends to facilitate AV nodal conduction in vivo. The actions of quinidine, procainamide, and disopyramide are very similar, and they are often collectively referred to as type I agents.

2. **Pharmacokinetics.** Quinidine is most frequently used as an oral preparation. Several oral formulations are available containing differing amounts of quinidine base (see Table 1). Quinidine sulfate is more rapidly absorbed than the gluconate salt. Quinidine is 80% bound to plasma albumin and is primarily (60% to 80%) **metabolized by the liver.** The hepatic metabolites and a small amount of unchanged quinidine are excreted in the urine. The metabolites have little if any antiarrhythmic action. Therapeutic concentrations depend on the assay method but appear to be between 2 and 5 μg/ml (using the double extraction procedure).

3. **Indications and toxicity.** Quinidine is useful for the prevention of both supraventricular and ventricular arrhythmias, related to both enhanced automaticity and reentrant mechanisms. Quinidine also may be useful for suppression of both premature atrial or ventricular beats that are symptomatic or to prevent the development of a sustained arrhythmia.

Quinidine is frequently used to convert atrial fibrillation or flutter to sinus rhythm and is useful in maintaining sinus rhythm after conversion. Since quinidine has an AV nodal vagolytic effect and can also slow the rate of atrial fibrillation/flutter (permitting less rate-dependent AV block), it has the potential of dangerously accelerating the ventricular rate when given alone. Therefore, quinidine therapy in patients with atrial fibrillation/flutter **should be preceded by adequate AV node blockade** with either digitalis, beta blockers, or verapamil.

Quinidine is beneficial in patients with the **WPW syndrome** because it slows conduction and prolongs refractoriness in the accessory pathway. Thus, in the WPW syndrome quinidine is useful in both reentrant tachycardias that utilize the accessory pathway and atrial fibrillation, where decreased conduction over the pathway slows the ventricular rate.

The therapeutic efficacy of quinidine is limited by the **high** (up to 30%) **incidence of side effects** with gastrointestinal intolerance (diarrhea, nausea, vomiting, anorexia, bloating) being most common. These side effects are generally, but not always, dose dependent. Some relief may be obtained with a different formulation of quinidine, and in some cases tolerance may develop. However, these side effects are the most frequent reason for discontinuing the drug. Large doses of quinidine may produce a distinct intoxication syndrome (cinchonism) consisting of impaired hearing, tinnitus, blurred vision, headache, and tremor.

TABLE 1. Characteristics of commonly used oral antiarrhythmic agents

Drug/preparation	% Bioavailability	Time to peak concentration (hr)	Effective plasma concentration	Usual dose	Primary route of metabolism	Elimination half-life (hr)
Quinidine						
Quinidine sulfate	80	1½	2–5 µg/ml	200–600 mg q6hr	Hepatic	5–7
Quinidine sulfate—sustained release	80	2–6		600–900 mg q8–12hr		
Quinidine gluconate	60–70	4		324–972 mg q6–8hr		
Polygalacturonate	75	2–4		275–825 mg q8–12hr		
Procainamide	85	1	4–10 µg/ml	250–1000 mg q3–4hr	Renal / Hepatic (NAPA)	2½–5 / 6–8 (NAPA)
Sustained release	85	2–3		500–2000 mg q6hr		
Disopyramide	90	2–3	2–5 µg/ml	100–300 mg q6hr	Renal	7
Sustained release	90	5		200–400 mg q12hr		
Tocainide	100	1	3.5–10 µg/ml	150–600 mg q6–8hr	Hepatic/renal	11–16
Propranolol	10–40 (first-pass effect)	1–2	40–100 ng/ml	10–80 mg q6hr	Hepatic	2–6
Verapamil	20 (first-pass effect)	2	Not established	40–120 mg q6–8hr	Hepatic	4–6
Diltiazem[a]	100	2	Not established	30–120 q8hr	Hepatic	4–6
Diphenylhydantoin	95	8–12	10–20 µg/ml	300–600 mg q.d. after loading	Hepatic	24

[a]Diltiazem has not been approved for therapy of cardiac arrhythmias at the present time.
NAPA, N = acetylated derivative of procainamide.

The QRS complex may widen because of the slowing of interventricular conduction caused by quinidine. When it is excessive (50% beyond control), QRS widening indicates cardiac toxicity and a need to discontinue therapy. At high levels quinidine may cause sinus arrest or conduction block. Quinidine also may prolong repolarization and the QT interval, which may lead to the appearance of a unique ventricular arrhythmia, torsades de pointes (see III. C. 7.). This arrhythmia can lead to syncope (perhaps the mechanism of "quinidine syncope") or sudden death. This may occur as a result of excessive dosage or individual susceptibility. Excessive **prolongation of the QT interval** may be an indication of individuals susceptible to this complication. The incidence is probably between 0.5% to 4% of patients receiving quinidine.

Occasionally quinidine can produce hypotension, especially when given parenterally. Contributing causes include a negative inotropic action and peripheral vasodilation. Less commonly, quinidine may produce drug fever, cutaneous reactions, and thrombocytopenia. These are usually idiosyncratic hypersensitivity reactions. When quinidine is administered to patients on chronic digoxin therapy, serum levels of digoxin can increase significantly, and there is increased danger of digoxin toxicity.

C. Procainamide

1. **Actions.** Procainamide acts similarly to quinidine, with effects most prominent in Purkinje and ventricular tissue. Its electrophysiologic effects may be less sensitive to changes in potassium concentration than quinidines'.

2. **Pharmacokinetics.** Procainamide may be administered intravenously (Table 2), intramuscularly, or orally. Absorption after oral administration is variable but averages 85%. Procainamide is 15% bound to plasma proteins. Normally, about half of the drug is cleared unchanged by the **kidneys.** Hepatic metabolism with the formation of the N-acetylated derivative (NAPA) accounts for the remainder. The elimination of the parent drug ranges between 2½ to nearly 5 hr. NAPA has antiarrhythmic action of its own and is cleared almost exclusively by renal mechanisms with an elimination half-life of 6 to 8 hr.

TABLE 2. *Characteristics of commonly used intravenous antiarrhythmic agents*

Drug	Therapeutic plasma concentration	i.v. dose	
		Loading	Maintenance
Procainamide	4–10 µg/ml	500–1000 mg (≤50 mg/min)	2–4 mg/min
Lidocaine	1.2–6 µg/ml	1–2 mg/kg suggested: 75 mg, then 50 mg q 5′ × 2	1–4 mg/min
Propranolol	40–100 ng/ml	2–10 mg (<1 mg/min)	Not established
Verapamil	Not established	0.075 mg/kg (0.150 mg/ kg in 30 min if necessary)	0.125 mg/min (after a rapid loading infusion of 0.375 mg/min × 30 min.)
Bretylium	Not established	5–10 mg/kg	1–2 mg/min
Diphenylhydantoin	10–20 µg/ml	500–1000 mg (<50 mg/5 min)	300–600 mg q.d.

Therapeutic levels for procainamide are suggested to be between 4 and 10 μg/ml although therapeutic success sometimes requires levels as high as 20 μg/ml. Interpreting therapeutic levels is confounded by the presence of NAPA at levels approaching or exceeding that of the parent compound. Often a combined therapeutic range of procainamide and NAPA is suggested from 10 to 30 μg/ml.

Since clearance of both procainamide and its metabolite are by renal mechanisms, drug dose must be reduced in patients with renal impairment. Assessment of serum concentrations is helpful in these patients.

3. **Indications and toxicity.** Procainamide has therapeutic effects very similar to quinidine. Clinically, it is most often used for the **termination or suppression of ventricular arrhythmias.** Intravenous procainamide may be used in patients with potentially life-threatening ventricular arrhythmias refractory to or intolerant of lidocaine. Procainamide may be used to treat supraventricular arrhythmias but is usually employed after quinidine has proved unsuitable. Procainamide delays conduction and prolongs refractoriness over the accessory pathway in patients with WPW syndrome. It may be the intravenous drug of choice in WPW patients with atrial fibrillation/flutter with predominant and rapid conduction over the accessory pathway.

Intravenous procainamide may produce serious hypotension or bradycardia especially when given rapidly or in doses exceeding 1 g. Administration rates should not exceed 50 mg/min. Significant hypotension or bradycardia is rare with oral administration. Like quinidine, procainamide may prolong the QRS and QT intervals. Procainamide may intensify conduction delay and should be **used cautiously in the presence of AV block.** Gastrointestinal **side effects** (nausea, vomiting, anorexia) are common. Drug fever, rash, neurologic manifestations (disorientation, depression, malaise) have been reported.

With prolonged use, **drug-induced lupus erythematosus** (LE) may develop. Since this is more common in patients who are slow acetylators of the drug, procainamide and not NAPA is probably responsible. Approximately 50% to 70% of those taking standard therapeutic doses will develop an elevated antinuclear antibody titer and positive LE cell preparation usually after 3 to 6 months of therapy. About one-third of these will develop a clinical lupus-like syndrome that requires discontinuing procainamide but usually resolves after therapy is stopped.

D. Disopyramide

1. **Actions.** Disopyramide is similar to both quinidine and procainamide in its electrophysiologic effects.

2. **Pharmacokinetics.** Disopyramide is most commonly administered orally. Most of the drug (50% to 60%) is excreted unchanged by the kidneys with an elimination half-life of approximately 7 hr.

3. **Indications and toxicity.** Disopyramide has a clinical spectrum similar to

quinidine and procainamide. It is effective for the prevention of both supraventricular[1] and ventricular arrhythmias. It is usually administered after patients have proved refractory or intolerant to quinidine and procainamide. Disopyramide has a **marked depressant effect on cardiac contractility.** The most serious side effect is a precipitation or worsening of cardiac failure, **especially in patients with left ventricular dysfunction.** It should be used cautiously in these patients. The most **common side effects** reflect the potent anticholinergic action of disopyramide with dryness of the mouth, blurred vision, and urinary hesitancy or retention occurring in a dose-dependent fashion. Gastrointestinal intolerance, hepatic toxicity, agranulocytosis, and marked QT prolongation with torsades de pointes have been reported.

E. **Lidocaine**

1. **Actions.** Lidocaine **shortens action potential duration** in Purkinje and ventricular tissue, and depresses automaticity in Purkinje tissue. Lidocaine decreases the rate of depolarization and slows conduction (like type I agents) only at potassium concentrations in the high physiologic range but not at low potassium concentrations. The effects of lidocaine appear to be **more marked in ischemic tissue.** Lidocaine has little consistent effect on AV nodal conduction, although it may shorten the refractoriness of the AV node in some individuals. It has a depressant action on conduction in the His-Purkinje system.

2. **Pharmacokinetics.** Lidocaine is usually administered intravenously. Under urgent conditions, therapeutic plasma levels (1.2 to 6 μg/ml) can be rapidly achieved by either a single bolus or rapid (over 20 min) loading infusion (1 to 2 mg/kg) or by smaller, repeated boluses (e.g., 50 to 75 mg initially, and then 50 mg every 5 min for 2 to 3 doses). After bolus administration plasma lidocaine levels rise initially then fall rapidly, reflecting plasma-to-tissue redistribution. Repeated, smaller boluses permit rapid achievement of therapeutic plasma concentrations while avoiding excessively high levels and is the preferred method of loading when conditions allow. The loading dose should be decreased by half in the presence of congestive heart failure. Maintenance therapy usually consists of infusions of 1 to 4 mg/min.

   Lidocaine is 60% bound to plasma proteins and is nearly completely **metabolized by the liver.** It is thus sensitive to drugs that affect hepatic blood flow or metabolism. It should be used cautiously, at lower maintenance doses, and with assessment of plasma levels in patients with hepatic disease. Elimination half-life is approximately 1½ hr.

3. **Indications and toxicity.** Lidocaine is primarily effective for the termination and prevention of serious ventricular arrhythmias. It is the **agent of choice to prevent VT or ventricular fibrillation (VF) in patients with acute myocardial infarction.** It also may be useful for ventricular arrhythmias associated with digitalis excess, anesthesia, or postcardioversion.

   It is of limited utility in patients with supraventricular arrhythmias. Lidocaine has the potential of enhancing AV nodal conduction and can therefore increase

[1]Not yet approved for this use.

the ventricular rate during atrial fibrillation/flutter. Its effect on accessory pathway conduction is uncertain. It has been advocated for atrial fibrillation in patients with the WPW syndrome, but this is controversial. Procainamide is probably the drug of choice to slow the ventricular rate in this setting.

Central nervous system manifestations are the most common **side effects** and are dose related. Somnolence or agitation, dizziness, confusion, depression, tremor, hearing loss, paresthesias, diplopia, and seizures can occur with over-dosage. Less frequently, hypotension and sinus arrest can occur. Complete heart block may be precipitated in patients with impaired conduction. Lidocaine may suppress the ventricular escape rhythm in patients with AV block. Myocardial depression is rare with lidocaine. Lidocaine does not prolong the QT interval at usual levels.

F. Tocainide

1. **Actions.** Despite documented efficacy, the availability of lidocaine as only an intravenous medication precludes its use in the chronic suppression of ventricular arrhythmias. Tocainide is a primary amine analog of lidocaine, lacking two ethyl groups that contribute to lidocaine's high first-pass hepatic metabolism. Tocainide is effective when administered orally and will probably soon be approved for clinical use. The electrophysiologic effects of tocainide are very similar to those of lidocaine. The actions of both drugs appear sensitive to the external potassium concentration.

2. **Pharmacokinetics.** Ingestion of tocainide is followed by rapid and complete absorption. Tocainide is approximately 50% bound to plasma proteins. An average of 35% of ingested tocainide is excreted unchanged in the urine. The remainder undergoes **hepatic metabolism** and conjugation with glucuronic acid before **renal excretion.** The metabolites do not have antiarrhythmic activity.

3. **Indications and toxicity.** Like lidocaine, tocainide is indicated for therapy of ventricular arrhythmias. It has been shown to be effective in suppressing premature ventricular beats, both chronic and those associated with acute infarction. Tocainide also exhibits **efficacy in preventing recurrent VT**, even in some patients refractory to other antiarrhythmic agents. Response to lidocaine may predict whether therapy with tocainide is likely to be successful.

At least some side effects occur in 35% to 60% of patients receiving oral tocainide and are concentration dependent. The incidence of **side effects** serious enough to warrant discontinuance is 10% to 16%. Tocainide may cause gastrointestinal intolerance (nausea, vomiting, anorexia), rash, or neurologic effects (tremor, dizziness, lightheadedness, ataxia, confusion, slurred speech, sleep disturbance, or paresthesias). Worsening or precipitation of congestive failure is not common with tocainide.

G. Beta Blockers

1. **Actions. Propranolol** is the prototypical beta-blocking agent and the one most frequently used for its antiarrhythmic action. Other beta-blocking agents differ in several respects that affect the incidence and nature of side effects and

dosing regimen (beta-receptor selectivity, lipid solubility, pharmacokinetics) but do not account for major differences in antiarrhythmic action. Propranolol directly **reduces the slope of the spontaneous diastolic depolarization in cells of the sinus node.** It also **prolongs conduction through the AV node,** but the effect is indirect. The action potential of AV nodal cells is dependent on the slow inward (Ca^{2+}) current. Catecholamines facilitate the magnitude of this slow current and thus beta blockade depresses AV conduction. At high levels, propranolol has some quinidine-like action. However, current evidence does not implicate this effect in the antiarrhythmic actions of propranolol at doses that are generally used clinically.

2. **Pharmacokinetics.** Propranolol may be administered intravenously or orally. Propranolol is nearly completely absorbed after ingestion but undergoes **significant first-pass hepatic metabolism** necessitating oral doses much higher, for a given effect, than when the drug is given intravenously. Intravenous propranolol is usually administered slowly (1 mg every 1 to 2 min) to effect. The usual dose required for beta blockade is 2 to 10 mg (maximum 0.15 mg/kg). It should be given cautiously to avoid hypotension, failure, or bradycardia.

Propranolol is highly bound (90% to 96%) to plasma proteins and is cleared by hepatic metabolism with an elimination half-life of 2 to 6 hr. This is increased in the presence of hepatic disease. The physiologic half-life of propranolol probably outlasts its pharmacokinetic half-life, and effects are often present 24 to 36 hr after discontinuing chronic administration.

3. **Indications and toxicity.** Propranolol, by increasing the degree of block at the AV node, is most useful in treating supraventricular arrhythmias. Propranolol may be effective both in terminating and preventing arrhythmias in which the AV node participates in the reentry circuit. It is useful in controlling the ventricular rate of atrial fibrillation or flutter. Propranolol also can be used **in combination with digitalis,** when digitalis alone provides insufficient rate control, especially with exercise. Propranolol is less effective for ventricular arrhythmias but may suppress premature ventricular beats or VT, especially when exercise-induced.

Propranolol has a **negative inotropic action** and may precipitate or worsen congestive failure **in patients with impaired ventricular performance.** It should be administered cautiously in these patients. Sinus bradycardia, asystole, or AV block can occur, especially in the presence of sinus or AV node disease. Isoproterenol and atropine are effective therapy if required.

Propranolol may cause **bronchospasm** in patients with bronchospastic pulmonary disease. **In patients receiving insulin,** beta blockade can inhibit epinephrine-induced glycogenolysis and mask the autonomic manifestations of hypoglycemia (tachycardia, diaphoresis, and tremor). **Propranolol has been suggested to worsen symptoms** in patients with intermittent claudication, Raynaud's phenomena, or (theoretically) vasospastic (Prinzmetal) angina. Other side effects include fatigue, lethargy, mental dullness, and sleep disturbance.

Selective beta blockers such as metoprolol[2] or atenolol[2] may be useful in place of propranolol in patients with bronchospastic disease or diabetes mellitus since they have less beta-2 blocking effect at low doses.

H. Calcium Channel Blockers: Verapamil and Diltiazem

1. **Actions.** All three available calcium-channel blockers (verapamil, diltiazem, nifedipine) have, in isolated tissue preparations, potent effects on the sinus and AV nodes. However, in man these direct effects are considerably modified by changes in sympathetic tone induced by the peripheral vasodilatation produced by the calcium-channel blockers. The degree of the vasodilatation is greatest for nifedipine and less for verapamil and diltiazem. Thus, only verapamil and diltiazem have clinically important antiarrhythmic effects. Both **prolong AV nodal conduction** without significant effects on heart rate. Conduction velocity and refractoriness of atrial, ventricular, and His-Purkinje tissue is not significantly affected.

2. **Pharmacokinetics.** Verapamil may be given intravenously or orally. Diltiazem is only available for oral use. **Both** are readily absorbed from the **gastrointestinal tract**, but **verapamil** undergoes **extensive first-pass metabolism in the liver.** Therapeutic levels are not well established.

   For intravenous use verapamil is usually administered as a single intravenous infusion of 0.075 mg/kg (approximately 5 mg for an adult patient) given over 2 min. If the desired effect is not obtained, a second dose of 0.150 mg/kg (approximately 10 mg for an adult) can be given after 30 min. When administered in this manner, maximum AV nodal slowing occurs 5 to 30 min after administration, returning to control values in approximately 2 hr. For a more prolonged effect repeated boluses may be given (every 2 to 4 hours as needed) or a sustained infusion may be utilized: a rapid loading infusion (0.375 mg/min for 30 min) followed by a maintenance infusion of 0.125 mg/min.

3. **Indications and toxicity.** Intravenous verapamil is probably the **drug of choice for PSVT** after simple vagal maneuvers have failed. It is also effective in slowing the ventricular rate in atrial fibrillation/flutter and ectopic atrial tachycardias. Verapamil is effective in terminating reentry tachycardias in patients with the **WPW syndrome.** However, it will not slow the ventricular rate in WPW patients during atrial fibrillation/flutter when conduction occurs over the accessory pathway. In fact, like digoxin, it may facilitate conduction over the accessory pathway and **can increase the ventricular rate.** It should not be used in this situation.

   Oral verapamil[3] (and probably diltiazem[3], although data are inadequate at present) is useful in slowing the ventricular rate in chronic atrial fibrillation and in the prophylaxis of recurrent, symptomatic PSVT. The overall incidence of **side effects** with verapamil use is 6% to 14%. Serious side effects requiring discontinuance are about one-tenth as common. Constipation, headache, nausea, and peripheral edema are most common. Verapamil has **intrinsic negative**

---

[2]Not approved for therapy of cardiac arrhythmias at the present time.
[3]Oral verapamil has not been approved for the chronic therapy of supraventricular arrhythmias. Diltiazem has not been approved for use in arrhythmias at the present time.

inotropic and peripheral vasodilating effects. While unimportant in the absence of congestive heart failure, this effect can become clinically significant in patients with serious ventricular dysfunction. Verapamil should be administered with caution in these patients. At high doses verapamil may produce sinus bradycardia (especially in patients with sinus node dysfunction), Mobitz I, or complete AV block. These are rarely clinical problems. Serious hypotension, bradycardia, and asystole can occur, especially when intravenous verapamil is given concomitantly with intravenous beta-blocker therapy. **Diltiazem** use is associated with a **lower incidence of side effects** (3% to 5%), with headaches, peripheral edema, and rash being most frequently reported.

I. Cardiac Glycosides

1. **Actions.** The cardiac glycosides are most frequently prescribed for the treatment of **cardiac failure.** They are discussed extensively elsewhere (see Chapter 6). The effect of the glycosides on cardiac arrhythmias is not completely understood. Digitalis preparations have a vagotonic effect on the AV node. The glycosides tend to enhance spontaneous diastolic depolarization and are potentially arrhythmogenic, especially at high levels.

2. **Pharmacokinetics. Digoxin** is the glycoside most frequently used and is available for oral and intravenous administration. **Ouabain** is sometimes utilized when a short-acting intravenous preparation is desired. Intravenous loading of digoxin may be accomplished by administering 0.5 to 1 mg over 4 to 24 hr, depending on the urgency (0.5 mg initially, then 0.25 mg every 2 to 4 hours for two doses).

   Bioavailability after ingestion of digoxin is variable (averaging 65%) owing to both patient and preparation factors. Oral loading (with 1 to 1.5 mg) also can be accomplished over a day or two. Daily maintenance therapy is 0.125 to 0.5 mg q.d. Digoxin is **metabolized primarily by the liver**, and the elimination half-life is 36 to 48 hr.

3. **Indications and toxicity.** The spectrum of clinical efficacy for digitalis is similar to the other antiarrhythmic agents whose predominant action is to enhance block at the AV node (beta blockers and the calcium-channel blockers). It may terminate or prevent reentrant arrhythmias involving the AV node and slows the ventricular response during atrial fibrillation/flutter, intra-atrial reentry, or ectopic atrial tachycardia. An exception to this observation is patients with the **WPW syndrome** and atrial fibrillation/flutter. In patients with WPW digoxin may accelerate conduction over the accessory pathway and increase the ventricular rate. Digoxin has limited utility for ventricular arrhythmias, but it is not generally considered the drug of choice for these arrhythmias.

   The cardiac glycosides **in excess** may be **arrhythmogenic.** Enhancement of the automaticity of cells with spontaneous diastolic depolarization may lead to ectopic atrial tachycardia, junctional tachycardia, and ventricular premature beats (often multiform) or VT. These ectopic tachycardias may coexist with high-grade AV block. The tendency for digoxin to cause **toxic arrhythmias** is increased in the presence of **hypokalemia and/or hypomagnesemia. Side** effects of digoxin also include gastrointestinal intolerance (nausea, vomiting) and neurologic symptoms (headache, malaise, visual symptoms).

J. Diphenylhydantoin

1. **Actions.** Diphenylhydantoin decreases the rate of initial depolarization in atrial tissue at high physiologic concentrations of potassium. In contrast to quinidine, it does not decrease the rate of initial depolarization nor slow conduction but does shorten refractoriness in Purkinje or ventricular tissues. Diphenylhydantoin also decreases spontaneous automaticity. It may limit the electrophysiologic effects of digitalis excess.

2. **Pharmacokinetics.** Oral and intravenous preparations are available. The drug is absorbed nearly completely, and equivalent loading doses (approximately 1,000 mg) are required for both routes of administration. Intravenous administration should be no faster than 50 to 100 mg every 5 min. Asystole, ventricular arrhythmias, or severe hypotension can occur with rapid intravenous administration. Oral loading can be achieved reasonably rapidly by administering a total dose of 1,000 mg the first day, followed by 500 mg for 1 or 2 days, prior to daily maintenance therapy of 300 to 600 mg q.d. (approximately 14 mg/kg).

   Diphenylhydantoin is **highly** (average 80%) **bound to plasma albumin.** Marked hypoalbuminemia leads to an increase in the proportion unbound (active). Metabolism is predominantly **hepatic**, with a very small amount excreted unchanged in the urine. Elimination half-life is about 24 hr. Clearance is decreased by hepatic disease and by drugs that can decrease its metabolism (coumadin, INH + PAS). Induction of hepatic microsomal enzymes by phenobarbital can increase the clearance rate.

3. **Indications and toxicity.** Diphenylhydantoin may be useful for supraventricular and ventricular arrhythmias related to digitalis intoxication. Its efficacy for other arrhythmias is uncertain, but it probably has a limited role in the therapy of ventricular tachycardia or premature beats.

   High grade AV block, asystole, and hypotension have been reported with intravenous use. Diphenylhydantoin has the potential for prolonging His-Purkinje conduction. High plasma levels may be associated with neurologic symptoms, including nystagmus (usually indicates plasma levels in excess of 20 μg/ml), confusion, drowsiness, ataxia, diplopia, and vertigo. **Other side effects** include gastrointestinal intolerance (nausea, vomiting, anorexia), macrocytic anemia, rash, and gingival and lymphoid hyperplasia.

K. Bretylium

1. **Actions. Action potential duration and refractoriness** of atrial, Purkinje, and ventricular tissues are **prolonged** by bretylium. It does not depress rapid depolarization or conduction velocity, nor does it affect automaticity. Bretylium increases the **fibrillation threshold** in cardiac tissue. In addition to these effects, bretylium also has marked **antisympathetic effects.** Initially it stimulates, but subsequently inhibits, release of norepinephrine from nerve endings.

2. **Pharmacokinetics.** Bretylium is suitable only for intravenous or intramuscular use. As yet, no analog has been approved for oral administration. Intravenous

loading is generally achieved with an initial bolus of 5 mg/kg (given over 15 min if conditions allow). Additional doses of 10 mg/kg can be given, at 15 to 30 minute intervals, up to a total of 30 mg/kg. Maintenance may be achieved by repeated boluses (5 to 10 mg/kg over 15 to 30 min) at 6- to 8-hr intervals or by continuous intravenous infusions (1 to 2 mg/min). Therapeutic plasma levels have not been adequately defined. Bretylium is primarily eliminated unchanged by **renal excretion**, with an elimination half-life that averages 10 hr.

3. **Indications and toxicity.** Bretylium is useful for VT or VF. It should be **reserved for life-threatening arrhythmias that are refractory to lidocaine and procainamide.** Bretylium (although it may produce hypertension initially) can cause subsequent **hypotension** that is exacerbated by upright posture. (Orthostatic hypotension has been a significant side effect of the oral analogs of bretylium currently under investigation.) In addition to the initial release of norepinephrine from nerve endings, bretylium also **inhibits uptake of norepinephrine and epinephrine** into adrenergic nerve endings. This may account for the increased responsiveness to sympathomimetic agents observed in some patients, with resulting hypertension and tachycardia. Nausea and vomiting may occur during bretylium use.

L. **Cardioversion**

1. **Actions.** Reentry arrhythmias, as previously described, depend on the availability of electrically excitable tissue in advance of the depolarization wave front. Cardioversion, by causing simultaneous depolarization of all cardiac tissue, produces refractory tissue in advance of the wave front, terminating the tachycardia. Theoretically, **all reentrant arrhythmias can be terminated** by cardioversion. In contrast, **arrhythmias** due to enhanced **automaticity** can be expected to **resume** after attempted cardioversion.

2. **Methods.** Present methods of cardioversion involve the delivery of a brief (2- to 5-msec) direct-current impulse from a previously charged capacitor. The electrical impulse is delivered to the heart through paddle electrodes coated with conducting electrode paste positioned across the anterior chest (one paddle in the region of the apex, the other at the level of the second or third interspace to the right of the sternum). With elective cardioversion, one paddle may be positioned posteriorly in the left infrascapular region. The anterior paddle is positioned just to the right of the sternum.

The energy stored by the capacitor is routinely measured in watt-sec (Wsec) (joules) and varies from 5 to 400 Wsec. The **energy delivered is typically somewhat less than the energy stored.** The extent of this discrepancy should be known. **Energy requirements for successful cardioversion depend on the arrhythmia.** In general, ventricular arrhythmias have higher energy requirements than do atrial arrhythmias. For fibrillation or flutter (both atrial and ventricular) the coarser the rhythm, the less the energy required for successful termination. Thus, coarse atrial flutter is generally quite easily terminated, often requiring only 25 Wsec or less. In contrast, fine VF may require the maximum energy available. Initial settings should be as low as possible, in keeping with the arrhythmia and the clinical situation. If unsuccessful, subsequent energy settings should be progressively higher.

To avoid delivery of the impulse during the vulnerable period of the cardiac cycle, thereby possibly precipitating VF, cardioversion should be **synchronized to the QRS complex.** Appropriate sensing and synchronization should be documented before cardioversion.

For elective cardioversion, patients should take nothing by mouth for 8 to 12 hr. They should have an adequate intravenous route, and their electrocardiogram (EKG) should be monitored. Normal serum electrolytes should be assured. Routinely, **digitalis therapy is withheld** for a day or two prior to cardioversion, because digitalis toxicity may predispose patients to serious ventricular arrhythmias postcardioversion. The use of lower energies may reduce the risk of postcardioversion arrhythmias in digitalis toxicity. Therapeutic digitalis levels probably do not pose an increased risk. Anesthesia is obtained by intravenous diazepam or a short-acting barbituate (e.g., methohexital). Respiratory suppression is a potential complication of these drugs, and appropriate precautions should be taken.

3. **Indications, contraindications, and complications.** Cardioversion is appropriate for the emergent or elective treatment of both supraventricular (atrial fibrillation or flutter, PSVT, tachycardias associated with the WPW syndrome) or ventricular (VT or VF) tachycardias. Specific indications are discussed below.

Cardioversion is not likely to be successful for arrhythmias due to enhanced automaticity (e.g., sinus tachycardia, nonparoxysmal junctional tachycardia) and is **potentially dangerous for patients with digitalis-induced arrhythmias.** Cardioversion is not the therapy of choice for tachycardias likely to recur, unless no other options exist. In atrial fibrillation resulting from a primary, uncorrected cause (e.g., hyperthyroidism) cardioversion probably should be delayed. When therapy of the underlying condition reduces the risk of recurrence, cardioversion may be attempted.

Cardioversion is **generally safe and well tolerated.** Skin erythema and muscle soreness are not uncommon, especially if higher energies are required or the paddle-electrode/paste-skin interface is less than optimal. **Skin burn** may be treated with a topical steroid after cardioversion. Muscle enzyme titers may rise postcardioversion, but evidence of myocardial injury or MB CPK elevation is infrequent. Transient arrhythmias are not uncommon after cardioversion. Lidocaine may be administered if ventricular arrhythmias persist. Serious ventricular arrhythmias are rare. Transient sinus arrest or bradycardia is occasionally observed after cardioversion. This may be because of a parasympathetic discharge after cardioversion and atropine (0.4 to 1 mg, i.v.) is helpful. Occasionally, postcardioversion patients manifest sinus node abnormalities not appreciated prior to reversion to sinus rhythm. Atropine, isoproterenol, or pacing may be required in these patients. Systemic and pulmonary emboli and pulmonary edema can occur.

III. MANAGEMENT OF TACHYARRHYTHMIAS

A. **General**   Intelligent management of cardiac arrhythmias requires not only a diagnosis of the arrhythmia, but also an appreciation of the clinical setting in which it occurs. The need for and urgency of therapy must be carefully assessed.

1. **Diagnosis** is the first step in appropriate management and is often possible by analysis of the electrocardiogram alone, which provides critical information on the rate, regularity, morphology, and AV relationship of the arrhythmia (Table 3).

   The **distinction between supraventricular** arrhythmias (conducted aberrantly) **and ventricular arrhythmias may be particularly difficult.** Features suggesting ventricular origin include left axis deviation, atypical bundle branch block morphology, QRS duration 140 msec or greater, capture or fusion beats, and evidence of AV dissociation. Termination of a tachycardia by carotid sinus pressure does not prove supraventricular origin, since VT also can, rarely, be terminated by vagal stimulation. The most important diagnostic feature is the AV relationship: AV dissociation is nearly pathognomonic for VT. If this information is unavailable from the surface EKG, then physical exam (variable S_1, cannon a waves), Lewis leads, an esophageal lead, or intracardiac atrial recording may be helpful. Under certain circumstances a particular arrhythmia may defy interpretation, and His bundle recordings are necessary for diagnosis. This is particularly true in patients with known or suspected preexcitation.

   Patients with episodic and infrequent symptoms of possible arrhythmic origin are difficult to assess. Ambulatory electrocardiography (Holter monitoring) or transtelephonic EKG transmission during symptoms may be helpful techniques in these patients.

2. **Electrophysiologic (EP) evaluation** involves the insertion (under local anesthesia) of electrode catheters for the purpose of recording intracardiac electrograms and the introduction of pacing stimuli. EP evaluation can include

   a. **Sinus node** assessment.

   b. **AV node** assessment.

   c. **His-Purkinje system** assessment.

   d. Studies of **spontaneous or induced tachycardia.**

   Reentrant arrhythmias are, in general, inducible by appropriately timed premature stimuli. Approximately 90% of reentrant supraventricular arrhythmias are inducible with EP testing. The incidence of inducible VT depends on the underlying cardiac disease but is generally high (making EP testing useful) with coronary artery disease, congestive cardiomyopathies, mitral valve prolapse, and primary electrical disease of the heart.

   EP testing is very helpful in determining the existence, location, and conducting properties of **accessory pathways.** It is often required to determine the nature of wide QRS tachycardias in association with the WPW syndrome. In the presence of an inducible arrhythmia, repeat EP studies can determine the efficacy of therapy. EP mapping can frequently locate the origin of a particular tachycardia (or component of the reentrant pathway) permitting a surgical approach.

3. Prior to selection of a specific therapy it is important to determine **whether therapy is warranted.** This is a problem, because **all antiarrhythmic agents are associated with significant side effects, toxicity, cost, uncertain efficacy, and significant potential for worsening arrhythmias.** Manifestations

TABLE 3. *EKG features of regular tachycardias*

Tachycardia	P morphology	QRS morphology	AV relationship	Characteristic response to CSM/or verapamil
Automatic SVT				
EAT	Often subtly different from SR	nl or aberrant	1:1[a]	Atrial—no change or ↓ Ventricular ↓
Nonparoxysmal JT	Retrograde (may be buried in QRS)	nl or aberrant	Usually 1:1; infrequently associated with retrograde block (AVD)	Atrial—may induce retrograde block Ventricular—may ↓
Reentrant SVT				
Sinus node reentry	Normal (sinus P)	nl or aberrant	1:1[a]	Atrial—may terminate or ↓ Ventricular ↓
Intra-atrial reentry	Different from sinus	nl or aberrant	1:1[a]	Atrial—no change Ventricular ↓
AVNRT	Retrograde (frequently buried in QRS)	nl or aberrant	Usually 1:1; may be retrograde block	Terminate or no change
APRT ("concealed")	Retrograde	nl or aberrant	1:1	Terminate or no change
Atrial Flutter	Flutter	nl or aberrant	1:1 or higher	Atrial—no change Ventricular ↓ (abrupt)
Ventricular tachycardia	May be retrograde	Wide	AVD or 1:1 (retrograde)	None (infrequently terminates)
WPW-APRT	Retrograde	nl or aberrant (wide)[b]	1:1	Terminate or no change

[a]Rapid SVT may be associated with AV block (i.e., 2:1, 4:1).

[b]The most common reentry tachycardia associated with the WPW syndrome utilizes the AV node and the His-Purkinje pathway for conduction from the atria to the ventricle. The accessory pathway conducts from the ventricle to the atria to complete the circuit. Thus, the morphology of the QRS is usually normal. Occasionally, the reentry circuit functions in the opposite direction, and activation of the ventricle takes place over the accessory pathway. The morphology of this reverse tachycardia is wide and abnormal.

CSM, carotid sinus massage; SVT, supraventricular tachycardia; EAT, ectopic atrial tachycardia; JT, junctional tachycardia; AVD, atrioventricular dissociation; AVNRT, AV node reentry tachycardia; APRT, accessory pathway reentry tachycardia; WPW, Wolff-Parkinson-White syndrome; SR, sinus rhythm.

of arrhythmias often warranting therapy include **symptoms and signs of inadequate cardiac output or uncomfortable palpitations.** Occasionally, asymptomatic arrhythmias are treated in order to prevent more serious arrhythmias.

4. It is important to clarify the **specific goals of therapy.** This may include **termination, prevention** of recurrence, or **amelioration** of a chronic arrhythmia or one likely to recur.

B. **Management of Supraventricular Tachycardias** Although selection of antiarrhythmic therapy is largely empiric, an understanding of the pathophysiologic mechanisms of arrhythmias and electrophysiologic characteristics of the antiarrhythmic agents allows intelligent drug selection. This philosophy is used in generating the following guidelines (Table 4).

1. **Sinus tachycardia** is rarely a primary cardiac dysrhythmia. More frequently, it is an appropriate **response to a noncardiac condition**, such as hypotension, hypovolemia, hypoxia, anemia, congestive failure, fever, pain, or anxiety. In general, therapy should be directed at the underlying cause. Occasionally, the tachycardia is deleterious in and of itself, and therapy may be indicated (e.g., in acute myocardial infarction, hyperthyroidism prior to definitive therapy). **Propranolol**, either intravenously or orally, is the drug of choice.

2. **PSVT.** Ninety percent of PSVTs are **reentrant arrhythmias** involving the AV node (AV node reentry tachycardia and concealed accessory pathway reentry tachycardia). Recommended management for these arrhythmias include:

   a. **Termination.** If poorly tolerated, cardioversion. If tolerated:

   (1) **Maneuvers designed to increase vagal tone.** Carotid sinus massage, gagging, and Valsalva maneuvers are often successful. These maneuvers should be repeated after subsequent pharmacologic therapy if necessary. PSVT may respond to rest, reassurance, and sedation. Clues to effective therapy in an individual patient can be obtained from a history of successful termination of previous attacks. Pharmacologic means to increase vagal tone are not as consistently effective as verapamil (see below) if simple maneuvers fail.

   (2) **Intravenous verapamil** administered as a single dose of 5 mg, i.v., is the drug of choice **if vagal maneuvers fail.** If this is ineffective, a 10-mg dose of verapamil can be administered 30 min later. This therapy is effective in 80% to 90% of patients with PSVT. Transient and mild **hypotension** frequently occurs 1 to 5 min after intravenous administration. Prolonged and marked hypotension is a potential side effect, and precautions must be taken should cardioversion be necessary. If necessary, intravenous fluids or pressor agents are generally effective. Because of its negative inotropic action, verapamil should be **used cautiously in patients with congestive heart failure.** Intravenous **propranolol** (0.5 to 3 mg, i.v.) is the second most effective drug but should **not** be given concomitantly with intravenous verapamil or in patients with cardiac failure or chronic obstructive pulmonary disease.

TABLE 4. Guidelines for management of supraventricular tachycardias[a]

Tachycardia	Termination	Prevention	Amelioration
Reentrant			
PSVT	If poorly tolerated cardioversion	Digoxin	
AVNRT	Vagal maneuvers	Type I agents	
APRT ("concealed")[c]	Intravenous verapamil (or propranolol)[b]	Verapamil or propranolol	
	Intravenous digoxin		
	Type I agents		
SNRT	Type I agents	Type I agents	
	Digoxin	Type I agents	
IART	Add quinidine		Digoxin, verapamil, and/or propranolol
Atrial fib/flutter[c]	Elective cardioversion		Digoxin, verapamil,[d] and/or propranolol
Acute & Paroxysmal			
Subacute			
Associated WPW	Vagal maneuvers	Digoxin	
Reentry tachycardias	Intravenous verapamil	Type I agents	
	Intravenous digoxin	Verapamil or propranolol	
	Type I agents		
AFib/flutter with antegrade AP conduction	Cardioversion, if necessary	Type I agents	IV procainamide
			Digoxin and verapamil **contraindicated**
Automatic			
EAT	Type I agents	Type I agents	Digoxin, verapamil, and/or propranolol

[a]See text for additional details. These guidelines may vary with the clinical situation.
[b]Intravenously propranolol is the second most effective drug, but should **not** be given concomitantly with intravenous verapamil.
[c]Occasionally, intra-atrial pacing may terminate atrial flutter. Atrial flutter is often difficult to control. Conversion of flutter to fibrillation by intra-atrial pacing or cardioversion often will reduce the ventricular rate.
[d]Digoxin and verapamil may facilitate AP conduction, accelerating the ventricular rate to dangerous levels.

PSVT, paroxysmal supraventricular tachycardia; AVNRT, atrioventricular node reentry tachycardia; APRT, accessory pathway reentry tachycardia; SNRT, sinus node reentry tachycardia; IART, interatrial reentry tachycardia; WPW, Wolff-Parkinson-White syndrome; AP, accessory pathway; EAT, ectopic atrial tachycardia; type I agents: quinidine, procainamide, disopyramide.

(3) **Digitalis preparations** may be given alone or with verapamil for termination of PSVT. Ouabain (0.25 to 0.5 mg, i.v., initially, and then 0.1 mg every 30 min, as needed, to a maximum of 1 mg) or digoxin (0.5 mg, i.v., initially, with 0.25 mg every 2 to 4 hr to a maximum of 1 to 1.5 mg) are probably equally effective.

(4) **Edrophonium chloride** (Tensilon®), a short-acting acetylcholinesterase inhibitor, increases vagal tone. Two to 5 mg may be administered as an intravenous bolus. Edrophonium should be **administered cautiously in patients** with hypotension, bronchospastic disease, or ischemic heart disease. No more than 10 mg should be given in 10 min. Vagal tone also can be increased by mild (20 to 50 mm Hg systolic) blood pressure elevation induced by intravenous **phenylephrine** (Neosynephrine®), 0.5 to 1 mg. This may be particularly helpful in patients who have normal or only slightly decreased pressure. (Significant hypotension may be an indication for cardioversion.) Phenylephrine is **contraindicated** in patients with hypertension, coronary artery disease, or hyperthyroidism.

(5) **Procainamide** may be used if the above are ineffective.

(6) **Elective cardioversion** may be used in patients refractory to pharmacologic therapy; however, cardioversion **after excess digitalis** may result in **serious ventricular arrhythmias.** Right atrial or ventricular pacing also can terminate these arrhythmias by introducing premature stimuli into the tachycardia or with overdrive pacing. This technique may be used safely in patients who have received digitalis.

b. **Prevention.** In some patients, avoiding caffeine, alcohol, nicotine, and overfatigue may limit the frequency of recurrence. Chronic pharmacologic prophylaxis should be reserved for patients in whom the disadvantages of the tachycardia (because of frequency, duration, or associated symptoms) outweigh the disadvantages of chronic drug therapy.

Digoxin has the advantage of once-a-day administration, moderate cost, and relative safety; it is generally well tolerated. However, patients who have the **WPW** syndrome and **atrial fibrillation** are **exceptions,** and are probably best not treated with digoxin. Propranolol may be added to digoxin if digoxin alone is ineffective. **Quinidine, procainamide, and disopyramide** are useful because they affect the AV node and also suppress premature stimuli that can initiate tachycardia. **Verapamil** (60 to 120 mg every 6 hr) or **propranolol** (20 to 80 mg every 6 hr) also are effective. Multiple drug combinations utilizing digoxin, a quinidine-like agent, and verapamil or propranolol may be necessary.

Very infrequently, patients are refractory or intolerant to drug therapy. Some of these patients may be candidates for **implantation of a pacemaker** capable of terminating the tachycardia. Surgical interruption of an accessory AV pathway or the His bundle also is an option for certain patients.

c. **Intra-atrial reentry tachycardia** would not be expected to be either terminated or prevented by drugs that slow AV nodal conduction (since the reentry circuit resides completely within atrial tissue). For both termination and prevention, quinidine, procainamide, or disopyramide are probably the most appropriate therapeutic choices. These arrhythmias may be difficult to suppress. In this case therapy designed to slow the ventricular response rate is most appropriate (see below).

3. Atrial fibrillation/flutter

a. **Termination.** If poorly tolerated, **cardioversion** is appropriate. If the arrhythmia is well tolerated, **digoxin** (and probably propranolol or verapamil) may be prescribed to decrease the heart rate. This will often terminate the tachycardia, especially if it is acute or paroxysmal in nature. The efficacy of these drugs in terminating the arrhythmia may be the result of hemodynamic improvement associated with the decrease in ventricular rate.

If this is ineffective and conversion to sinus rhythm is considered possible and appropriate, then **reestablishing sinus rhythm** by pharmacologic or electrical means may be attempted (see Fig. 1). **Quinidine** (or procainamide or disopyramide) is then administered to convert the patient to sinus rhythm or, failing that, to maintain sinus rhythm after cardioversion. Intravenous **procainamide** may also terminate atrial fibrillation/flutter (after digitalization) but is probably without advantage compared to rapid oral loading with quinidine or procainamide.

Atrial flutter occasionally may be converted to sinus rhythm by rapid intra-atrial **pacing** techniques. This approach is valuable if digitalis toxicity is a possibility.

b. **Prevention.** Quinidine, procainamide, or disopyramide are most effective. They usually are prescribed in combination with digoxin to prevent rapid ventricular rates should atrial fibrillation recur.

c. **Amelioration.** In some patients sinus rhythm cannot be chronically maintained, or atrial fibrillation is paroxysmal. **Rate control** is then the goal of chronic therapy. Drugs that have a prominent slowing effect on the AV node are indicated. **Digoxin** is usually the drug of choice. If additional slowing is required, then **oral verapamil or propranolol** may be combined with digoxin. Since digoxin has a rate-slowing effect that is less pronounced during exercise, the addition of a second drug frequently is indicated in patients who have a marked increase in rate with exercise.

Atrial flutter may be especially difficult to slow, and intra-atrial pacing or cardioversion at low energies may convert the flutter to atrial fibrillation. This usually is associated with a decreased rate.

4. Ectopic atrial tachycardia and multifocal atrial tachycardia. Automatic tachycardias are most effectively **terminated** and **prevented** by quinidine, procainamide, or disopyramide in usual doses. Cardioversion is unlikely to be effective. These arrhythmias tend to be refractory, and therapy to decrease the ventricular rate may be desirable.

Amelioration: Discontinuing potentially aggravating pharmacologic agents (e.g., beta agonists) may slow the intrinsic rate of the tachycardia. Propranolol is rarely successful in slowing or terminating the atrial arrhythmia. If the ventricular rate is rapid, propranolol, verapamil, or digoxin may be used to produce AV node block and decrease the ventricular rate. However, digoxin in excess or in the presence of hypokalemia may cause an ectopic atrial tachycardia. This should be suspected when the tachycardia coexists with AV block or frequent premature ventricular contractions (PVCs). Despite the tachycardia, the ventricular rate may be slow and require atropine or ventricular pacing (see below). If hypokalemia is present, careful placement of K+ under EKG monitoring is required to avoid worsening of AV block.

Multifocal atrial tachycardia results when two or more atrial ectopic foci are accelerated so that ectopic P waves with different configurations and different cycle lengths become manifest. These patients often have serious chronic pulmonary disease, congestive failure, or coronary artery disease. Again, digitalis excess may play a causal role.

Multifocal atrial tachycardia is often refractory to antiarrhythmic agents, although quinidine or diphenylhydantoin may be effective. **Therapy** should be directed toward treatment of the underlying disease, correction of hypoxia, and elimination of potentially exacerbating pharmacological agents. Selection of an agent to control the ventricular rate may be complicated by the possibility of digitalis toxicity and the contraindication of propranolol in patients with bronchospasm. Verapamil may be helpful but has not been adequately tested. Rate control is often difficult, perhaps because these patients are usually ill and under increased sympathetic tone. Even in patients in whom digitalis is not contributing to the arrhythmia, evidence of digitalis toxicity often precedes rate control.

5. **Nonparoxysmal junctional tachycardia.** This arrhythmia usually is seen in association with digitalis toxicity, myocardial infarction, rheumatic fever, or after cardiac surgery. Treatment is rarely required, and the arrhythmia is **usually short-lived.** If **digitalis toxicity** is the cause, it is important to recognize this, withhold digoxin, and **correct hypokalemia** if it exists.

6. **Supraventricular arrhythmias associated with WPW syndrome.** The typical **reentrant arrhythmias** with antegrade conduction through the AV node and retrograde conduction over the accessory pathway or the reverse tachycardia with antegrade conduction over the accessory pathway and retrograde conduction over the AV node are both effectively terminated by verapamil. Therapy is in general comparable to that for PSVT. Effective prophylactic agents include quinidine-like antiarrhythmic agents, digoxin, propranolol, and verapamil, alone or in combinations.

During **atrial fibrillation/flutter in patients with the WPW syndrome**, conduction can occur over two pathways. The accessory pathway may permit very rapid ventricular rates.

   a. **Termination:** If poorly tolerated, cardioversion is indicated. The drug of choice is **intravenous procainamide** to slow accessory pathway conduction and perhaps to terminate fibrillation. Lidocaine's role is uncertain.

   b. **Digoxin and verapamil are contraindicated because they can potentially facilitate accessory pathway conduction**, increase the ventricular rate,

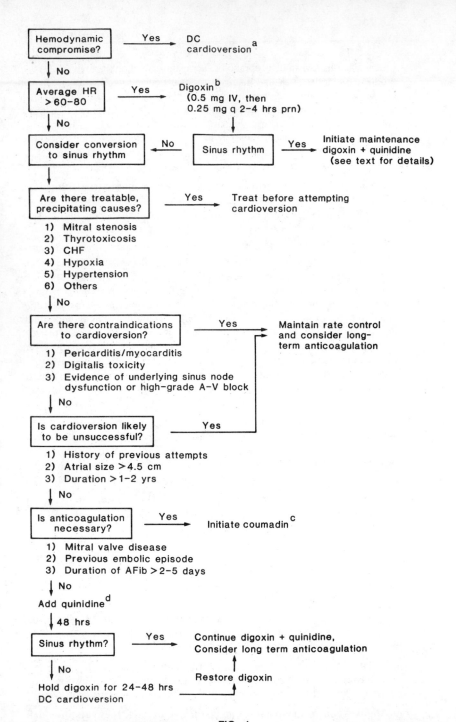

FIG. 1

and cause VF. Preventive therapy is probably most effective with quinidine, procainamide, or disopyramide.

7. **Premature atrial contractions** are very frequent even in individuals without organic heart disease. They usually are benign and rarely require therapy. Occasionally, therapy is indicated because of uncomfortable symptoms or to prevent sustained and more serious supraventricular arrhythmias. Quinidine, procainamide, or disopyramide in the usual oral doses are the drugs of choice. Infrequently, propranolol alone or combined may be beneficial.

C. **Management of Ventricular Arrhythmias** The effective management of ventricular arrhythmias is frequently confusing and frustrating. The difficult decisions are often not with what to treat but whether to treat and how to determine drug efficacy (end point).

1. **Indications for therapy.** The specific goals of therapy are to prevent life-threatening arrhythmias and symptomatic events (even if not life-threatening). The disadvantages of antiarrhythmic therapy have been outlined, but it is important to emphasize that in 10% to 15% of patients ventricular arrhythmias may be aggravated by antiarrhythmic therapy. What may initially be a benign ventricular arrhythmia may, with therapy, become life-threatening. Thus, it is **critical to balance the risks and complications** of antiarrhythmic therapy against the consequences of not treating a particular arrhythmia in a given patient.

a. **PVCs** are ubiquitous. There is no convincing evidence that they indicate an increased risk of arrhythmic death in patients **without evidence of organic heart disease.** Therefore, in the absence of significant symptomatology, therapy does not appear warranted.

In patients with **chronic organic heart disease** the occurrence of premature ventricular beats epidemiologically identifies a population at increased risk both for sudden (presumably arrhythmic) and nonsudden death. However, their incidence in this population is very high, and the available data does not permit adequate assessment of the risk in any given individual. It appears, however, that patients with frequent (greater than an average of 10 per hr) premature ventricular beats tend to be those with repetitive forms (see below) and are at significantly increased risk. Unfortunately, there is no convincing evidence that suppression of PVCs in these patients decreases their incidence of sudden death. Therapy should be individualized and may be indicated, especially in the presence of documentation or symptoms suggestive of more malignant arrhythmias.

FIG. 1. Suggested management of patient with atrial fibrillation. [a]Serious ventricular arrhythmias can occur if cardioversion is attempted in patients with digitalis intoxication. Fifty to 100 Wsec is usually sufficient to cardiovert patients with atrial fibrillation. If initial attempts are unsuccessful, higher energies should be used on subsequent attempts. [b]Propranolol or verapamil can be used instead of or in addition to digoxin for rate control. Intravenous propranolol and verapamil should not be used in combination (see text for additional details). [c]Therapeutic anticoagulation is required for 2 to 3 weeks before and for 2 weeks after cardioversion. [d]Approximately 10% to 20% of patients may convert to sinus rhythm with quinidine. DC, direct current; HR, heart rate; CHF, congestive heart failure; AV, atrioventricular; AFib, atrial fibrillation.

In the setting of an **acute myocardial infarction**, premature ventricular beats (especially if early, repetitive, multifocal, or frequent—5 or more per min) have been considered a warning of potential VF. However, up to 60% of patients with an acute infarction may manifest "warning" premature ventricular beats without subsequently developing VF. Moreover, a significant percentage of patients who do develop fibrillation do so without a prodrome of warning arrhythmias. Therefore, **prophylactic lidocaine administration** is recommended in patients with documented or suspected acute infarction unless their age or clinical status makes lidocaine toxicity more likely. Procainamide is probably an effective alternative to lidocaine therapy. Suppression of all premature ventricular beats does not appear necessary to prevent development of VF.

b. **Nonsustained ventricular tachycardia (NSVT).** Variously defined, NSVT is most appropriately viewed as a self-terminating arrhythmia of a duration too short to be associated with hemodynamic compromise (usually < 15 to 30 sec). Documentation of NSVT does not necessarily imply the presence or risk of a sustained arrhythmia. The requirement for therapy in patients without organic heart disease, in patients with non-coronary artery disease (e.g., cardiomyopathy, mitral valve prolapse), and patients with chronic coronary artery disease, in the absence of symptoms is uncertain and controversial. EP testing (especially in patients with subtle symptoms) may identify individuals at risk for sustained arrhythmias.

In patients with a **recent myocardial infarction**, NSVT on a predischarge Holter even if brief, asymptomatic, and infrequent, may be associated with a high (up to 38%) 1-year mortality owing to sudden death. Antiarrhythmic therapy is probably indicated in these patients for at least 6 to 12 months.

c. **Sustained ventricular tachycardia.** Even when well tolerated, sustained ventricular tachycardia is a serious arrhythmia and should be treated. VT is, more often than realized, the initial rhythm of sudden death. Degeneration into VF frequently occurs before monitoring is available.

d. **Sudden death syndrome.** The risk of recurrence in patients successfully resuscitated from an episode of sudden cardiac arrest depends on the association of the arrest with an acute myocardial infarction. In the presence of acute infarction the risk of recurrence is low (2% in the subsequent year), and specific antiarrhythmic therapy probably is not indicated. In the absence of associated infarction, the 1-year recurrence rate is high (22% to 50%) and indicates an underlying propensity for life-threatening arrhythmias. Therapy is recommended in these patients.

2. **Appropriate end points for therapy.** Since no universally effective agent is available for the therapy of ventricular arrhythmias, selection of an effective agent remains empiric and depends on the choice of therapeutic end point.

a. **Documented therapeutic blood level.** Although initial studies suggested that patients with stable, therapeutic plasma levels of an antiarrhythmic agent had a lower incidence of recurrent sudden death than patients with subtherapeutic levels, the efficacy of this approach has not been confirmed in adequate clinical trials. The observation that a significant proportion of patients are refractory to conventional agents makes it unlikely that this technique is adequate for a given individual with a malignant ventricular arrhythmia. Initiation of a conventional antiarrhythmic agent and documentation of therapeutic plasma levels may be a reasonable first therapeutic option in patients with well tolerated ventricular arrhythmias.

  b. Suppression of monitored arrhythmias. Suppression of PVCs may not be an adequate therapeutic end point for the prevention of lethal arrhythmias because

  (1) Suppression of PVCs may not correlate with suppression of more malignant arrhythmias.

  (2) Suppression of PVCs may require much higher levels of antiarrhythmic agents (with a greater incidence of side effects) than are necessary to suppress serious arrhythmias.

  (3) Since PVC frequency shows tremendous spontaneous variation, a large (85% to 90%) decrease is required to confirm drug effect.

  (4) In some patients extended monitoring fails to reveal even PVCs between episodes of sustained arrhythmias.

  Suppression of repetitive forms may be correlated with suppression of more malignant arrhythmias. Failure to suppress couplets and NSVT in patients with sustained ventricular arrhythmias probably predicts clinical failure. However, several studies have implied that elimination of these repetitive forms does not guarantee a good clinical outcome.

  Suppression of clinical arrhythmia is the goal of effective therapy. However, it may occur too infrequently and too variably to be a practical guide to therapy. An empiric approach is appropriate if episodes are sufficiently frequent to allow assessment of pharmacologic therapy, especially if episodes are well tolerated.

  c. Inability to reinduce the ventricular arrhythmia during an EP restudy while on therapy may be a good predictor of a successful clinical outcome, although a controlled comparison of this approach to other, noninvasive means for determining drug efficacy (e.g., suppression of repetitive forms) has not been carried out. EP methods are useful for patients with sustained VT in the presence of chronic coronary artery disease, cardiomyopathy, mitral valve prolapse, or primary electrical abnormalities. It also appears to be an effective approach in patients successfully resuscitated from a cardiac arrest who have inducible VF or VT.

3. Premature ventricular beats: Specific therapy. For suppression of symptomatic palpitations, quinidine, procainamide, or disopyramide are the most efficacious agents. Tocainide also is useful, but experience with this agent is limited. Occasionally, propranolol (especially for exercise-induced PVCs or in mitral valve prolapse), digitalis or diphenylhydantoin are helpful. It should be remembered that the **goal of therapy is suppression of symptoms and not obliteration of all PVCs.** Overaggressive therapy should be avoided. After therapeutic intervention, evaluation is advised to assure that aggravation of the ventricular arrhythmia by the antiarrhythmic agent has not occurred.

In patients **with acute infarctions**, prophylactic treatment with lidocaine has been shown to reduce the incidence of VF. Rapid intravenous loading can be accomplished by an initial 75-mg bolus, followed by a 50-mg bolus after 5 min, and a third 50-mg bolus 5 min after the second. Stable plasma levels can be maintained by an intravenous infusion of 2 to 4 mg/min. Careful observation to prevent lidocaine toxicity, especially in the elderly, is required. Plasma concentrations may be helpful.

4. **VT: Specific therapy**

   a. **Termination.** In the presence of hemodynamic emergency, **immediate cardioversion** is indicated. Occasionally a chest thump, if initiated early, is effective. Repeated cardioversion at higher energies should be delivered if necessary. If unsuccessful, cardioversion also can be repeated after administration of lidocaine or bretylium. Appropriate therapy includes correction of any contributing cause (hypokalemia, hypoxia, acidosis). VT that is well tolerated is not an indication for immediate cardioversion. Pharmacologic termination should be attempted.

   If cardioversion is ineffective, or if the tachycardia is well tolerated, **intravenous lidocaine** in full-loading doses can be administered. If lidocaine is ineffective or contraindicated, **intravenous procainamide** may be used. Up to a maximum of 750 to 1,000 mg may be administered intravenously (at a rate that should not exceed 50 mg/min) if significant hypotension, widening of the QRS (150% baseline), or marked QT-interval prolongation does not limit therapy. If termination of VT is not accomplished, elective cardioversion should be considered. **Bretylium** may be effective in terminating VT. However, in the setting of previous drug therapy, bretylium administration runs the risks of hypotension and myocardial depression.

   Occasionally when pharmacologic therapy is ineffective or VT is recurrent, **intracardiac ventricular pacing** may be effective in terminating the tachycardia. Premature stimuli or burst (overdrive) pacing may be effective. These techniques have the potential for accelerating the tachycardia or causing VF.

   b. **Prevention.** Quinidine, procainamide, disopyramide, or tocainide may be effective therapy for patients with recurrent VT. These agents are often prescribed sequentially and empirically until an effective agent is found. The failure of one of these agents does not preclude success with another. All have the potential of exacerbating the ventricular arrhythmia. Occasionally, an antiarrhythmic agent may worsen the arrhythmia at low doses but may successfully prevent recurrence at higher doses.

   Infrequently, propranolol, digoxin, or diphenylhydantoin are effective, or combination therapy is required. Unfortunately, many patients are refractory to conventional antiarrhythmic agents. Some may respond to newer, investigational agents. It is important to document that apparent drug failure is not the result of nontherapeutic drug levels because of poor absorption. Patients refractory to antiarrhythmic agents may be candidates for pacemaker therapy (investigational antitachycardia devices) or a surgical approach designed to modify the tachycardia.

5. VF: Specific therapy

a. Termination. Immediate cardioversion is the treatment of choice. Cardiopulmonary resuscitation should be initiated if there is any delay in cardioversion. If cardioversion is ineffective, it should be repeated after the administration of lidocaine and/or bretylium as necessary.

Lidocaine should be administered if the initial attempt at cardioversion is unsuccessful. **Bretylium** as an intravenous bolus of 5 to 10 mg/kg, with subsequent doses up to a maximum of 30 mg/kg, may facilitate cardioversion or may rarely spontaneously convert VF to sinus rhythm.

b. Prevention. VF may occur in circumstances in which recurrence is unlikely, and chronic preventive therapy is not required. Fibrillation occurring in association with an acute myocardial infarction is an example. Recurrent VF is treated in a manner analogous to recurrent VT. For patients refractory to antiarrhythmic therapy, surgery or an automatic implantable defibrillator (at present an investigational device) is an option.

6. Accelerated idioventricular rhythm (AIVR) rarely requires therapy and generally has been considered a benign ventricular arrhythmia. This impression of benignity may not be completely accurate, but in general AIVR is a self-limited, well tolerated arrhythmia usually associated with infarction or digitalis excess. If the loss of the atrial contribution to cardiac output is significant, atropine or AV sequential-pacing can be considered. Lidocaine may suppress the ectopic focus.

7. Torsades de pointes is a unique ventricular arrhythmia with a distinct morphology seen in association with QT-interval prolongation. Characteristically, the amplitude of the QRS complexes varies, and the polarity appears to spiral around the baseline. This arrhythmia is rapid and may terminate spontaneously or have a fatal outcome. Recognition is important because antiarrhythmic drugs (especially quinidine, procainamide, disopyramide) frequently prolong the QT interval and may either aggravate or cause torsade. The treatment of choice is withdrawal of offending agents and overdrive atrial pacing. Isoproterenol infusions also will shorten the QT interval until overdrive pacing can be instituted.

IV. MANAGEMENT OF BRADYARRHYTHMIAS

A. General Chronic bradyarrhythmias may present with symptoms of chronically inadequate cardiac output (congestive failure, renal dysfunction, impaired cerebral function) or intermittent symptoms of pre- or frank syncope. Pharmacologic therapy is, in general, inadequate for the chronic management of the bradyarrhythmias. **Cardiac pacing usually is indicated** for relief of symptoms or for prophylaxis against serious exacerbations of the bradycardia.

B. Specific Therapies

1. Sinus node dysfunction. Asymptomatic sinus bradycardia or sinus pauses probably do not require therapy. If necessary to prevent or eliminate symptoms, therapy can be rapidly initiated with atropine (0.5 to 2 mg, i.v., every 3 to 4 hr) or isoproterenol infusion (0.25 to 2 mg/min). **Temporary pacing** may be necessary.

Permanent pacing is indicated for symptomatic sinus node dysfunction in the absence of transient or reversible etiologies (e.g., antihypertensive therapy with clonidine, guanethidine, methyldopa; beta-blocker therapy; sinus node dysfunction associated with ischemia or infarction).

Sinus node dysfunction may manifest with inappropriate and symptomatic suppression after episodes of tachycardia (tachy-brady syndrome). This may occur in **patients with coexisting atrial disease** where episodes of recurrent paroxysmal atrial fibrillation or atrial tachycardia are followed by prolonged pauses following reversion to sinus rhythm. Many of these patients require permanent pacing, since therapy to slow the ventricular rate during atrial fibrillation often exacerbates the sinus node dysfunction.

2. **AV node block.** First-degree AV block does not require therapy. Most episodes of persistent second-degree Mobitz type I (Wenckebach) block are drug induced (e.g., digitalis, propranolol, verapamil). Although infrequently required, atropine or isoproterenol will decrease conduction block in the AV node. Rarely will pacing be required because of symptomatic bradycardia. **High-grade AV block** may occur with AV node fibrosis, and is most commonly manifested during atrial fibrillation. An inappropriately slow ventricular rate that produces symptoms warrants **permanent pacing**, if transient and reversible causes can be excluded. High-grade AV block may also be due to **hypervagotonia** and may be seen in association with hypersensitive carotid sinus syndrome, swallow syncope, or glossopharyngeal neuralgia. The hypersensitive carotid sinus syndrome may produce faintness or loss of consciousness with carotid sinus pressure. The hypotension may be due to sinus slowing, AV block, peripheral vasodilation, or a combination of these factors. If symptoms are due to a decrease in heart rate, permanent pacing is indicated.

3. **Infranodal block.** Most commonly, progressive fibrosis of the fascicular bundle branch system produces partial or complete block in the His-Purkinje system. If significant involvement of all fascicles of the distal conducting system occurs, then complete heart block will occur. Symptoms may reflect the slow intrinsic rate of the escape mechanism or the intermittent failure of the relatively unreliable subsidiary pacemaker (presyncope, Stokes-Adams attacks). Occasionally significant bradycardia can result in a tendency for serious ventricular arrhythmias. Symptomatic patients with **third-degree heart block** should be permanently paced. Temporary pacing is probably indicated in these patients until a permanent pacemaker can be inserted. Asymptomatic complete heart block may be an indication for permanent pacing because of the unreliable escape pacemakers.

In the event of fibrosis or degeneration of the right bundle branch and either the anterior or posterior fascicle of the left bundle or of both fascicles of the left (chronic bifascicular bundle branch block), conduction depends on the remaining fascicle. Statistically, the risk of complete heart block is low (approximately 1% to 5%), and the **prognosis** for these patients is good. Partial involvement of the remaining fascicle probably indicates a group of patients at higher risk for the development of complete heart block. This may be clinically inapparent, or it may present as coexisting first-degree AV block or intermittent failure of the remaining fascicle to conduct (Mobitz type II second-degree block). **His bundle recording** (see above) may permit distinction of patients with intact conduction through the remaining fascicle and those in whom conduction is impaired. Permanent pacing may be indicated in the latter.

4. **Conduction disease associated with myocardial infarction.** Sinus bradycardia is common in association with myocardial infarction, especially early in the course and with inferior infarctions. Contributing causes include sinus node ischemia, hypervagotonia secondary to pain or intracardiac reflexes, and drugs with a vagotonic (e.g., morphine) or depressive (e.g., sedatives) effect. Sinus bradycardia is not a poor prognostic sign and rarely requires therapy. When **symptomatic**, atropine or temporary pacing are appropriate choices.

In general, conduction block within the AV node is seen in conjunction with inferior infarction and disease of the right coronary artery. High-grade block usually progresses from lesser degrees of block, and is associated with a satisfactory escape rhythm. **Block is almost always transient.** The mean duration of high-grade AV block is 2 to 3 days and ranges up to about 14 days. Atropine and/or temporary pacing may be necessary if symptoms warrant. These patients do not appear to be at higher risk than other patients with comparable infarctions.

Infranodal block most commonly occurs in association with **anterior infarction.** Unlike conduction delays in the AV node secondary to inferior infarctions, the bundle branch conduction abnormalities often persist or recur intermittently after the acute phase of the infarction, and complete heart block can occur suddenly. **High-grade block** (complete heart block or Mobitz type II block) is an indication for pacing. **New bundle branch block or bifascicular disease** (left bundle branch block or right bundle branch block with either left anterior or left posterior fascicular block) in association with acute anterior infarction indicates a group of patients with a significant risk of progression to high-grade block (approximately 10% to 30%), who also should be temporarily paced. The risk is especially high with accompanying first-degree AV block (approximately 40%).

Bifascicular involvement due to anterior infarction indicates extensive myocardial damage, and there is a **high peri-infarction mortality**, even with temporary pacing. There is also a high incidence of sudden death in the year after infarction. Some of this mortality may be due to recurrent high-grade block, but the degree to which this mortality can be reduced by permanent pacing is uncertain. Current recommendations for permanent pacing in this group of patients are controversial but probably should include those who have manifested transient high-degree block with their infarction.

C. **Cardiac Pacemakers**   Cardiac pacemakers have changed dramatically in the last few years. Commonly available pacemakers now include devices that sense and pace in the atrial as well as ventricular chamber (preserving AV synchrony and physiologic rate flexibility); that have programmable rate, output, and sensing characteristics (permitting noninvasive adjustment of these parameters for changing physiologic conditions); and that can transmit important information from the pacemaker to an external telemetry device. In addition, there are automatic or externally triggered pacemakers that can terminate or prevent tachycardias as discussed above. Description of these capabilities are beyond the scope of this chapter, but pacing indications and basic considerations are discussed.

Cardiac pacemakers may be used for either therapeutic or prophylactic reasons in the treatment of bradyarrhythmias (see Table 5). Symptomatic bradyarrhythmias usually are an indication for pacing no matter what the etiology of the bradyarrhythmia. **Temporary** pacing is indicated if the cause of the bradycardia is transient or reversible or may be used until permanent pacing can be achieved.

Permanent cardiac pacing is appropriate to prevent or minimize symptoms, most commonly in association with complete heart block, Mobitz type II block, highgrade block (either persistent or recurrent) in the AV node, or in association with sinus node dysfunction. Many cardiologists also utilize permanent pacing prophylactically in asymptomatic patients with complete heart block, or patients who have manifested transient high-grade block in association with an acute myocardial infarction.

Demand pacing, where the pacemaker generates a stimulus only if spontaneous activity is not detected for a certain preset interval, is most frequently utilized. Temporary pacing may be safely accomplished by the percutaneous (or by cutdown) introduction of a transvenous pacing wire using fluoroscopic and/or electrocardiographic guidance to position the lead. Attention to radiographic position, paced QRS morphology and axis, pacing and sensing thresholds, and intracardiac electrograms is useful to assure appropriate position and function initially as well as to follow serially to anticipate or evaluate potential complications. Permanent pacing may be accomplished with either endocardial (transvenous) or epicardial

TABLE 5. *Indications for cardiac pacing*

Temporary

Therapeutic
  For symptomatic bradycardias in association with
    Sinus node dysfunction
    High-grade AV block (e.g., AF with slow ventricular response, hypersensitive carotid sinus
      syndrome)
    Mobitz type II block
    Complete heart block
    Other
  Either transient (drug-induced, in association with acute MI) or until permanent pacing is
    established
Prophylactic
  Preexisting LBBB prior to right heart catheterization
  In association with acute anterior MI with
    Complete heart block
    Mobitz II block
    Incomplete trifascicular block

Permanent

Therapeutic
  For symptomatic bradycardias of any origin if unassociated with transient or reversible
    cause
Prophylactic
  Complete heart block or Mobitz type II block
  Transient high-grade block in association with acute MI

AV, atrioventricular; AF, atrial flutter; MI, myocardial infarction; LBBB, left bundle branch block.

TABLE 6. *Characteristics of selected ventricular-demand pacemakers*

Pacemakers	Magnet response	End-of-life characteristics
Most nonprogrammable pacemakers	72 bpm	<65 bpm (10% ↓)
Medtronic Spectrax (5984)	100 bpm × 3 beats, then programmed rate	10% ↓ in expected rate
Pacesetter Programalith	5% below programmed rate	10% below programmed rate
Telectronics Optima–MP	100 bpm	≤85 bpm (15% ↓)
CPI Microlith P	100 bpm	≤90 bpm (10% ↓)
Intermedics Cyberllth	90 bpm	≤81 bpm (10% ↓)
Cordis Multicor Gamma	Same as programmed rate	Elective replacement 3% ↓ Mandatory replacement 6% ↓

bpm, beats per minute.

(surgical implantation) leads. Lead dislodgement (with loss of pacing and/or sensing function), perforation, battery depletion, and infection are **potential complications.** Implanted demand pacemakers may be converted to a fixed rate, asynchronous mode, to assess appropriate pacing function by positioning an external magnet over the implanted generator. Battery depletion is signaled by a change in the pacing rate (Table 6). The reader is referred to the bibliography for a more detailed discussion of cardiac pacemakers.

BIBLIOGRAPHY

Gallagher, J. J. (1982): Mechanisms of arrhythmias and conduction abnormalities. In: *The Heart*, 5th ed., edited by J. W. Hurst, pp. 489–519. McGraw-Hill, New York.

Gallagher, J. J., Pritchett, E. L. C., Sealy, W. C., Kasell, J., and Wallace, A. G. (1978): The preexcitation syndromes. *Prog. Cardiovasc. Dis.*, 20:285.

Hindman, M. C., Wagner, G. S., JaRo, M., Atkins, J. M., Scheinman, M. M., DeSanctis, R. W., Hutter, A. H. Jr., Yeatman, L., Rubenfire, M., Pujura, C., Rubin, M., and Morris, J. M. (1978): The clinical significance of bundle branch block complicating acute myocardial infarction 2. Indications for temporary and permanent pacemaker insertion. *Circulation*, 58:689.

Varriale, P., and Naclerio, E. A., eds. (1979): *Cardiac Pacing: A Concise Guide to Clinical Practice*. Lea and Febiger, Philadelphia.

Wellens, H. J. J., Bar, F. W. H. M., and Lie, K. I. (1978): The value of the electrocardiogram in the differential diagnosis of a tachycardia with a widened QRS complex. *Am. J. Med.*, 64:27.

Woosley, R. L., and Shand, D. G. (1978): Pharmacokinetics of antiarrhythmic drugs. *Am. J. Cardiol.*, 41:986.

8.

Acute Respiratory Failure

Talmadge E. King, Jr.

8.

Acute Respiratory Failure

Acute respiratory failure (ARF) is a common life-threatening situation that requires **immediate treatment.** It occurs when the respiratory system is unable to adequately exchange oxygen and carbon dioxide between the environment and the tissues of the body adequately. The result is an inability of the system to meet the metabolic demands of the body. ARF is a physiologic state not a disease entity and as such is defined by analysis of arterial blood gases. The following are useful guidelines: **a Pao$_2$ less than 50 mm Hg (hypoxemia), a Paco$_2$ greater than 50 mm Hg (hypercapnia), and a decrease in the arterial pH to 7.30 (acidemia) when breathing room air.**

The successful management of patients with ARF requires a **high index of suspicion** because the clinical manifestations are nonspecific and often occur when gas exchange is markedly impaired. Furthermore, the decision to institute life-saving measures (oxygen therapy, intubation, assisted ventilation, cardiopulmonary resuscitation, chest tube thoracostomy, etc.) may be required before a detailed clinical evaluation and laboratory investigation can be obtained. Therefore, **successful management of ARF requires the clinician simultaneously to: assess the condition of the patient; understand and institute the many general measures valuable to prevent the physiologic effects of ARF; begin specific treatment aimed at the primary precipitating event or disease process; and predict and prevent the many serious complications that arise frequently in this clinical setting.**

I. DIAGNOSIS

A. Major Causes   Table 1 contains a list of the **major causes** of ARF. ARF may occur abruptly (minutes, hours, or days) in persons with previously normal lungs, or it may be superimposed on patients with a history of chronic respiratory insufficiency—i.e., chronic obstructive pulmonary disease (COPD). There are two primary types of ARF: failure of oxygenation (**hypoxemia**) or failure of ventilation (**hypercapnia**). Both processes may be present in a given patient, but usually one type predominates.

B. History and Physical Examination

   1. The **time course** over which the patient's condition deteriorated is important. In addition, a history of cough, sputum production, chest pain, shortness of breath, or fever should be elicited.

   2. Careful observation of the patient, noting in particular **general appearance** and **mental status**, is important.

   a. The manifestations of **hypoxemia** resemble those of alcohol intoxication— disorientation, confusion, apprehension, impaired cognitive function, and personality changes (sometimes frankly combative behavior). Tachypnea, tachycardia, and hypertension are frequently present. **Cyanosis**, when present, is helpful to the diagnosis because it suggests a severe degree of arterial oxygen desaturation (i.e., Pao_2 <50 mm Hg and O_2 saturation <80%. However, cyanosis is a notoriously **unreliable sign** because:

(1) Detection requires natural not artificial lighting.

(2) More than 5 g/100 ml of reduced hemoglobin is required to detect cyanosis of the mucous membranes (central); therefore, it may not be recognized in an anemic patient.

(3) Depressed cardiac output and vasospasm may cause peripheral (nail bed) cyanosis in the presence of normal arterial blood saturation.

  b. The symptoms of acute or subacute **hypercarbia** resemble those of an anesthetic—somnolence, headache, disorientation, confusion, lethargy. Common physical findings include asterixis, engorgement of retinal veins or papilledema, hypotension, diaphoresis, myoclonus, seizures, and eventually coma. It should be noted that **depression of consciousness in the presence of ARF is an extremely ominous clinical finding, often indicative of potentially lethal degrees of hypoxemia, hypercapnia, and acidemia.**

3. **Abnormalities in the respiratory rate or pattern of breathing** are sensitive indicators of the presence of respiratory dysfunction. A **normal respiratory rate is almost never present** with ARF. Furthermore, **signs of respiratory muscle fatigue** are important because they often herald the onset of ARF and carbon dioxide retention. These signs include:

  a. Difficulty swallowing (weakness of muscles of the pharynx and larynx).

  b. Dyspnea with tachypnea.

  c. Use of accessory muscles of respiration.

  d. Paradoxical movements of the chest and abdomen (inspiratory muscle fatigue).

  Chest-abdomen asynchrony exists when the normal, smooth, synchronous, outward movement of the chest and abdomen during inspiration is replaced by:

  a. A change in breathing pattern such that chest excursions are much greater than abdominal excursions.

  b. Inward movement of the abdomen during inspiration (in severe cases).

4. Careful examination of the **cardiovascular system** is essential. The most important initial points to establish are:

  a. Evidence of right or left heart failure (neck vein distention, S_3, loud second heart sound that is widely but physiologically split, peripheral edema of the legs).

  b. The presence of pulsus paradoxus (i.e., a drop in discrepancy between the first intermittent systolic Korotkoff sounds and the pressure at which all sounds are heard; >10 mm Hg is abnormal).

C. Arterial Blood Gases

  1. Indications. Analysis of arterial blood gases should be obtained as soon as possible in any patient with symptoms or signs of ARF, regardless of the

TABLE 1. *Causes of acute respiratory failure*

Location of disease	Examples
Central nervous system	
Brain	Sedative overdose
	Craniocerebral trauma
	Cerebrovascular accidents
	Sleep-apnea-hypersomnolence syndrome
Spinal cord and muscles	Spinal cord trauma, cervical vertebral fracture
	Myasthenia gravis
	Guillain-Barré syndrome
	Poliomyelitis
Pulmonary system	
Upper airways	Foreign body aspiration
	Laryngospasm or edema
	Vocal cord tumor
	Cricoarytenoiditis in rheumatoid arthritis
Chest wall	Flail chest
	Kyphoscoliosis
	Ankylosing spondylitis (rarely)
Lower airways and lungs	COPD (bronchitis, asthma, emphysema, or cystic fibrosis)
	Severe pneumonias (particularly viral)
	Adult respiratory distress syndrome (see Table 3)
Cardiovascular system	Pulmonary edema

clinical judgment regarding the severity of the patient's respiratory illness. It is frequently the only mechanism available to differentiate life-threatening situations requiring immediate treatment from less urgent changes in oxygenation, ventilation, or acid-base balance. Measurements should be made following an acute clinical change in a critically ill patient; to monitor the effects of therapy, especially when a change is made; and serially to assess the progression of or recovery from ARF.

2. **Blood gas interpretation.** Clinically, the level of ventilation as determined by the **partial pressure of carbon dioxide** (normal $Pa_{CO_2} = 35$ to 45 mm Hg) is of first importance. A low Pa_{CO_2} indicates hyperventilation, and an elevated Pa_{CO_2} indicates hypoventilation. Neither abnormality may necessarily require correction unless the magnitude results in a significant acid-base disturbance (i.e., chronic alveolar hypoventilation in a COPD patient with renal compensation may not require immediate treatment) or if it occurs acutely in association with shock or cardiac arrhythmia.

Importantly, **the detrimental effects of hypercapnia are mediated through its effect on pH. Arterial pH** (normal = 7.35 to 7.45) and bicarbonate concentration (normal = 22 to 28 mmol/liter) are useful adjuncts in the differentiation between acute or chronic problems (renal compensation requires hours to days) and in determining the presence or absence of concomitant metabolic disorders (see Chapter 2).

a. Hypoxemia is frequently first identified or suspected by finding a reduced Pa_{O_2} (normal = 85 to 95 mm Hg at sea level breathing room air). The four mechanisms of abnormal gas exchange in the lung resulting in hypoxemia are ventilation-perfusion imbalance, hypoventilation, right-to-left shunt, and diffusion impairment (see Table 2). One or more of these mechanisms may be present in a patient with respiratory failure.

b. In addition, appropriate interpretation of an abnormal arterial P_{O_2} requires consideration of the **oxyhemoglobin dissociation curve** because it expresses the relationship between Pa_{O_2}, O_2 saturation ($Sa_{O_2}\%$), and O_2 content (Fig. 1). Significant points on the curve:

(1) The O_2 content relates the saturation, hemoglobin concentration, and amount of oxygen that can be combined with hemoglobin and dissolved oxygen: O_2 content = (saturation × hemoglobin × 1.39 ml of O_2 per gram of hemoglobin) + 0.003 ml of O_2 per 100 ml of blood for each mm Hg of P_{O_2}.

(2) Above a P_{O_2} of 60 mm Hg the curve is fairly flat, with >90% saturation; therefore, in the management of hypoxemia it is not necessary to strive for a much higher Pa_{O_2}.

(3) Below a Pa_{O_2} of 60 mm Hg it is extremely important that every effort be made to increase the Pa_{O_2} (mechanical ventilation with or without positive-end expiratory pressure or high levels of inspired O_2), since even a small rise in Pa_{O_2} may result in a significant increase in O_2 content.

TABLE 2. *Mechanisms of arterial hypoxemia*

Abnormal gas exchange	Diseases	Pa_{CO_2}	$P(A-a)O_2{}^a$	Response of Pa_{O_2} to O_2 therapy
Alveolar hypoventilation	Central nervous system depression or neuromuscular disease	↑	Normal	↑
Ventilation-perfusion inequality	COPD Interstitial lung disease Asthma	NC	↑	↑
Right-to-left intrapulmonary shunt	Cardiogenic and noncardiogenic edema Severe pneumonia Massive and submassive pulmonary embolism Cardiopulmonary bypass surgery Atelectasis	NC	↑	NC[b]
Diffusion impairment	? During exercise in patients with pulmonary fibrosis or emphysema	NC	↑	↑
Reduced atmospheric oxygen	High altitude	↓	Normal	↑

[a]See section II.A.l.b.
[b]If shunt fraction > 25% of cardiac output.
NC, no change.

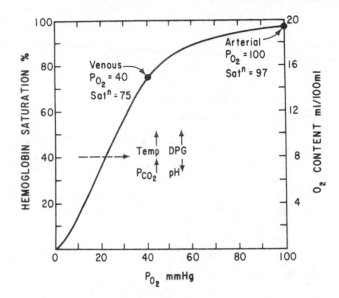

FIG. 1.   Oxyhemoglobin dissociation curve. The degree to which oxygen combines with hemoglobin depends on the level of PO_2. **Key points:** The shape of the O_2 dissociation curve has several physiologic advantages; i.e., it facilitates the loading of PO_2 in the face of a fall in alveolar PO_2, and the steep portion of the curve allows the peripheral tissues to withdraw large quantities of O_2 despite small drops in capillary PO_2. The position of the curve depends on temperature, pH, PCO_2 and level of 2,3 diphosphoglycerate (DPG) inside red cells. Factors that shift the curve to the right facilitate the unloading of O_2, and those that shift the curve to the left result in improved loading of O_2. An increase in PCO_2 and temperature and a decrease in pH and increase in DPG shift the curve to the right. Changes in these parameters in the opposite direction shift the curve to the left. (From West, J. B. 1977: *Pulmonary Pathophysiology—the Essentials*, p. 22. Williams & Wilkins Company, Baltimore, with permission.)

    c. Major changes in management are best made when performed in the context of the **trend** in arterial blood gases rather than from a single blood gas result. However, **acute, severe hypoxemia** ($PaO_2 < 50$ mm Hg and $SaO_2\% < 75$) should be aggressively treated because it will result in cyanosis, changes in mental status, cardiovascular depression (shock, hypotension), lactic acidemia, coma, and hypoxic brain death. Furthermore, **progressive respiratory acidosis (pH ≤ 7.20)** in the face of appropriate oxygen administration requires mechanical ventilation.

    d. Common errors in blood gas interpretation:

        (1) Although it is assumed that the PaO_2 reflects a low arterial blood content, there can be significant arterial hypoxemia due to **anemia** or **carbon monoxide poisoning** with a normal PaO_2.

        (2) It must be understood that the PaO_2 does not necessarily reflect **tissue oxygen delivery**, which depends on blood flow (total cardiac output and regional blood flow), hemoglobin concentration, and the oxygen saturation of arterial blood. Consequently, the **major goal** of management is to provide adequate tissue oxygenation because it is tissue hypoxia that results in metabolic acidosis, hypotension, cardiac arrhythmias, and cardiopulmonary arrest.

(3) **Venous blood obtained** rather than arterial blood.

(4) The **patient's status not noted**:

(a) Level of inspired oxygen increased but not recorded ($Pao_2 = F_{Io_2} \times 5$) or reduced atmospheric oxygen as a result of altitude (Pao_2 at sea level is about 90 mm Hg, whereas it is approximately 70 mm Hg at 5,280 ft above sea level).

(b) The patient's temperature is abnormal—**hypothermia** causes falsely high Pao_2 and $Paco_2$ and low pH values, and **hyperthermia** lowers Pao_2 and $Paco_2$ and increases the pH compared with the true values expected in vivo.

(c) Age of patient (the older the patient, the lower the expected Pao_2).

(d) Position of the patient when sample obtained (supine position lowers Pao_2 by 5 to 10 mm Hg).

(e) Hemoglobin concentration.

(5) **Technical errors:** blood contaminated by air (bubbles or unsealed syringe), blood stored too long before analysis, errors in calibration, handling of the specimen, or instrument failure.

D. **Other Tests**   Only after it is clear that no immediate management measures are required should the following tests be performed: chest roentgenograms (including previous films if available); routine laboratory data (CBC with differential, electrolytes: bicarbonate, sodium, chloride, potassium, inorganic phosphate, and magnesium); electrocardiogram; sputum Gram stain and cultures of blood, urine, and sputum; other studies (e.g., bedside spirometry, lung scans, angiograms, emergency bronchoscopy, etc.).

II. **MANAGEMENT OF ARF**   The goal of the initial evaluation of any patient suspected of having ARF should be to **determine the primary disorder** and/or to **distinguish the primary type of respiratory failure** present (i.e., oxygenation versus ventilation failure) because most therapeutic decisions are based on correction of these processes.

A. **Hypoxemic ARF: Pathophysiology**

1. The **basic mechanisms** of abnormal gas exchange leading to arterial hypoxemia (Pao_2 values below 60 mm Hg or arterial oxygen saturation below 90%) and their response to oxygen therapy are listed in Table 2. Admixture of abnormally desaturated venous blood (especially in patients with impaired gas exchange and decreased cardiac output) is an additional mechanism lowering Pao_2.

2. Several **nonpulmonary factors** affect gas exchange: hemoglobin content and affinity for oxygen (arterial oxygen desaturation), blood flow to tissues (cardiac output and regional distribution), and carbon dioxide production.

3. In order to manage patients with respiratory failure successfully, the clinician must understand how to **evaluate the efficiency of gas exchange** in the lungs and the adequacy of tissue oxygenation. Arterial blood gases are a relatively insensitive measure of the overall gas exchange efficiency because that factor depends on the overall ventilation (the partial pressure of oxygen in the alveolus—PA_{O_2}; matching of alveolar ventilation and blood flow; and diffusion across the alveolocapillary membranes and hemoglobin affinity for oxygen) as well as other nonpulmonary factors that alter the mixed venous Pa_{O_2} and Pa_{CO_2}.

a. **The partial pressure of alveolar oxygen** (PA_{O_2}) can be determined by the **alveolar gas equation**:

$$PA_{O_2} = PI_{O_2} - \frac{PA_{CO_2}}{R}$$

The partial pressure of the inspired oxygen (PI_{O_2}) = (barometric pressure − water vapor pressure)×fraction of inspired oxygen (FI_{O_2}). The barometric pressure equals 760 mm Hg at sea level, and the water vapor pressure equals 47 mm Hg. The FI_{O_2} breathing room air equals 0.21, and the respiratory exchange ratio

$$R = \frac{carbon\ dioxide\ production}{oxygen\ consumption}$$

is assumed to be 0.8. The partial pressure of alveolar carbon dioxide (PA_{CO_2}) is approximately equal to the arterial CO_2 (Pa_{CO_2}); therefore, the Pa_{CO_2} obtained from the arterial blood gases is substituted for the PA_{CO_2}. Consequently, a normal person living at sea level should have a PA_{O_2} of 100. Measurement of the PA_{O_2} is useful because it can be used to determine if hypoventilation is present and because it is required in the calculation of the alveolar-arterial oxygen gradient.

b. The **alveolar-arterial oxygen gradient** is calculated by the formula:

$$P(A-a)O_2 = PA_{O_2} - Pa_{O_2}$$

Therefore, a normal person living at sea level should have a $P(A-a)O_2$ of less than 20 mm Hg when breathing room air; i.e., the $PI_{O_2} = (760$ mm Hg − 47 mm Hg)×21 = 150 mm Hg, and since the PA_{CO_2} is assumed to equal the Pa_{CO_2} (normal is 40 mm Hg and is obtained from measurement of the arterial blood gases), and R equals 0.8, the $PA_{O_2} = 150 - 40/0.8 = 100$ mm Hg. Therefore, if the Pa_{O_2} is normal, then the $P(A-a)O_2 = 100 - 90 = 10$ mm Hg. The alveolar-arterial oxygen gradient is widened by ventilation-perfusion ($\dot{V}/\dot{Q}$) inequality, or increasing right-to-left shunt. Serial calculation of the $P(A-a)O_2$ is often useful in following the patient's clinical course. Since changes in the FI_{O_2} will cause a variation in the $P(A-a)O_2$ without any change in the amount of lung disease, the measurement should be made at the same FI_{O_2}. In the presence of shunt, increasing FI_{O_2} results in progressive widening of $P(A-a)O_2$ gradient; whereas in patients with $\dot{V}/\dot{Q}$ imbalance the change occurs in a curvilinear fashion in response to increasing FI_{O_2}: initially widening of the $P(A-a)O_2$ gradient and then a decline at higher FI_{O_2}.

c. Measurement of the **physiological shunt** or **venous admixture** ($\dot{Q}s/\dot{Q}t$) is another useful parameter in clinical practice because:

(1) Shunting is not improved by high inspired O_2 ($FI_{O_2} = 100\%$) and thus distinguishes itself from the other three causes of hypoxemia.

(2) When the shunt fraction exceeds 25%, little benefit accrues from increasing the inspired fraction of oxygen above 50% (the risk of oxygen toxicity markedly increases when the FI_{O_2} exceeds 50%) and frequently in patients with true shunt [atelectasis, severe airspace edema—i.e., adult respiratory distress syndrome (ARDS)], the FI_{O_2} can be lowered without a significant decline in the Pa_{O_2}.

The true physiological shunt is best quantitated while the patient is breathing 100% oxygen; however, this sometimes causes absorption atelectasis. Therefore, measurement at the level of FI_{O_2} being used is appropriate and reasonably accurate:

$$\frac{\dot{Q}s}{\dot{Q}t} = \frac{Cc_{O_2} - Ca_{O_2}}{Cc_{O_2} - C\bar{v}_{O_2}}$$

where $\dot{Q}s$ = shunt blood flow; Qt = cardiac output; Cc_{O_2}, Ca_{O_2}, and $C\bar{v}_{O_2}$ = the O_2 content in pulmonary end-capillary, arterial, and mixed venous blood. The O_2 content of end-capillary blood is assumed to equal the alveolar P_{O_2} (see II. A.). The $C\bar{v}_{O_2}$ is measured from a sample of blood obtained with a catheter in the pulmonary artery (usually assumed to be 4.5 to 5.0 ml/100 ml of blood). The Ca_{O_2} is usually calculated using the measured Pa_{O_2} and saturation (see I. C. 2.). The normal value for the $\dot{Q}s/\dot{Q}t$ is less than 5% and can rise to >50% in patients with severe respiratory disease.

d. The goal of therapy is to maintain **adequate tissue oxygenation**, but unfortunately, no satisfactory method exists for assessing the adequacy of tissue oxygenation.

(1) The **total clinical picture** (heart, brain and renal function) is more important than any single parameter for assessing whether or not the patient is being adequately oxygenated at the tissue level.

(2) The **mixed venous oxygen tension** ($P\bar{v}_{O_2} = 35 - 45$ mm Hg) or saturation ($Sv_{O_2} = 65 - 75\%$) is an additional measurement that can provide an indication of the oxygen delivery—oxygen consumption relationship. Mixed venous blood is obtained from a flow-directed, balloon-tipped catheter placed within the pulmonary artery. It is important that the Sv_{O_2} be measured directly rather than calculated from the $P\bar{v}_{O_2}$ because the oxyhemoglobin dissociation curve (Fig. 1) is steep in the normally encountered range of Sv_{O_2}. Small errors in the measurements of $P\bar{v}_{O_2}$ will be magnified in the calculation of the Sv_{O_2}. Furthermore, the $P\bar{v}_{O_2}$ is primarily affected by Pa_{O_2}, cardiac output, and tissue utilization of oxygen, but the Sv_{O_2} depends on the position of the oxygen-hemoglobin dissociation curve as well. A fall in Sv_{O_2} implies anemia, arterial oxygen desaturation, and/or decreased cardiac output; however, a normal or high value does not exclude these disturbances. Occasionally, the Sv_{O_2} appears inappropriately high for the clinical picture (i.e., septic

shock with lactic acidosis). Three mechanisms may be operative in this situation:

(a) The tissues are not capable of extracting oxygen from blood.

(b) "Peripheral shunts" exist such that there is contamination of mixed venous blood by arterial blood.

(c) There is abnormal distribution of blood flow such that areas with low oxygen extraction ratios receive a disproportionate share of the cardiac output.

If the $P\bar{v}_{O_2}$ is less than 30 mm Hg or SvO_2 is less than 40%, tissue hypoxia and lactic acidosis are likely, which portends a poor prognosis in respiratory failure, myocardial infarction, and septic shock.

B. **Causes of Hypoxemic Respiratory Failure**   Multiple conditions can cause a primary failure of oxygenation without hypercapnia. In practical terms patients can be divided into two groups based on the severity of the hypoxemia: **Mild-to-moderate hypoxemia secondary to widespread $\dot{V}/\dot{Q}$ mismatching** (i.e., pulmonary embolism, pneumonia, asthma); these patients usually respond to modest concentrations of supplemental oxygen (24% to 40%) (see III. A.); and **severe hypoxemia** unresponsive to high FI_{O_2} because of severe $\dot{V}/\dot{Q}$ mismatching or right-to-left shunt—i.e., pulmonary edema either cardiogenic (increased microvascular pressure with pulmonary artery wedge pressure >18 mm Hg) or noncardiogenic (capillary leakage with pulmonary artery wedge pressure <12 mm Hg) (see Table 2).

1. **"Cardiogenic" pulmonary edema**

   a. **Diagnosis.** Pulmonary edema is a medical emergency resulting from an abnormal accumulation of fluid in the extravascular spaces and tissues of the lung. It occurs most commonly in patients with a previous history of ischemic, valvular, or hypertensive cardiovascular disease and left ventricular failure. Tachypnea, dyspnea, orthopnea, diaphoresis, diffuse moist rales, left-sided gallop rhythm, hepatojugular reflux, and/or neck vein distention are useful clinical manifestations. The chest X-ray usually reveals cardiomegaly, bilateral pleural effusions, prominent pulmonary vessels with perfusion redistribution and Kerley B lines (short, linear, horizontal markings near the pleural surface in the lower lung zones caused by interlobar septal edema), or air space densities in a perihilar distribution. The hypoxemia present in this syndrome usually results from $\dot{V}/\dot{Q}$ inequality. In addition, a low cardiac output frequently complicates acute myocardial infarction and thus reduces the mixed venous O_2 and aggravates the hypoxemia.

   b. **Management.** The major goal of therapy is to **relieve the tissue hypoxia** by therapy aimed at the combined problems of impaired oxygen delivery and increased work of breathing. **Oxygen therapy** is provided, usually with nasal cannula (4 to 6 liter/min) and/or a tight fitting face mask ($FI_{O_2} = 50\%$ to 60%). Recheck arterial blood gases in 15 to 30 min. Bronchodilators (aminophylline—see Chapter 9) should be started if diffuse wheezing is present.

Improved pulmonary congestion is obtained by elevation of the head of bed, keeping feet dependent unless systemic hypotension is present; and using rotating tourniquets applied to three extremities and maintained for approximately 20 min; if longer use is required, the tourniquets should be released in succession every 10 to 15 min sequentially (this may cause increased peripheral vascular resistance). Institute drug therapy, especially **diuretics** (furosemide 20 to 40 mg, i.v., can be repeated within 5 to 10 min at twice the initial dose to a total dose of 200 mg) and **morphine** (3 to 5 mg, i.v., slowly); avoid when hypotension or obtundation is present, and repeat 2 to 3 times at 10-min intervals unless complications occur. Cardiac performance can be improved by **digitalis** if evidence of cardiomegaly is present, in the absence of acidosis or hypokalemia. **Vasodilators** are useful when hypertension is present.

Correct underlying or associated problems, especially acidosis, electrolyte imbalances, arrhythmias, hypotension or hypertension, renal failure, anemia, or pleural effusions. Often a major management decision is to distinguish cardiogenic from noncardiogenic pulmonary edema. Therefore, the **pulmonary vascular pressures** should be measured in any patient where doubt exists (balloon flotation catheter). If these immediate measures do not result in improvement or if ventilatory failure ensues, intubation and mechanical ventilation should be considered.

2. **Neurogenic pulmonary edema** commonly follows head trauma, cerebrovascular accidents, and heroin abuse. The mechanism remains to be elucidated. Treatment is mainly directed at correction and management of the CNS lesions. Supplemental oxygen therapy and/or mechanical ventilation is frequently required.

3. **High-altitude pulmonary edema** is most often encountered in natives of high altitudes who reascended after at least 1 to 3 weeks at a lower altitude. In normals the risk is greatest in persons less than 21 years of age, following rapid ascent to high altitude (>8,000 ft) or if heavy physical exertion is undertaken on arrival at high altitude. The **clinical presentation** is characterized by dyspnea with exertion followed by tachypnea at rest. Acute mountain sickness (headache, insomnia, lassitude, anorexia, nausea, vomiting, lightheadedness, Cheyne-Stokes respiration during sleep, depression, oliguria, irritability, and chest discomfort) and high-altitude cerebral edema (like acute mountain sickness but with severe neurologic manifestations including hallucinations, seizures, or coma) are sometimes present. Death can occur within 8 hr because of hypoxemia (severe, widespread pulmonary edema) and CNS dysfunction. The **pathophysiology** is unclear, but intrapulmonary shunting is present and the wedge pressures remain normal.

Suggested **preventive measures:**

a. Above 10,000 ft, a slow ascent (~1,000 feet/day) is advocated.

b. Avoid prolonged heavy physical exertion.

c. Avoid sedatives and hypnotics.

A prior history of high-altitude pulmonary edema does not predict recurrences. **Treatment** is based mainly on prompt recognition, institution of oxygen therapy, and immediate descent of 2,000 to 3,000 ft. Not uncommonly, death occurs during sleep because of the added effects of hypoventilation. Diuretic therapy may be extremely hazardous in these volume-contracted persons, and other drugs (digitalis, isoproterenol, corticosteroids, naloxone) have not been proven to be beneficial.

4. **ARDS** (noncardiogenic pulmonary edema secondary to increased vascular permeability) is a common form of hypoxemic ARF that occurs following a variety of catastropic insults or risk factors (Table 3). It results in a **high mortality**: >75% of patients requiring an $F_{I_{O_2}}$ >0.5 to maintain adequate oxygenation. The hypoxemia of ARDS is caused by $\dot{V}/\dot{Q}$ **imbalances and intrapulmonary shunting** (often exceeding 50%) in association with a **reduction in the functional residual capacity** (i.e., air remaining in the lungs at the end of a normal expiration).

   a. **Diagnosis** of ARDS depends on the clinical setting (catastrophic event) in the absence of underlying chronic lung disease or left heart failure (wedge pressure >18 mm Hg). Clinically, the patients are in respiratory distress (tachypnea >20/min, labored breathing, diaphoresis, and variable degrees of mental disorientation), and their chest roentgenogram reveals a patchy bilateral interstitial and/or alveolar pattern that progresses to diffuse, con-

TABLE 3. *Disorders associated with the development of the adult respiratory distress syndrome (ARDS)*

Inadequate tissue perfusion (shock)	Inhaled toxic agents
Septic	Oxygen toxicity
Cardiogenic	Smoke inhalation
Hemorrhagic	Corrosive chemicals (especially
Anaphylactic	oxides of nitrogen)
Trauma	Infectious causes
Pulmonary contusion	Gram-negative sepsis
Nonpulmonary, multisystem	Viral pneumonia
(including head	Bilateral pneumonia
injury)	(staphylococcal or streptococcal)
Fat emboli	Fungal pneumonia
Burns	*Pneumocystis carinii*
Liquid aspiration	Miliary tuberculosis
Gastric contents (pH < 2.5)	Legionnaires' pneumonia
Near drowning (fresh and salt	Hematologic disorders
water)	Massive blood transfusions
Hydrocarbon fluids	Disseminated intravascular
Drugs	coagulation
Narcotic drug abuse (especially	Post-cardiopulmonary bypass
overdoses)	Other miscellaneous
Heroin	Pancreatitis
Methadone	Uremia
Propoxyphene	Paraquat ingestion
Other drugs	Radiation pneumonitis
Barbiturates	Amniotic fluid emboli
Thiazides	Eclampsia
Colchicine	Air emboli
Ethchlorvynol (Placidyl®)	Increased intracranial pressure
Salicylates	Seizures
Chlordiazepoxide (Librium®)	Diabetic ketoacidosis
Dextran 40	Carcinomatosis

fluent, homogeneous infiltrates throughout both lung fields. The characteristic finding on arterial blood gases is an uncorrectable hypoxemia (Pa_{O_2} $\leqslant$50 mm Hg on room air and not improved with $F_{I_{O_2}}$ $\geqslant$0.6). Other physiologic findings include pulmonary capillary wedge pressure <12 mm Hg, total respiratory compliance <40 cc/cm H_2O (an expression of lung distensibility defined as the volume change per unit change in the transpulmonary pressure, usually >20 to 30 cc/cm H_2O), increased shunt fraction ($\dot{Q}s/\dot{Q}t$) and increased dead-space ventilation (V_D/V_T).

b. **Management.** Because no marker for the risk of ARDS exists, **prevention** requires keen vigilance and aggressive prophylactic measures in the face of conditions associated with ARDS (Table 3); i.e., preventing gastric aspiration, restoration of circulating blood volume after shock, treating sepsis as early as suspected, providing adequate nutrition, and using blood filters for blood transfusions exceeding 4 units. After the development of ARDS, management is empirical and **supportive** aimed primarily at **maintaining tissue oxygenation** by support of the respiratory and circulatory systems and treatment/control of the underlying primary problem.

Oxygen therapy should be provided such that the Pa_{O_2} is maintained above 60 mm Hg. In ARDS this may be obtained only following intubation and mechanical ventilation with the use of positive end-expiratory pressure (PEEP). Because tissue oxygenation is dependent on several factors, a low cardiac output, anemia, or factors that alter oxygen demand (pain, fever, labored breathing, agitation) should be corrected or minimized. The avoidance of oxygen toxicity (100% $F_{I_{O_2}}$ for greater than 18 to 24 hr) is essential.

Endotracheal intubation and **mechanical ventilation** should be instituted when progressive hypoxemia unresponsive to high $F_{I_{O_2}}$ is present ($F_{I_{O_2}}$ $\geqslant$60% and Pa_{O_2} $\leqslant$60 mm Hg), if hypercapnia and/or metabolic acidosis appears, if the patient becomes obviously fatigued and can no longer sustain the work of breathing, or if shock develops. **The key to knowing when to intubate and ventilate is a matter of clinical judgment based on close monitoring (Table 4).**

The goals of mechanical ventilation are to improve arterial oxygenation (and thereby improve tissue oxygenation), decrease the work of breathing, and allow the use of nontoxic levels of inspired O_2 ($F_{I_{O_2}}$ $\leqslant$50%). When mechanical ventilation is instituted, the tidal volume should be set at 10 to 15 ml/kg and the inspired oxygen at 100%. An arterial blood gas measurement should be obtained in 15 to 30 min after the onset of therapy and the $F_{I_{O_2}}$ adjusted to maintain a Pa_{O_2} $\geqslant$60 mm Hg at an $F_{I_{O_2}}$ of $\leqslant$50%. If hypoxemia persists and cardiac output appears clinically stable, a trial of PEEP should be instituted. PEEP usually is instituted at 3 to 4 cm H_2O and increased by 2 to 5 cm H_2O increments until satisfactory oxygenation is obtained. High levels of PEEP (>15 cm H_2O) are rarely required, and it has been suggested that intermittent mandatory ventilation (IMV) be used with PEEP in an effort to minimize hypocarbia and to avoid the depression in cardiac output and barotrauma associated with the high mean intrathoracic pressure (see III. D.).

TABLE 4. *Indications for mechanical ventilation*

Underlying process	Useful parameters or manifestations
Inadequate Ventilation	
Apnea (cardiopulmonary arrest, drug overdose, CNS process)	Absolute indication
Chronic obstructive pulmonary disease (COPD) Immediately on presentation (usually a clinical decision) During conservative management	Impaired mental status; pH<7.25; P_{O_2}<40 mm Hg on supplemental oxygen; respiratory rate: >40/min or <20/min Progressive mental deterioration; pH<7.25
Status asthmaticus (during vigorous medical therapy)	Cardiopulmonary arrest Clinical deterioration: mental obtundation, coma, advancing fatigue and impending exhaustion; progressive hypercapnia and acidemia
Neuromuscular weakness or sedative overdose	Asynchronous breathing Respiratory rate >40/min Inspiratory force < −20 cm H_2O Vital capacity <15 ml/kg Pa_{CO_2} >50 and/or pH <7.30
Head trauma	Apnea or disordered breathing pattern Need for hyperventilation (Pa_{CO_2} = 25–30 mm Hg for 24–48 hr) to reduce cerebral blood flow (edema)
Inadequate Oxygenation	
Adult respiratory distress syndrome (ARDS)	Severe hypoxemia unresponsive to high $F_{I_{O_2}}$ (i.e., need for PEEP) Progressive fatigue; cardiovascular compromise

Other therapeutic modalities to consider in ARDS include **skillful fluid management** aimed at maintaining adequate perfusion and oxygen delivery to vital organs. Unfortunately, one commonly walks a tightrope between administering fluid to treat hypovolemia and reduced cardiac output (usually unmasked by the institution of PEEP) and administering diuretics (to manage overt evidence of fluid overload and fluid retention) or vasoactive drugs (to maintain cardiac output when central blood volume is lowered to reduce the pulmonary wedge pressure and edema—usually inotropic agents such as dopamine or dobutamine in combination with nitroprusside, which reduces peripheral vascular resistance). Therefore, frequent physical examination and monitoring aimed at hemodynamic function (mental status, systemic blood pressure, urine output, electrolytes and acid-base status) are mandatory. The use of the flow-directed balloon-tipped catheter offers an important tool for monitoring pulmonary vascular pressures (especially pulmonary capillary wedge pressure), cardiac output, and mixed venous oxygen tension. **Crystalloid infusions** (200 ml over 15 to 30 min) rather than colloid solutions are recommended for volume replacement. Colloid therapy has not been shown to be superior to crystalloid infusion; it is expensive (up to 50 times more than isotonic salt solution) and may increase extravascular lung water. Blood transfusions should be administered if the hemoglobin falls below 10 g. Regardless of the type of fluid used, the pulmonary vascular pressures should be closely monitored to prevent the sequelae of overzealous therapy or hypovolemia.

Sedation and/or **paralysis** is **rarely** indicated in the management of ARDS (or other causes of ARF) because it is important to monitor clinical status. Frequently, restlessness indicates an inappropriate ventilator set-up or malfunction or an acute change in the patient's status (hypoxia, acidosis, or hypercapnia) rather than the need for sedation or paralysis. **Correction of factors that might interfere with gas exchange**—large pleural effusions, gastric distention (air or ascitic fluid)—should not be overlooked. **Left ventricular failure** may be a contributing factor in ARDS and should be managed appropriately. Correct **hypocapnia** since it can cause a decrease in cardiac output and cerebral blood flow as well as increases in the frequency of cardiac arrhythmias (decrease minute ventilation, add dead space, use IMV).

Corticosteroids have no proven benefit in the management of ARDS or any of the common associated conditions leading to ARDS (aspiration pneumonia, chest trauma) and are probably contraindicated in others (infections). Despite this, pharmacologic doses of corticosteroids (methylprednisolone, 30 mg/kg in divided doses over 24 hr for no longer than 48 hr) have been recommended by some physicians. Because **infection** is a frequent cause of ARDS, broad-spectrum antibiotic coverage should be given when it is suspected. Appropriate cultures should be obtained and the regimen discontinued or adjusted based on the results (culture and sensitivity). Prophylactic antibiotics are not indicated except in selected severely immunocompromised patients. Adequate **nutritional support** should be provided. **Complications** are extremely common; therefore, they should be anticipated and managed promptly (see Table 5).

C. Hypercapnic-Hypoxemic ARF

  1. **Pathophysiology.** Hypercapnia results from inadequate alveolar ventilation, increased CO_2 production, or a combination of the two. Hypoventilation is the major cause of an elevated $Paco_2$. **Ventilatory failure** is diagnosed by finding hypercapnia ($Paco_2$ >48 mm Hg), respiratory acidosis (pH <7.35), and hypoxemia (Pao_2 <60 mm Hg), unless the patient received supplemental oxygen prior to drawing the arterial blood gases (e.g., in the ambulance or emergency room). This can occur in previously healthy individuals **without** specific lung disease or in persons **with** previous lung dysfunction. The mechanisms responsible for diminished ventilation include: altered control of breathing; neuromuscular or musculoskeletal abnormalities; and proximal or distal airflow obstruction. It is useful conceptually and therapeutically to divide conditions leading to hypercarbia into two groups: those resulting from de-

TABLE 5. *Complications associated with acute respiratory failure and its management*

Complications associated with intubation and extubation
  Insertion trauma (laryngeal injury)
  Improper tube placement (esophagus or right mainstem)
  Cuff complications (tracheal stenosis, erosion or dilation; tracheoesophageal fistula, erosion of the innominate artery)
  Postextubation obstruction (supraglottic or subglottic edema)
  Gastric aspiration
  Airway obstruction (mucus, endotracheal tube)
  Endotracheal tube dislodgement (extubation)
Complications of ventilatory and monitoring procedures
  Pulmonary barotrauma (pneumothorax, pneumomediastinum, subcutaneous emphysema)
  Acid-base disturbances (alkalosis)
  Cardiovascular problems
    Arrhythmias (multifocal atrial tachycardia)
    Hypotension and low cardiac output
  Machine failure (patient disconnected, alarms malfunction)
  Flow directed, balloon-tip catheterization
    Pulmonary infarction
    Pulmonary hemorrhage
    Arrhythmias
  Deconditioning (respiratory muscle failure)
Metabolic complications
  Syndrome of inappropriate antidiuretic hormone (SIADH)
  Electrolyte imbalances
    Hypokalemia and hypochloremia
    Severe hypophosphatemia and hypomagnesemia
Renal
  Fluid retention
  Renal failure
Gastrointestinal
  GI hemorrhage
  Ileus
  Gastric distension
  Pneumoperitoneum
Infection
  Sepsis
  Nosocomial pneumonia
Hematologic
  Anemia
  Thrombocytopenia
  Disseminated intravascular coagulation
Other problems
  Pulmonary embolism
  Drug toxicity (theophylline, digitalis)
  Oxygen toxicity
  Malnutrition
  Psychiatric disturbances ("ICU psychosis," depression, agitation)

creased minute ventilation and those resulting from severe $\dot{V}/\dot{Q}$ mismatch (COPD and asthma).

2. ARF secondary to decreased minute ventilation

a. The most **common causes** of depression of minute ventilation are head trauma, generalized intracranial disease, and drugs. Most of the diseases associated with this syndrome have characteristic signs and symptoms that allow their identification as the precipitating event. The major clinical point is that rapid diagnosis often depends in part on recognition of the conditions capable of producing insufficient respiratory function (Table 1). **Drug overdose** (hypnotics and opiates) is often diagnosed by its presentation (young, previously healthy patient) or history suggestive of acute, massive ingestion (empty medicine bottles or commercial products), partially digested pills in gastric lavage, previous suicide attempts, needle marks, and pupillary responses (pinpoint pupils). **Head trauma or another intracranial process** that produces ARF is usually associated with other gross neurologic abnormalities. Disorders that alter respiratory **neuromuscular function** (e.g., Guillain-Barré syndrome, myasthenia gravis) or **chest wall movement** (e.g., kyphoscoliosis) are characterized by a chronic or subacute clinical course, generalized muscular weakness, and an associated precipitating event (e.g., infection, sedation). The clinical findings associated with respiratory muscle fatigue are detailed above (see I. B. 3.).

  b. **Management.** If the patient is **alert and cooperative**, providing **supplemental oxygen** (3 to 4 liter/min via nasal prongs, or 30% to 40% oxygen by mask) may be adequate. In this situation it is extremely important that the patient be monitored carefully in an intensive care unit (ICU). **Monitoring** should include frequent **arterial blood gas analysis** (a P_{CO_2} >45 mm Hg indicates increased possibility of respiratory arrest); examination for signs of worsening respiratory muscle fatigue; measurement of the **ventilatory reserve** (vital capacity less than 1.0 L is an ominous sign; peak inspiratory force less than 15 mm Hg indicates muscle weakness in an alert, cooperative patient); calculation of the $P(A - a)_{O_2}$ (normal means neuromuscular weakness or CNS depression; widened means associated or superimposed lung disease, e.g., aspiration pneumonia, COPD). **Aminophylline** in therapeutic doses increases diaphragmatic contractility by 15% to 20%.

  If the patient is **stuporous or comatose and has a depressed gag reflex and shallow respiration** then control of the airway (i.e., endotrachial intubation) is of extreme importance. Care must be taken to clear secretions and watch for aspiration. Supplemental oxygen delivered by several assisted breaths should be administered before attempted intubation, to avoid exaggerating the hypoxemia. When opiate overdose is suspected (coma, pinpoint pupils, respiratory depression), intubation followed by naloxone is indicated. (Marked vomiting and pulmonary aspiration can follow the administration of naloxone.)

  Mechanical ventilation (see III. D.) is required in most cases of ARF due to hypoventilation, especially if apnea or overt respiratory muscle failure is present. At least 12 to 14 hr of complete ventilator support is required to restore respiratory muscle contractility. Extubation should not be undertaken before careful evaluation of respiratory muscle strength. Overzealous ventilation leading to hypocapnia is to be avoided, since seizures and arrhythmias can occur in this setting.

  It is critically important that all other metabolic (hypoxia, acidosis, electrolyte deficiencies), circulatory (shock, heart failure), and infectious processes be corrected.

Ventilatory support may be required for prolonged periods, especially in patients with neuromuscular disease. Therefore, careful attention should be applied to supportive care (see III. D.). Artificial ventilation should not be instituted in patients with progressive neuromuscular disease in the absence of an acute reversible cause for the respiratory failure. Use of a rocking bed or body respirator may allow adequate alveolar ventilation so that these patients may return to the home environment. Electrophrenic pacing is occasionally useful in patients with Ondine's curse (central hypoventilation).

3. **ARF secondary to COPD.** Asthma (see Chapter 9) and COPD are frequent causes of ARF. In both situations patients are functionally stable until **acute deterioration is precipitated by some further insult:** left ventricular failure, acute pulmonary embolism, pneumonia, pneumothorax, respiratory depression (caused by excessive oxygen therapy, sedative hypnotic or narcotic analgesic drugs), surgery (especially of chest and abdomen), a change in medical regimen (stopping the medication), or occasionally malnutrition (patients bedridden for months who slowly slip into ARF).

a. Strict criteria for the **diagnosis** of ARF in patients with COPD is difficult to define: hypoxemia (Pao_2 $\leq$ 60 mm Hg), hypercapnia ($Paco_2$ >50 mm Hg), respiratory acidosis (pH <7.35), associated with a worsening of the patient's respiratory symptoms compared to baseline. Knowing the patient's **baseline** is extremely important (especially previous arterial blood gases and mental/physical function), since it may be very difficult to distinguish an acute exacerbation superimposed on chronic respiratory insufficiency. The onset of ARF is usually heralded by progressive dyspnea, often associated with productive cough, followed within hours or days by impaired judgment, insomnia, agitation, and physical signs of labored breathing, bronchospasm, and respiratory muscle fatigue. Occasionally, patients present with depressed mentation and inappropriately decreased respiratory rate because of respiratory depression (sedative drugs or high inspiratory oxygen en route to the hospital).

b. The **management** of ARF secondary to COPD requires a conservative approach if at all possible (i.e., avoidance of an artificial airway and mechanical ventilation). The **basic principles of therapy** are: apply immediate life-saving measures (treat hypoxemia and improve airflow); monitor in intensive care unit; determine and correct the precipitating factors; treat the underlying condition; and, avoid complications.

Prevention of ARF requires an appropriate awareness on the part of the patient and physician of the major impact the many seemingly minor insults can have.

Oxygen therapy is the cornerstone of therapy. **Death or irreversible brain damage results within minutes when severe hypoxemia is present, whereas hypercapnia may be well tolerated (or produce narcosis) and result in no significant tissue injury. Therefore, patients must not be allowed to remain hypoxemic or have a sudden discontinuance of supplemental oxygen therapy because of a fear of hypercapnia.**

The appropriate amount of oxygen is that which satisfies tissue oxygen needs (usually a Pao_2 ≥60 mm Hg) without worsening the respiratory acidosis and/or further depressing sensorium. Therefore, oxygen therapy should be initiated at low Fi_{O_2} either by nasal prongs (1 to 2 liter/min) or Venturi face mask (24% or 28% Fi_{O_2}). The former is preferred because it is better tolerated by the patient and less likely to be removed to talk, eat, drink or receive a medication aerosol. Arterial blood gas levels should be measured at frequent intervals, usually every 30 min for the first 1 to 2 hr or until it is certain that the Pao_2 is adequate and severe hypercapnia with acidosis is not developing. Higher flows or Fi_{O_2} are given until the Pao_2 exceeds 50 to 60 mm Hg. **It is important that management not be discontinued because of the almost expected rise in $Paco_2$ that will occur with oxygen administration.** However, if the patient experiences progressive hypercapnia (especially in the presence of asynchronous breathing), profound acidemia (pH <7.25), or mental obtundation (poor arousal, stupor, or coma) despite adequately administered oxygen, then an artificial airway and mechanical ventilation are required.

c. **Relief of airflow obstruction. Bronchodilator therapy** (see Chapter 9) should be instituted early in the management of patients with ARF to improve airway resistance. An inhaled beta-sympathomimetic agent, such as metaproterenol or albuterol, is extremely effective and can be administered by metered-dose or hand-held nebulizer [intermittent positive pressure breathing (IPPB) is not necessary]. Oral or parenteral sympathomimetics may also be helpful. **Intravenous theophylline** is recommended in the treatment of ARF because, in addition to its effects on the airways, it has been shown to improve respiratory muscle contractility, increase mucociliary clearance, improve the ventilatory response to hypoxemia, improve right ventricular ejection fraction, and increase the glomerular filtration rate. Its bronchodilator effect appears to be additive with sympathomimetic agents. If no evidence of improvement is associated with these drugs, they should be discontinued—especially in elderly patients, in whom significant side effects are common. Occasionally, inhaled bronchodilators will cause a transient fall in the Pao_2 because of a worsening of the $\dot{V}/\dot{Q}$ match. **Corticosteroids** in pharmacologic doses have been advocated for COPD patients with refractory ARF. The rationale is that corticosteroids will reduce airway edema and inflammation. Methylprednisolone 2 mg/kg/24 hr (or its equivalent in other steroid preparations) in four divided doses, for 48 to 72 hr, appears reasonable. **Atropine sulfate** (0.02 mg/kg, aerosolized in a fluid volume of 2 to 3 ml, every 4 to 6 hr) occasionally is used in patients with severe chronic airflow limitation unresponsive to beta agonists. Maximum effect occurs at 60 min following the dose.

Management of tracheobronchial secretions should include the following:

(1) Mechanical removal using **postural drainage and percussion** and nasal tracheal suctioning (cautiously as hypoxemia, reflex bronchospasm, and cardiac arrhythmias have been reported); this should follow bronchodilator therapy and be discontinued if not effective (i.e., increased volume of sputum or subjective changes in dyspnea) after 12 to 24 hr.

(2) Adequate **hydration** to enhance mucus flow.

(3) Broad spectrum **antibiotic therapy** (ampicillin, erythromycin, or tetracycline, 250–500 mg every 6 hr) is often useful. Routine antimicrobial testing should be performed before starting antibiotic therapy in an attempt to identify a specific pathogen.

d. **Other therapeutic measures: Adequate hydration** is needed to maintain venous return and cardiac output, especially in presence of pulmonary hypertension. Digitalis is of questionable value in the management of cor pulmonale in the absence of left ventricular dysfunction and may be associated with an increased incidence of arrhythmias. **Aggressive diuresis**, even in the presence of severe hepatic congestion and marked peripheral edema, should be avoided. **Posthypercapnic, hypokalemic metabolic alkalosis** frequently occurs and should be anticipated in an effort to prevent arrhythmias and decreased respiratory drive.

Respiratory stimulants have been advocated as temporary adjuncts in the management of ARF because they increase minute ventilation, tidal volume, and respiratory frequency and may acutely lower $PaCO_2$ (e.g., doxapram via continuous intravenous infusion in ICU). Unfortunately, these effects result in an increase of energy expenditure and work of breathing, which may be detrimental in COPD patients. Furthermore, most patients with unstable COPD or asthma already have increased central drives to breathe, and further stimulation would be ineffective.

Intubation and mechanical ventilation (see III.) are not required in the majority of patients aggressively treated as outlined above. **Progressive deterioration of mental status and/or severe acidemia, especially in an uncooperative, exhausted patient, are the major indications for ventilatory support, not the level of $PaCO_2$.**

A large endotracheal tube (8 mm internal diameter or greater) is required because of the frequent need for suctioning of thick secretion in these patients. **At least 24 to 48 hr of ventilation** should be given before weaning or extubation to allow recovery of the respiratory muscles. Withdrawal of mechanical ventilation is discussed in section III.

A frequent error in management is **hyperventilation: the goal should be to maintain the patient's baseline arterial blood gases** because these patients are frequently hypercapnic and have developed appropriate renal compensation. Failure to follow this principle frequently results in alkalosis (pH >7.50) with its attendant problems (decreased cardiac output, impaired cerebral blood flow, predisposition to cardiac arrhythmias); and prolonged ventilation because of difficulty in weaning.

III. **GENERAL PRINCIPLES OF RESPIRATORY THERAPY**   The basic aims of therapy for acute respiratory failure are to provide adequate tissue oxygenation and to reverse the disease process that led to the failure. The first decision is whether mechanical ventilation is required or oxygen therapy will suffice.

A. **Oxygen Therapy**   The basic principle guiding the use of oxygen is that **it should be administered at the lowest concentration necessary to achieve satisfactory levels of PaO_2 (usually 50 to 60 mm Hg).** This cautious use of oxygen protects against pulmonary oxygen toxicity and the suppression of the hypoxic drive to breath (especially in decompensated COPD). **No matter what the method of administration or level of F_{IO_2} used, management must be guided by analysis of arterial blood gases.**

1. **Methods of oxygen administration**

   a. **Nasal cannulas** (prongs) deliver humidified oxygen at rates of 0.5 to 10 liters/min (usually only flows up to 5 to 6 liter/min are tolerable) and are perhaps the best choice for most applications requiring low F_{IO_2} therapy. Continuous flow (through one or two prongs) fills the nasopharynx or oropharynx with oxygen so that this method works in mouth breathers as well as in patients with an occlusive nasogastric tube or bronchoscope in the nostril. Nasal prongs are particularly valuable because of the high acceptance rate by patients, and they allow uninterrupted oxygen therapy while talking, eating, coughing, taking medication, or during suctioning procedures. Oxygen supplied at rates of 1 to 4 liter/min results in an F_{IO_2} of about 25% to 30%, depending on the patient's minute ventilation.

   b. **Masks. Face masks** can be used to provide higher F_{IO_2} than nasal cannulas and open tents but are much more uncomfortable and less stable than other methods. In fact, patients often cannot tolerate these devices because they elicit a "smothering" sensation, and they are discarded when the patient is agitated, dyspneic, asleep, or eating. This can be hazardous because it will occasionally result in a precipitous fall in Pa_{O_2}.

   Simple masks can provide an F_{IO_2} of approximately 40% at 6 liter/min to 60% at 8 liters/min, depending on the patient's ventilation.

   The **Venturi mask** is an air-entrainment mask that delivers a precise concentration of oxygen (24%, 28%, 31%, 35%, 40%, and 50%). The oxygen enters the mask through a narrow jet, and it entrains a constant flow of air that enters via surrounding holes. It is useful in patients with decompensated COPD with CO_2 retention where more precise control of the F_{IO_2} is desirable. In practice, this method is no more useful than nasal prongs and not as well tolerated by patients.

   Partial rebreathing masks make possible the delivery of higher concentrations of oxygen (35% to 60%), provided the reservoir bag is kept properly inflated by a continuous flow of oxygen. Adequate oxygen flow reduces carbon dioxide accumulation (9 to 10 liter/min).

   Nonrebreathing masks are similar to partial rebreathing masks, but they have a one-way expiratory valve that prevents rebreathing of expired gas. These masks can deliver a F_{IO_2} in the range of 60% to 100%, depending on the flow of oxygen (12 to 15 liter/min), degree of fit around the face, patient cooperation, and ventilation. Only rarely will this form of therapy work for more than a few hours, at which time endotracheal intubation will be required to manage most patients with severe hypoxemic ARF.

   c. **The T-tube** (T-piece) is used to deliver oxygen (F_{IO_2} 21% to 100%) in spontaneously breathing patients intubated with an endotracheal or tracheostomy tube, usually as a part of the weaning from mechanical ventilation. Rebreathing of room air can be eliminated by extending the expiratory side of the T-piece and increasing the inspired gas flow to two to three times the patient's minute ventilation.

d. **Other means** of supplementing F_{IO_2}: The **tracheostomy mask or collar** is a small, open-domed hood that creates a tentlike area over the tracheostomy orifice and provides high humidity and additional F_{IO_2}. The **face tent** provides high humidity and can substitute for a face mask if the patient cannot tolerate having his nose covered. It is often used in conjunction with nasal prongs to provide a higher F_{IO_2} and humidity in the postextubation period. **Oxygen tents** are no longer used.

Hyperbaric oxygen (100% O_2 at pressures greater than atmospheric) is used in the management of severe carbon monoxide poisoning and in decompression.

2. **Complications of oxygen therapy**

a. The fear of significantly **increasing hypercapnia and acidemia** by oxygen administration is well founded but need not be crippling. Modest increases in Pa_{CO_2} can be considered an expected adaptive response and is usually well tolerated. The chance of a patient requiring intubation and **mechanical ventilation** is markedly reduced by the following: avoiding uncontrolled or injudicious use of oxygen; avoiding sedatives or other medication that might lead to respiratory or cough suppression; and once oxygen is started, **never discontinue**, even in the face of hypercapnia—i.e., add mechanical ventilation but do not discontinue oxygen.

b. The use of **humidified gas** will prevent drying of secretions.

c. **Oxygen toxicity** is characterized by progressive dyspnea, chest pain, cough, and progression of diffuse pulmonary infiltrates. Susceptibility varies between individuals but is increased if exposure to >50% oxygen lasts longer than 48 hr. Atelectasis (denitrogenation) and convulsions (especially with hyperbaric oxygen therapy) are other complications of prolonged exposure to oxygen at levels of 50% or greater.

B. **Airway Care and Secretion Management** Adequate secretion clearance and maintenance of a patent airway are significant problems in the management of all forms of ARF.

1. Adequate **hydration** and **humidification** of oxygen-enriched gases are extremely important in preserving mucociliary function and reducing sputum viscosity. Excessive hydration is to be avoided, since it will add to the cardiovascular stress common in ARF.

2. The patient should be instructed how to perform an **effective cough**: From a sitting position in a chair or edge of the bed if possible, bend forward and take several slow, deep breaths followed by two or three coughs in rapid succession while contracting abdominal muscles; then a deep breath, repeating the cycle (splinting of the chest will help reduce incisional pain). **Expectorants** and **mucolytic agents** have limited value in most patients, especially if they are well hydrated and taught to cough effectively.

3. **Physiotherapy.** Several techniques are available, including **postural drainage, chest percussion, turning side-to-side at periodic intervals and incentive**

spirometry, the purpose of which is to reduce the work of breathing by removing secretions and improving airflow and gas exchange. Only patients with thick, tenacious secretions that are difficult to clear or those with large sputum volumes should be considered for this therapy. The **order** for these procedures should include the objectives, anatomic localization of the disease process, and the frequency and length of therapy. The effectiveness of these procedures should be documented, and if ineffective, they should be discontinued after 12 to 24 hr. Results are optimized by giving bronchodilator therapy before chest physiotherapy. **Complications** are uncommon but include worsening hypoxemia (caused by positioning with the abnormal lung dependent) and bronchospasm.

4. **Suctioning** is not as effective as a spontaneous cough, but it is often necessary in patients who cannot clear their secretions. Sterile techniques and adequate preoxygenation are important. Complications include mucosal bleeding, life-threatening hypoxemia, cardiac arrhythmias, bacteremia, and cardiac arrest.

C. Artificial Airways

1. **Types of artificial airways**

   a. **Oropharyngeal airway** is easily inserted and should be used in an unconscious, spontaneously breathing patient with airway obstruction. Its basic purpose is to hold the tongue away from the posterior wall of the pharynx. Use in an alert, responsive patient might induce severe retching and vomiting.

   b. **Nasopharyngeal airway** is a soft rubber or plastic tube that can be advanced easily through a patent naris until the tip is in the posterior pharynx behind the tongue. It is reasonably well tolerated in a responsive patient and allows the passage of air into the lower pharynx and larynx.

   c. **Oral esophageal obturator airway** is a tube approximately 37 cm in length that is open at the top and has a blind end at the bottom. The lower blind end is inserted into the esophagus and an inflatable cuff is blown up to occlude the esophagus. The upper end is attached to a specially designed face mask, and several side holes in the tube allow the egress of air from the interior of the tube to the pharynx. This type of airway is used primarily in emergency departments or by trained paramedics. Hazards include laceration and rupture of the esophagus, tracheal intubation, and gastric distention. Aspiration is particularly a problem when this airway is being removed; therefore, endotracheal intubation should be performed before removal.

2. **Tracheal intubation** should be performed by either the oral or nasal route in an emergency situation. An emergency tracheostomy should be avoided unless upper airway obstruction is present.

   a. **Indications for endotracheal intubation:**

      (1) Cardiopulmonary resuscitation with need for complete control of the airway.

      (2) Need for mechanical ventilation.

      (3) Protection of the airway from the aspiration of gastric contents.

(4) Control of airway secretions.

(5) Complete upper airway obstruction.

b. **Routes of tracheal intubation: Orotracheal tubes** are easier to insert in an emergency situation and are particularly useful when secretion control is a problem because a larger-size tube can be used. Unfortunately, this type of placement is uncomfortable, impairs swallowing, impairs oropharyngeal hygiene, and is difficult to stabilize for long periods.

Nasotracheal tubes are much better tolerated and should be inserted when long-term ventilatory management is expected. They are easy to stabilize, allow oral hygiene, and cannot be bitten or chewed. A tube with an internal diameter >7.5 mm should be inserted whenever possible. Smaller tubes kink and obstruct easily; they make suctioning difficult and may make weaning difficult because of the high resistance to flow.

Tracheostomy should be performed as an "elective" procedure after stabilization of the acute situation, following prolonged (2 to 4 weeks) endotracheal intubation, or as an emergency if complete upper airway obstruction (tumor, foreign body) is present.

c. **Cuff care.** Successful management of intubated patients requires attention to airway management (see III. B.). In addition, the use of an endotracheal tube with a high-volume, low-pressure cuff allows a good seal of the airway with a reduction in pressure damage to the tracheal mucosa. The cuff should be inflated until no leak of air is heard during inspiration (using the stethoscope over the trachea). Slowly remove air until a small leak ("minimal" air-leak technique) occurs (i.e., the patient's expired tidal volume may fall 50 to 100 ml as the air escapes around the tube). The **cuff pressure** should be checked and maintained at less than 25 mm Hg. Use of this approach will significantly reduce postextubation tracheal problems, and it makes periodic cuff deflation unnecessary and probably contraindicated, since that does not reduce the chance of tracheal complications and predisposes the patient to aspiration.

d. **Complications.** See Table 5.

D. **Mechanical Ventilation**

1. **Indications** (see Table 4). Mechanical ventilation is required whenever the patient is unable to maintain adequate alveolar ventilation. It is more difficult to determine when (and if) mechanical ventilation is indicated in other situations—e.g., hypoxemic ARF in the presence of normal alveolar ventilation; when there is excessive work of breathing required to maintain a normal $Paco_2$; or prophylactically in patients with imminent ARF. The decision for intubation and ventilation is often based on the clinical appearance and is verified by analysis of arterial blood gases. Furthermore, the decision must take into account whether or not the process causing ARF is reversible. General guidelines for the institution of mechanical ventilation in several common situations are provided in Table 6.

2. **Types of ventilators.** There are two types of positive pressure ventilators.

a. **Pressure-cycled** machines allow the flow of gas from the respirator to

TABLE 6. *Guidelines for the initiation and management of mechanical ventilation*

Establish an airway
  Provide emergency airway management
    Artificial ventilation without intubation (see III. C.)
      Airway control
      Head tilt maneuver
      Oral or nasopharyngeal airway
      Positive pressure ventilation (mouth-to-mouth or bag-to mask) with supplemental oxygen
      Clear airway of any obstructing foreign material
      Seek to treat underlying or associated diseases
    Endotracheal intubation required (see III. C. 2.)
      Preoxygenate and preventilate patient
      Assemble and check necessary equipment
      Provide anesthesia, sedation, or muscle relaxation as required
      Select proper route of intubation and type of tube
        (cuffed; >7.5 mm internal diameter)
      Intubate and ventilate with a resuscitation bag while checking tube placement (auscultate
        the chest)
      Stabilize the endotracheal tube and clear secretions
        (sterile technique)
      Obtain chest X-ray (to check tube placement and exclude
        complicating process, e.g. pneumothorax)
      Move to ICU; never leave patient unattended
Mechanical ventilator (if required)
  Select type of ventilator (see III. D.)
  Select ventilator settings:
    Mode: Assist/control or IMV (see III.D.)
    F_{IO_2}: 100% initially, then adjust to keep $Pao_2 \geqslant 60$ mm Hg
    Tidal volume: 10–15 ml/kg; and rate: 8–15/min
    Adjust inspiratory flow rate; inspiratory to expiratory time
      (I/E ratio), if necessary
    Adjust alarms and pressure limits
    Obtain arterial blood gases in 15–30 min and readjust ventilator
      accordingly (including adding PEEP or CPAP)
Long-term ventilator care:
  Anticipate and prevent complications (see Table 5)
  Provide supportive care and airway management (see III. B.)
  Monitor respiratory and hemodynamic function (see III. D. 5.)
  Wean and extubate when appropriate (see III. D. 8.,9.)

ICU, intensive care unit; IMV, intermittent mandatory ventilation; PEEP, positive end-expiratory pressure; CPAP, continuous positive airway pressure.

continue until a preselected airway pressure is reached. The tidal volume delivered by these machines varies with changes in airway resistance and lung compliance and therefore exposes the patient to considerable risk.

b. **Volume-cycled ventilators** provide flow until a specific preset volume has been delivered. This feature, along with its power to ventilate difficult patients and its flexibility (controls to vary pressure, flow, and respiratory rate, controlled oxygen concentration settings, and appropriate alarms for high and low pressure, low F_{IO_2} and electrical failure), makes this the ventilator of choice in most hospital settings. The major drawback to volume-cycled ventilators is that they can produce high transpulmonary pressures, which may significantly impair venous return and cause hypotension.

3. **Mode of mechanical ventilation.** IMV and assisted mechanical ventilation are the most common ventilator modes in current use.

a. **Controlled mechanical ventilation**—i.e., a machine set to deliver a certain number of breaths per minute that cannot be increased by the patient's efforts to take more breaths—is rarely used today. It usually requires paralysis or heavy sedation and must be closely monitored, since the physician must make the adjustments necessary to meet any increase in patient demand. This method is useful as a mode of ventilation at home (high cervical cord injury) or during transport.

b. **Assist/control ventilation** is the most popular mode of mechanical ventilation because the patient initiates the inspiratory cycle of ventilation, thereby setting his or her own cycling rate, yet each breath is delivered by the ventilator. Furthermore, the ventilator is set at a certain rate, and if the patient ceases to breathe, this set value is the actual rate of breaths delivered. Most often the machine backup rate is set at 12 to 15 or just below the frequency set by the patient, so that if apnea or inability to trigger occurs, ventilation will not abruptly decline. Two significant problems may be encountered with this mode: respiratory alkalosis is common when a tachypneic patient is ventilated with assist/control; and respiratory muscle weakness may result from prolonged disuse. (Malnutrition, electrolyte imbalances, and the catabolic effects of ARF all contribute to respiratory muscle dysfunction in ARF.)

c. **IMV** has grown in popularity in many centers. Originally proposed as a weaning technique, it recently has been used as a means of providing continuous ventilatory support.

Technique: The patient is connected simultaneously to a circuit that enables spontaneous breathing and mechanically ventilated breaths timed to coincide with spontaneous efforts. This forces the patient to provide respiratory effort and thus can be a form of graded exercise.

Patients predisposed to the development of **hypocarbia** (those who "fight the ventilator" despite ventilator adjustments or sedation) often can be better managed by this method. IMV allows the patient to set his or her own Pa_{CO_2}, and the machine insures a minimum minute ventilation.

Patients who are **hemodynamically unstable** (decreased cardiac output despite adequate fluid management) on assist/control because of increased mean intrathoracic pressure [especially when PEEP or continuous positive airway pressure (CPAP) is required] may show improvement in the IMV mode.

IMV is **contraindicated** in patients having frequent apneic episodes or rapidly changing neurologic or metabolic status; in patients receiving paralytic agents or large doses of sedatives; and in patients with such high mandatory machine breaths (>15 breaths/min) that the patient's efforts are ineffective.

When IMV is instituted, attention should be paid to the **ventilator circuitry** to ensure a set-up that will minimize the work of breathing (usually a **"continuous-flow, closed circuit" IMV**). If the patient's inspiratory efforts result in a deflection of >2 cm H_2O in the negative direction on the ventilator's airway pressure manometer, it suggests that significant respiratory work is required to breathe through the circuit; therefore, the circuitry should be changed or the ventilator changed to the assist/control mode.

d. Positive pressure ventilation

    (1) Intermittent positive pressure breathing (IPPB) describes a gas-delivery system where the pressure at the airway during inspiration is greater than atmospheric and returns to atmospheric level (zero) during expiration (i.e., expiration is passive). In the past this was prescribed as a method to deliver an aerosolized bronchodilator or to encourage deep breathing in a cooperative patient too weak to inhale deeply. IPPB may cause impaired venous return (i.e., depressed cardiac output) and gastric distention. It is contraindicated in patients with pneumothorax, mediastinal or subcutaneous emphysema, hypotension or shock, tracheoesophageal fistula, or recent gastrectomy, and in patients who are comatose or otherwise unable to protect their airway. **IPPB has no role in the treatment of ARF.**

    (2) CPAP connotes ventilatory support using a pressure greater than atmospheric at the airway opening throughout a **spontaneous** respiratory cycle (usually via tight-fitting face mask or endotracheal tube in a spontaneously breathing patient). The pressure is obtained by passing humidified and warmed gas at a high continuous flow rate (20 to 50 liter/min) to a distensible inspiratory reservoir bag and then to the patient. It acts by increasing the functional residual capacity. A form of CPAP has been used successfully in the management of severe hypoxemia that accompanies the infant respiratory distress syndromes and in selected cases of ARDS. Complications include gastric distention, vomiting, aspiration, facial discomfort, skin erosion, and hypotension.

    (3) PEEP is a continuous expiratory pressure threshold imposed during mechanical ventilation; i.e., the volume of gas in the patient's chest at the end of expiration [the functional residual capacity (FRC)] is increased. This has proved to be a valuable adjunct in the management of ARDS. PEEP **improves oxygenation** in ARDS by recruitment of collapsed alveoli and by stabilizing and expanding fluid-filled alveoli (redistribution of pulmonary edema fluid) so that gas exchange is improved. PEEP does not decrease lung water. PEEP is **contraindicated** in patients with ARF secondary to COPD (emphysema, chronic bronchitis or asthma) and in patients with localized disease such as lobar pneumonia or unilateral pulmonary edema, pneumothorax, bronchopleural fistula, or severe hypovolemia.

    The **adverse effects** of PEEP should be understood and anticipated:

    (a) A **reduction in cardiac output** is common and results primarily from the impedance to venous return induced by the high intrathoracic pressure; at high levels of PEEP left ventricular dysfunction may also play a role.

(b) **Barotrauma** with pneumothorax is common in ARDS with or without PEEP.

(c) **Oxygen delivery** may fall via three mechanisms: decreased cardiac output, increased venous admixture (especially in patients with nonhomogeneous disease), and increased noncapillary shunt flow (intracardiac shunt).

(d) **Increased cerebral venous and intracranial pressure** secondary to impedence of venous return.

(e) **Increased work of breathing** (especially with spontaneous breathing).

(f) **Fluid retention and decreased urinary output** (probably mediated through the release of antidiuretic hormone (ADH) and changes in intrarenal perfusion).

(g) The **sudden withdrawal or lowering of PEEP** during mechanical ventilation may result in a severe worsening of gas exchange that occasionally cannot be reversed for several hours afterward.

Furthermore, the abrupt withdrawal of PEEP can cause a sudden redistribution of intravascular volume to the intrathoracic vessels and promote pulmonary edema and shunting, as well as a rebound increase in intracranial pressure. Therefore, patients who have demonstrated a positive response to the institution of PEEP should have it withdrawn cautiously (5 cm H_2O over 6 hr) to avoid the above complications. A **"PEEP trial"** is characterized by:

(a) Established mechanical ventilation with hemodynamic stabilization (i.e., hypovolemia treated).

(b) All other ventilatory variables kept constant (especially tidal volume and F_{IO_2}).

(c) PEEP added in increments starting at 3 to 5 cm H_2O (note: recruitment of collapsed alveoli by PEEP may take 30 min or longer).

(d) The effect of PEEP on oxygenation and hemodynamics monitored following each change (15 to 30 min).

The role of early or prophylactic PEEP remains to be determined. The goals of PEEP therapy are basically those of mechanical ventilation in general (see above). PEEP should be **withdrawn** only when the patient is stable, has an adequate Pao_2 (on an F_{IO_2} of $\leq 40\%$), and improved lung compliance (≥ 25 ml/cm H_2O).

(4) **High-frequency positive-pressure ventilation (HFPPV)** is an experimental method of ventilation in which small tidal volumes (approaching the patient's anatomical dead space) are delivered, using high respiratory frequency (60 to 120 cycles/min). Airway pressure is significantly less than in other forms of positive-pressure ventilation. Its clinical application remains to be elucidated.

4. **Respiratory and hemodynamic monitoring in acute respiratory failure** is extremely important since complications are frequent under the best of cir-

cumstances, and appropriate monitoring will increase ability to detect (and treat) these complications.

a. **Respiratory monitoring.** **Bedside measurements** should include:

(1) Repeated physical examination (pulse and respiratory rate, breathing pattern, chest examination).

(2) Daily body weight (good guide to fluid balance).

(3) Measurement of intake and output (good estimate of renal perfusion).

(4) Following serum electrolytes.

(5) Daily chest roentgenograms (tube placement, vascular catheter position, fluid overload, localized lung hyperinflation, atelectasis, pneumonia, pneumothorax).

(6) Electrocardiograms (continuous monitoring is essential since serious arrhythmias are common).

(7) Serial hematocrit (every 4 hr if hemorrhage suspected) and hemoglobin measurements (needed to calculate oxygen content of the blood).

(8) Analysis of arterial blood gases.

The **efficiency and adequacy of oxygenation** should be assessed routinely (see II. A.). The role of **mass spectrometry**, continuous **analysis of inspired and expired gas**, and **transcutaneous gas measurements** in routine clinical management needs further evaluation.

The **adequacy of ventilation** is primarily determined by serial measurement of the **$Paco_2$** but **tidal volume** (<5 ml/kg is extremely poor) and the **ratio of dead space to tidal volume** (V_D/V_T) also are helpful. The V_D/V_T (normal $= 0.2$ to 0.4) is a measure of that portion of the tidal volume that is not participating in gas exchange. The formula used clinically is:

$$\frac{V_D}{V_T} = \frac{Paco_2 - P_{\bar{E}CO_2}}{Paco_2}$$

where V_D = dead space; V_T = tidal volume; $Paco_2$ = arterial carbon dioxide tension; and $P_{\bar{E}CO_2}$ = mean expired carbon dioxide tension, obtained by collecting a 3-min specimen of expired gas.

An increased V_D/V_T can suggest pulmonary embolism, or excessive mean airway pressure causing a redistribution of blood flow so that regions of the lung are ventilated but not perfused (e.g., shock or hypovolemia); or it might explain a high ventilatory requirement.

Evaluating respiratory mechanics and ventilatory reserve is essential in assessing the patient's course, especially as it relates to the patient's continued need for ventilatory assistance. **Vital capacity and inspiratory force** (the maximal pressure below atmospheric pressure that a patient can generate against an occluded airway) provide useful data. A vital capacity <10 ml/kg, respiratory rate >25/min, and an inspiratory force <20 cm H_2O generally indicate a need for continued ventilatory assistance. Serial measurement of the **airway pressure** (peak pressure as measured on the ventilator manometer during inspiration) can be useful. An increase usually heralds a change in the patient and should be investigated. In addition, one can serially measure "compliance" (defined as the forces resisting expansion of the lung, equal to volume change per unit pressure change) and arrive at a more specific indication of the cause for the respiratory distress.

Static compliance ($C = \Delta V/\Delta P$) is a measure of the elastic properties of the lung and chest wall and will decrease (curves shift more to the right) in the presence of a tension pneumothorax, atelectasis, pulmonary edema, and pneumonia. It is obtained by plotting the relationship between the change in **static airway pressure** (i.e., the outflow of the ventilator is momentarily occluded at the end of inspiration by pinching the expiratory tubing or dialing in expiratory retard and the pressure dial will show a momentary plateau at which no air is flowing) and **tidal volume.** Both determinations are usually obtained over a range of tidal volumes, 400 to 1,000 ml, and a "static compliance curve" is generated. When PEEP is being used, it must be subtracted from the peak and plateau pressures before calculation of the compliance. The normal compliance of the lung is 200 ml/cm water, and in mechanically ventilated patients it is about 80 to 100 ml/cm water (includes lung and chest wall).

Dynamic compliance is a measure reflecting the flow-restrictive properties of the airway and would be expected to decrease in the presence of conditions increasing flow resistance (e.g., bronchospasm and mucus plugging). This is not truly the dynamic compliance because it measures both compliance and resistance components. It is obtained similar to the static compliance except that the **peak pressure** obtained at each tidal volume is used to generate the pressure-volume curve. If a patient becomes hypoxemic without changes in compliance curves, then pulmonary embolism should be suspected. (**Note:** These pressure-volume measurements are not the same as those obtained in a physiology laboratory, which are usually measured during a single breath.)

b. **Hemodynamic monitoring.** The **goal** of the management of ARF is to sustain and/or improve tissue oxygenation. Unfortunately, the therapy often alters those factors responsible for maintaining adequate tissue oxygen delivery (i.e., cardiac output and arterial oxygen content). Therefore, hemodynamic monitoring via a flow-directed, balloon-tipped catheter is frequently required because it allows measurement of pulmonary vascular pressures, cardiac output, and mixed venous oxygen tension (Pv_{O_2}) and saturation (Sv_{O_2}). This is especially true when PEEP is being used, because it has been shown that in hypovolemic patients (wedge pressure $\leqslant 5$ to 8 mm Hg) the Pa_{O_2} may increase, but its effect is limited by a significant decline in cardiac output and systemic oxygen transport. Furthermore, monitoring the **wedge pressure** is sometimes the only means to identify and prevent fluid overload and left ventricular failure (wedge pressure > 18 to 20 mm Hg). In this regard, the wedge pressure should be kept as low as possible while maintaining adequate cardiac output.

The measurement of the wedge pressure may be a problem when PEEP is used because the positive alveolar pressure is transmitted to the pulmonary microvasculature, and if it exceeds the left atrial pressure, the measured wedge pressure may be artificially high. Thus, if the wedge pressure is higher than the pulmonary artery diastolic pressure or if an increase in wedge pressure follows an increase in the level of PEEP, then the measured wedge pressure is artifactually increased. In this instance, the wedge pressure should be measured with the PEEP off (not more than 15 sec) to provide a better estimate of the true left ventricular pressure. Occasionally, mechanical ventilation causes significant respiratory artifacts. For this reason, a calibrated oscilloscope or graphic printout of the wedge pressure is required to obtain an accurate wedge pressure. Usually, simultaneous measurement of airway and vascular pressures are made, and the wedge measurement is taken at end-expiration. If the respiratory artifact is excessive the catheter has to be moved to a flow-dependent portion of the lung.

The "auto-PEEP" phenomenon—i.e., the spontaneous development of PEEP at the alveolar level in severely obstructed, mechanically ventilated patients secondary to "air trapping"—recently has been reported as a cause of severe depression in cardiac output as well as falsely elevated wedge pressures. It can be detected by occluding the expiratory port at the end of the set exhalation period.

5. Supportive care of patients during mechanical ventilation (see III. B.)

   a. Good nursing care is essential in the management of ARF. The **prevention of skin ulcers and joint immobility** should be a priority. Furthermore, patients should be given **graded exercise training** (standing, sitting, and/or walking) as soon as possible, so that withdrawal from ventilatory support is facilitated.

   b. Often **effective communication** is not carried out in these critically ill patients (especially by physicians!). Every effort should be made to establish and maintain a frame of reference with the outside world (calendar, radio, clock, frequent reminders of the day and time) and to educate patients regarding treatment (especially when changes such as weaning are being made).

   c. It is not uncommon for patients requiring mechanical ventilation to develop a severely compromised **nutritional status.** Conventional intravenous dextrose solutions provide only 400 to 600 calories per day. Often weaning is rendered difficult, if not impossible, because of malnutrition-induced inspiratory muscle fatigue. Thus, it is important to maintain a high caloric intake (see Chapter 21). A **high carbohydrate load** may result in as much as a 20% increase in CO_2 production. During periods of weaning this may add a significant ventilatory load, making spontaneous ventilation difficult. In this event a larger portion of the caloric intake should be provided by lipids, thereby reducing carbon dioxide production.

6. Numerous **complications** are associated with or caused by the management of acute respiratory failure. Table 5 provides a list of these problems, which should be reviewed frequently in an effort to anticipate and prevent as many as possible.

"Fighting the respirator" is a problem frequently encountered in ventilator management. It reflects on patient management and **not** on the patient. During the initial phases of mechanical ventilation, if the patient with ARF is alert or begins to improve, agitation is the rule (i.e., fear, anxiety, disorientation, inability to speak, etc.). In these instances calm, sympathetic (but firm) reassurance by the nurse or physician usually will solve the problem. If the agitation persists, care must be taken to make sure that the patient and the ventilator are properly interfaced. Attention to the ventilator and some experimentation—i.e., inspiratory flow rate, cycling frequency, triggering sensitivity and endotracheal tube—often will identify the problem, and the **ventilator** can then be properly adjusted to match the patient's needs.

However, the occurrence of sudden agitation and fighting of the ventilator in a previously calm patient suggests a significant change in clinical status and requires rapid assessment at the bedside. The most common problems encountered are: ventilator malfunction; complication of mechanical ventilation (pneumothorax, pulmonary edema, pulmonary embolism, pneumonia, etc.); airway obstruction (mucous plugging, atelectasis, bronchospasm); and, endotracheal tube malfunction (migration to region of vocal cords or above, kinking, cuff failure, secretion build-up, etc.).

Proper management requires the following steps: recognize the situation as acute clinical change rather than an annoyance; perform rapid bedside analysis; disconnect patient from the ventilator and "bag" (manual ventilation with self-inflating resuscitation bag); check vital signs (hypotensive?) and auscultate chest (equal breath sounds? wheezing?); check ventilator (all tubing connected? water in tubing? settings unchanged?) and check monitoring equipment; suction the airway and check status of endotracheal tube; obtain arterial blood gases; and **talk to the patient** (Are you getting enough air? Are you in pain? Do you need something else?). Only after completing this evaluation and trying various adjustments should sedation and paralysis be considered. In fact, muscle paralysis should be considered a last resort in ventilator management. Sedation with diazepam (2 to 5 mg, i.v., every 5 to 20 min) or morphine is preferred.

7. **Weaning from mechanical ventilation.** This is probably the most difficult management decision facing the ICU team caring for a patient on a ventilator. Strictly speaking, weaning means the **gradual withdrawal** over hours to days of ventilatory support. In some patients (drug overdose) weaning and extubation occur rapidly as the patient regains consciousness. In other patients, especially those with COPD and ARDS, where prolonged mechanical ventilation was required, weaning may take several days or weeks to accomplish, with many aborted attempts before successful extubation. Furthermore, a patient who meets the requirements for weaning may not meet those for extubation—i.e., chronic aspiration or severe obtundation (following head trauma) requiring prolonged tracheostomy.

   a. **Guidelines for weaning:** The patient should be **clinically improved**, with correction of associated disorders that may interfere with successful weaning (e.g., fluid overload, severe pain requiring analgesics or sedatives, electrolyte disturbances especially alkalemia, hypophosphatemia, and hypokalemia). The patient should be **alert** and cooperative, with **stable vital signs** and **intact gag reflexes.**

Patient's **physiologic function** should be compatible with "weanability," as follows: $Pa_{O_2} \geq 60$ mm Hg and $F_{I_{O_2}} \leq 50\%$ on the ventilator, with PEEP ≤ 5 cm H_2O; acceptable Pa_{CO_2} and pH; for patients with chronic hypercapnia prior to mechanical ventilation, this means a Pa_{CO_2} and pH similar to baseline; and adequate measures of ventilatory reserve and inspiratory muscle strength. Although some patients should be weaned even if these criteria are not met (e.g., COPD), the following are general guidelines:

(1) **Vital capacity** ≥ 10 to 15 ml/kg body weight and **tidal volume** >5 ml/kg body weight predict adequate spontaneous lung inflation and effective cough.

(2) **Maximum peak inspiratory pressure** greater than -25 cm H_2O indicates adequate muscle strength and neuromuscular coordination for spontaneous ventilation.

(3) **Minute ventilation** (V_E) of less than 10 liter/min and **maximum voluntary ventilation** (MVV) greater than $2 \times V_E$ suggest that the patient is able to increase ventilation in response to a further increase in demand, i.e., increased CO_2 production.

(4) An **alveolar-arterial oxygen gradient** [$P(A - a)O_2$] of less than 350 mm Hg on $F_{I_{O_2}}$ of 100% or a $Pa_{O_2} \geq 60$ mm Hg on an $F_{I_{O_2}} \leq 40\%$ suggests that adequate oxygen delivery will be maintained even if Pa_{O_2} falls initially.

b. **Methods of weaning**

(1) **Traditional or T-tube technique:** Initiate weaning **early in the morning** when full staff is available. Make sure the patient fulfills the **criteria outlined above** and understands the purpose of the procedure. **Do not give analgesics or sedations**, if possible. **Suction and position appropriately** (sitting or semiupright). Obtain **baseline** vital signs and arterial blood gases. **Attach T-piece** with same $F_{I_{O_2}}$ and humidification (unless Pa_{O_2} marginal, then increase $F_{I_{O_2}}$ by at least 10%). **Observe and reassure patient.** Do not leave the patient unattended. Monitor vital signs frequently.

Obtain arterial blood gases after 15 to 30 min. If patient begins to fail (i.e., intolerable dyspnea, hypotension (>20 mm Hg), tachycardia (>30/min), depressed mental status, or arrhythmia), obtain arterial blood gas if possible and return patient to ventilator. If the patient tolerates the initial T-tube trial (1 to 2 hr), **extubation** may be performed in selected cases. Most often the patient is given progressively longer weaning periods until off ventilator for 4 to 6 hr without problems. Most patients with COPD require repeated short trials (often only 5 to 15 min followed by return to ventilator). At night the patient is returned to the ventilator and allowed to rest. After a while the patient will be able to tolerate longer periods (4 to 6 hr) without mechanical ventilation, and then extubation should be considered. When using any weaning technique care should be taken not to exhaust the patient.

(2) **IMV technique** allows the patient to be slowly withdrawn from the

mechanical ventilator without manipulation of the tubing. (See III. D.). The fixed ventilator rate is reduced by one to two breaths per minute at 1- to 2-hr intervals according to how well this is tolerated by the patient. It is useful to follow similar parameters as outlined above. Arterial blood gases should be obtained at frequent intervals. The major **disadvantages** of this procedure are: IMV can increase the work of breathing; unnecessarily prolong the weaning period because the rate is not adjusted properly; and, most importantly, it gives the staff a false sense of security, and the patient is **not** watched carefully (because the patient is on the ventilator) with potentially disastrous results.

c. **The "unweanable" patient.** Most patients can be withdrawn successfully from ventilatory support when the principles outlined above are followed. Weaning failure often occurs because basic principles of assessment are not employed, and the patient is not ready for weaning since the underlying disease process has not been resolved. Other common causes of weaning failure include the following:

(1) **Respiratory muscle failure. Neuromuscular dysfunction** (e.g., myasthenia or myasthenia-like syndrome) was inapparent before weaning trial started. (Aminoglycosides rarely cause such weakness and should be stopped if possible.) **Electrolyte imbalances** are common and need to be corrected before weaning (especially depletion of potassium, calcium, phosphate, and magnesium). **Malnutrition** is common, and a period of hyperalimentation (either oral or parenteral) may be required before weaning can be attempted. Semistarvation causes both muscular weakness and depressed ventilatory drives.

(2) **Alkalosis** (pH >7.45) is the most common cause of depressed drive to breathe. In such patients respiratory alkalosis and metabolic alkalosis (diuresis and gastric suctioning) are common. Occasionally patients with chronic CO_2 retention are hyperventilated during ventilatory support and develop a reduced Pa_{CO_2} and a slower fall in bicarbonate. When weaning is tried, the patient cannot sustain this level of Pa_{CO_2}, and a sudden retention of CO_2 occurs, leading to a mixed respiratory acidosis and occasionally inducing cardiac arrhythmias and cardiac arrest. Therefore, chronic CO_2-retainers should be ventilated at levels consistent with their baseline arterial blood gases, and when discontinued from the ventilator, the $F_{I_{O_2}}$ should not be excessive.

(3) The continued need for **narcotic analgesics** and other sedating drugs will depress ventilation and make weaning difficult. In some patients extubation actually decreases agitation and the need for sedatives.

(4) Patients with very **high ventilatory requirements** (minute ventilation >10 liter/min and normal Pa_{CO_2}) may not be able to sustain respiration for prolonged periods. Therefore, causes of high CO_2 production (hyperalimentation and sepsis) or increased dead-space ventilation (pulmonary emboli or ARDS) should be sought and managed. Measurement of CO_2 production and calculation of the V_D/V_T ratio can help gauge the relative contribution of these two problems.

(5) If a patient is being ventilated with an **endotracheal tube** less than 7 mm internal diameter, this may need to be changed (preferably ≥8 mm internal diameter) because it increases the work of breathing.

(6) **Other problems** that affect tissue oxygen delivery should be corrected—fever, anemia, heart failure, hypovolemia, infection.

8. **Extubation.** This is the final step facing the patient after successful weaning from mechanical ventilation. Successful extubation requires a cooperative patient who understands the procedure and is reassured that reintubation will be instituted if necessary. If possible, extubation should be performed early in the day when staff is at full strength. A person expert in intubation (and the equipment necessary) should be readily available. The patient should be suctioned carefully (through the airway and above the cuff) and positioned appropriately (semierect). Vital signs and baseline arterial blood gases should be known. The patient should be hyperventilated with two or three deep breaths and the cuff deflated with the suction catheter in the trachea. Extubation should be performed quickly and high-humidity oxygen administered. Vital signs should be rechecked and evidence of laryngospasm noted (inspiratory stridor). Arterial blood gases should be obtained in 15 to 30 min.

Reintubate if patient develops mental obtundation, uncontrolled laryngospasm, or progressive hypoxemia, hypercarbia, or acidosis. **Postextubation complications** include hoarseness, difficulty swallowing, and rarely, severe glottic edema causing laryngospasm (treat with racemic epinephrine 0.5 ml in 3 ml saline via aerosol).

BIBLIOGRAPHY

Bone, R. C. (1982): Symposium on adult respiratory distress syndrome. *Clin. Chest Med.*, 3:1–215.

Bone, R. C. (1983): Symposium on respiratory failure. *Med. Clin. North Am.*, 67:549–750.

Dorinsky, P. M. and Whitcomb, M. E. (1983): The effect of PEEP on cardiac output. *Chest*, 84:210–216.

Hudson, L. D. (1981): Adult respiratory distress syndrome. *Semin. Resp. Med.*, 2:99–172.

Kryger, M., Bode, F., Antic, R., and Anthonisen, N. (1976): Diagnosis of obstruction of the upper and central airway. *Am. J. Med.*, 61:85–93.

Luce, J. M., Pierson, D. J., and Hudson, L. D. (1981): Intermittent mandatory ventilation. *Chest*, 79:678–685.

Meehan, R. T., and Zavala, D. C. (1982): The pathophysiology of acute high altitude illness *Am. J. Med.*, 73:395–403.

Pierson, D. J. (1982): Acute respiratory failure. In: *Pulmonary Emergencies*, edited by S. A. Sahn. Churchill Livingstone, New York.

Sahn, S. A., Lakshminarayan, S., and Petty, T. L. (1976): Weaning from mechanical ventilation. *JAMA*, 235:2208–2212.

Staub, N. C. (1974): Pulmonary edema. *Physiol. Rev.*, 54:678–811.

Stauffer, J. L. (1982): Tracheal intubation. In: *Pulmonary Emergencies*, edited by S. A. Sahn. Churchill Livingstone, New York.

Timms, R. M., Kvale, P. A., Anthonisen, N. R., et al. (1981): Selection of patients with chronic obstructive pulmonary disease for long-term oxygen therapy. *JAMA*, 245:2514–2515.

West, J. B. (1977): *Pulmonary Pathophysiology—The Essentials*. Williams and Wilkins, Baltimore.

Wood, L. D. H. and Prewitt, R. M. (1981): Cardiovascular management in acute hypoxemic respiratory failure. *Am. J. Cardiol.*, 47:963–972.

9.

Pulmonary Diseases

Talmadge E. King, Jr.

9.

Pulmonary Diseases

I. CHRONIC AIRFLOW OBSTRUCTION The most common lung diseases are those caused by chronic airflow obstruction. Asthma, chronic bronchitis, emphysema, cystic fibrosis, and bronchiectasis constitute the majority of these processes. Because they so often occur together, **chronic bronchitis** (chronic cough and sputum production for 3 months out of a year during 2 consecutive years) and **emphysema** (destruction of pulmonary parenchyma with loss of elastic recoil) are usually grouped together under the term **chronic obstructive pulmonary disease (COPD).**

A. Clinical Presentation COPD is a clinical syndrome characterized by breathlessness and objective evidence of airflow obstruction on spirometry. Most patients develop symptoms (cough, recurrent infection, or dyspnea) between ages 30 and 50. However, most will have had minor symptoms (e.g., smoker's cough) for years prior to presentation. Cigarette smoking is the most important risk factor.

   1. The **diagnosis** of COPD depends on the stage of the disease at the time of **presentation**; i.e., productive cough, dyspnea with exertion, bronchospasm, recurrent "colds," are common early manifestations.

   2. Spirometry usually reveals limitation to expiratory airflow at all lung volumes; i.e., forced expiratory volume in one second (FEV_1) is reduced, and the ratio of the FEV_1 to the forced vital capacity (FVC) is also reduced (<75%).

   3. The **chest radiograph** may be helpful in the diagnosis of **emphysema** as suggested by hyperinflation, flattening of the hemidiaphragms, avascularity of the lungs, enlargement of the retrosternal space, and the presence of bullae; **bronchitis** is indicated by increased bronchovascular markings, increase in the size of the pulmonary arteries, and cardiac enlargement.

   4. Arterial blood gases in patients with mild to moderate COPD will usually have a low Pa_{O_2} and normal or slightly low Pa_{CO_2}. The $P(A-a)O_2$ gradient (see Chapter 8) is widened, secondary to abnormal matching of ventilation and perfusion.

B. Management Therapy of COPD is primarily directed at controlling the symptoms, predisposing factors, and complications. Although chronic bronchitis and emphysema can be treated by similar regimens, it is an error to oversimplify the management. Care should be taken to identify the predominant pathophysiologic process, especially those components of the disease that are potentially reversible (e.g., bronchospasm, inflammation, and airway secretions). Patients with emphysema frequently do not have reversible bronchospasm and are not hypoxemic until late in the course. On the other hand, the true bronchitic frequently has significant reversible bronchospasm, moderate-to-severe hypoxemia, hypercapnia, and pulmonary hypertension.

Patients with COPD may present with several clinical pictures: **early** management for breathlessness or cough; during an **acute exacerbation** manifested by worsening dyspnea, fatigue, productive cough (usually thick, tenacious sputum), wheezing, hypoxemia, and signs of cor pulmonale; and, full-blown **respiratory failure.** The management of acute respiratory failure secondary to COPD is discussed in Chapter 8 (section II. B.). The following emphasizes the key principles of **long-term management.**

1. **Patient education** is unquestionably the most important aspect of any treatment protocol. The patient must be taught the basics of respiratory anatomy and physiology, as well as how to deal with the psychological stresses of a chronic illness. **Smoking cessation** must be stressed at every visit to every patient regardless of age. The cessation of smoking will result in a definite beneficial response (decrease cough and sputum) and can make the difference between a relatively normal life span and premature death in those patients susceptible to the ill effects of smoking.

2. Measures must be taken to **reduce the work of breathing** caused by airway obstruction.

   a. **Relieve the bronchospasm:**

      (1) **Bronchodilators** are the mainstay in the management of reactive airway disease. Since most patients with COPD have some component of bronchospasm complicating their disease, all patients should be given a **defined trial of bronchodilators.** Appropriate subjective and objective evaluation of the results and side effects of bronchodilators is essential. Furthermore, the drugs should be withdrawn if some modification in dyspnea, bronchopulmonary secretions, or pulmonary function cannot be demonstrated (see Asthma).

      (2) **Corticosteroids** (prednisone 20 to 40 mg p.o. q.d.) should be prescribed in patients with

         (a) Bronchospasm refractory to optimal bronchodilator therapy.

         (b) Sputum and blood eosinophilia (with sputum eosinophilia being a better indicator of steroid responsiveness).

         (c) Improvement in the FEV_1 of 30% or more above the baseline value in response to inhaled bronchodilator, or an increase in the FVC following a trial course of the drug.

         (d) Improvement in exercise tolerance and subjective parameters.

         Following the response to steroids (by spirometry 3 to 4 weeks after instituting therapy) is absolutely essential. Responders should be continued on the lowest effective steroid dose (usually 20 mg/day), and it should be discontinued in nonresponders. Inhaled corticosteroids have no documented role in COPD but are occasionally employed in steroid responders in an attempt to avoid the many complications of systemic therapy.

   b. **Reduce the secretions:**

      (1) Remove all possible **irritants**.

(2) **Oral hydration** should be encouraged.

(3) **Antibiotics** are important agents in the treatment as well as the prophylaxis of acute purulent exacerbations of chronic bronchitis. However, most exacerbations appear to be initiated by viral infections and then become secondarily infected by bacteria. Therefore, the self-administration of antibiotics is desirable and safe in the properly instructed patient (change in the color or consistency of sputum). Ampicillin, tetracycline, erythromycin, or trimethoprim-sulfamethoxazole are the agents of choice. When pneumonia is present, intravenous antibiotics should be guided by: the clinical presentation; radiographic appearance; and, the predominant organism on sputum Gram stain and culture (blood or sputum).

(4) **Chest physiotherapy** (postural drainage and percussion) is recommended for patients with chronic bronchitis who produce large amounts of secretions (>30 ml of sputum daily). Supplemental oxygen should be used during the procedure to prevent hypoxemia.

(5) **Physical conditioning** and **breathing retraining** (pursed-lip breathing and abdominal augmentation) are important modalities because they improve exercise performance. This response evokes a general sense of well-being, increased motivation, and a positive self-image.

3. **Oxygen therapy.** There is no question of the importance of oxygen therapy in acute respiratory failure. Furthermore, there is increasing evidence that **long-term controlled oxygen therapy** will improve exercise tolerance, alleviate pulmonary hypertension, cor pulmonale, and secondary polycythemia, and improve the cognitive function and general well-being of hypoxemic COPD patients. Thus, long-term oxygen therapy is beneficial when: (a) severe and persistent hypoxemia (PaO_2 55 mm Hg or less) is present at rest or (b) there is clinical evidence of chronic hypoxemia (mental impairment, markedly deteriorating exercise capacity, pulmonary hypertension, cor pulmonale, or right ventricular failure) and sleep hypoxemia. Oxygen therapy should be instituted only after the patient has received aggressive management to improve the hypoxemia, directed at secretions, bronchospasms, and infection. **Continuous therapy** is more efficacious than nocturnal therapy, especially in those patients with severely altered pulmonary and cerebral function. A minority of COPD patients will have only sleep hypoxemia. These patients usually have unexplained erythrocytosis or rarely cor pulmonale. Therefore, measurement of PaO_2 during sleep or continuous monitoring of oxygen saturation is required to identify nocturnal hypoxemia.

4. **Additional treatment modalities:**

   a. **Sedatives** and **tranquilizers** should be avoided because of the potential respiratory depression that can occur.

   b. **Immunization** against influenza and pneumococci is recommended for patients with COPD.

   c. **Diuretics** and **digitalis** should be avoided except when left ventricular failure is present. Care must be taken to treat any underlying metabolic problems (especially electrolyte imbalances) before these agents are utilized.

    d. Repeated **phlebotomy is rarely indicated in the management of secondary polycythemia if appropriate oxygen therapy is instituted.**

    e. Intermittent positive-pressure breathing (IPPB) has no documented role in the management of ambulatory or hospitalized COPD patients.

5. Hospitalization. Because patients with COPD have frequent episodes of acute exacerbation, it is often difficult to decide when to hospitalize them. No firm rules can apply but useful guidelines for hospital admission include:

    a. Any patient with impaired mental status.

    b. The presence of fever, chest pain, marked fatigue, or exhaustion, new changes on the chest roentgenogram, presence of dehydration, and/or hypotension.

    c. Severe tachypnea and a normal $PaCO_2$ or marked CO_2 retention compared to previous arterial blood gases.

    d. Any patient living alone or with no one available to supervise him closely.

When evaluating a patient, it is important to get information from the family regarding the baseline level of function (mental and physical). Also, previous arterial blood gas measurements (especially baseline, asymptomatic values), pulmonary function tests, and response to treatment should be sought, since they can often guide current management.

C. Cor Pulmonale Complicating COPD Chronic hypoxemia and acidosis cause pulmonary hypertension that can lead to right heart failure. In addition to treatment directed at infection and bronchospasm, **oxygen therapy** is the critical treatment in decompensated COPD with progressive cor pulmonale. Digitalis and diuretics have only a limited role in management because of the potential complications (cardiac arrhythmias and respiratory depression caused by diuretic-induced metabolic alkalosis). Pulmonary thromboembolism is a frequent cause of clinical deterioration in this setting. Severe polycythemia (hematocrit>70%) occasionally complicates cor pulmonale, and phlebotomy may be indicated to reduce the afterload on the right ventricle.

II. SLEEP APNEA HYPERSOMNOLENCE SYNDROME

A. Diagnosis Disordered respiratory function during sleep has been increasingly recognized over the last decade. Two major categories have been defined: **Obstructive apnea** (cessation of breathing for>10 sec) characterized by no flow of air at the nose or mouth, although cyclic respiratory efforts persist (and often increase in intensity), and snoring is frequently present. Less commonly, **central apneas** are manifested by the absence of any respiratory efforts. Both situations, obstructive and central apneas, result in alveolar hypoventilation, oxygen desaturation (decrease >4% is considered abnormal), and sleep deprivation. Most often these occur in some combination.

Diagnosis of this syndrome frequently requires a searching inquiry. Nocturnal insomnia, personality and intellectual changes, sexual dysfunction, daytime somnolence, morning headache, noisy snoring, unexplained pulmonary and systemic hypertension, and enuresis are associated problems that will sometimes alert the physician to this syndrome. Massively obese patients, those with COPD, men, postmenopausal women, and patients with anatomic variations that cause obstruction of the hypopharynx (e.g, hypognathia, pharyngeal or lingual tonsil hypertrophy, etc.) are predisposed to this problem.

B. Treatment   Treatment of this syndrome is important since many of the manifestations are reversible. **Obstructive sleep apnea** requires measures that will maintain the patency of the upper airway during sleep. **Weight reduction** is the primary mode of therapy in morbidly obese patients. **Agents that enhance ventilatory responsiveness**—e.g., medroxyprogesterone acetate (20 mg three times a day) or protriptyline (20 mg, p.o., at bedtime)—have met with limited success in a few patients with obstructive sleep apnea. The application of continuous positive pressure by a **face mask** has been reported to be a useful method to keep the upper airway open. However, when life-threatening cardiorespiratory events occur during sleep, **tracheostomy** is required. **Surgical correction** (i.e., removal of tonsillar and adenoid tissue) may improve the syndrome.

In patients with **central apneas**, diaphragmatic pacing via the phrenic nerve or a rocking bed may be helpful. The long-term efficacy of this approach remains to be fully evaluated. Patients with **primary alveolar hypoventilation** occasionally respond to medroxyprogesterone. **Sedatives** and **alcohol should be avoided** in these patients.

III. ACUTE ASTHMA AND STATUS ASTHMATICUS

A. Pathophysiology   Asthma is a chronic disease characterized by episodic shortness of breath (usually accompanied by wheezing and cough) due to hyperirritable airways and reversible airflow obstruction. The airflow obstruction is caused by bronchial smooth muscle spasm, mucosal edema, mucus hypersecretion, and subsequent narrowing and plugging of the bronchial tree. Most episodes of acute asthma resolve uneventfully following the institution of therapy. However, severe respiratory failure and sudden death can occur. Most symptomatic asthmatic episodes are precipitated by nonallergenic stimuli, such as viral respiratory infection, environmental irritants (sulfur dioxide), exercise, and cold air. In some patients, environmental allergens, emotional distress, and drugs (aspirin) will tend to precipitate symptoms. Also, a rising number of occupationally related agents are being recognized as causes of acute attacks. "All that wheezes is not asthma," therefore; other processes should be considered, including pulmonary edema, large-airway obstruction (tumor or foreign body), anaphylaxis, pulmonary embolism, and vocal cord dysfunction. The keys to successful management of asthma are: an organized approach aimed at **recognizing the severity** of an attack; and appropriate **administration of specific** (and adequate) **therapy** known to reverse the majority of episodes.

B. Diagnosis of Acute Asthma   Most patients with acute asthma are readily recognized. What may not be obvious is the severity of the attack. Fortunately, most patients will not experience a life-threatening attack. **Oxygen** should be promptly administered in all patients with an acute attack (2 to 6 liter/min by nasal prongs) to treat the hypoxemia that frequently accompanies these attacks.

1. **History. How and when did the episode start?** A rapid progression suggests severe disease. **Have there been previous attacks of severe asthma and is this similar or different?** The majority of patients who have an acute attack will have experienced similar episodes. **Can precipitating factor(s) be identified?** Respiratory tract infection or a recent change in drug regimen are found commonly. **What medications has the patient been taking?** Are aspirin or other drugs likely to have induced the attack? Also, it is important to record the specific medications (and quantity) the patient has taken to control this attack. **Any known allergies? Are there other diseases present that might require an alteration in therapy, especially cardiac disease?**

2. **Physical examination.** Rapid assessment aimed at the following should be performed initially: temperature; respiratory rate and effort (accessory muscles, signs of inspiratory muscle fatigue; see Chapter 8); blood pressure (hypertension common during acute attack, pulsus paradoxus > 20 mm Hg suggest severe asthma); chest examination (rales suggest cardiac failure; wheezing does not correlate with severity; unilateral wheezing may represent endobronchial lesion or pneumothorax); mental status (impaired consciousness suggests cerebral hypoxia or acidemia).

3. **Laboratory examination**

   a. **Bedside spirometry,** FVC and FEV_1, should be performed immediately, if available, and the patient can cooperate. **Peak expiratory flow rate** (PEFR) obtained using a peak flow meter or gauge is also helpful (<100 liter/min is correlated with severe obstruction). These values are useful as a baseline indication of severity (Table 1) and can be used to determine therapeutic response.

   b. **Arterial blood gases** are probably required only when the asthmatic attack is severe—i.e., PEFR or FEV_1 less than 70% of predicted. A $Pao_2 \leqslant 60$ mm Hg suggests severe airflow obstruction. The $Paco_2$ is decreased and the pH increased in most symptomatic patients. Therefore, a $Paco_2$ in the normal range (35 to 45 mm Hg), associated with a pH<7.35, suggests severe airflow obstruction with impaired alveolar ventilation and inspiratory muscle fatigue.

TABLE 1. *Indicators of severe asthmatic attack*

History of previous status asthmaticus
Disturbances of consciousness; obvious exhaustion; silent chest; severe dyspnea; accessory-muscle use; moderately severe wheezing
Poor airflow: $FEV_1 \leqslant 0.5$ liter; FVC < 1.0 liter; PEFR < 100 liter/min
Abnormal arterial blood gases:
    $Pao_2 \leqslant 55$ mm Hg (or central cyanosis)
    $Paco_2 \geqslant 45$ mm Hg and/or pH <7.35
Pulsus paradoxus (>15 to 20 mm Hg); respiratory rate >30 breaths/min; pulse rate > 120 beats/min
Complications present: EKG abnormalities, pneumothorax, pneumomediastinum
Inadequate response to bronchodilator therapy within 15 min

c. **Other tests.** A **chest roentgenogram** is probably needed only when admission to the hospital is planned to exclude pneumonia, pneumothorax, pneumomediastinum, mucoid impaction, and atelectasis. Other routine tests (complete blood count, sputum smears, electrocardiogram) should be obtained as clinically indicated.

C. **Treatment**   After the initiation of oxygen therapy to relieve the hypoxemia, management is directed at the so-called "ABCs of asthma": intravenous aminophylline, beta-adrenergic medications, and corticosteroids.

1. **Acute asthma**

a. **Oxygen** 2 to 6 liters/min is required because bronchodilators can cause worsening of V/Q mismatch leading to a fall in the Pao_2.

b. **Intravenous fluids** (200 to 300 ml/hr) may be required to prevent or treat dehydration, loosen secretions, prevent mucus impaction, and maintain intravascular volume.

c. **Bronchodilator therapy.** Recent studies suggest beta-adrenergic medications as the first-line drug for controlling asthma. If the patient can tolerate **inhaled** therapy, **one** of the following can be given:

(1) **Albuterol** (metered-dose inhaler 0.09 mg/puff) two inhalations every 4 to 6 hr.

(2) **Metaproterenol sulfate** 0.3 ml diluted in 2.5 ml saline or water via nebulizer; or two inhalations via metered-dose inhaler every 4 to 6 hr.

(3) **Isoetharine mesylate** 0.5 ml in 2.5 ml saline or water every 2 to 4 hr via a nebulizer.

In the emergency room, these drugs can be repeated (once or twice) within 15 to 30 min if no improvement occurs.

In severely dyspneic patients, **parenteral sympathomimetic therapy** is preferred:

(1) **Epinephrine** (0.3 ml to 0.5 ml of 1:1,000 solution) is given subcutaneously and may be repeated two or three times at 15- to 30-min intervals if no improvement occurs; **or,**

(2) **Terbutaline sulfate** (0.25 to 0.5 mg) subcutaneously every 4 to 6 hr; in acute situations it may be repeated after 15 to 30 min.

These drugs (even the beta-2 agents) must be used cautiously in elderly patients because of the potential for serious **adverse reaction** (myocardial ischemia, arrhythmias, and systemic hypertension). **No more than one drug should be used at a time.** Furthermore, extreme care should be taken if the patient has used beta-adrenergic agents earlier in the course of the acute episode. Tachyphylaxis may occur in patients given excessive amounts of beta-adrenergic agents. The patient who fails to respond to beta-adrenergic medication should be given aminophylline.

Intravenous aminophylline (a form of theophylline) has long been one of the mainstays of asthma therapy. This drug alone will control many episodes but is considered to be less effective in the initial therapy of an acute attack compared to inhaled or parenteral beta-adrenergic agents. However, there appear to be therapeutic advantages in combining theophylline and an oral beta-adrenergic agonist in the treatment of asthma.

If the patient is currently **taking a theophylline preparation**, then:

(1) A theophylline level should be obtained immediately.

(2) Aminophylline should be started at an i.v. infusion rate of 0.2 to 0.8 mg/kg/hr while awaiting the results (once the level is known, adjustments can be made in the level of infusion). If the patient is **not taking a theophylline preparation**, then give a **loading dose**, 3 to 6 mg/kg, i.v., over 20 min; start maintenance infusion, 0.2 to 0.8 mg/kg/hr.

The maintenance dose and infusion rate should be lower in patients with congestive heart failure (0.2 mg/kg/hr), liver disease, advanced age, or severe COPD (0.4 mg/kg/hr), or in those concurrently taking those medications that decrease theophylline clearance, such as cimetidine, erythromycin, or propranolol. Smokers (0.8 mg/kg/hr) and children require increased infusion rates.

Theophylline toxicity generally correlates with the serum levels. Therefore, a blood level should be measured after 24 hr of constant infusion and the dosage adjusted to achieve a level of 10 to 20 μg/ml.

d. If no improvement occurs after 1 to 2 hr of intravenous aminophylline (and beta-adrenergic therapy), then intravenous **corticosteroids** should be instituted (hydrocortisone 100 mg every 6 hr or its equivalent). Inhaled corticosteroids should not be used in the acute management of asthma. If there is no improvement after 6 to 12 hr, the corticosteroid doses can be doubled until control has been established. This form of acute therapy has limited side effects and occasionally is effective in breaking an acute asthmatic episode. **Long-term, high-dose corticosteroid therapy should be avoided.** Therefore, after the acute episode is controlled, oral prednisone should be administered (50 to 100 mg/day) and rapidly tapered over a week or two, as tolerated.

e. **Other therapeutic modalities. Antibiotics** should be administered (e.g., tetracycline 250 to 500 mg q.i.d.) when fever, pneumonia, or purulent sputum is present. Sputum cultures should be obtained and the regimen adjusted if appropriate. **Physiotherapy** (chest percussion and suctioning) may be useful if the patient cannot raise secretions. However, some patients may not tolerate these procedures. **Sedation** should be **avoided**, since the agitation will resolve with effective management of the bronchospasm.

Effective **inhaled bronchodilator therapy** requires **trained personnel** (including the prescribing physician) who know how to give inhaled therapy and can demonstrate the proper technique. Success depends on the **dose** of aerosol administered and the **site** of aerosol deposition in the lungs. It usually takes 5 to 15 min for aerosol preparations to exert a bronchodilatory effect; therefore, pulmonary function tests should not be obtained before that time. The following method of inhalation with a **metered aerosol device** is suggested:

(1) Encourage patient to empty his or her lungs as fully as possible through forced expiration.

(2) The inhaler should be shaken well and placed into the wide-open mouth (it can be placed between the lips, but care must be taken to avoid occluding the mouthpiece or obstructing air flow).

(3) The patient should inhale a puff of the aerosol using a **slow, deep** inhalation, and then hold his breath for about 10 sec before exhaling.

(4) Slow exhalation through pursed lips or through the nose is preferred.

(5) After 10 to 15 min of rest the procedure should be repeated.

Excessive use of aerosols should be discouraged.

Care should be taken to avoid aspirin-containing compounds, acetylcysteine, ultrasonic nebulizers, IPPB, inhaled corticosteroids, cromolyn sodium, sedatives, transtracheal aspiration, and cool mist.

2. **Status asthmaticus** is an acute attack of asthma unresponsive to conservative therapy. It is a serious, life-threatening illness requiring hospitalization and intensive therapy. In fact, many patients with status asthmaticus have been symptomatic for several days or even weeks, and a few represent inadequately managed patients who have made several trips to the emergency room with incomplete resolution of the airflow obstruction. The presence of a **silent chest** in a symptomatic asthmatic is an ominous sign (see Table 1).

The **therapy of status asthmaticus** must be tailored to each individual, but basically it involves the management principles presented above for acute asthma. **Inhaled atropine** (1 mg via nebulizer every 3 to 4 hr) also may be helpful, especially in patients with severe cough. Other modalities have been tried, such as **intravenous isoproterenol** (0.1 μg/kg/min), **rectal ether, general anesthesia**, and **bronchopulmonary lavage**.

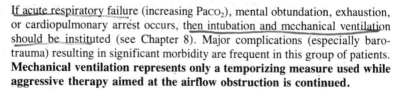 If acute respiratory failure (increasing Paco$_2$), mental obtundation, exhaustion, or cardiopulmonary arrest occurs, then intubation and mechanical ventilation should be instituted (see Chapter 8). Major complications (especially barotrauma) resulting in significant morbidity are frequent in this group of patients. **Mechanical ventilation represents only a temporizing measure used while aggressive therapy aimed at the airflow obstruction is continued.**

3. **Chronic asthma management.** Care must be taken to identify and avoid the known **precipitating factors.** The drug regimen should be adjusted appropriately. If the patient failed to respond to a single agent, then an additional bronchodilator should be added (e.g., poor response to an inhaled beta agonist requires the addition of a theophylline preparation). If the patient required a beta-adrenergic agent, theophylline, and corticosteroids, then this regimen should be continued following the acute episode and the corticosteroids withdrawn over days or weeks. If the patient develops worsening symptoms during corticosteroid withdrawal, an alternate-day therapeutic regimen should be attempted. Furthermore, **inhaled corticosteroids** (beclomethasone) may be

used and occasionally will allow the withdrawal of orally administered corticosteroids, thereby reducing the systemic side-effects of corticosteroid therapy.

Cromolyn sodium is not used in the management of acute asthma but is useful as prophylaxis for both extrinsic and intrinsic asthma (especially exercise- or cold-induced asthma).

4. **Allergic bronchopulmonary aspergillosis** is a disease that occurs in asthmatics because of the colonization of the tracheobronchial tree by *Aspergillus fumigatus*, leading to a hypersensitivity reaction. It is characterized by asthma, eosinophilia, shifting pulmonary infiltrates, markedly elevated serum IgE, serum precipitins, and positive skin test reactivity to *Aspergillus* antigen. Mucoid impaction leading to proximal bronchiectasis occurs with progressive disease. Systemic corticosteroids are the mainstay of therapy.

5. **Anaphylaxis** is an IgE-mediated life-threatening syndrome triggered by a drug, a food, diagnostic agents (e.g., iodinated contrast materials), or an insect bite. Symptoms vary from mild skin reactions to acute upper airway obstruction (laryngeal edema or laryngospasm), status asthmaticus, or vascular collapse (occasionally in the absence of respiratory symptoms). Management consists mainly of epinephrine (0.2 to 0.5 ml of 1:1,000 dilution subcutaneously or intramuscularly) every 15 to 30 min as necessary (usually 2 to 3 doses). In severe cases intravenous epinephrine (1 ml bolus of 1:1,000 every 3 to 5 min to a total dose of 5 to 10 mg) and massive fluid replacement may be required. Sublingual or endotracheal administration of epinephrine can be effective when an intravenous line cannot be established. Antihistamines and corticosteroids should be administered to patients with severe symptoms. Aminophylline is indicated for bronchospasm, and intubation and ventilation for respiratory failure. Shock requires appropriate measures including fluids and vasopressors (dopamine, 2 to 50 μg/kg/min). Hospitalization for 6 to 12 hr of observation is required in any patient with an anaphylactic or anaphylactoid (release of chemical mediators by nonantigenic agents) reaction.

IV. INHALATION INJURY OF THE LUNGS

A. **Pulmonary Aspiration** Pulmonary aspiration is a common complication in medical and surgical patients. **Prevention** is the key to management. Conditions that predispose to aspiration include altered consciousness (alcoholism, drug abuse, use of sedatives, cardiopulmonary arrest, general anesthesia, strokes), dysphagia (esophageal disorders), and mechanical disruption of defense barriers (nasogastric tubes and tracheostomies). The aspiration syndromes can be divided into three forms based on the pathophysiologic features, the clinical presentation, and the therapeutic approach.

1. **Aspiration of gastric contents (chemical pneumonitis).** This form usually occurs in patients with altered consciousness or impaired cough or gag reflex. The **onset is usually acute** (1 to 5 hr) and is manifested by fever, dyspnea, tachypnea, and diffuse rales. In approximately one-third of patients, cough, cyanosis, bronchospasm and apnea occur and are particularly **ominous signs**. Moderate to severe **hypoxemia** is common. The chest roentgenograms may be normal immediately following the acute event and progress to localized or diffuse alveolar infiltrates (including ARDS). Prominent **interstitial changes**

may result from chronic aspiration. The severity of the injury depends on the **quantity** of material aspirated and the **pH** of the aspirated material (i.e., pH<2.5 causes acid injury). The pH of normal fasting gastric juice is between 1.5 and 2.4.

The majority of patients recover with conservative **airway** and **fluid manage-ment,** particularly if care is taken to prevent a recurrence. **Oxygen therapy** to prevent hypoxemia and **inhaled bronchodilators** to manage bronchospasm are frequently required. A small number progress to severe respiratory distress (ARDS) and require aggressive ventilatory management (see Chapter 8). Emer-gency **bronchoscopy** may be required to remove particulate material. Corti-costeroids and prophylactic antibiotics have not been proved to be beneficial. However, superimposed bacterial pneumonia in patients with acid aspiration carries considerable morbidity and mortality. Therefore, the recurrence of fever, purulent sputum, leukocytosis, new or expanding pulmonary infiltrates, unexplained clinical deterioration, increasing hypoxemia, and pathogens in sputum should prompt appropriate antimicrobial therapy.

2. **Aspiration of foreign bodies** is most common in children. Other causes of upper airway obstruction include infection, tumor, trauma, laryngeal edema or laryngospasm (see Chapter 8). The manifestations and management deci-sions are based primarily on the site of obstruction. **Large objects** (e.g., a meat chunk) can obstruct the larynx (at the level of the vocal cords), trachea, or mainstem bronchus and produce symptoms of asphyxia ("cafe coronary"). Management requires rapid identification of the problem and utilization of the **Heimlich maneuver** (four back blows followed by four manual thrusts—i.e., a quick upward thrust over the abdomen causing a sudden elevation of the diaphragm and forcing air through the trachea). If the necessary equipment is available, an attempt can be made to remove the foreign body by **direct visualization with a laryngoscope**. Removal by sweeping with the index finger across the posterior pharynx should be attempted but has the risk of impacting the material deeper into the airway. If this fails, an emergency tracheostomy is required.

   Smaller objects may migrate to more distal sites within the tracheobronchial tree (especially down the right mainstem bronchus). Patients usually present with hoarseness or cough. Occasionally, involvement of the major bronchi leads to severe dyspnea, cyanosis, and localized wheezing. The chest roent-genograms usually will show atelectasis or obstructive emphysema. Failure to remove the obstructing object within 2 to 3 weeks may result in recurrent pneumonitis, bronchiectasis, lung abscesses, and/or empyema (see below). **Bronchoscopy** is frequently successful in removing most objects. Some pa-tients aspirate large volumes of **inert fluids** (barium, saline, nasogastric feed-ing solutions) causing: transient, self-limited hypoxemia; and, simple mechanical obstruction. **Immediate tracheal suctioning** usually results in rapid resolu-tion, and further therapy should be aimed at prevention.

3. **Aspiration of infected material** is the most common form of aspiration pneumonia and is frequently insidious in onset, being recognized primarily by the clinical course in a susceptible host (preexisting gingivodental disease, episode of unconsciousness—i.e., seizure—alcoholic or debilitated patients).

The presentation is usually indistinguishable from that of common bacterial pneumonias (see Chapter 10). Often the chest reveals infiltrates in dependent pulmonary segments (especially right upper lobe posterior segment or right lower lobe superior segment). Late in the course (1 to 2 weeks after aspiration) patients may have necrotizing pneumonia, lung abscess and/or empyema formation.

Treatment is initially empirical based on whether the aspiration was **community-acquired** (penicillin 2 to 3 million U/day, or clindamycin) or **hospital-acquired** (coverage for aerobic or mixed aerobic-anaerobic infection, e.g., clindamycin plus an aminoglycoside) and must be confirmed and adjusted based on appropriate cultures [sputum (usually transtracheal aspirate to avoid oral flora), blood, and/or pleural fluid].

4. **Lung abscess** frequently is one of the late complications of pulmonary aspiration. The presentation often is insidious, with weight loss, low-grade fever, and copious foul-smelling sputum production being the prominent findings. **Diagnosis** requires

   a. Appropriate identification of the infecting agent (cultures of material obtained from transtracheal aspiration, blood, pleural fluid, and occasionally transthoracic needle aspiration).

   b. Exclusion of other causes of cavitary lung disease [tuberculosis, fungal infection, carcinoma, cavitary infarction (i.e., bland or septic embolism or vasculitis), infected cyst or bullae, etc.].

   c. Fiberoptic bronchoscopy to exclude an obstructing endobronchial lesion (tumor or foreign body).

   Therapy demands: **drainage** of the involved lung (postural drainage, steam inhalation, rarely transthoracic needle aspiration or tube drainage); and, **antibiotic therapy.** Penicillin is usually adequate. Patients with **mild symptoms** and no major medical problems can be given parenteral penicillin (procaine penicillin 600,000 U i.m. every 6 hr or aqueous penicillin G 5 to 10 million U/day, i.v., in divided doses) or oral penicillin (500 mg p.o. every 6 hr). Those given parenteral penicillin can be switched to oral penicillin if clinical improvement occurs over several days and continued on oral therapy until resolution of the cavity. In patients with **severe** symptomatic disease, therapy with intravenous aqueous penicillin (2 million U, i.v. every 4 hr) may be required for 5 to 10 days. If **empyema** is present, chest tube drainage is required (occasionally, thoracotomy with rib resection is necessary to drain loculated areas of pus). It should be noted that fever may persist for several days to 3 weeks despite adequate therapy, and it may take several more weeks for resolution of the cavity.

B. **Near-Drowning** Drowning is the third most common cause of accidental deaths in the United States. The majority of these victims aspirate water and other impurities. Therefore, treatment of near-drowning victims requires **management of the airway and treatment of the asphyxia** (hypoxemia, hypercarbia, and severe metabolic acidosis). Basic cardiopulmonary resuscitation (CPR) should be instituted immediately. **Endotracheal intubation** and **mechanical ventilation** with 100% oxygen should be instituted as soon as possible (PEEP should be considered if hypoxemia persists). Metabolic acidosis is almost always present; therefore, immediate intravenous therapy with **sodium bicarbonate** is important. Arterial blood gases should be obtained to guide further therapy. Management similar to that described for ARDS is needed (see Chapter 8). **Hypothermia** is frequently present and should be corrected. Severe hypothermia has a protective effect on central nervous system function; therefore, patients may have a remarkable recovery if aggressive resuscitative efforts are applied. The role of prophylactic antibiotics (pulmonary infection) and corticosteroids (cerebral edema) in the management of these patients is unclear.

C. Toxic Injury, Thermal Injury, and Smoke Inhalation

1. **Toxic injury** secondary to accidental exposure to high concentrations of irritant gases (e.g., nitrogen dioxide, chlorine, carbon dioxide, phosgene, sulfur dioxide, cyanide, ammonia, and hydrogen sulfide) is becoming a significant problem in our industrialized society. The major clinical manifestations are those associated with acute noncardiogenic pulmonary edema (see Chapter 8). Management is mainly supportive, and hospitalization is required in any patient with suspected lower respiratory tract injury, because latent periods of up to 12 to 24 hr may occur before the onset of chest symptoms. Furthermore, patients may recover from the acute episode only to develop bronchiolitis obliterans 2 to 6 weeks later. This complication may be aborted with high-dose steroids if begun immediately on recurrence of cough and dyspnea.

2. **Thermal injury and smoke inhalation.** The major causes of lung injury owing to smoke inhalation are thermal injury and inhalation of toxic fumes and particulate matter. The clinical presentation in smoke inhalation may range from mild cough and irritation to pulmonary edema or coma. Furthermore, the complications of smoke inhalation vary temporally but are fairly predictable. **Carbon monoxide poisoning** (see below) occurs early (0 to 8 hr) and is believed to be the major cause of death at the scene of the fire. **Thermal injury** causes capillary disruption, mucosal edema, and hemorrhage, which can produce upper airway obstruction (0 to 8 hr) requiring endotracheal intubation. Stridor is an ominous finding. **Toxic fumes** (and thermal injury) can cause bronchospasm, stridor, airway plugging (desquamated tissue and secretions), and atelectasis (0 to 24 hr). **Noncardiogenic pulmonary edema** (leading to ARDS) is a dreaded complication that usually manifests itself after 24 to 96 hr. Finally, **pneumonia** occurs in a minority of cases, usually after 4 to 5 days.

3. **Management** (see Chapter 8). **Airway management is the first priority.** Supplemental oxygen should be given to all victims until the situation is accurately defined.

Once in the emergency room or hospital, careful examination for evidence of **conjunctivitis** (suggests exposure to high concentration of irritant gases), signs of **thermal injury** (burns of face, singed nasal hairs, pharyngeal erythema), alterations of **mental status** (obtundation, confusion, or agitation suggest tissue hypoxia, which may be a manifestation of carbon monoxide poisoning or abnormal gas exchange), and signs of **pulmonary edema** (rales, abnormal chest X-ray) should be frequently sought.

Antibiotics should be given only when evidence of infection is suspected. Prophylactic antibiotic use is to be discouraged. **Corticosteroids** may be used on a **short-term** basis (24 to 48 hr) in the management of upper airway obstruction, pulmonary edema, or severe bronchospasm.

D. Carbon Monoxide Poisoning

1. **Clinical manifestations and diagnosis.** This colorless, odorless, but highly toxic gas binds avidly to hemoglobin (>210 times greater than oxygen) so that oxygen transport in the body is markedly impaired and tissue hypoxia results. The manifestations are related primarily to the level of carboxyhemoglobin present. Associated diseases, especially cardiac disease and other factors that influence oxygen demand and delivery, also determine the severity of the clinical findings. **Diagnosis** depends on **measurement of the carboxyhemoglobin levels or oxygen content.** Oxygen saturation should be measured directly and not calculated, since the arterial Pa_{O_2} usually is normal. At carboxyhemoglobin levels of **20% to 30%**, headache, nausea, vomiting, weakness, dizziness, and diminished visual acuity are prominent symptoms. At levels ⩾**40%** there is little correlation between the symptoms and signs and the blood carboxyhemoglobin level. Characteristically, the manifestations are related to the **brain** (coma, seizures, ataxia, diffuse and fluctuating neurologic deficits) and the **cardiac system** (syncope, EKG abnormalities, myocardial ischemia/infarction). A level >**60%** is associated with coma and death.

2. **Treatment.** The half-life of carboxyhemoglobin is 4 to 6 hr, but increased alveolar ventilation and high inspired oxygen concentrations will significantly alter the displacement of carbon monoxide. Therefore, the immediate institution of **oxygen** therapy (preferably 100% oxygen) is mandatory; this will improve tissue oxygen delivery and shorten the half-life of carboxyhemoglobin to 40 to 50 min. Intubation and mechanical ventilation may be required if the patient is hemodynamically unstable and/or hypoventilation is present. **Hyperbaric oxygen** will hasten the removal of carbon monoxide and should be utilized in the treatment of life-threatening cerebral or coronary hypoxia. Appropriate steps should be taken to manage any factor that will reduce tissue oxygen delivery or increase tissue oxygen demand (e.g., anemia, hypothermia, hypotension, fever, metabolic acidosis).

V. PULMONARY EMBOLISM

A. Diagnosis

1. Pulmonary embolism (PE) is the most common cause of death among the recognized pulmonary diseases. Unfortunately, the **clinical diagnosis** of PE is extremely difficult and unreliable. A high index of suspicion is important and requires an understanding of the many conditions that predispose to venous thrombosis: elderly patient, prolonged bed rest, congestive heart failure, venous insufficiency, recent pelvic or hip surgery, carcinoma, and oral contraceptive use.

2. The **signs and symptoms** of PE are dictated by the size and extent of the embolic episode and by the preexisting cardiopulmonary reserve. **Massive PE** is often characterized by syncope, chest pain, acute dyspnea, hypotension, and signs of pulmonary hypertension. With medium-size PE, pleuritic chest

pain, dyspnea, low grade fever, hemoptysis, pleural friction rub, diffuse wheezing, or findings of pleural effusion are present. Occasionally, patients with recurrent small emboli present with slowly progressive cor pulmonale. Clinical evidence of deep venous thrombosis is absent in most patients with PE. Importantly, the most consistent clinical findings, **tachypnea** and **tachycardia**, are found in less than 50% of patients with PE.

3. When PE is suspected, the diagnosis must be pursued in a logical sequence. **Routine laboratory tests** should be obtained to eliminate the many competing diagnoses.

   a. **Arterial blood gases** usually reveal mild to moderate hypoxemia, with a widened $P(A-a)O_2$ gradient, and hypocarbia. However, a normal arterial blood gas does not exclude the diagnosis.

   b. The **electrocardiogram** is usually normal, but an S_1-Q_3 pattern, evidence of right ventricular strain or right atrial abnormalities (P pulmonale), may be present. However, tachycardia and nonspecific ST-T wave changes are most commonly present.

   c. The **chest roentgenogram** is usually normal or may have varying combinations of subtle or gross findings, including elevated hemidiaphragm, regional oligemia, pleural effusion, pleural-based infiltrate (Hampton's hump), changes in the size of the pulmonary arteries, and right ventricular enlargement. Pneumothorax should be excluded.

   d. The next diagnostic test is usually **ventilation-perfusion lung scans.** A normal perfusion scan excludes the diagnosis of PE and should be performed initially. If a perfusion defect is present, then the ventilation scan is performed, paying particular attention to the views that clearly showed the perfusion defects. Matched ventilation-perfusion defects are characteristic of parenchymal diseases, whereas "mismatched" defects (i.e., ventilation is normal in zones of reduced perfusion) are characteristic of vascular obstruction. Therefore, a high-probability scan (>87% frequency of PE) is characterized by perfusion defects substantially larger than the radiographic abnormalities, one or more large segmental defects, or two or more moderate-size ventilation-perfusion mismatches, without a corresponding radiographic abnormality.

   e. **Pulmonary angiography** should be performed whenever doubt exists as to the correct diagnosis or when major therapy is contemplated (i.e., thrombolytic therapy, inferior vena caval ligation, or embolectomy). A normal angiogram excludes the diagnosis of PE. The combined morbidity and mortality from pulmonary angiography is 1% to 2%.

B. Treatment

1. Pulmonary embolism is a complication of venous thrombosis, therefore, **prevention** is the key to successful management of PE. High-risk patients should be carefully monitored for the development of deep venous thrombosis. Useful techniques include fibrinogen leg scanning, impedance plethysmography, and contrast venography. Prophylactic therapy is effective in preventing venous thrombosis in selected high-risk patients (e.g., low-dose heparin 5,000 U, s.c., every 12 hr).

2. **Supportive care** aimed at the treatment of hypoxemia (oxygen therapy), hypotension, and reduced cardiac output is of first importance.

3. **Anticoagulation**

   a. **Heparin** is the drug of choice in the vast majority of patients with PE. It prevents further clot formation but cannot prevent detachment of preexisting venous thrombi. The ideal heparin regimen for PE is unknown. A useful regimen is to begin anticoagulation with a large intravenous bolus (5,000 to 20,000 U) followed by a continuous infusion of 1,000 to 1,500 U/hr, or enough to prolong the whole-blood clotting time or the activated partial thromboplastin time (PTT) two times control. Full-dose heparin is usually maintained for at least 7 days. Most patients are maintained on anticoagulation therapy for at least 3 months. Warfarin (adequate to prolong the prothrombin time 1½ to 2½ the control value) or subcutaneous heparin (7,500 U every 12 hr) are the two options for prolonged anticoagulation protection.

   b. In the presence of contraindications to anticoagulation (high risk of bleeding), recurrent emboli despite adequate anticoagulation, or severe embolization such that a recurrence might be fatal: **surgical interruption of the inferior vena cava** is indicated. This is accomplished by vena caval plication, clipping, ligation, or the insertion of a Mobin-Uddin umbrella or a Greenfield filter.

   c. **Thrombolytic therapy** warrants consideration in patients with: massive pulmonary emboli (greater than two lobar arteries involved; pulmonary emboli accompanied by shock; submassive pulmonary emboli superimposed on underlying cardiopulmonary dysfunction leading to physiologic decompensation; and, in iliofemoral thrombosis to prevent chronic postphlebitic problems. It does not replace the heparin therapy but is instituted for 24 to 48 hr before heparin to accelerate clot resolution. **Absolute contraindications** include active internal bleeding and cerebrovascular disease or a surgical procedure within the previous 2 months. Thrombolytic therapy is administered by giving a **loading dose** followed by a constant infusion dose intravenously. **Therapeutic monitoring** is performed by measurement of the whole-blood euglobulin lysis time, the thrombin time, or the PTT 4 to 6 hr after institution of the thrombolytic agent (to identify and confirm activation of the fibrinolytic system). Further laboratory monitoring is not required once systemic fibrinolysis has been established. The PTT should be measured before starting anticoagulation. These thrombolytic agents are extremely expensive and have not been proved to have a positive impact on morbidity, mortality, or recurrence.

   d. **Acute embolectomy** is indicated in patients with angiographically proved massive embolism and persistent shock despite medical therapy. Selected patients with chronic pulmonary emboli may benefit from thromboendarterectomy (available in specialized centers).

VI. **PLEURAL EFFUSION**

A. **Diagnosis**

1. Pleural fluid is usually radiographically evident when 300 to 500 ml has

accumulated within the pleural space. A **lateral decubitus X-ray** often will identify smaller quantities and will distinguish loculated from free-flowing fluid. **Ultrasonography** is usually helpful in the identification and localization of loculated effusions as small as 5 to 10 ml.

2. The initial step in the evaluation of a pleural effusion is careful examination of fluid obtained by **thoracentesis** in an effort to separate **transudates** (caused by altered Starling forces, e.g., congestive heart failure, cirrhosis, and hypo-proteinemia) from **exudates** (caused by inflammatory reactions, e.g., infection, pulmonary infarction, connective tissue diseases, and malignant processes). **Exudates** can be defined by finding any two of the three following criteria: a pleural fluid LDH greater than 200 IU/dl, a ratio of pleural fluid to blood LDH greater than 0.6, and a ratio of pleural fluid to blood protein greater than 0.5.

3. **Other tests** useful in determining the specific etiology of an exudate include the following:

   a. **Glucose** tends to be low (<40 mg%) in infections (empyema) and may be strikingly low (<30 mg%) in rheumatoid arthritis.

   b. Pleural fluid **acidosis** (pH<7.30) has been found in empyemas, rheumatoid pleurisy, tuberculosis, carcinoma, and esophageal rupture. It is most useful in distinguishing benign (pH>7.3) from complicated parapneumonic effusion.

   c. An elevated **amylase** (two times serum amylase) suggests acute pancreatitis, pancreatic pseudocyst, esophageal rupture, or carcinoma.

   d. **Stains** and **cultures**—look for infectious organisms (aerobic and anaerobic bacteria, tuberculosis, and fungi).

   e. **Cell count** and **differential**. Grossly bloody fluid suggests trauma, pulmonary embolism with infarction, malignancy, or postcardiac injury syndrome. Pus establishes the diagnosis of empyema. Leukocyte counts greater than 1,000/mm³ occur most often in exudates. Mononuclear cell predominance suggests pulmonary embolus with effusion, tuberculosis pleuritis, or malignant effusion. The presence of eosinophils makes the diagnosis of tuberculosis unlikely.

   f. **Lipids.** Chylous effusions contain a high percentage of neutral fats and fatty acid and stain positively with sudan III.

   g. **Cytology** is positive in approximately 60% of patients with documented pleural malignancy. A large volume of fluid is required for adequate cytological examination.

   h. **Pleural biopsy,** with a Cope or Abrams needle, is indicated in the setting of an undiagnosed exudative pleural effusion. The yield is highest in effusions where there is a mononuclear predominant cell differential, i.e., tuberculosis, carcinoma, or lymphoma.

B. **Treatment**

1. Treatment of a pleural effusion should be directed at the **underlying etiology**. Only rarely is manipulation of the pleural space required.

2. **Acute pleural fluid accumulation** occasionally will produce acute dyspnea, most often secondary to pleural pain rather than significant hypoxemia (unless severe parenchymal disease is also present). If the effusion is large, partial removal (500 to 1,500 ml) will provide symptomatic relief by improving the mechanical advantage of the inspiratory muscles. Occasionally, rapid removal of large volumes of fluid will produce ipsilateral pulmonary edema. Oxygen therapy should be provided for patients undergoing thoracentesis.

3. Bacterial pneumonias have an associated pleural effusion approximately 40% of the time. Approximately 10% of these **parapneumonic effusions** require tube thoracostomy for their resolution. Therefore, any patient with a moderate-to-large parapneumonic effusion should have a diagnostic thoracentesis (30 to 50 ml). Immediate tube thoracostomy is indicated if a parapneumonic effusion contains gross pus, is positive for organisms, has a glucose <40 mg/dl or a pH below 7.20. In some patients with chronic empyema, an open thoracostomy drainage procedure or a decortication is required because of inadequate drainage or development of a thick peel over the visceral pleura that prevents reexpansion of the lung.

4. **Malignant pleural effusions** most often result from secondary tumor involvement of the visceral or parietal pleura. They also may be caused by mediastinal lymph node infiltration, obstructive pneumonitis, atelectasis, thoracic duct involvement, hypoproteinemia, and mediastinal irradiation. Management of the underlying malignancy (systemic chemotherapy) will control some effusions. Symptomatic malignant effusions should be drained initially by thoracentesis and/or tube thoracostomy. Recurrences are best managed by prolonged chest tube drainage alone or with instillation of a **sclerosing agent. Tetracycline** is the most effective sclerosing agent. **Nitrogen mustard**, 10 mg in 50 ml sterile water, also has been recommended.

The following procedure is recommended:

   a. Chest tube drainage should be instituted for at least 24 hr or until minimal drainage (≤50 ml/day) occurs and the lung is fully expanded. ᵥ

   b. Instill **tetracycline hydrochloride** (10 mg/kg body weight diluted in 50 cc of saline); occasionally air is also instilled (~200 cc) to ensure maximum contact of sclerosing agent with pleura.

   c. Clamp the chest tube for 2 hr while repositioning the patient frequently (i.e., prone, supine, and in right and left lateral positions).

   d. Unclamp the chest tube and allow drainage to occur for the next 24 to 48 hr or until drainage is minimal.

Demerol® may be given 30 min before the procedure to reduce the pain frequently induced by this procedure. Fever and leukocytosis are other common side effects.

VII. HEMOPTYSIS

A. **Causes** Hemoptysis is the coughing up of blood and frequently reflects a serious underlying disease. There are numerous causes of hemoptysis. **Blood-streaked sputum** is frequently seen in chronic bronchitis and upper respiratory infection and is an early finding in lung cancer. **Massive** hemoptysis most commonly occurs in pulmonary tuberculosis (both active and inactive), bronchiectasis, and lung abscess. Other causes include bronchiolitis, mycetomas, cystic fibrosis, congenital heart disease, pulmonary bullae, and bronchogenic carcinoma (less than 8% of all cases). Pulmonary arteritis, Goodpasture's syndrome, idiopathic pulmonary hemosiderosis, Wegener's granulomatosis, mitral stenosis, and pulmonary embolus are other conditions giving rise to hemoptysis (usually mild to moderate in degree). Death from hemoptysis is most often due to asphyxiation, not exsanguination.

B. Evaluation of the Patient   The initial evaluation is directed at determining the site, severity, and cause of the bleeding.

1. The **severity** of the bleeding can be assessed by:

   a. Determining whether circulatory or respiratory insufficiency is present (systemic hypotension, respiratory distress, diffuse rales and rhonchi, etc.).

   b. Measuring the **rate** of bleeding by collecting the blood (massive hemoptysis has been defined as greater than 600 ml within 48 hr).

   c. Measuring the arterial blood gases (severe hypoxemia denotes markedly abnormal gas exchange), and serial hemoglobin levels may suggest the need for blood transfusions.

2. The **site** of bleeding is best determined by **fiberoptic bronchoscopy** during the bleeding episode. Rigid bronchoscopy is required when massive hemoptysis occurs and is useful for clearing the airway of clots and occluding the bronchus from which the bleeding is arising. Occasionally, it is difficult to tell if the blood is arising from the upper respiratory tract or from the gastrointestinal tract. However, a careful history, examination of the upper respiratory tract, and examination of the blood (true hemoptysis contains frothy blood and is bright red in color) will often clarify this situation. The **chest roentgenogram** may indicate the site and even the etiology of bleeding. However, aspiration of blood may obscure the radiologic signs.

3. The **cause** of the bleeding is best approached by attention to the history and physical examination (e.g., smoking history, trauma, valvular heart disease, signs of an infectious disorder, hematuria, other bleeding sites, bleeding profile, etc.).

C. Management

1. **Massive hemoptysis** is a medical emergency that can result in hypotension, anemia, cardiovascular collapse, and asphyxiation. **Supportive measures** aimed at maintaining vital functions are important (volume replacement, oxygenation, vasopressors, etc.). **Control of the airway** with endotracheal intubation should be carried out swiftly if required. The patient should be positioned with bleeding side down to prevent aspiration of blood into the contralateral lung. **Localization of the bleeding site(s)** is an absolute preoperative requisite, and **prompt surgical resection** is the treatment of choice. Contraindications to surgery include diffuse lung disease causing diffuse bleeding, coagulation abnormalities (e.g., anticoagulant therapy) that may be associated with diffuse bleeding, inoperable lung cancer, and lung disease of such severity that the patient might not have adequate pulmonary reserve to survive resection of functioning

lung tissue (i.e., a predicted $FEV_1 > 1.0$ liter after the procedure). Known cardiac disease that can cause hemoptysis should be corrected first (e.g., mitral stenosis requires mitral valve replacement rather than lung resection). In inoperable patients, the bleeding can be controlled by tamponade of the bronchial segment with a Fogarty balloon catheter or by embolization of the arterial supply to the bleeding segment. The latter technique is usually unsuccessful because the systemic bronchial circulation is the source of the bleeding.

2. In patients with **mild to moderate** hemoptysis, conservative management may suffice, as follows:

  a. Position with bleeding lung down.

  b. Mild sedation to facilitate patient cooperation must be used cautiously since suppression of the cough may occur and the signs of respiratory failure may be obscured.

  c. Control of the airway with endotracheal intubation if necessary.

BIBLIOGRAPHY

Acute Asthma and Status Asthmaticus

Cugell, D. W. and Fish, J. E. (1978): Beta$_2$ adrenergic agents and other drugs in reversible airway disease. *Chest*, 73 (Suppl):913–1022.

Kelsen, S. G., Kelsen, D. P., Fleegler, B. F., et al. (1978): Emergency room assessment and treatment of patients with acute asthma: Adequacy of the conventional approach. *Am. J. Med.*, 64:622–628.

Paterson, J. W., Woolcock, A. J., and Shenfield, G. M. (1979): Bronchodilator drugs. *Am. Rev. Respir. Dis.*, 120:1149–1188.

Rose, C. C., Murphy, J. G., and Schwartz, J. S. (1984): Performance of an index predicting the response of patients with acute bronchial asthma to intensive emergency department treatment. *N. Engl. J. Med.*, 310:573–577.

Shim, C. S., and Williams, M. H., Jr. (1983): Relationship of wheezing to the severity of obstruction in asthma. *Arch. Intern. Med.*, 143:890–892.

Chronic Airflow Obstruction

Hudson, L. D. and Pierson, D. J. (1981): Comprehensive respiratory care for patients with chronic obstructive pulmonary diseases. *Med. Clin. North Am.*, 65:629–645.

Petty, T. L. and Zwillich, C. (1980): The 22nd Aspen Lung Conference: Chronic obstructive pulmonary disease. *Chest*, 77 (Suppl):269–330.

Inhalation Injury of the Lungs

Bartlett, J. G., Gorbach, S. L. The triple threat of aspiration pneumonia. *Chest*, 68:560–566.

Lakshminarayan, S. (1982): Inhalation injury of the lungs. In: *Pulmonary Emergencies*, edited by S. A. Sahn. Churchill Livingstone, New York.

Pulmonary Embolism

Cheely, R., McCartney, W. H., Perry, J. R., et al. (1981): The role of noninvasive tests versus pulmonary angiography in the diagnosis of pulmonary embolism. *Am. J. Med.*, 70:17–22.

Moser, K. M. and Fedullo, P. F. (1983): Venous thromboembolism: Three simple decisions (Part 1 and 2). *Chest*, 117–121; 256–260.

Sleep Apnea Hypersomnolence Syndrome

Cherniack, N. S. (1981): Respiratory dysrhythmias during sleep. *N. Engl. J. Med.*, 305:325–330.

10.

Infectious Diseases

Martin J. Blaser and Richard T. Ellison III

10.

Infectious Diseases

I. ANTIMICROBIAL AGENTS

A. General Guidelines The selection of antimicrobial therapy must be based on the nature of the presumed or established infection, the condition of the host, and the characteristics of the antimicrobial agents.

1. **Cause of infection.** Appropriate efforts should be made to establish the definitive cause of an infection **before** initiating therapy, as antimicrobial therapy may interfere with diagnostic studies. Gram stains of appropriate specimens; cultures for bacteria, mycobacteria, fungi, chlamydiae, viruses; serology; and specialized tests for microbial antigens all may be utilized for **diagnosis** depending on the clinical situation. In many instances, diagnostic cultures also should be accompanied by antimicrobial-susceptibility testing to optimize antimicrobial therapy.

2. **Site of infection.** Although most antimicrobial agents achieve therapeutic concentrations in the bloodstream and soft tissues, there is **wide variation in drug concentration** achieved in specific sites of the body because of differences in water and lipid solubility, drug metabolism, and interactions with membrane transport systems. Of major concern is **antibiotic penetration across the blood-brain barrier** into brain parenchyma and the cerebrospinal fluid (CSF). Also important, although not as critical, is antibiotic penetration into urine, bone, peritoneum, and bile. Antimicrobial penetration into these areas is summarized in Table 1.

3. **Status of the host**

   a. **Severity of illness and general condition of host.** The severity of illness influences the rapidity and mode of antimicrobial therapy. Ease of venous access, amount of muscle mass, and the presence and absence of gastrointestinal disturbances also will influence the mode of drug administration. In general, **severe illness** is treated with intravenous therapy both to obtain therapeutic drug concentrations as rapidly as possible and to reach drug concentrations not achievable by other delivery systems. **Milder infections** may be treated with either oral agents or intramuscular injections.

   b. **Renal dysfunction.** The kidney is the major site for excretion of many antimicrobial agents, and to avoid potential toxicity these agents may require a **modification of dose and dosing interval** in patients with renal impairment. Further, several agents are directly nephrotoxic and can exacerbate renal failure. As there appears to be a correlation between the **creatinine clearance** and the handling of most antimicrobial agents, direct

TABLE 1. *Antibiotic penetration to body sites*[a]

Site	Excellent	Adequate	Inadequate
Bile	Clindamycin[b]	Penicillins	Vancomycin
	Lincomycin	Cephalosporins[b]	
	Erythromycin	Aminoglycosides	
	Rifampin	Chloramphenicol	
	Tetracyclines	Sulfonamides	
		TMP-SMX	
Bone	Penicillin	Isoniazid	
	Cephalosporins	Aminoglycosides	
	Clindamycin	Metronidazole	
	Lincomycin	Erthromycin	
	Sulfonamides	TMP-SMX	
Brain	Chloramphenicol	Penicillin G	
	Metronidazole	Lincomycin	
Cerebrospinal fluid	Chloramphenicol	Ampicillin	Aminoglycosides
	Sulfonamides	Carbenicillin[c]	First-generation
	TMP-SMX	Nafcillin	cephalosporins
	Pyrazinamide	Cefotaxime	Second-generation
			cephalosporins
	Isoniazid	Cefoperazone	Ketoconazole
	Rifampin	Tetracycline	
	Ethambutol	Amphotericin[d]	
	Metronidazole		
	Moxalactam		
	Vidarabine		

[a]Antibiotic concentrations achieved with usual routes of administration.
[b]Except with complete biliary obstruction.
[c]Not adequate for enteric gram-negative–rod meningitis.
[d]Adequate levels for cryptococcal and coccidioidomycosal disease.
TMP-SMX, trimethoprim-sulfamethoxazole.

measurement of the clearance can guide modification of antimicrobial therapy. An approximation of the creatinine clearance can be obtained by the following formula:

$$\text{Creatinine clearance (ml/min)} = \frac{140 - \text{age}}{\text{serum creatinine (mg\%)}}$$

Agents that require major adjustments of dose in patients with renal failure are usually intrinsically nephrotoxic and should have dosage modified for any reduction in creatinine clearance. Other agents usually do not require dose adjustment unless the creatinine clearance is less than 20 ml/min or the patient is on dialysis. Modifications for specific agents are summarized in Table 2. The use of serum drug assays is particularly important in patients with renal impairment to provide optimal drug concentrations.

c. **Hepatic dysfunction.** With severe dysfunction, drugs that either undergo hepatic metabolism or are hepatotoxic should be avoided. The major agents in this category are chloramphenicol, isoniazid, rifampin, pyrazinamide, and ketoconazole.

d. **Pregnancy and puerperium.** In general, the use of any antimicrobial agent should be **avoided** in pregnant and lactating women. However, penicillins and cephalosporins have been used frequently without apparent adverse effects. **Tetracyclines are specifically contraindicated**, and aminoglycosides, chloramphenicol, and sulfonamides are relatively contraindicated.

4. **Basic principles of antimicrobial therapy.** Antimicrobial therapy should be considered in the following three settings: **Initial empiric therapy**—broad-spectrum antimicrobial therapy directed against the potential pathogens in a severely ill patient, based on a clinical presentation in which therapy cannot be delayed for results of diagnostic tests. Thus, initial therapy is based on knowledge of the typical pathogens causing infection at a given site (see specific disease states) and preliminary laboratory studies. **Specific empiric therapy**—antimicrobial therapy directed against a confirmed pathogen while awaiting results of antimicrobial susceptibility tests. **Specific therapy**—narrow-spectrum antimicrobial therapy directed against a confirmed pathogen based on defined susceptibility to antimicrobial agents.

Given a choice of agents with comparable toxicity, for **severe infections** it is preferable to use an agent that is bactericidal toward the target microbe as opposed to an agent that inhibits microbial growth without killing (bacteristatic). With agents of comparable efficacy the **least toxic** agent should be used. When directing therapy toward a specific microbe, the agent with the narrowest possible antimicrobial spectrum should be chosen.

B. **Antimicrobial Susceptibility Testing**   For mild infections it may not always be necessary to determine antimicrobial susceptibilities, but for severe illnesses susceptibility testing should generally be utilized whenever the infecting microorganism is identified; exceptions to this are when it is technically difficult to test susceptibility, as with fungal illness, or when the pathogen has been universally susceptible to an antibiotic, as with streptococcal illness.

A microbe has been considered "sensitive" to a given agent when the therapeutically achievable antibiotic concentrations are at least eightfold greater than the antibiotic concentration that inhibits the microbe's growth in vitro. As urine antibiotic concentrations can be much higher than those achieved in serum, bacteria can therefore be "resistant" to a given antibiotic in the bloodstream but "sensitive" to it in the urine.

Using both this concept of susceptibility and pharmacokinetic data, a **standard drug concentration** has been defined for each antimicrobial agent to delineate antimicrobial susceptibility to that agent. Clinical microbiology laboratories determine the susceptibility of a given microorganism to different antimicrobial agents either by disc-diffusion tests (Kirby-Bauer) or measurement of **minimal inhibitory concentrations** (MIC) of the agents in broth, and then report susceptibility based on the defined standards. The clinician should interpret these data in relation to the site of infection and his knowledge of drug penetration to that location.

Additional antimicrobial susceptibility testing should be considered with infections for which maximum antimicrobial effect is desired (e.g., endocarditis, osteomyelitis) or when there is unexplained clinical failure. These tests include

TABLE 2. *Antibiotic dosing in renal or hepatic failure*

Drug	Dose change with renal failure GFR (ml/min) >50	10–50	<10	Dose change with liver failure	Effect of dialysis
Penicillins					
Amoxicillin	None	q 6–12 hr	q 12–24 hr	None	Significant (50%)
Ampicillin	None	q 6–12 hr	q 12–24 hr	None	Significant (40–80%)
Carbenicillin	q 8–12 hr	q 12–24 hr	q 24–48 hr	None	Significant (20–40%)
Cloxacillin	None	None	None	None	Insignificant
Cyclacillin	None	q 6–12 hr	q 12–24 hr	None	Significant (70–80%)
Dicloxacillin	None	q 4–8 hr	None	None	Insignificant
Methicillin	None	None	q 8–12 hr	None	Insignificant
Nafcillin	None	None	None	Decrease in severe liver disease	Insignificant
Oxacillin	None	None	None	Possible decrease with severe liver dysfunction	Insignificant
Penicillin G	None	q 8–12 hr	q 12–18 hr	None	Significant
Ticarcillin	q 8–12 hr	q 12–24 hr	q 24–48 hr	None	Significant
Cephalosporins					
Cefaclor	None	50–100% normal dose	25–33% normal dose	None	Insignificant
Cefamandole	None	25–50% normal dose	10–25% normal dose	None	Significant
Cefazolin	None	50% normal dose	25% normal dose	None	Significant
Cefoperazone	None	None	q.12 hr	Decrease in severe hepatic disease	None
Cefotaxime	None	None	q 8hr	None	None
Cefoxitin	q 8 hr	q 8–12 hr	q 24–48 hr	None	Significant
Ceftizoxime	q 8hr	q 8–12 hr	q 24–48 hr	None	Significant
Cefuroxime	None	q 8–12 hr	q 24 hr	None	Significant
Cephadroxil	q 8 hr	q 12–24 hr	q 24–48 hr	None	Significant
Cephalexin	None	q 6–12 hr	q 12–24 hr	None	Significant
Cephaloridine	Avoid Nephrotoxic	Avoid	Avoid	None	Significant

Antibiotic					
Cephalothin	None	None	q 8–12 hr	Decrease may be warranted in moderate to severe hepatic disease	Significant
Cephapirin	None	None	q 6–12 hr	Possible decrease in severe hepatic disease	Significant
Cephradine	None	50% normal dose	25% normal dose	None	Significant
Moxalactam	None	50% normal dose	25% normal dose q.12 hr	None	Significant
Aminoglycosides Amikacin	Dosage changes similar to kanamycin			None	Significant (22 ml/min)
Gentamicin	75–100% normal dose	35–75% normal dose	25–35% normal dose	None	Significant (26–48 ml/min)
Kanamycin	75% normal dose	35–50% normal dose	25% normal dose	None	Significant (30–40 ml/min)
Neomycin	None	q 8–12 hr	q 12–36 hr	None	Significant (30–50 ml/min)
Streptomycin	q 24 hr	q 24–48 hr	q 48–96 hr	None	Minimal (17 ml/min)
Tobramycin	Same recommendations as for gentamicin			None	Significant (50–60 ml/min)
Other agents Vancomycin	q 24–72 hr	q 72–240 hr	q 240 hr	None	Insignificant
Chloramphenicol	None	None	None	Decrease necessary in moderate to severe hepatic disease	Significant
Clindamycin	None	None	None	Decrease necessary in moderate to severe hepatic disease	Insignificant
Lincomycin	q 6 h	q 6–12 h	q 12–24 hr	Decrease necessary with moderate to severe hepatic disease	Slight
Erythromycin	None	None	None	Decrease necessary in patients with moderate to severe hepatic disease	Insignificant

TABLE 2. *(Continued)*

Drug	Dose change with renal failure GFR (ml/min)			Dose change with liver failure	Effect of dialysis
	>50	10–50	<10		
Tetracyclines					
Doxycycline	None	None	None	Decrease	Insignificant
Minocycline	None	None	None	Decrease	Slight
	May have some antianabolic effects that require dosage interval increases				
Tetracycline	Avoid	Avoid	Avoid	None	Slight
Sulfonamides					
Sulfamethoxazole	q 12 hr	q 18 hr	q 18–24 hr	Decrease may be necessary in severe hepatic disease	Significant (22 ml/min)
Sulfasalazine	None	None	None	Decrease in moderate to severe hepatic disease	—
Sulfisoxazole	None	q 8–12 hr	q 12–24 hr	Decrease may be necessary in severe hepatic failure	Moderate
Trimethoprim	q 12 hr	q 18 hr	q 18–24 hr	None	Significant
Metronidazole	None	q 8–12 hr	q 12–24 hr	Decrease in severe hepatic failure	Moderate
Antituberculosis					
Ethambutol	None	50% normal dose q 24 hr or 100% q 36 hr	25% normal dose q 24 hr or 100% q 48 hr	None	Significant
Isoniazid	None	None	66–100% normal dose	Decrease may be necessary in moderate to severe hepatic disease	Significant (20–49 ml/min)

Drug				
Rifampin	None	None	Patients with liver dysfunction or biliary obstruction may accumulate rifampin	Insignificant
Antifungals				
Amphotericin B	None	q 36–48 hr	Monitor closely for accumulation	Insignificant
Flucytosine	q 12–24 hr	q 24–48 hr	None	Significant (60–100 ml/min)
Miconazole	None	None	Decrease may be necessary in severe hepatic insufficiency	Insignificant
Antiviral agents				
Amantadine	Accumulation in renal failure anticipated Dosage changes with decreasing renal function may be necessary	None	None	Slight
Interferon	No dosage modification seems necessary		Accumulation in liver failure would not be anticipated	—
Vidarabine (ara-A)	Accumulation of ara-A in renal insufficiency warrants close monitoring and dosage adjustment		Probably none	—
Acyclovir	Accumulation in renal failure warrants close monitoring and dosage adjustment		Probably none	—

aModified from Anderson, R. J., Schrier, R. W., and Ganbertoglio J. G., eds. (1981): Clinical Use of Drugs in Patients with Kidney and Liver Disease, with permission.

GFR, glomerular filtration rate.

determinations of the minimal bactericidal concentrations (MBC) of antimicrobial agents and serum bactericidal activity.

C. Antibiotic Agents

1. Cell-wall-active agents

a. Beta-lactam antibiotics. This class of antibiotics, which includes both the **penicillin and cephalosporin** families, is bactericidal. They share a four-member beta-lactam ring and mimic a D-alanyl-D-alanine linkage, a universal component of bacterial cell walls, allowing inhibition of bacterial enzymes integral for cell-wall synthesis. **Variations in the spectrum of activity** of these agents are related to differences in: penetration to active sites within the bacterial cell wall; inhibition of the bacterial enzymes involved in cell-wall synthesis; and, susceptibilities to bacterial beta-lactamase enzymes that destroy the beta-lactam structure.

(1) Penicillins. Penicillin G, benzathine penicillin, procaine penicillin, and penicillin V are active against most strains of nonenterococcal streptococci, *Streptococcus pneumoniae*, beta-lactamase-negative staphylococci, and the gram-positive bacilli, excluding *Nocardia* species, occasional strains of diphtheroids, and *Listeria monocytogenes*. Although penicillin-resistant *Neisseria gonorrhoeae* are being seen increasingly in Asia, in the United States more than 98% of *N. gonorrhoeae* and all *Neisseria meningitidis* strains are susceptible. The spirochetes *Treponema pallidum* and *Leptospira* and *Borrelia* species, and the Lyme arthritis agent are all sensitive to penicillin, as are most anaerobic bacteria excluding *Bacteroides fragilis*. The enterococcal streptococci are susceptible to a combination of penicillin and aminoglycosides. (For dosages see Table 3.)

Penicillin G penetrates across serosal membranes and inflamed meninges, into brain parenchyma and bone. The **primary route of excretion** is by renal tubular secretion. Probenicid can partially block this secretion and may be used therapeutically to prolong the half-life of these agents.

Penicillin G and these closely related compounds are among the **least toxic** of all antibiotics and remain the **drugs of choice** when treating infections with susceptible organisms. **Hypersensitivity reactions**, including anaphylaxis and serum sickness, are the most common severe adverse reaction; anaphylaxis has an incidence of approximately 1 to 5 per 10,000 courses of therapy. Coomb's-positive hemolytic anemia, interstitial nephritis, and convulsions with extremely high dosage (>20 million U/day) are other rare toxicities.

Semisynthetic beta-lactamase-resistant penicillins. This group of antibiotics—**oxacillin, nafcillin, methicillin, cloxacillin, and dicloxacillin**—differs from penicillin G in being resistant to the action of staphylococcal beta-lactamase. They have spectra of activity comparable to penicillin G against most bacteria and also are effective against most strains of staphylococci. However, per gram they are not as active as penicillin G against other nonstaphylococcal bacteria, particularly the enterococci. Recently, *Staphylococcus aureus* and *Staphylococcus epidermidis* strains resistant to both this group of agents and all other present beta-lactam antibiotics have been recognized. Infection with these pathogens requires treatment with vancomycin.

The distribution and routes of excretion of these agents are comparable to that of penicillin G. All are highly protein bound and have longer serum half-lives than penicillin G. All may evoke the same hypersensitivity reactions as penicillin G and are contraindicated in penicillin-allergic patients.

Extended spectrum penicillins include ampicillin, amoxicillin, cyclacillin, and bacampicillin, a group of semisynthetic penicillins that retain the spectrum of penicillin G but have additional activity against some gram-negative bacilli such as *Hemophilus* species, community-acquired *Escherichia coli*, *Salmonella* species, and *Proteus mirabilis*. They are destroyed by beta-lactamases and therefore are not active against beta-lactamase-producing strains of *Staphylococcus*, *Hemophilus influenzae*, *N. gonorrhoeae*, or *Pseudomonas* species. Usually, they are not active against hospital-acquired aerobic gram-negative bacilli. These agents share a distribution in the body similar to that of penicillin G and a predominant renal route of excretion with **high urinary concentrations**. Therapeutic concentrations of these antibiotics also are achieved in bile.

Although they have the same likelihood of hypersensitivity reactions as penicillin G, three of these agents—ampicillin, amoxicillin, and bacampicillin—also show an **increased incidence of macular rashes**, particularly in patients with infectious mononucleosis. The rashes are not hypersensitivity reactions and are not a contraindication to continuing therapy. These agents can induce self-limited gastrointestinal disturbances with nausea, vomiting, and diarrhea; however, usage also may provoke pseudomembranous colitis.

Antipseudomonal penicillins—carbenicillin, ticarcillin, piperacillin, azlocillin, and mezlocillin—are semisynthetic penicillins with a basic spectrum of activity similar to that of ampicillin but with increased activity toward the aerobic gram-negative bacilli and, particularly, *Pseudomonas aeruginosa*. None is active against beta-lactamase-producing *S. aureus*. **Carbenicillin and ticarcillin** are active against some *Proteus* and *Enterobacter* species that are ampicillin resistant and against *B. fragilis* when used in high doses. They are therapeutically effective against serious *Pseudomonas* infections when used with an aminoglycoside. **Azlocillin** has a comparable spectrum but has more activity against some *P. aeruginosa* isolates. **Piperacillin and mezlocillin** are active against a broader range of gram-negative bacilli including many additional strains of *Klebsiella pneumoniae* and *Serratia* species. Piperacillin and azlocillin have comparable antipseudomonal activity. Because of the potential emergence of resistant gram-negative bacilli, these agents usually are used in conjunction with an aminoglycoside.

TABLE 3. *Use of penicillins*

Agents	Usual dosage and route of administration	Specific advantages	Specific disadvantages and adverse effects
Basic penicillins			
Penicillin G	600,000–1,200,000 U q 6 hr, i.m., or 8–24,000,000 U/day, i.v., in q 2–4-hr doses		
Procaine penicillin G	600,000–1,200,000 U q 6 hr, i.m.	Prolonged half-life	Procaine reaction (severe anxiety immediately after injection)
Benzathine penicillin	600,000–1,200,000 U, i.m.	Antispirochetal serum concentrations for 14 days after i.m. injection	
Penicillin VK	Child <5: 125 mg, p.o. q 6 hr Child >5, adult 250–1,000 mg, p.o., q 6 hr	Acid stable allowing oral administration	
Semisynthetic penicillinase-resistant penicillins			
Oxacillin	500 mg, p.o., q 4–6 hr 1–2 g, i.m. or i.v., q 4 hr		Interstitial nephritis, hepatitis (1.5%)
Cloxacillin	500 mg, p.o., q 6 hr	2 × peak concentration of oxacillin after oral dose	
Nafcillin	1–2 g, i.v. or i.m., q 4 hr		Erratic oral absorption, neutropenia (3%)
Methicillin	1–2 g, i.v. or i.m. q 4 hr		Interstitial nephritis, neutropenia (0.1–7%)
Extended-spectrum penicillins			
Ampicillin	250–1,000 mg, p.o., q 6 hr in adults 1.0–2.0 g, i.v. or i.m. q 4 hr		Food decreases oral absorption
Amoxicillin	250–500 mg, p.o. q 6 hr	Food does not change absorption	
Bacampicillin	0.4–0.8 g, p.o. q 12 hr	Food does not alter absorption, metabolized to ampicillin	Expensive
Hetacillin	0.25 g, p.o. q 6 hr; 150 mg/kg/day, i.v. in q 6 hr doses	Metabolized to ampicillin	
Antipseudomonal penicillins			
Carbenicillin	24–40 g/day, i.v. in q 4 hr doses		Platelet dysfunction, high Na$^+$ content
Indanyl carbenicillin	0.5–1.0 g, p.o. q 6 hr	Acid stable, allowing oral treatment of *Pseudomonas* urinary tract infection	Does not achieve therapeutic concentration in serum

TABLE 3. *(Continued)*

Agents	Usual dosage and route of administration	Specific advantages	Specific disadvantages and adverse effects
Ticarcillin	18–24 g/day, i.v. in q 4 hr doses		Platelet dysfunction, high Na+ content
Azlocillin	18–23 g/day, i.v. in q 4 hr doses	Increased antipseudomonal activity	
Mezlocillin	18–24 g/day, i.v. in q 4 hr doses	Broad activity against enterobacteriaceae	
Piperacillin	18–24 g/day, i.v. in q 4 hr doses	Broad activity against enterobacteriaceae and increased antipseudomonal activity	

Distribution and excretion of these drugs are similar to that of penicillin G and ampicillin. However, the CSF penetration across inflamed meninges is not adequate for routine treatment of gram-negative rod meningitis. In addition to the hypersensitivity reactions of the penicillin family, **adverse effects** related to these agents include a reversible qualitative platelet dysfunction, rare neutropenia, and seizures with high dosage. Carbenicillin and ticarcillin contain 4.7 mEq/g and 5.2 mEq/g sodium, respectively, which can contribute to congestive heart failure. However, since ticarcillin is given in half the dose of carbenicillin, sodium overload is not as great a concern. Piperacillin, mezlocillin, and azlocillin each contain 1.98 mEq/g sodium.

(2) **Cephalosporins.** The term cephalosporin is now commonly used to include a family of semisynthetic beta-lactam antibiotic agents that have been derived from the natural compound cephalosporin C. They have been most usefully grouped into therapeutically similar compounds by considering them as "generations" of antibiotic agents. Regardless of generation, **all penetrate well** into bone, soft tissue, and placenta and across serosal and synovial membranes. Of the currently available cephalosporins only **cefuroxime and the third-generation agents** penetrate the blood-brain barrier in any appreciable concentration. All but cefoperazone have a predominantly **renal mode of excretion**, and all share a 10% to 15% incidence of cross-reactivity for hypersensitivity reactions with the penicillin compounds. The usual route of administration and dosage of this class are shown in Table 4.

First generation cephalosporins currently available are **cephalothin, cephapirin, cephalexin, cepharadine, and cefadroxil.** These agents are active against all gram-positive cocci except for the methicillin-resistant staphylococci and the enterococci. **Although methicillin-resistant staphylococci may appear susceptible to cephalosporins by in vitro susceptibility tests, infections with these microorganisms will not respond to cephalosporin therapy.** Most aerobic and anaerobic gram-positive bacilli except *Nocardia* and some *Listeria* strains are susceptible. The *Neisseria* species and most community-acquired aerobic gram-negative bacilli, including *E. coli, Salmonella* species,

TABLE 4. *Use of cephalosporins*

Agents	Usual dosage and route of administration	Specific advantages	Specific disadvantages and adverse effects
First-generation cephalosporins			
Cephalothin	2–12 g/day, i.v./i.m. q 4–6 hr		i.m. administration painful, false-positive Clinitest
Cefazolin	1–6 g/day, i.v./i.m. q 6–8 hr	Peak level 4 × cephalothin with comparable dose, and longer half-life	
Cephapirin	2–12 g/day, i.v./i.m. q 4–6 hr	Comparable to cephalothin	
Cepharadine	2–12 g/day, i.v./i.m./p.o. q 4–6 hr	Available in both oral and parenteral form	Less active against *H. influenzae*, false-positive Clinitest
Cephaloridine		None	Should be avoided because of significant nephrotoxicity
Cephalexin	1–4 g/day, p.o. q 4–6 hr	Most experience for oral therapy	
Cefadroxil	1–2 g/day, p.o. q 12–24 hr	Prolonged serum half-life	
Second-generation cephalosporins			
Cefamandole	1.5–12 g/day, i.m./i.v. q 4–6 hr	More active against *H. influenzae*, and selected gram-negative bacilli	i.m. administration painful, disulfiram-like effect, expensive
Cefaclor	0.75–4.0 g/day, p.o. q 8 hr	Active against *H. influenzae*	Expensive
Cefoxitin	3–12 g/day, i.m./i.v. q 4–6 hr	More active against *B. fragilis*, *N. gonorrhoeae* and selected gram-negative bacilli	Expensive
Cefuroxime	2.25–9.0 g/day, i.m./i.v. q 8 hr		
Third-generation cephalosporins			
Cefotaxime	2–12 g/day, i.v./i.m. q 4–6 hr	More active against gram-negative bacilli, good CSF penetration	Vitamin K–dependent coagulopathy, expensive
Moxalactam	2–12 g/day, i.v./i.m. q 6–8 hr	More active against gram-negative bacilli, good CSF penetration	Vitamin K–dependent coagulopathy, disulfiram-like effect, expensive
Cefoperazone	2–12 g/day, i.v./i.m. q 6–8 hr	More active against gram-negative bacilli, longer half-life	Vitamin K–dependent coagulopathy, disulfiram-like effect, expensive
Ceftizoxime	2–12 g/day, i.v./i.m. q 6–8 hr	Similar to cefotaxime	Vitamin K–dependent coagulopathy, expensive

ampicillin-sensitive *Shigella* species, and *Pasturella multocida*, are susceptible. These cephalosporins are usually active against the *Klebsiella* species, and have further synergistic activity with the aminoglycosides against these bacteria. Some anaerobic gram-negative bacilli are susceptible, but *B. fragilis* isolates are uniformly resistant. The spirochetes *T. pallidum* and *Leptospira* are susceptible. First-generation cephalosporins are inactive against most other classes of microorganisms. There is only minimal CNS penetration of these agents, and **they should not be used to treat meningitis or brain abscess.** They are generally nontoxic except for **hypersensitivity reactions**, which include rashes, eosinophilia, and Coomb's-positive hemolytic anemia. They may be associated with gastrointestinal disturbances, including pseudomembranous colitis, and nephrotoxicity has been noted with both cephalothin in combination with an aminoglycoside and cephaloridine as single agent. There are no indications for the use of cephaloridine.

Second-generation cephalosporins—cefamandole, cefoxitin, cefaclor, and cefuroxime—have expanded activity against gram-negative enteric bacilli. **Cefamandole, cefaclor, and cefuroxime** are more active against *E. coli, K. pneumoniae, Enterobacter* species, *Providencia* species, *Proteus* species, *Morganella morgagni*, and beta-lactamase-producing *H. influenzae*. **Cefoxitin** has a similar spectrum of activity except for *H. influenzae* and has more activity against anaerobic bacteria, including *B. fragilis*. The activity of this group against gram-positive bacteria is no better than the first-generation agents. None is active against *P. aeruginosa*.

As with the first-generation agents, **cefamandole, cefoxitin, and cefaclor do not adequately penetrate the central nervous system (CNS), and they cannot be used for treatment of meningitis.** Cefuroxime penetrates the CNS and has been approved for treatment of meningitis, but there is only limited clinical experience with the agent in this setting. **Adverse reactions** seen with these agents are similar to those of the first-generation cephalosporins, but there is an increased propensity for coagulopathy owing to suppressed vitamin K production. Cefamandole can cause a disulfiram-like reaction.

Third-generation cephalosporins currently available are **cefotaxime, moxalactam, cefoperazone, and ceftizoxime.** They have improved activity against the beta-lactamase-producing *N. gonorrhoeae, H. influenzae*, and enteric gram-negative bacilli. They have both broader spectra of activity and more intrinsic activity against each susceptible organism (lower MIC). Activity against *P. aeruginosa* is variable, and the use of any of these agents for hospital-acquired enteric gram-negative bacilli should be guided by in vitro susceptibility testing. They have significantly less activity against gram-positive bacteria than the first-generation cephalosporins. Moxalactam has activity against anaerobic bacteria comparable to cefoxitin.

Therapeutic antibiotic concentrations are achieved in bile and CSF with usual dosage. This has allowed these antibiotics to be used for **treat-**

ment of gram-negative bacillary meningitis. There has been more experience treating meningitis with cefotaxime and moxalactam than with cefoperazone or ceftizoxime, and these **latter agents are not approved for this use at this time.** **Adverse reactions** with these agents include hypersensitivity reactions, prolongation of the prothrombin time due to inhibition of vitamin K production (particularly with moxalactam), an increased propensity for superinfections with resistant organisms (particularly *Candida albicans* and enterococci), and disulfiram-like reactions with moxalactam and cefoperazone.

b. **Vancomycin** is a bactericidal agent that irreversibly binds to the mucopeptide portion of the bacterial cell wall of susceptible bacteria by a different mechanism from that of the beta-lactam antibiotics. It is active against all gram-positive cocci including methicillin-resistant *S. aureus* and multidrug-resistant *S. pneumoniae*. It usually is not bactericidal for the enterococci at therapeutically achievable concentrations but is synergistically active in conjunction with aminoglycosides. Gram-positive aerobic and anaerobic bacilli including *Bacillus anthracis*, diptheroids, and *Clostridium* species are susceptible.

Vancomycin is poorly absorbed from the gastrointestinal tract and **must be administered intravenously** for systemic therapy. The usual adult dose is 500 mg, i.v. every 6 hr, in patients with normal renal function. Normally 80% to 90% of vancomycin is excreted unchanged by the kidneys, and there is minimal biliary excretion or in vivo metabolism. The half-life is markedly prolonged **with renal insufficiency**, and vancomycin is not removed by hemodialysis or peritoneal dialysis. A single dose of 15 mg/kg every 7 to 10 days can be given to anuric patients to maintain serum drug levels in a range from 8 to 25 µg/ml. Serum concentrations greater than 50 µg/ml 1 hr after intravenous administration should be avoided.

Vancomycin **diffuses rapidly** into soft tissue, bone, and body fluids. Although it does not penetrate normal meninges, therapeutic CSF concentrations are achieved in meningeal inflammation.

Initial preparations of vancomycin in the 1960s may have been impure and were associated with nausea, flushing, nephrotoxicity, phlebitis, eosinophilia, and maculopapular rashes. The recent preparations have not been associated with these complications. **Ototoxicity** and **nephrotoxicity** may develop with serum concentrations of 50 µg/ml. Nephrotoxicity may be more frequent when vancomycin is used in association with an aminoglycoside.

2. Agents that inhibit protein synthesis

a. **Aminoglycosides.** The aminoglycoside antibiotics include **neomycin, kanamycin, streptomycin, gentamicin, tobramycin, amikacin, and netilimicin.** They share a common bactericidal mechanism of irreversible binding to bacterial ribosomal proteins. Differences in the spectrum of activity of these antibiotics are the result of both differing bacterial uptake of the agent and differing susceptibilities of the agents to R-plasmid-mediated inactivating enzymes.

These antibiotics have similar spectra of **activity** and pharmacokinetic properties. All have some activity against *S. aureus*, but other gram-positive bacteria are usually resistant. Streptococcal species, including enterococci, are resistant to the aminoglycosides alone but show synergistic sensitivity to the combination of an aminoglycoside and either a basic penicillin, an ampicillin-like agent, or vancomycin. The aminoglycosides are most active against aerobic gram-negative bacilli, including the *Enterobacteriaceae*, *P. aeruginosa*, and such less common pathogens as *Yersinia pestis* (the cause of plague), *Francisella tularensis* (the cause of tularemia), and *Brucella* species. The mycobacteria also are susceptible to agents of this class, but essentially all other microorganisms are resistant.

All of these drugs have minimal (1%) absorption after oral administration and require intramuscular or intravenous administration (Table 5). The half-life of these agents in persons with normal renal function is approximately 2 hr. All are rapidly excreted by the kidney, and dosage modification is required with renal insufficiency; all are removed by hemodialysis or peritoneal dialysis. There is **good penetration** across serosal and synovial membranes, into bile, and across the placenta. Pulmonary concentrations are usually less than 40% of serum levels, and there are only minimal CSF levels even with inflamed meninges.

TABLE 5. *Use of aminoglycosides*

Agents	Usual dosage and route of administration	Specific advantages	Specific disadvantages and adverse effects
Streptomycin	1 g/day, i.m. q.d. or b.i.d.	Drug of choice for brucellosis, plague, tularemia, first-line agent for *M. tuberculosis*	Most enteric gram-negative bacilli are resistant
Kanamycin	15 mg/kg/day, i.m./i.v. q 6–12 hr		In-hospital enteric gram-negative bacilli are frequently resistant
Neomycin	4–12 g/day, p.o.	Treatment of hepatic coma	3% systemic absorption, diarrhea
Gentamicin	Initial 2 mg/kg; maintenance 3–5 mg/kg/day, i.m./i.v. q 8–12 hr		
Tobramycin	Initial 2 mg/kg; maintenance 3–5 mg/kg/day, i.m./i.v. q 8–12 hr	May have less nephrotoxicity and ototoxicity than gentamicin	
Amikacin	Initial 7.5 mg/kg; maintenance 15 mg/kg/day, i.m./i.v. q 8–12 hr	Aminoglycoside of choice when gentamicin resistance is prevalent	
Netilimicin	Initial 2 mg/kg; maintenance 3–5 mg/kg/day, i.m./i.v. q 8–12 hr	May be less nephrotoxic and ototoxic than gentamicin	

The aminoglycosides have a low toxic-to-therapeutic ratio, and **therapy should be monitored with serum drug assays.** Peak serum levels 30 min after intravenous administration or 1 hr after intramuscular administration should not exceed 10 μg/ml for **gentamicin, tobramycin,** or **netilimicin;** 30 μg/ml for **amikacin;** or 40 μg/ml for **kanamycin and streptomycin. Nephrotoxicity** can be produced by all of these agents, with neomycin the most nephrotoxic and streptomycin the least. The nephrotoxicity appears to be dose related and is potentiated by "loop" diuretics, advanced age, hypotension, or the recurrent use of a cephalosporin or vancomycin. **Ototoxicity** also is a dose-related effect of all aminoglycosides. Vestibular dysfunction is more frequently associated with streptomycin, gentamicin, and tobramycin, auditory toxicity with kanamycin and amikacin. Ototoxicity also can be potentiated by loop diuretics and advanced age. A rare complication of these agents is neuromuscular blockade, which is enhanced with preexisting myasthenia gravis or concurrent use of neuromuscular blocking agents.

b. **Chloramphenicol** is a bacteriostatic antibiotic that reversibly inhibits bacterial protein synthesis and has a broad spectrum of activity. It is generally active against gram-positive cocci and bacilli, although some strains of enterococci, *S. aureus, S. pneumoniae,* and *Nocardia* are resistant. Most aerobic and anaerobic gram-negative bacteria are sensitive to chloramphenicol, including community-acquired enteric gram-negative bacilli, *Neisseria* species, *H. influenzae, Brucella,* and *B. fragilis.* Occasional strains of *Salmonella, Shigella, B. fragilis* and hospital-acquired gram-negative bacilli can be resistant.

Chloramphenicol can be administered orally or parenterally. The usual adult dosage is 1 to 3 g/day, every 6 hr. It is **distributed widely** in the body and penetrates well into bone, placenta, brain, eye, across serosal and synovial membranes, and into CSF. It is metabolized to an inactive nontoxic form in the **liver** and excreted in the urine.

A reversible dose-related **bone marrow suppression** can occur with anemia, leukopenia, and thrombocytopenia in as many as one-third of patients treated with chloramphenicol. This occurs more frequently in patients with hepatic dysfunction and at daily doses greater than 2 g. Irreversible **fatal aplastic anemia** occurs with a frequency between 1 in 11,500 to 1 in 21,600 treatment courses. **Additional toxicities** include the gray syndrome (circulatory collapse in premature infants and newborns), optic neuritis, coagulopathy resulting from vitamin K deficiency, hypersensitivity reactions, and gastrointestinal disturbances.

c. **Clindamycin and lincomycin** reversibly block bacterial protein synthesis by binding to ribosomal proteins. They have comparable spectra of activity, although clindamycin is the more active. They are effective against most gram-positive cocci except the enterococci but less so than the beta-lactam antibiotics and vancomycin. They can be used for these pathogens in the penicillin- and cephalosporin-allergic patient, although therapy should be guided by susceptibility testing. Almost all the aerobic gram-negative bacteria are resistant. The anerobic gram-negative bacilli, including *B. fragilis,* are susceptible. They are not effective against mycobacteria, mycoplasmas, rickettsiae, or fungi, but clindamycin is active against the malarial pathogens *Plasmodium falciparum* and *P. vivax*, and against *Babesia microti*. Both agents can be administered either orally or parenterally. The usual adult dose for clindamycin is 150 to 450 mg, p.o., every 6 hr, or 150 to 900 mg, i.v., every 6 hr; for lincomycin, 500 mg, p.o., every 6 to 8 hr, or 600 to 1,200 mg, i.v., every 8 to 12 hr. Both antibiotics **penetrate well** into soft tissue and bone and cross placental, synovial, and serosal membranes. They do not achieve therapeutic CSF concentrations. They undergo **hepatic metabolism** and are excreted in the urine. Dosage reduction should be considered with severe hepatic disease.

The major **toxicity** of these agents is gastrointestinal, with diarrhea occurring in up to 7% of treated patients. Much less frequently pseudomembranous colitis owing to *Clostridium difficile* will develop (see II. C. 6.). Hypersensitivity reactions, minor elevations of aspartate aminotransferase (SGOT), jaundice, and neutropenia are rare adverse effects.

d. **Erythromycin** is a bacteriostatic agent that binds to bacterial ribosomal proteins. It is active against most gram-positive bacteria and many *Nocardia* isolates, but strains of enterococci and *S. aureus* can be resistant. It is less active against these bacteria than are the beta-lactam antibiotics or vancomycin. Erythromycin is active against some gram-negative bacteria including *N. gonorrhoeae, Bordetella pertussis, Campylobacter jejuni* and *Legionella* species, but most gram-negative bacteria are resistant. It is active against *T. pallidum, Chlamydia trachomatis*, mycoplasmas, and epidemic and scrub typhus.

Erythromycin can be administered orally or parenterally. The usual dosage is 500 mg, p.o., every 6 hr, but oral administration can be increased to 1 g, p.o., every 6 hr. For serious infections, 300 to 1,500 mg, i.v., every 6 hr, can be administered. Erythromycin is **broadly distributed** in the body, crossing all membranes well except for the meninges. Adequate CSF concentrations are not achieved. Erythromycin undergoes significant metabolic inactivation, apparently in the **liver**, and is excreted into the bile. Dosage modification should be considered with severe hepatic dysfunction.

Mild nausea, vomiting, and diarrhea are the most frequent **side effects** and are dose related. Ototoxicity and skin rashes occur quite rarely. Cholestatic jaundice develops with erythromycin estolate at a frequency of 1 per 1,000 courses but does not occur with other erythromycin preparations.

e. **Tetracyclines.** The tetracyclines are primarily bacteriostatic compounds that bind to bacterial ribosomal proteins. When initially introduced, they had activity against most gram-positive bacteria, but a high prevalence of resistant staphylococcal and streptococcal strains has developed, and the tetracyclines are third-line agents against these pathogens. They are active against a variety of aerobic gram-negative bacteria, including *E. coli, Klebsiella, Yersinia, Brucella, P. multocida, F. tularensis, H. influenzae, N. meningitidis*, and *N. gonorrhoeae*, but most hospital-acquired gram-negative bacilli and the *Bacteroides* species are resistant. The spirochetes *T. palli-*

dum, Borrelia, and *Leptospirae,* and the Lyme arthritis agent are all susceptible to tetracyclines as are the *Mycoplasma* species, rickettsiae, and chlamydiae.

The tetracyclines can be administered orally or parenterally. Dosages are given in Table 6. They **penetrate well** into all body cavities and fluids, and adequate CSF concentrations are achieved across inflamed meninges. **Minocycline and doxycycline** are the most lipophilic and have the best penetration into the CNS. These agents are excreted through the urine and bile.

The most common **side effects** are mild gastrointestinal disturbances, vaginal yeast infections, and photosensitivity. Tetracyclines are deposited in the teeth and bone of growing children and cause discoloration of teeth in children exposed when less than 6 to 7 years of age, or in utero when exposed after the first trimester of pregnancy. For this reason and because of an association with "acute fatty liver of pregnancy" when given intravenously, they should be used **very carefully in pregnant women**. They should not be administered to patients with renal insufficiency, as they can exacerbate preexisting renal disease. Hepatotoxicity can rarely develop.

3. Agents that inhibit DNA or RNA synthesis

a. Rifampin is a bactericidal agent that binds to RNA polymerase, thus inhibiting RNA and protein synthesis. Its spectrum of activity is quite broad, but its use is limited by the rapid development of microbial resistance when it is administered alone. It is active against most gram-positive bacteria, including methicillin-resistant *S. aureus, Neisseria* species, and *Brucella* and *Legionella* species. It is highly active against *Mycobacterium tuberculosis,* therapy for which is its major clinical indication, and is also active against some of the atypical mycobacteria and *M. leprae.*

TABLE 6. *Use of tetracyclines*

Agents	Usual dosage and route of administration	Specific advantages	Specific disadvantages and adverse effects
Tetracycline and chlortetracycline	0.25–0.5 g, p.o. q 6 hr		i.m. administration painful and not recommended
Oxytetracycline	0.5–1.0 g, i.v./i.m. q 12 hr		i.v. administration associated with thrombophlebitis
Demeclocycline	150 mg, p.o. q 6 hr or 300 mg, p.o. q 12 hr		Nephrogenic diabetes insipidus (invariable at dose of 1200 mg/day)
Doxycycline	100 mg, p.o./i.v. q 12 hr	Safer to use in patients with renal failure	
Methacycline	150 mg, p.o. q 6 hr or 300 mg, p.o. q 12 hr		
Minocycline	100 mg, p.o. q 12 hr	Safer to use in patients with renal failure, alternate agent for meningococcal prophylaxis	Vestibular toxicity (30–89%)

Rifampin is well absorbed after oral administration and has been administered in dosage of 8 to 20 mg/kg/day, either q.d. or b.i.d. Usually, it is given as 600 mg, p.o., q.d. before breakfast. It is **broadly distributed** in the body, penetrating all tissues well. Therapeutic CSF concentrations are easily achieved across inflamed meninges. It is excreted through both the liver and kidneys with the hepatic route predominant.

Rifampin causes a harmless red discoloration of body fluids that may be mistaken for blood. Important **toxicities** include hepatotoxicity in up to 20% of patients, particularly in patients receiving concurrent hepatotoxic drugs or those with preexisting liver disease or alcoholism. Thrombocytopenia, anemia, hypersensitivity reactions (including interstitial nephritis, drug fever, and "influenza syndrome"), and gastrointestinal disturbances also may develop.

b. **Sulfonamides** are a class of bacteriostatic antimicrobial agents that act by blocking folate metabolism. The development of acquired bacterial resistance has greatly restricted their in-hospital use. They remain active against some strains of gram-positive cocci, the actinomyces and *Nocardia* species, community-acquired enteric gram-negative bacilli, some *N. meningitidis* isolates, and the malaria and *Toxoplasma* strains. The spectra of activity of the sulfonamides are so similar that only one agent is used for standard susceptibility testing.

The sulfonamides are usually administered orally, although parenteral preparations of sulfadiazine are available. The dosage varies with the preparations. Adult dosage of the short-acting agents, including sulfadiazine and "triple sulfas," is 2 to 3 g initially and 1.0 g every 6 hr subsequently. For the longer-acting agent, sulfmethoxazole, the dosage is 2 g initially followed by 1.0 g every 12 hr. Eliminated predominantly through the **kidneys** with minimal bilary excretion, the short- and medium-acting sulfonamides achieve significantly higher urinary concentrations than the longer-acting agents. All of these agents are **well distributed** in the body. The short-acting agents achieve therapeutic CSF concentrations across normal meninges, and there is significant placental transfer.

The sulfonamides have some uncommon but significant **adverse effects**, including hypersensitivity reactions, drug fever, photosensitization, Stevens-Johnson syndrome, periarteritis nodosa, systemic lupus erythematosus, blood dyscrasias (agranulocytosis, hemolytic anemia in G6PD-deficient persons), hepatotoxicity, and nephrotoxicity (primarily the result of crystalluria). Teratogenicity has been noted in laboratory animals but has not been reported in humans.

c. **Trimethoprim-sulfamethoxazole** (TMP-SMX) is a fixed 1:5 combination of trimethoprim, an inhibitor of the enzyme dihydrofolate reductase important in folate metabolism, and a medium-acting sulfonamide. Although both agents may be used alone, the combination has a synergistic bactericidal effect against a variety of microorganisms, including most nonenterococcal gram-positive cocci, the majority of the gram-negative bacilli, and *N. meningitidis, N. gonorrhoeae, H. influenzae, H. ducreyi, Nocardia, Chla-*

mydia, and some atypical mycobacteria. TMP-SMX also is active against *Pneumocystis carinii*. *Pseudomonas* isolates are resistant.

TMP-SMX is well-absorbed after oral or intravenous administration. The usual adult dosage is 160 mg trimethoprim and 800 mg sulfamethoxazole, p.o., every 12 hr. For serious infections such as *Pneumocystis carinii* pneumonia, a maximum dose of 20 mg/kg/day of trimethoprim should be used either orally or parenterally. A peak serum sulfamethoxazole concentration of 100 μg/ml should be obtained. Trimethoprim alone is available for urinary tract infection (UTI) or the prevention of traveler's diarrhea; the usual adult dosage is 100 mg, p.o., every 12 hr.

Both agents are **distributed well** throughout the body, with good bone, soft tissue, and CSF penetration. Trimethoprim is particularly concentrated in prostatic tissue. The primary route of excretion of both agents is **renal**, with minimal biliary elimination.

Adverse effects associated with TMP-SMX are uncommon but include all the toxicities associated with sulfonamide therapy. Skin rashes and gastrointestinal disturbances each occur independently with a frequency of 3.5%. Megaloblastic anemia, hepatotoxicity, and nephrotoxicity all have been noted rarely.

d. **Metronidazole** is a microbial agent with activity derived from its intracellular reduction to a toxic molecule by enzymes essential for anaerobic growth. It is currently the most active agent available against the **obligate anaerobic bacteria**, including *Bacteroides* and *Clostridia* species. It has less activity against microaerophilic organisms and gram-positive anaerobic cocci and has no activity against most other microorganisms except the protozoa *Trichomonas vaginalis, Entamoeba histolytica*, and *Giardia lamblia*.

Metronidazole is well absorbed after oral or rectal administration and may also be given intravenously. The usual dosage for metronidazole varies with the clinical setting. Anaerobic infections are treated with an initial 15 mg/kg dose and 7.5 mg/kg every 6 hr subsequently. Trichomoniasis and giardiasis may be treated with 250 mg every 8 hr for 7 to 10 days; trichomoniasis also may be treated with a single 2-g dose. Amebiasis is treated with 750 mg every 8 hr for 7 to 10 days.

The major route of excretion is **renal**, although **hepatic** metabolism occurs and dosage should be modified for severe hepatic insufficiency. The drug is **distributed well** throughout the body, with bactericidal levels achieved in bone, abscess cavities, brain, CSF, and bile.

Metronidazole has **relatively few adverse effects**. It may induce a disulfiram-like reaction, a metallic taste, or minor gastrointestinal disturbances. Less frequently, it produces reversible neutropenia or CNS side effects. Of potential concern is an association between metronidazole and carcinogenicity in laboratory animals. To date there has been no evidence of an increased frequency of cancer or birth defects among humans treated with metronidazole, although the predicted frequency of such events makes it unlikely that it would appear yet.

4. Agents used predominantly for mycobacterial infections

a. **Isoniazid** is a bactericidal agent that is exclusively active against mycobacteria. It appears to inhibit synthesis of mycolic acids essential for these organisms, although the exact mechanism of action remains to be defined. Isoniazid is administered orally in a dose of 5 to 8 mg/kg/day, typically 300 mg in a single dose. With severe illness, the dosage may be increased to 10 mg/kg/day. It also may be administered twice weekly at 15 mg/kg in certain standardized antituberculous regimens.

Isoniazid is metabolized by acetylation in the **liver** and excreted in the urine. It is **well distributed** in all body fluids and tissues, including CSF and areas of caseous necrosis. It has **relatively little toxicity.** The major adverse effect is hepatitis with asymptomatic transaminase elevation developing in up to 20% of patients. Overt hepatitis develops in only 1% of treated patients, with an increased frequency seen in patients over 35 years of age, alcoholics, and those receiving concurrent rifampin. Additional infrequent toxicities include fever, maculopapular rashes, and reversible peripheral neuropathy owing to induction of pyridoxine deficiency. This final effect is rare and occurs only at doses greater than 10 mg/kg/day. It can be reversed with supplemental pyridoxine administration without altering the antimycobacterial efficacy. Rarely, psychosis, confusion, convulsions, and muscle twitchings can occur.

b. **Rifampin** (see C.3.a.).

c. **Ethambutol** is a mycobacteriostatic agent that appears to inhibit RNA synthesis. It is administered orally with a usual initial dosage of 25 mg/kg/day, which can be decreased to 15 mg/kg/day for daily therapy or increased to 50 mg/kg/day for twice-weekly therapy. It is predominantly **excreted through the kidney**, and dosage should be modified for severe renal insufficiency or dialysis. Detailed information on distribution in the body is unavailable, but it appears that only very low CSF concentrations can be achieved.

The **major toxicity** of ethambutol is a dose-related optic neuritis that is reversible if recognized shortly after onset. Additional extremely rare side effects include peripheral neuritis, nephrotoxicity, and allergic reactions.

d. **Pyrazinamide** is a bactericidal agent active against intracellular mycobacteria through an undefined mechanism of action. It is active only against *M. tuberculosis*. There is nearly total absorption after oral administration, and the recommended dosage is 30 mg/kg/day. It is **excreted by the kidney** after metabolism in the body. Distribution in the body has not been completely defined, but CSF penetration appears to be adequate. Pyrazinamide can produce hepatitis, hyperuricemia, gastrointestinal discomfort, hypersensitivity reactions, and arthralgias.

e. **Para-aminosalicylic acid** (PAS) is a bacteriostatic agent that inhibits folate synthesis in mycobacteria. The usual orally or intravenously administered adult dosage is 10 to 20 g/day in one or two doses. PAS is **excreted through the kidney**, and the dosage should be modified for renal failure. It is **distributed well** throughout the body except for the CSF. PAS may cause gastrointestinal irritation, fever, skin rashes, hepatitis, neutropenia, hemolytic anemia (in G6PD deficient individuals), and sodium overload.

5. **Systemic antifungal agents**

a. **Amphotericin B** is a fungicidal agent that disrupts the integrity of the plasma membrane of susceptible fungi by binding to an ergosterol component. It is active against *Cryptococcus neoformans, Candida* species, *Torulopsis glabrata*, and the agents of spirotrichosis, North and South American blastomycosis, histoplasmosis, coccidioidomycosis, aspergillosis, and mucormycosis. It can act synergistically with 5-flucytosine (5-FC) against *Candida* species and *C. neoformans* by promoting its penetration into the fungi. In vitro testing suggests that miconazole and ketoconazole can antagonize amphotericin B by blocking synthesis of the ergosterols to which it binds.

Amphotericin B is a relatively insoluble compound that is poorly absorbed after oral or intramuscular administration. It is given by slow intravenous infusion over 4 to 6 hr as a colloid suspension in 5% dextrose. It is light sensitive and precipitates in the presence of salt; its use is associated with both **local phlebitis and systemic reactions** such as chills, fever, hypotension, and arrhythmias during the infusion. Heparin (500 to 1,000 U) and hydrocortisone (5 to 25 mg) may be added to the infusion to diminish these reactions. Patients who have had reactions on prior doses may benefit from premedication with an antihistamine, antiemetic, or antipyretic. A **test dose** of 1 mg must be given by slow infusion to observe for severe febrile or hypotensive reactions. Immediately thereafter, a dose of 5 to 10 mg can be given, followed by daily infusions incrementally increased by 10 to 20 mg/day until a dose of 0.5 to 1.0 mg/kg/day is achieved. The dose should not exceed 50 mg/day. Many patients will not be able to tolerate this dosage because of nephrotoxicity and should receive reduced daily doses or alternate-day therapy. Amphotericin B is conventionally given to a total dose of 1.0 to 2.0 g, depending on the clinical situation. It may be administered **intrathecally or intraventricularly** in gradually increasing doses to a maximum of 0.3 mg two to three times per week, **intraperitoneally** at a concentration of 1 μg/ml, or as **bladder irrigation** with 50 mg in 1,000 ml sterile water infused daily. **Such usages require consultation with a physician who has had experience with this drug.**

The distribution and excretion of amphotericin B are unknown although it appears to be stored in **body fat**. It **penetrates poorly** into body fluids, and CSF levels are low. Amphotericin B is a **very toxic agent** used only because there are no other comparable agents available. **Adverse reactions** are frequent during intravenous administration and include fever, chills, headache, and gastrointestinal disturbances. Thrombophlebitis is common. Nephrotoxicity always accompanies amphotericin B administration, but therapy usually can be continued if the serum creatinine remains less than 3 mg%. Early toxicity is reversible if the agent is withheld for several days, and amphotericin B can be reinstituted at a lower daily dosage or on an alternate-day regimen. Additional toxicities include anemia, renal tubular acidosis, and severe pulmonary reactions when the agent is administered concurrently with granulocyte transfusions.

b. **5-Flucytosine.** 5-FC interferes with fungal nucleic acid synthesis. Activity is limited to the pathogenic yeasts (*C. neoformans, Candida* species, and *Torulopsis* species) and *Asperigillus* species. It should not be used as single-drug therapy, as resistant organisms can emerge during therapy. 5-FC is administered orally at a usual dosage of 37.5 mg/kg every 6 hr. Ninety percent of an oral dose is **excreted unchanged in the urine**, and the dosage should be lowered with renal failure or dialysis. 5-FC drug assays are available through referral laboratories and should be used to maintain peak levels between 50 and 75 μg/ml. 5-FC is **distributed to all body tissues and fluids**, including CSF.

Toxicities include skin rashes, nausea, vomiting, leukopenia, thrombocytopenia, hepatotoxicity, and enterocolitis. The bone marrow and hepatic toxicities are both dose related and occur more frequently with serum levels ≥ 100 μg/ml. The agent is teratogenic in laboratory animals and is **contraindicated in pregnancy.**

c. The **imidazoles** are a family of antifungal agents that inhibit synthesis of ergosterol, an essential component of the fungal cell membrane. The family includes **clotrimazole, miconazole, and ketoconazole**, but only the latter two can be used systemically. **Miconazole** and **ketoconazole** have similar spectrums of activity, being active in vitro against strains of *C. neoformans, Candida* species, *Histoplasma capsulatum, Paracoccidioides brasiliensis, Blastomyces dermitides, Coccidioides immitis, Sporotrichium schenkii,* some *Aspergillus* species, the dermatophytes, and *Petriellidium boydii* (an amphotericin-B–resistant fungus). Studies of the clinical efficacy of these agents are limited, and in most instances they should be considered second-line antifungal agents.

Miconazole is poorly absorbed from the gastrointestinal tract and is available only as an intravenous preparation or a topical cream. The intravenous dosage is 400 to 1,200 mg, i.v., every 8 hr after a trial dose of 200 mg. **Ketoconazole** achieves adequate serum concentrations with oral administration; however, an acid milieu is required, and achlorhydria, cimetidine, and antacids decrease absorption. The usual adult dosage is 200 to 400 mg/day given once a day with a mildly acidic liquid.

The imidazoles are metabolized to inactive compounds in the liver, and dosage does not require adjustment for renal insufficiency. Relatively little is known about the penetration of the imidazoles into body tissues and fluids. **Miconazole** has poor penetration into urine, sputum, and CSF. If it is used for fungal meningitis, then intrathecal or intraventricular therapy should be considered. **Ketoconazole** has poor penetration into urine, bone, and CSF and is not efficacious for infections in these sites.

The imidazoles are significantly **less toxic than amphotericin B. Miconazole** has been associated with pruritus, skin rashes, phlebitis, thrombocytosis, hyperlipidemia, and hyponatremia. Acute cardiorespiratory arrest has been reported with the first intravenous dose, and it is recommended by the manufacturer that a trial dose of 200 mg (in at least 200 ml D_5W) be administered over 60 min with a physician present. **Ketoconazole** has been associated with nausea, pruritus, gynecomastia, rash, and cholestatic hepatitis. Hepatic enzyme studies should be evaluated periodically in patients on long-term therapy.

6. **Antiviral agents.** Relatively few nontoxic chemotherapeutic approaches to treating viral infection currently exist. At present there are no broad-spectrum antiviral agents. Current agents block viral metabolic pathways that are unique to a single virus or a single class of viruses.

a. **Amantadine and rimantadine** appear to inhibit the penetration of the **influenza A virus** into susceptible cells. Activity is limited to influenza A viruses, and these agents are effective in both treatment and prophylaxis. They can reduce the severity and duration of fever and the intensity of other influenzal symptoms. Prophylaxis is effective only during the period of administration.

Amantadine and rimantadine are well absorbed orally. The usual adult dosage for amantadine is 200 mg/day given in two doses; for rimantadine, 100 to 200 mg/day in two doses. These agents are **excreted unchanged in the urine**, and their dosage should be adjusted with severe renal insufficiency.

Approximately 5% of patients treated with amantadine develop **mild reversible CNS effects** that most frequently include lightheadedness, difficulty concentrating, and insomnia. Rarely, vision disturbances, ataxia, anorexia, skin rashes, and urinary frequency have been noted. Rimantadine has been less frequently associated with the same reactions. These agents should be used **with more caution** in patients with epilepsy or severe cerebral atherosclerotic disease.

b. **Vidarabine (adenine arabinoside;** ara-A) inhibits viral DNA replication and is clinically effective against active **herpes simplex** and **herpes zoster-varicella** virus infections, although it has no effect on latent infection. Ara-A can be administered as a 3% **topical** ophthalmic ointment or **intravenously**. Oral absorption is poor, and intramuscular administration produces pain and muscle necrosis. Ara-A is given in a dose of 10 to 15 mg/kg/day in a single 12-hr infusion. It is relatively insoluble and cannot be given in a concentration greater than 0.7 mg/ml. It is compatible with all common intravenous solutions but not with blood, plasma, or plasma expanders.

Ara-A is rapidly metabolized to a less active ara-hypoxanthine that is **renally excreted**. The dosage should be decreased in patients with renal failure. The distribution of ara-A has not been adequately studied, but clinically it has been effective for treatment of **encephalitis and disseminated infections.**

The **major toxicities** related to ara-A include fluid overload and cerebral edema in susceptible patients—owing to the large fluid volume required for administration—anorexia, nausea, vomiting, megaloblastic anemia, leukopenia, tremors, and thrombophlebitis. Coma and death have been reported in several patients with chronic renal failure. The drug should be **avoided in pregnancy.**

c. Acyclovir blocks viral DNA replication and is clinically effective for **herpes simplex** and **herpes zoster-varicella** viral infections. It is converted to an active form by viral thymidine kinase; resistant herpes viruses lacking this enzyme have been noted. Like ara-A, it blocks active viral replication but does not affect latent herpes viruses.

Acyclovir is currently available as both a 5% **topical** ointment and an **intravenous** preparation. Topical acyclovir is applied to lesions every 3 hr for 7 days. The intravenous dose of acyclovir is 5 mg/kg every 8 hr for herpes simplex infections or 5 to 10 mg/kg every 8 hr for herpes zoster infections.

Acyclovir is **excreted predominantly through the kidney**, and dosage reduction with renal failure may be necessary. It is **well distributed** throughout the body, including the CSF and is the drug of choice for disseminated herpes simplex and herpes zoster infections. At present there are no data available on the use of acyclovir for CNS disease, and ara-A should be used for these infections. Acyclovir appears to be a **relatively nontoxic** agent, although intravenous treatment has been associated with reversible elevations of serum creatinine and aspartate aminotransaminase. Cutaneous irritation after extravasation from a vein can occur.

II. TREATMENT OF INFECTIOUS DISEASES

A. Approach to the Patient Suspected of Having an Infection

1. **Diagnosis.** Proper diagnosis is the key to treatment of infectious diseases, as it is for all aspects of medicine. Particular emphasis should be placed on obtaining a **history** relevant to the following symptoms: fever, rigors, and local as well as general manifestations of inflammation, including pain, swelling, redness, warmth, and loss of function. Since any organ system can be involved and any symptom can be produced by infection, careful history taking will provide the correct diagnosis in at least 75% of cases. Important **physical findings** include fever, the signs of local inflammation, and purulence. Few **laboratory tests** are of value, but among those that are most useful are the total and differential white blood cell counts, microscopic examinations of involved body fluids, and radiographic examinations of involved areas. An important diagnostic goal is to **differentiate between infection**, which should be treated, **and colonization**, which usually should not.

2. **Principles of infectious disease management. Drain appropriate infections.** Some infections—such as urinary tract infections, gastroenteritis, and pneumonia—drain spontaneously. The role of the physician is to encourage drainage from naturally draining sites or to permit drainage from deep sites by surgical intervention. **In hospital practice, failure to respond to antimicrobial therapy is most often due to failure to provide adequate drainage.**

Maintain function of diseased organs. Supportive therapy, such as ventilation, is often necessary until the infected organ can return to function. **Ad-**

minister antitoxins. Toxins can disable or kill before antibiotics are effective. Illnesses for which antitoxins are necessary include botulism, tetanus, and diphtheria. Passive or active immunization for such viral diseases as rabies may be life-saving. **Remove foreign bodies.** In most cases, infection cannot be eradicated when contaminated foreign bodies (e.g., sequestra, catheters) are left in place. **Alleviate precipitating factors.** Underlying conditions such as hyperglycemia, neutropenia, and immunosuppression make the treatment of infections difficult, and should be reversed as quickly as possible. **Isolate infected patients** to prevent the spread of pathogens to other patients or hospital employees. Every hospital has an infection-control policy mandating requirements for respiratory, skin and wound, enteric, blood and secretion, and complete isolation. Such procedures should be rigorously enforced. If a communicable disease (such as tuberculosis) is suspected, isolate the patient until the disease has been excluded.

Use of antimicrobial agents: In most cases bactericidal agents are not necessary. The exceptions are endovascular infections, endocarditis, osteomyelitis, bacterial meningitis, and rapidly progressive infections (such as streptococcal bacteremia) in which host defenses are not adequate. There are several circumstances in which the use of more than one antimicrobial agent may be indicated:

a. Empiric broad-spectrum therapy for suspected bacterial infection in a patient too ill to await culture results (e.g., septic shock).

b. Documented or suspected polymicrobial infections for which a single agent is not sufficient (e.g., ruptured abdominal viscus).

c. When antimicrobial synergy is necessary, as in cryptococcal meningitis, enterococcal endocarditis, and suspected or documented gram-negative infection in neutropenic hosts.

d. To prevent emergence of drug resistance, as in some mycobacterial infections.

Antimicrobial therapy of most infections should be continued until the infection has been eradicated. Usually a decision on the duration of treatment is based on established precedents. Table 7 contains guidelines for the duration of therapy in several common conditions; however, individual judgments are most important.

Use of antipyretic therapy: Fever should be treated only if its continued presence compromises host functions. It is a cardinal sign of infection and a valuable indicator of the state of infection in most situations. To obscure a fever may needlessly prolong the time necessary for diagnosis and to assess response to therapy. **Follow-up cultures** are rarely helpful. Before ordering follow-up cultures the physician must answer the question: "What can I learn from the culture results that will influence therapy?"

B. Pneumonia "Captain of the men of death," pneumonia occurs both in previously healthy persons and in patients debilitated by a wide variety of chronic conditions. In all age groups, in all parts of the world, pneumonia is one of the leading causes of morbidity and mortality. A large number of microbial agents cause pneumonia.

TABLE 7. *Guidelines on duration of antimicrobial therapy
for common infectious problems*

Condition	Specific diagnosis	Duration (days)
Pneumonia	Pneumococcal	10
	Gram-negative	21–28
	Lung abscess	42–90
	Tuberculosis	180–270
Endocarditis	Viridans streptococcal	28
	Enterococcal	42
	Staphylococcal	28–42
Meningitis	Bacterial	14
	Cryptococcal	42
Urinary tract	Cystitis	1ᵃ or 5–10
infection	Pyelonephritis	10–14
Osteomyelitis	Staphylococcal	42
Peritonitis	Spontaneous	10–14
	bacterial	
Genital tract	Pelvic inflammatory	10–21
Pharyngitis	Streptococcal	1ᵃ or 10
Arthritis	Staphylococcal	28–42

ᵃSingle-dose therapy.

Although there is considerable overlap between the two groups, pneumonia may be thought of as either community or nosocomially acquired.

1. **Diagnosis.** The diagnosis of pneumonia is based on the constellation of symptoms (fever, cough, dyspnea, chest pain) and signs (temperature elevation, tachypnea, signs of consolidation) present.

   a. **Chest X-ray.** An infiltrate on chest X-ray confirms the presence of pneumonia in a patient whose clinical signs and symptoms are compatible, but chest X-ray findings are nonspecific and may be present in a variety of other pulmonary conditions. Early in the course of pneumonia no infiltrates may be present. **The upper airways have resident bacterial flora; therefore, with few exceptions, sputum examination is not helpful unless an infiltrate is present on chest X-ray.** Chest X-ray also may detect lung abscesses (pneumatocoeles), cavities, and effusions. Specialized techniques, including lordotic films for demonstrating apical tuberculosis, lateral decubitus films for demonstrating effusions, and tomograms for demonstrating calcifications in coin lesions, are often valuable.

   b. **Sputum examination** may yield important clues to the etiology of pneumonia. Specimens may be either **expectorated** sputum, a **nasotracheal aspirate**, or a **transtracheal aspirate**. An adequate specimen contains fewer than 10 epithelial cells per low-power field. If expectorated or nasotracheally acquired specimens are inadequate, transtracheal aspiration should be considered. **Complications** of a transtracheal aspiration include tracheal hemorrhage, pneumomediastinum, and vagal reactions; however, these are rare in the hands of clinicians experienced with this technique.

   A sputum specimen should always be examined by Gram stain, and adequate specimens should be cultured for aerobic bacterial pathogens. Gram stain will indicate the predominant bacterial flora and the presence or absence of polymorphonuclear leukocytes. In general, smears with epithelial cells represent oral secretions and need not be cultured. If clinical circumstances warrant, viral, mycoplasma, or anaerobic cultures (only from transtracheal aspirates) should be obtained.

c. **Blood cultures. All patients sufficiently ill with pneumonia for sputum cultures to be obtained must have blood cultures done.** Because sputum has a normal flora, isolation of bacteria, even if the predominant species, does not always indicate the etiologic agent; thus, the diagnostic power of the sputum culture is limited. Isolation of bacteria from a site that has no normal flora, such as the bloodstream or pleural fluid, provides the most certain indication of the etiology of pneumonia.

d. **Leukocyte count.** Elevation of the peripheral blood leukocyte count is a nonspecific finding. However, leukocytosis with a shift to immature polymorphonuclear forms suggests bacterial infection. Normal or low leukocyte counts suggest viral or atypical pneumonias. Overwhelming bacterial sepsis may depress the leukocyte count, but blood smears show a marked shift to young cells.

e. **Serology.** Acute-phase and convalescent-phase serum samples should be frozen at $-20°C$ from patients for whom the etiology of pneumonia is not certain within 48 hr after admission to the hospital, or in whom there is suspicion on a clinical or epidemiologic basis that an unusual pathogen is present. Specific bacterial, fungal, or viral etiologies can be documented by using antibody titers, although the information is usually obtained too late to be of help for that particular patient.

2. **Supportive measures.** Maintaining **adequate oxygenation** is the primary goal. When respiratory distress is suspected, documentation of the extent of compromise can be obtained by monitoring **arterial blood gases**. Initially, supplemental oxygen should be administered by **nasal prongs**. The degree of respiratory compromise determines the nature of procedures necessary to maintain oxygenation (e.g., **intubation and ventilation**). **Pleuritic pain**, if severe, should be treated with oral analgesics or intercostal nerve blocks. **Pleural effusions** must be tapped for diagnostic purposes; if empyema or a sterile loculation is present, **chest tube drainage** is essential. Cough-suppressing medications usually are not necessary unless coughing is causing persistent pain, exhaustion, or respiratory compromise. Many patients with pneumonia are volume depleted; thus, maintenance of **intravascular hydration** is essential.

3. **Community-acquired pneumonia** (Fig. 1). Use of empiric or specific antimicrobial therapy depends on the clinical status of the patient. Those without preexisting compromise who appear well ("walking pneumonia") often have viral infections and may require no specific treatment. Those patients with probable bacterial pneumonia of mild to moderate severity can be treated with oral agents, including penicillin VK 250 mg, p.o., q.i.d.; erythromycin 250 mg, p.o., q.i.d.; tetracycline 250 mg, p.o., q.i.d.; or cephalosporins (including cefadroxil 500 mg, p.o., b.i.d., or cephalexin 250 mg, p.o., q.i.d.) for 10 days. Severely ill patients should be hospitalized and treated with parenteral

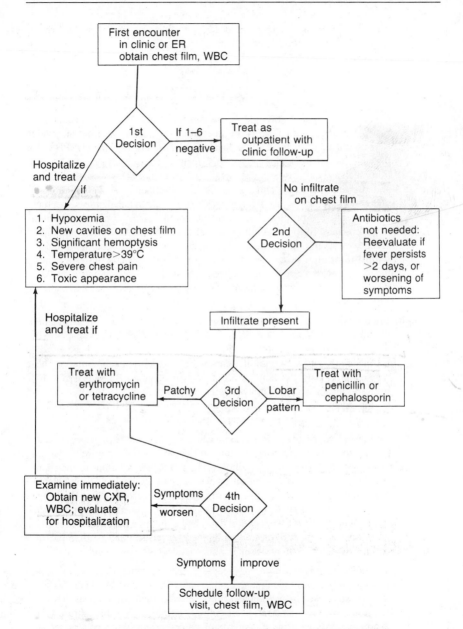

FIG. 1. Approach to community-acquired lower respiratory infections.

agents, depending on the specific bacterial etiology suspected or confirmed. Therapy for community-acquired aspiration pneumonia with anaerobic organisms is discussed in Chapter 9. The antibiotic therapy for other common community-acquired pneumonias is as follows.

a. **Viral pneumonia.** Viruses are the most common causes of acute pneumonia, but since they are usually mild, affected persons do not seek medical attention. The usual etiologic agents are influenza A and B and adenoviruses. **Influenza can largely be prevented** by annual vaccination, which is recommended by the United States Public Health Service (USPHS) for the elderly and for high-risk patients, including those with chronic conditions such as heart disease, chronic obstructive pulmonary disease (COPD), and diabetes mellitus. During outbreaks of influenza A, amantadine (or rimantadine) may be used for prophylaxis or treatment of the same high-risk patients. For prophylaxis, treatment should be started when an outbreak is documented in the community (hospital or nursing home) and should be given as 100 mg, p.o., b.i.d. Treatment at the same dose should begin within 48 hr after onset of symptoms and should continue until 48 hr after the symptoms have remitted. In uncomplicated viral pneumonia, antibiotic therapy is not indicated, although patients should be observed for bacterial superinfections.

b. **Pneumococcal pneumonia.** For uncomplicated infections the **treatment of choice** is procaine penicillin G 600,000 U, i.m. every 12 hr. After defervescence, penicillin VK 250 mg, p.o., every 6 hr, may be used to complete a 10-day course. Patients with multilobar pneumonia or those who are seriously ill should be treated with aqueous penicillin G 1 to 2 million U, i.v., every 4 hr. Penicillin-allergic patients can be treated with erythromycin 500 mg, every 6 hr, or cephalosporins. Multiple drug-resistant pneumococci are rare but can be treated with vancomycin.

c. **Legionnaires' disease.** Pneumonia caused by *Legionella pneumophilia* and related species is surprisingly common as a community-acquired infection, especially in older men who smoke. The **diagnosis** is based on the identification of organisms in sputum or pleural fluid by culture (using selective media), by direct fluorescent microscopy, or by serology. **Erythromycin** 500 mg, i.v., every 6 hr, for 21 days is recommended. Symptomatic improvement may require several days, and radiologic improvement is much more delayed. For seriously ill patients either tetracycline or rifampin may be added. Relapses may occur in spite of adequate treatment.

d. *Mycoplasma pneumoniae* may cause patchy or lobar pneumonia. **Diagnosis** is based on clinical suspicion, usually in patients less than 30 years old whose chest X-ray indicates more disease than the clinical condition suggests, or by demonstration of cold agglutinins in serum, culture of the agent, or serologic testing. **Agents of choice** are erythromycin or tetracycline 500 mg, p.o., every 6 hr, for 7 to 10 days.

e. *Staphylococcus aureus.* Pneumonia is not commonly caused by this organism except after viral (influenza, measles) infections or as a complication of right-sided staphylococcal endocarditis. **Treatment of choice** is a penicillinase-resistant penicillin, such as methicillin or oxacillin, 1 to 2 million U, i.v., every 4 hr. Rare penicillin-sensitive isolates can be treated with penicillin G; methicillin-resistant isolates should be treated with vancomycin. After defervescence, oral agents may be used to complete 4 weeks of therapy.

f. *Hemophilus influenzae.* This agent is usually seen in patients with COPD. **Ampicillin is the treatment of choice** and is given as 500 mg, p.o., q.i.d., for patients with mild infections, and 2 g, i.v., every 4 hr, for severe infections, for 10 days. If beta-lactamase–mediated resistance is present, alternative treatments include chloramphenicol, cefamandole, and TMP-SMX.

g. *Klebsiella pneumoniae.* This is an uncommon pathogen except in alcoholic patients. Treatment of choice is **cephalothin** or an equivalent first-generation cephalosporin given as 2 g, i.v., every 4 hr, and an aminoglycoside. After defervesence, treatment with an oral agent should complete a 21- to 28-day course.

h. **Other agents.** Uncommon causes of acute pneumonia and their treatments include: *C. psittici* (psittacosis, in bird handlers), tetracycline 500 mg, p.o., every 6 hr for 14 to 21 days; *Coxiella burnetti* (Q fever, in sheep or cattle workers), tetracycline or chloramphenicol 500 mg, p.o., every 6 hr for 14 to 21 days; *Y. pestis* (plague, in endemic areas), streptomycin 500 mg, i.m., every 12 hr, and tetracycline 500 mg, i.v., every 6 hr, plus strict respiratory isolation); *F. tularensis* (tularemia, in persons with rabbit, rodent, tick, or deer-fly exposure), streptomycin 500 mg, i.v., every 6 hr for 14 days; *Nocardia asteroides* (nocardiosis), sulfadiazine 2 g, p.o., every 6 hr, or TMP-SMX for 6 to 8 weeks; *Histoplasma capsulatum* (histoplasmosis pneumonia, in endemic areas), amphotericin B 1.5 to 2 g total dosage; and *Coccidioidomycosis immitans* (coccidioidomycosis pneumonia, in endemic areas), amphotericin B 1.5 to 2 g total dosage.

4. **Nosocomial pneumonia. Hospitalized patients** are at increased risk for pneumonia because of underlying diseases, instrumentation (bronchoscopy and endotracheal intubation), prior antimicrobial therapy, immunosuppression, neurologic deficits interfering with clearance mechanisms, and malnutrition. Because a variety of agents cause nosocomial pneumonia, **broad-spectrum empiric treatment** is indicated. Therapy should include an aminoglycoside (for gram-negative coverage) and a first-generation cephalosporin or semisynthetic penicillin (for gram-positive including *S. aureus* coverage). The particular agents used should be based on a review of local susceptibility patterns of hospital-acquired pathogens. Other antimicrobial agents may be added, depending on the clinical circumstances.

a. **Gram-negative bacteria.** These are by far the most common nosocomial pathogens. The most common agents are *E. coli, Klebsiella* species, *P. aeruginosa, Proteus, Acinetobacter, Enterobacter*, and *Serratia* species. **Empiric therapy** should be with an aminoglycoside, and **specific therapy** should be based on antimicrobial susceptibility reports. In addition to aminoglycosides, these microorganisms are commonly susceptible to third-generation cephalosporins, antipseudomonal penicillins, and chloramphenicol. **Empyema** is common and must be drained when present. Because these are necrotizing pneumonias, therapy should be continued for at least 3 weeks. Despite antimicrobial therapy, mortality is high, in large part due to the underlying illnesses of these patients.

b. Fungi. Patients on long-term antibacterial therapy in the hospital are at high risk for developing fungal pneumonia or disseminated fungal infection. Most common causes are *C. albicans*, other *Candida* species, *Torulopsis*, and *Aspergillus* species. Therapy is with amphotericin B; consultation should be sought.

c. *Legionella pneumophilia* and related organisms. See II. B. 3. b.

5. Pneumonia in immunocompromised hosts. Although there is overlap with community-acquired and other nosocomially acquired pneumonias, the agents causing pneumonias in immunocompromised hosts are often significantly different. Clinical signs and sputum examination are often not helpful in diagnosing these pneumonias, **bronchoscopy** (with brush biopsy) or **open-lung biopsy** is often necessary to make a specific etiologic diagnosis. **Empiric therapy** for pneumonias should include an aminoglycoside and a first-generation cephalosporin. Other therapy will be based on clinical impression or identification of specific etiologic agent.

a. *Pneumocystis carinii*. **TMP-SMX** for at least 2 to 3 weeks is the **treatment of choice.** Seriously ill patients should be given TMP 5 mg/kg and SMX 25 mg/kg, i.v., every 6 hr. Those with less serious illnesses may be treated with TMP-SMX, 1 double-strength tablet every 12 hr. In patients not responding, allergic to, or unable to tolerate oral TMP-SMX, the **alternative** (more toxic) treatment is pentamidine isethionate, which may be obtained from the Centers for Disease Control.

b. Cytomegalic inclusion virus (CMV). Although CMV infections are common, they are rarely fatal. No specific therapy is available at present.

c. *Nocardia*. See II. B. 3. h.

d. *Cryptococcus neoformans*. **Treatment of choice** is amphotericin B (0.3 mg/kg/day, i.v.) plus flucytosine (37.5 mg/kg, p.o., every 6 hr) for 6 weeks.

6. Pneumonia in the acquired immune deficiency syndrome (AIDS). The most common **causes** of pneumonia are *P. carinii*, CMV, *Mycobacterium avium-intracellulare* species, *M. tuberculosis*, *Cryptococcus*, and *Nocardia*. **Diagnosis** is based on sputum examination for acid-fast bacilli (AFB) and cultures. In the absence of a diagnosis, open or brush biopsy may be needed to diagnose *Pneumocystis*. Multiple infections may occur. AIDS patients often develop acute febrile responses to TMP-SMX.

C. Gastrointestinal Infections   After acute respiratory infections, gastrointestinal infections are the most common illnesses for which patients seek medical attention. A wide variety of bacterial, viral, and parasitic agents may cause such infections, but diagnosis of the etiologic agent and specific antimicrobial therapy is not always necessary. The **majority of infections are self-limiting** and require supportive care only (Fig. 2). Diagnosis and specific treatment for several important etiologies

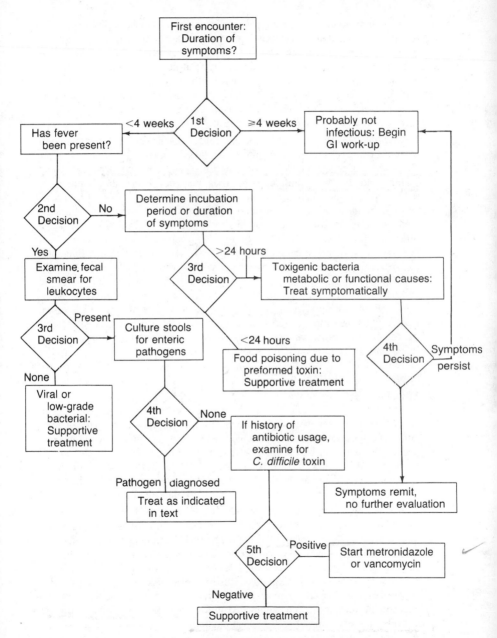

FIG. 2.   Approach to acute diarrheal illness.

are listed below. However, for all patients with acute diarrheal diseases, fluid status must be evaluated, since significant volume depletion may not be readily apparent. **Hypovolemic shock** and concomitant **electrolyte abnormalities** are responsible for the majority of the occasionally fatal infections. Serious consideration should be given to hospitalizing patients with orthostatic hypotension for the purpose of fluid and electrolyte repletion. For patients with mild or no apparent hypovolemia, electrolyte-rich oral fluids, such as juices and soft drinks, should be strongly encouraged for the duration of illness.

1. **Campylobacter infections.** *C. jejuni* and related species are the most common bacterial causes for acute gastrointestinal illnesses in the United States. After a prodrome of fever and myalgias lasting for several hours to days, abdominal cramps and diarrhea commence; diarrhea may be watery, bile-stained, or bloody. Although infection is usually self-limiting within 7 days, life-threatening infections can occur. Severe or persistent infection may mimic inflammatory bowel disease, which should not be diagnosed until *Campylobacter* infection has been excluded. A history of fever or the presence of fecal leukocytes or blood are important **diagnostic clues**. Presumptive diagnosis can be made by visualizing characteristic vibrio-forms on Gram stain or darkfield microscopy of fecal specimens. A definitive diagnosis calls for fecal culture, which requires that the laboratory has appropriate methods for isolation. Patients with persistent illness, bloody diarrhea, or high fever should be treated with erythromycin (250 mg, p.o., q.i.d., for 5 to 7 days). Alternative treatments are oral tetracycline or clindamycin. For systemic *Campylobacter* infections or bacteremia, chloramphenicol or gentamicin are indicated. For systemic infections caused by *C. fetus*, therapy for 4 weeks may be necessary to prevent relapses.

2. **Shigella infections.** In the United States, shigellosis is primarily a disease of preschool-age children and their parents, male homosexuals, and travelers to developing countries; however, any population group may be affected. **Characteristic symptoms** are fever and bloody diarrhea, but milder symptoms can occur. **Diagnosis is based on fecal culture.** Although most patients are ill for less than 1 week, antimicrobial therapy both shortens the duration of symptoms and decreases the likelihood of person-to-person spread. Thus most symptomatic patients should receive antimicrobial treatment; the **agent of choice** is 1 double-strength TMP-SMX (160/800) tablet, p.o., every 12 hr.

3. **Salmonella infections.** Most *Salmonella* infections in the United States are manifest as acute gastroenteritis, but occasionally septicemia, focal infection, or enteric fever occurs. Gastroenteritis caused by *Salmonella* cannot be distinguished from that due to *Campylobacter* or *Shigella*. On occasion, blood cultures of patients with *Salmonella* gastroenteritis are positive. **Supportive treatment** is indicated for most patients because use of antibiotics does not shorten the duration of uncomplicated illness. Antibiotic treatment prolongs convalescent excretion of the organism in stools.

Septicemia and focal infections are the next most common manifestations of *Salmonella* infections and the diagnosis is made by isolating *Salmonella* from blood or deep tissue sites. The most typical presentations of focal infections are osteomyelitis, abscesses, and endovascular infections. **Therapy for ab-**

scesses includes adequate drainage and 2 to 3 weeks of systemic antimicrobial agents. **Treatments of choice** include ampicillin 1 g, i.v., every 4 hr; chloramphenicol 500 mg, i.v., every 6 hr; or TMP-SMX (160/800), i.v., every 12 hr. Therapy for intravascular infections should be at least 4 to 6 weeks, and surgery to remove an infected focus may be necessary.

About 300 cases of **typhoid fever** (caused by *Salmonella typhi*) are reported annually in the United States; paratyphoid (*S. paratyphi* A or B) is less common. Foreign travel or immigrants from developing countries account for most cases. Typhoid and the other enteric fevers present with fever and prostration. These are systemic infections, and constipation is more common than diarrhea. During the first week of illness, blood cultures are usually positive and fecal cultures are negative. As the illness progresses, stool cultures become positive and blood cultures are negative. Other diagnostic aids include urine or bone marrow cultures. Serologic tests to demonstrate antibody to *Salmonella* O and H antigens have little role in diagnosis due to lack of specificity. The **treatment of choice** is chloramphenicol 50 mg/kg/day in 4 to 6 divided doses until the patient is afebrile, then 30 mg/kg/day for the remainder of a 2-week course. **Alternative treatments** are TMP-SMX (160/800) taken once every 12 hr, or amoxicillin 1 g, p.o., q.i.d., especially if the patient has come from an area in which resistance to chloramphenicol is prevalent. Approximately 10% of treated patients develop a relapse, which is usually milder, within the first 14 days posttherapy. Convalescent excretion of the organisms may persist for up to 6 months, but a chronic carrier state is uncommon except in persons with preexisting biliary tract disease.

4. **Yersinia infections.** *Y. enterocolitica* is a less common cause for acute diarrheal disease in the United States. Symptoms are similar to those produced by *Campylobacter, Shigella,* or *Salmonella,* and **diagnosis** is based on fecal culture. Special media or cold enrichment are necessary for isolation. Some patients present with **mesenteric adenitis,** a syndrome indistinguishable from acute appendicitis. The diarrhea and the adenitis are usually self-limiting. For those patients with fever, bloody diarrhea, or persistent syndromes, antimicrobial treatment with **tetracycline** 500 mg, p.o., q.i.d., for 10 days, or **TMP-SMX** taken every 12 hr for 7 days, is indicated.

5. **Giardia infections.** *Giardia lamblia* is a protozoan that causes a subacute syndrome of diarrhea, flatulence, abdominal bloating, and belching of foul air with a "rotten-egglike" odor. Vomiting and fever are uncommon. Symptoms may last for days to weeks. Groups at increased risk are persons who drink untreated water from streams, live in small mountain towns, are traveling, are male homosexuals, have contact with young children at day-care centers, or have immunoglobulin deficiencies. **Diagnosis** is made by identifying cysts or trophozoites in feces, duodenal contents, or small-bowel biopsy. Negative fecal examinations may require the latter two procedures. The **treatment of choice** is quinacrine 100 mg, p.o., t.i.d., or metronidazole 250 mg, p.o., t.i.d., for 5 to 7 days. A second course of therapy is sometimes necessary.

6. **Clostridium difficile infections.** *C. difficile,* either endogenous or nosocomially acquired, will increase in concentration in the bowel lumenal contents of patients treated with antibiotics or antineoplastic agents, or those who have

had bowel manipulation or instrumentation. Although virtually all antibiotics have been associated with overgrowth of *C. difficile*, most cases have resulted from the use of penicillins, clindamycin, cephalosporins, and combinations of other broad-spectrum agents. Overgrowth results in production of at least two pathogenic toxins. **Clinical manifestations** range from asymptomatic toxin production to diarrhea to a fulminant "pseudomembranous colitis" resulting in bloody diarrhea, fever, and abdominal pain. **Diagnosis** is based on identification of toxin in feces; but isolation of *C. difficile* from feces, although nonspecific, is a sensitive indicator of etiology. Treatment consists of **discontinuing the antimicrobial agents** when possible and, if significant symptoms persist, therapy with vancomycin 125 mg, p.o., q.i.d., or metronidazole 500 mg, p.o., t.i.d., for 10 days. Cholestyramine 1 g, p.o., q.i.d., for 10 days will bind toxin, but relapses may occur after cessation. Since cholestyramine binds vancomycin, these agents should not be used together.

D. Meningitis   Meningitis is most often caused by bacterial or viral agents. Most viral infections have a benign outcome. However, with bacterial infections, if treatment is delayed, permanent neurologic sequelae or death are nearly universal. When meningitis is suspected clinically on the basis of fever, headache, or change in mental status, diagnostic procedures and institution of therapy should be done immediately (Fig. 3). **Therapy must begin within 30 min of considering the diagnosis of bacterial meningitis.**

1. Diagnosis

a. Lumbar puncture. The diagnosis of meningitis is based on examination of fluid obtained at lumbar puncture. When meningitis is suspected, funduscopic examination should exclude papilledema, and then lumbar puncture is performed. If papilledema is present and bacterial meningitis is strongly suspected, either a small-gauge needle should be used to withdraw 1 to 3 ml of fluid or antibiotics should be started empirically. Arrangements should then be made for emergency **computerized axial tomography** (CAT). CSF should be stained and a cell count done, and then sent for culture, with protein, glucose, and VDRL determinations in all cases. The glucose level in the blood should be determined concurrently. If CSF findings are not suggestive of meningitis, then CAT scanning and other diagnostic procedures may be done.

b. Cultures. CSF specimens should be immediately plated to allow the growth of organisms difficult to culture, such as *N. meningitidis* (meningococcus). When meningococcal meningitis is suspected, warmed culture media should be available at the bedside and after inoculation placed in a candle jar. All patients should have **blood** cultures performed. If CSF examination suggests viral infection (e.g., predominant lymphocytosis), specimens of CSF, **throat washings**, and **feces** should be frozen at − 70°C until they can be cultured for viral isolation.

c. CSF examination. Total and differential **cell counts** should be done. CSF should be centrifuged and the sediment Gram-stained. If negative, acridine orange, India ink (cryptococcus), and AFB stains should be considered. CSF protein usually is elevated in inflammatory conditions of the meninges

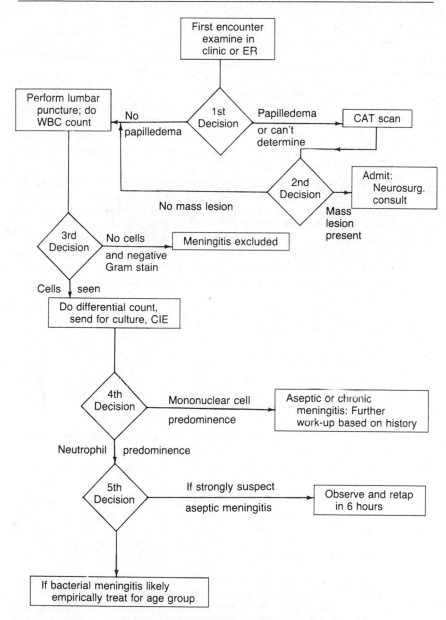

FIG. 3. Approach to suspected meningitis.

and CNS. Glucose concentrations less than 50% of the serum glucose suggest bacterial, tuberculosis, mumps, or lymphochoriomeningitis (LCM) virus meningitis.

d. **Counterimmunoelectrophoresis (CIE).** CIE and related techniques (latex agglutination and coagglutination) can be used to detect polysaccharide capsular antigens in CSF, serum, or urine. These techniques can yield a **rapid diagnosis** when Gram stains or cultures are negative or if prior antibiotic therapy suppresses bacterial growth. Detectable capsular antigens are of *S. pneumoniae, H. influenzae* type B, *N. meningitidis* groups A, C, Y, and W135, and *C. neoformans*.

2. **Empiric therapy** with an antibiotic that penetrates the blood-brain barrier (Table 1) should be given immediately after the lumbar puncture until an acute pyogenic infection has been excluded. In the rare situations (such as awaiting a CAT scan) in which waiting for lumbar puncture would delay initiation of therapy, treatment should begin immediately and lumbar puncture performed as soon as possible. Empiric therapy depends on the **age** of the patient and whether any **predispositions** such as previous trauma, immunosuppression, or pneumonia are present. *H. influenzae* and *N. meningitidis* are the **major pathogens in children** under 5; *S. pneumoniae* and *N. meningitidis* in **adults**; and in the immunosuppressed, *L. monocytogenes* and gram-negative bacilli are important. Empiric therapy for community-acquired acute pyogenic meningitis in adults is **penicillin G.** For hospitalized or debilitated patients, especially if gram-negative bacilli are seen on CSF examination, a **third-generation cephalosporin** such as cefotaxime should be added. In most cases, intrathecal therapy is not indicated. **Supportive therapy** includes maintenance of respiration with mechanical ventilation if necessary, control of seizures, and restriction of fluid intake to minimize cerebral edema. **Corticosteroids** may be used to reduce cerebral edema or progressive neurologic deterioration (e.g., during basilar tuberculosis meningitis) if necessary, once appropriate antibiotics have been started.

3. **Specific antimicrobial therapy.** The treatment for specific microorganisms is as follows:

a. *S. pneumoniae.* Aqueous penicillin G 2 million U, i.v., every 2 hr for 14 days is optimal. For penicillin-allergic patients, chloramphenicol 1 g, i.v., every 6 hr, may be substituted. Because relative resistance of pneumococci to penicillin is emerging, all CSF isolates should be tested for susceptibility using an oxacillin disk.

b. *N. meningitidis* requires the same dosage of penicillin as for *S. pneumoniae*. Chloramphenicol is alternative therapy. Because of the transmissibility of meningococci to previously healthy hosts, patients with meningococcal infections should be placed in **respiratory isolation** for the first 24 hr of antimicrobial therapy. Household members and hospital personnel in close contact with untreated patients should receive **prophylaxis with rifampin** 600 mg, p.o., b.i.d., for 2 days to eradicate nasopharyngeal carriage. If the organism is susceptible, prophylaxis with sulfadiazine 1 g, p.o., b.i.d. for 2 days, or minocycline 100 mg, p.o., b.i.d. for 2 days, can be used.

c. *H. influenzae.* Because beta-lactamase production is becoming more prevalent in certain areas, **chloramphenicol** 25 mg/kg/day, i.v., every 6 hr, is now the **agent of choice** for initial therapy for *H. influenzae* meningitis. If isolates are beta-lactamase negative, then ampicillin (50 mg/kg, i.v., every 4 hr, for children and 2 g, i.v., every 6 hr, for adults) can be used to complete a 10-day course.

d. *L. monocytogenes.* This gram-positive rod is the fourth most common cause for meningitis in adults, especially those immunosuppressed or elderly. CSF Gram stain is often negative, or *Listeria* may be confused with diphtheroids, which are often commensals. The **treatment of choice** is ampicillin 2 g, i.v., every 4 hr, or penicillin G 2 million U, i.v., every 2 hr, and gentamicin 3 mg/kg/day in 3 divided doses in a patient with normal renal function.

e. *S. aureus* is an **uncommon cause** of meningitis except after head trauma, neurosurgical procedures, or staphylococcal bacteremia. **Oxacillin** 3 g, i.v., every 4 hr for 14 days is the antibiotic of choice.

f. **Gram-negative bacilli.** These are **uncommon causes** of meningitis except in neonates or other immunologically compromised hosts and after head trauma or neurosurgical procedures. Initial treatment is cefotaxime 2 g, i.v., every 4 hr, or moxalactam 4 g, i.v., every 4 hr; but if the isolate is susceptible, use of ampicillin, chloramphenicol, or TMP-SMX is indicated.

3. **Prosthetic device meningitis.** Infections of prosthetic devices such as shunts, reservoirs, and intracranial pressure monitors usually are caused by *S. aureus*, *S. epidermidis*, or (less often) gram-negative bacilli. **Initial therapy** should be with vancomycin 500 mg, i.v., every 6 hr. If gram-negative bacilli are present on stain, cefotaxime or moxalactam should be given. Therapy should be modified on the basis of culture and antimicrobial susceptibility results. Curing most of these infections requires removal of the foreign body.

E. **Osteomyelitis** Infections of bone are becoming increasingly common as survival of patients with vascular disease is prolonged and as a result of orthopedic procedures in which foreign bodies are used. **Three major types** of osteomyelitis are recognized: hematogenous; secondary to a contiguous source of infection; and, resulting from vascular insufficiency. The diagnosis should be considered in patients with pain localized over a bone, chronic drainage, or persistent fever. **Radiographic changes**, including periosteal elevation and lytic or sclerotic lesions of bone, may lag 2 to 3 weeks behind clinical manifestations. **Bone scans** may show lesions early but often do not differentiate between a primary focus in bone or in the overlying soft tissues. **Definitive diagnosis** is based on isolating the organism from a biopsy of affected bone or from the bloodstream in a patient with clinical or radiographic findings compatible with osteomyelitis.

1. **Hematogenous.** In **adults**, hematogenous osteomyelitis is most often due to *S. aureus*, whereas in **children** *H. influenzae*, *S. pyogenes*, and *S. pneumoniae* also are important. *Salmonella* can cause osteomyelitis in persons with hemoglobinopathies. Virtually every clinically relevant bacterium or fungus has been found to cause osteomyelitis. Treatment, based on the causative organism

and its susceptibilities, should be with a **bactericidal antibiotic** at a high dose for at least 6 weeks. Such therapy usually will cure this type of osteomyelitis.

2. **Contiguous infection.** Osteomyelitis may develop in the adjacent bone after local trauma, fractures (and placement of orthopedic fixation or prosthetic devices), or infections of soft tissue, sinuses, or urinary tract. *S. aureus, S. epidermidis*, and *S. pyogenes* are most common, but because of proximity to the veins draining the urinary tract, lower vertebral osteomyelitis is often caused by enteric gram-negative rods. **Diagnosis** must be based on deep bone cultures, as sinus tracts to the skin are colonized with a variety of bacteria that frequently differ from the underlying pathogen. Successful treatment depends on **eradication of the contiguous focus**, which usually requires removal of all foreign bodies, as well as **antibiotic-mediated sterilization of bone.** Pieces of devitalized bone (sequestra) must be removed for cure. Nevertheless, chronic osteomyelitis is difficult to cure, and **chronic suppressive therapy** is often the only option after a 6- to 8-week course of high-dose parenteral therapy has failed.

3. **Vascular insufficiency.** Patients with long-standing diabetes mellitus or atherosclerotic peripheral vascular disease are at high risk for developing osteomyelitis in their feet due to vascular insufficiency and anesthesia. In addition to high-grade gram-positive pathogens, infections due to gram-negative rods, group B streptococci, fungi, and anaerobes often occur. Such patients usually are not bacteremic or febrile unless an overlying cellulitis is present. **Amputation** of the affected area usually is required for cure. **Definitive therapy** is based on susceptibilities of organisms isolated from deep culture sites. If bone culture is not possible due to local or underlying disease, empiric initial therapy should include gram-positive, gram-negative, and anaerobic coverage. **Chronic antibiotic suppression** could be an alternative to amputation.

F. **Infective Endocarditis**   Although infective endocarditis (IE) may be caused by a wide variety of microorganisms, gram-positive cocci including viridans streptococci, group D streptococci (*S. faecalis* and others), and staphylococci (*S. aureus* and *S. epidermidis*) account for more than 90% of infections. Two overlapping syndromes exist: **subacute bacterial endocarditis (SBE) and acute bacterial endocarditis (ABE).** Fungal endocarditis usually is subacute. Untreated SBE leads to demise in weeks or months, whereas ABE causes death within days. In general, viridans and group D streptococci cause SBE; *S. aureus* and the pneumococcus cause ABE. SBE usually occurs as a result of seeding of low-grade pathogens, such as viridans streptococci, onto a valve or endocardium with a prior anatomical defect; whereas ABE, caused by pyogenic cocci, may affect previously normal valves. **Left-sided endocarditis predominates** except in intravenous-drug abusers and patients with infected central venous catheters. Dental and genitourinary tract procedures are frequent causes for seeding of valves. Less common pathogens of endocarditis, including gram-negative bacteria and fungi, occur in intravenous-drug abusers, hospitalized patients with intravenous lines and prior antibiotic therapy, and persons with prosthetic valves.

1. **Diagnosis.** IE should be suspected in patients who either have known antecedent valve disease or have recently been instrumented and who present with fever, a new or changing heart murmur, and evidence of peripheral emboli-

zation. **Diagnosis** is made in a person with a suggestive clinical setting who has repeated positive blood cultures. Three sets of blood cultures taken over a 1-hr (for ABE) or 6-hr (for SBE) period will detect greater than 95% of patients ultimately found to have IE. Exceptions include patients who have received prior antibiotics, in whom the culture may turn positive after 1 to 2 weeks or not be positive at all, or those with IE caused by fastidious gram-negative organisms and fungi (especially *Aspergillus*). **Echocardiography** may be used to ascertain the extent of valve damage, hemodynamic compromise, or propensity for embolic foci, but it has a high false-negative rate. It can neither confirm nor exclude the diagnosis of IE.

2. **Treatment.** Because phagocytic cells have little or no effectiveness against organisms in endocardial lesions, **high-dose, long-term antibiotic therapy** is essential. **Bactericidal agents must be used.** Adequacy of therapy is based on clinical response and maintenance of trough serum bactericidal activity at 1:8 dilution. **Early valve replacement surgery is indicated for progressive congestive heart failure, major systemic emboli, and resistant sepsis.** Valve replacement is most frequently necessary in prosthetic valve, fungal, and staphylococcal endocarditis. Persistance of low-grade fever or development of drug rashes or fever are common and are not necessarily indications for discontinuing antibiotic therapy.

a. **Empiric therapy.** While awaiting blood culture results in cases of suspected endocarditis, empiric antibiotic therapy is necessary. For **SBE, therapy of choice** is penicillin G 2 million U, i.v., every 2 hr, plus streptomycin 500 mg, i.m., every 12 hr. For culture-negative endocarditis, diagnosed on the basis of fever, changing murmur, and/or peripheral embolic phenomena, this regimen should be continued for 4 weeks unless clinical status worsens. **ABE** is empirically treated with oxacillin 2 g, i.v., every 4 hr; penicillin G 1 million U every 2 hr, and an aminoglycoside. For **prosthetic valve endocarditis,** therapy of choice is vancomycin 500 mg, i.v., every 6 hr, penicillin G, and an aminoglycoside as above.

b. **Viridans and nonenterococcal group D streptococci.** Isolation of *S. bovis* should initiate procedures to exclude a neoplastic or inflammatory process in the gastrointestinal tract. **Treatment of choice** is penicillin G 2 million U, i.v., every 2 hr for 4 weeks, with streptomycin 500 mg, i.m., every 12 hr for 2 weeks. Patients at increased risk for streptomycin toxicity may be treated with penicillin alone. For patients allergic to penicillin, **alternative therapies** are vancomycin 500 mg, i.v., every 6 hr, or cephalothin 2 g, i.v., every 4 hr, for 4 weeks. Desensitization to penicillin is another alternative.

c. *Steptococcus faecalis* **and other group D enterococci.** All streptococci with MICs to penicillin G ≥ 0.1 µg/ml must be treated with **penicillin and an aminoglycoside** for synergy. Isolates with high-level resistance (MIC 1:2000) to aminoglycosides will not benefit from synergy. For penicillin-allergic patients, vancomycin is substituted for penicillin, but because both vancomycin and aminoglycosides are nephrotoxic and ototoxic, serum levels should be carefully monitored.

d. *Staphylococcus aureus.* Treatment of choice is **oxacillin** 2 g i.v., every 4 hr for 6 weeks. For patients with slow resolution of sepsis, blood cultures should be repeated and examinations should be done to identify abscesses. In the absence of positive findings either rifampin or gentamicin can be added. Aortic valve staphylococcal endocarditis frequently requires **valve replacement** for cure. Tricuspid valve endocarditis is more benign, and 4 weeks of therapy is usually sufficient.

    e. Pneumococcus and *Streptococcus pyogenes* (group A beta-hemolytic). Penicillin G 1.6 to 2.0 million U, i.v., every 4 hr for 4 weeks should be given.

3. Prosthetic valve endocarditis (PVE). Both prosthetic heterograft and mechanical valves may become infected. Cases occurring within 1 month of surgery (early) are most often caused by *S. epidermidis, S. aureus, Candida* species, and gram-negative bacilli. Later cases are caused both by these organisms and streptococci. Almost all cases of mechanical valve PVE are associated with valve ring abscess, and as with all infections with foreign bodies in place, **removal of the foreign body** is often necessary for cure. Antibiotic treatment is based on the specific sensitivities of the organism and should be continued for 6 weeks.

4. Prophylaxis. Populations at risk for SBE include persons with rheumatic heart disease, prosthetic valves, congenital heart disease (including calcific aortic stenosis, idiopathic hypertrophic subaortic stenosis, and the mitral valve prolapse "murmur-click" syndrome). Persons with intravascular or articular prostheses also should receive prophylaxis. Standard prophylactic regimens have been developed by the American Heart Association, as follows:

    a. Dental procedures. Parenteral therapy is preferred with aqueous penicillin G 1 million U mixed with procaine penicillin G 600,000 U given intramuscularly 30 to 60 min before the procedures. For patients with rheumatic heart disease who regularly receive penicillin prophylaxis and for patients with prosthetic valves, streptomycin 1 g, i.m. also is given. Penicillin V 500 mg, p.o., every 6 hr, is then given for 8 doses. Alternatively, oral therapy is penicillin V 2 g given 30 to 60 min before the procedure, then 500 mg every 6 hr for 8 doses. For penicillin-allergic patients, parenteral therapy is vancomycin 1 g, i.v., given over 60 min, begun 60 to 90 min before the procedure, followed by erythromycin 500 mg, p.o., every 6 hr for 8 doses. Oral therapy is erythromycin 1 g, p.o., 30 to 120 min before the procedure, followed by 500 mg, p.o., every 6 hr for 8 doses.

    b. Gastrointestinal and genitourinary (GU) procedures. Prophylaxis is required before cystoscopy and colonoscopy. For patients with prosthetic valves, prophylaxis should be considered before ureteral catheterization, sigmoidoscopy, dilatation and curretage of the uterus, insertion or removal of an intrauterine device, or gastrointestinal biopsies. Prophylaxis is either aqueous penicillin G 2 million U, i.m. or i.v., or ampicillin 1 to 2 g, i.m. or i.v., plus gentamicin 1.5 mg/kg, i.m., 30 to 60 min before the procedure, then repeated every 8 hr times two. For penicillin-allergic patients use vancomycin 1 g, i.v., infused over 60 min, plus gentamicin, and repeat once 12 hr later.

G. Urinary Tract Infections (UTI)   Major clinical syndromes are cystitis, pyelonephritis, prostatitis, and urethritis. **Bacteriuria** is common in the first two conditions and is usually greater than 10^5 bacteria/ml, but symptomatic infection can result from 10^3 bacteria/ml as well. **Diagnosis** is suggested by symptoms (dysuria, urgency, frequency, fever) and signs (superpubic or flank tenderness, pyuria). A specific etiologic diagnosis is based on bacterial isolation from a promptly cultured, uncontaminated specimen, either a clean-voided midstream or a catheter-obtained urine specimen.

1. **Cystitis** is a common problem of young women (Fig. 4) but rare in young men. Because UTI in men suggests either an anatomic defect or obstruction in the urinary tract, diabetes mellitus, or another host defect, the first episode requires a complete GU evaluation. Women having episodes less often than every 6 to 12 months do not require evaluation. **Chronic cystitis** occurs in patients with residual urine caused by obstruction or neurogenic bladder dysfunction, or in those with indwelling catheters. Community-acquired UTI usually is caused by *E. coli* susceptible to most antibiotics. Recurrent or nosocomial UTI is more often caused by other gram-negative bacilli, including *Klebsiella*, *Proteus*, *Serratia* and *Pseudomonas* species that may be resistant to multiple antibiotics. Therapy is as follows: Young, reliable, nonpregnant women with no known predisposition should be treated with **single-dose amoxicillin 3 g or double-strength TMP-SMX**. Because of good response to single-dose therapy (and cost) urine culture is not routinely indicated, but a follow-up contact must be assured. **Longer oral regimens** should be given to pregnant women, women with abnormal anatomy or function, and males with UTI. Urine culture may be indicated. Treatment should be for 7 days with sulfisoxazole, ampicillin, amoxicillin, tetracycline, cephradine, or cephalexin. Tetracycline should be avoided during pregnancy. Failure to respond may indicate the need for GU evaluation. In chronic UTI the presence of an indwelling catheter makes eradication of infection impossible. Such patients should be treated only for symptomatic episodes with short (5-day) courses of antibiotics to suppress the infection. Closed catheter systems diminish the number of symptomatic episodes, but prophylaxis is not helpful. Long-term broad spectrum therapy encourages the emergence of resistant organisms. **Prophylaxis for young women with recurrent UTI**: 1 tablet of TMP-SMX nightly or prior to intercourse diminishes frequency of episodes. Postintercourse voiding also should be encouraged.

2. **Pyelonephritis** may occur either as an extension from cystitis, in which case it is relatively easy to resolve, or as a result of urinary tract obstruction or anatomic defect. Occasionally, pyelonephritis occurs as a result of hematogenous spread. **Empiric treatment** should be with ampicillin 1 g, i.v., every 4 hr, and/or an aminoglycoside, pending culture results. When clinical toxicity of infection has diminished, oral therapy can be used to complete a 10-day course. If obstruction is present, cure will not be possible without removing the cause. On very rare occasions, struvite stones caused by *Proteus* infections will dissolve with long-term antibiotic therapy. Renacidin infusions also have been used to dissolve struvite stones or to prevent recurrence after surgical removal.

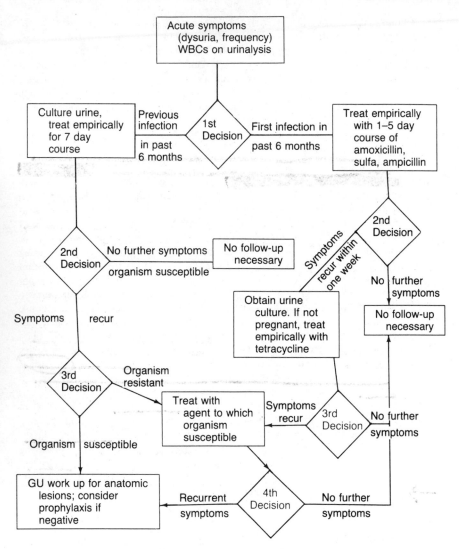

FIG. 4. Approach to urinary tract infection in a young woman.

3. **Prostatitis must be differentiated from prostatosis.** The latter is not infectious in origin, but symptoms may be similar to prostatitis. **Acute** bacterial prostatitis frequently is caused by the enteric gram-negative bacilli and should be treated empirically with oral TMP-SMX, ampicillin, or cephalosporin pending culture results. Duration of therapy is 2 weeks, and sitz baths are an important adjunct. **Chronic** bacterial prostatitis should be treated with an

antimicrobial agent to which the pathogen is susceptible and which penetrates the prostatic secretions (TMP-SMX, erythomycin with bicarbonate, tetracycline) for at least 3 months.

4. **Urethritis** usually is a sexually transmitted disease caused by *N. gonorrhoeae, C. trachomatis*, and genital mycoplasmas *(Ureaplasma urealyticum)*. **Diagnosis of nongonococcal urethritis** (NGU) is based on the presence of neutrophils on urethral smear and the absence of gonococci on smear or culture. **Treatment** of NGU is with tetracycline 500 mg, p.o., q.i.d. for 7 days. If there is only one sexual partner, the partner should be treated simultaneously. **Relapses** are common and should be treated with a second course of tetracycline. Subsequent relapse should be treated with erythromycin 500 mg, p.o., q.i.d. for 7 days.

H. **Sexually Transmitted Diseases** Sexually transmitted diseases are epidemic in the United States. The risk for both heterosexuals and homosexuals increases in relation to the number of partners and the nature of practices, including oral-genital, genital-anal, and oral-anal intercourse. Diseases involve the genital organs, the bowel, skin, and systemic sites. A wide variety of bacterial (including *N. gonorrhoeae, T. pallidum, C. trachomatis*, and enteric pathogens), viral (herpes simplex, hepatitis A and B, cytomegalovirus), and protozoan *(E. histolytica, G. lamblia)* agents may be sexually transmitted. In Table 8 the USPHS recommendations for treatment of several of these diseases are indicated.

AIDS is a syndrome of opportunistic infections and/or Kaposi's sarcoma occurring in persons who are not normally at risk because of immunosuppression. **Population groups at risk** include male homosexuals, intravenous-drug abusers, recipients of blood products, persons from Haiti and other areas in the Caribbean and heterosexual contacts and children of these high risk groups. Infecting agents include bacteria *(M. tuberculosis, M. avium-intracellulare*, and *Nocardia)*, fungi *(C. neoformans, C. albicans)*, protozoa *(Toxoplasma gondii, Cryptosporidia, P. carinii)*, and viruses (herpes simplex, cytomegalovirus). **Treatment** for AIDS at present involves supportive and antimicrobial therapy for the infections actually present in the patient. Mortality is high and reflects the degree of immunosuppression. Hospitalized patients with AIDS should be under needle and secretion precautions to diminish the possibility of transmission. To date no nosocomical transmission of AIDS is known to have occurred.

I. **Tuberculosis** Tuberculosis causes chronic infection of the lung and, less often, of lymph nodes, kidney, bone and joints, or meninges, as well as disseminated disease. The **etiologic agent** is *M. tuberculosis*, but other nontuberculous (atypical) mycobacteria may produce identical pulmonary disease. **Diagnosis** is based on the symptoms (including cough, fever, weight loss, and hemoptysis), signs of chronic pulmonary infection, and the recognition of AFB on sputum smear. **Any patient suspected of having active pulmonary tuberculosis should be placed in immediate respiratory isolation until the diagnosis has been ruled out.** Hospitalization is not required for many persons with tuberculosis but may be useful for initiating therapy to render the patient noninfectious and to explain the necessity for compliance with therapy.

1. **Uncomplicated pulmonary tuberculosis. Tuberculosis should never be**

TABLE 8. *Treatments for sexually transmitted diseases*

Infection	Treatment	Comments
Syphilis Early (<1 yr)	Benzathine penicillin G 2.4 million U i.m. Tetracycline 500 mg, p.o. q.i.d. × 15 days[a]	Single-dose treatment for primary, secondary, and early latent
Late (≥1 yr)	Benzathine penicillin G 2.4 million U, i.m. q week × 3 Tetracycline 500 mg p.o. q.i.d. × 30 days[a] Erythromycin 500 mg, p.o. q.i.d. × 30 days[a]	Includes late latent and cardiovascular
Neurosyphilis	Aqueous penicillin G 2–4 million U, i.v. q 4 hr × 10 days followed by benzathine penicillin G 2.4 million U, i.m. q week × 3, or benzathine penicillin alone for 3 weeks as specified	
In pregnancy	As above	Penicillin-allergic patients should be treated with erythromycin not tetracycline
Gonorrhea Urethritis	Aqueous procaine penicillin G 4.8 million U, i.m. × 1 Amoxicillin 3.0 g, or ampicillin 3.5 g, p.o. with probenecid 1.0. g, p.o. Tetracycline 500 mg, p.o. q.i.d. × 7 days or doxycycline 100 mg, p.o. b.i.d × 7 days Spectinomycin 2 g., i.m. Cefoxitin 2 g, i.m. plus probenicid 1 g, p.o.	 Will also treat concurrent chlamydia For penicillinase-producing isolates For spectinomycin-resistant, penicillinase-producing isolates
Pharyngitis	Procaine penicillin G, tetracycline, doxycycline, TMP (720 mg)/SMX (3600 mg), p.o., q.d. × 5	As for urethritis For penicillinase-producing spectinomycin resistance
Salpingitis Mild	Cefoxitin (2 g, i.m.) amoxicillin (3 g, p.o.), ampicillin (3.5 g, p.o.), or procaine penicillin G (4.8 million U, i.m.), each with probenecid 1 g, p.o., followed by doxycycline 100 mg, p.o. b.i.d. × 14 days	Outpatient treatment
Severe	Cefoxitin 2 g, i.v. q 6 hr plus doxycycline 100 mg, i.v. q 12 hr, followed by doxycycline 100 mg, p.o. b.i.d.; or clindamycin 600 mg, i.v. q 6 hr plus an aminoglycoside followed by clindamycin 450 mg, p.o. q 6 hr or doxycycline 100 mg, i.v. q 12 hr plus metronidazole 1 g, i.v. q 12 hr followed by both drugs orally	In-hospital treatment, parenteral treatment for at least 4 days and 14-day course completed by oral regimen

TABLE 8. *(Continued)*

Infection	Treatment	Comments
Disseminated	Amoxicillin (3 g, p.o.) or ampicillin (3.5 g, p.o.) each plus probenicid 1 g, p.o. followed by 500 mg, p.o. q 6 hr of either for 7 days; or aqueous penicillin 2.5 million U i.v. q 6 hr until improvement, then p.o. amoxicillin or ampicillin until improvement, then ampicillin to complete course	High-dose in-hospital parenteral therapy usually not necessary
In pregnancy	Amoxicillin or ampicillin plus probenecid	As for urethritis
	Spectinomycin 2 g, i.m.	For penicillin-allergic patients
Herpes genitalis	Acyclovir	Moderately effective for treatment of primary disease
Trichomoniasis	Metronidazole 2 g, p.o.	Not to be given to pregnant women; male partner also should be treated
Candida vaginitis	Nystatin vaginal tablets q.d. × 7 days	
	Miconazole cream b.i.d. × 3 days	
	Clotrimazole cream b.i.d. × 3 days	
Bacterial vaginosis ("Nonspecific vaginitis")	Metronidazole 500 mg, p.o. b.i.d. × 7 days for severe cases	Ampicillin may be used during pregnancy
Hemophilus ducreyi	TMP/SMX (160/800), p.o.	Single-day treatment

*a*For patients allergic to penicillin refer to comments column.

treated with **fewer than two drugs.** Current recommendations are for **isoniazid** (INH) 300 mg, p.o., q.d., and **rifampin** 600 mg, p.o., q.d. for 9 months. After daily therapy for 2 to 8 weeks, directly supervised twice-weekly treatment (INH 15 mg/kg and rifampin 600 mg) may be used, especially in those individuals likely to be noncompliant. For patients from areas in which INH resistance is common, initial therapy should include ethambutol 15 mg/kg/day until susceptibility results are known.

2. **Extrapulmonary tuberculosis.** Although there are no controlled studies evaluating the efficacy of short-course chemotherapy for treatment of extrapulmonary tuberculosis, there is little reason to believe that short-course chemotherapy would not be effective, especially since extrapulmonary tuberculosis involves fewer organisms than pulmonary tuberculosis. Thus, short-course (9-month) therapy may be used for extrapulmonary tuberculosis. However, for those patients in whom the risk of relapse is high, such as those who are immunosuppressed or who have silicosis, longer therapy should be considered. **Prednisone treatment** 1 mg/kg/day in combination with antimicrobial

agents may be indicated for tuberculous meningitis, pericarditis, and pleuritis to diminish initial toxicity, with gradual tapering of steroids over a 1-month period.

3. **Retreatment of tuberculosis.** Relapses may be due to resistant organisms. Patients who have been treated previously for tuberculosis should be treated with at least two drugs not previously used, pending the results of sensitivity testing.

4. **Preventive therapy** (INH 300 mg, p.o., q.d.) for 1 year will diminish the incidence of tuberculosis occurring in several population groups. Preventive therapy is indicated in those instances in which this benefit outweighs the potential risk of drug toxicity. These groups include:

   a. **Household contacts** of patients with active pulmonary tuberculosis, who are at high risk whether or not their PPD skin tests are positive on initial examination (treatment can be stopped if the PPD remains negative 3 months later).

   b. **Persons with positive PPDs** and evidence on chest X-ray of previous reactivation disease such as apical scarring.

   c. Persons with documented **PPD skin test conversion to positive** within the previous 2 years.

   d. **Groups for whom chemoprophylaxis may be indicated** in individual cases, including PPD reactors with normal chest X-rays who are under the age of 35, are immunocompromised, have diabetes mellitus or silicosis, or have had a gastrectomy.

5. **Nontuberculous mycobacteriosis.** Infections with nontuberculous mycobacteria such as *M. kansasii* and *M. avium-intracellulare* occur predominantly in **middle-age men with preexisting lung disease.** The clinical manifestations are indistinguishable from those caused by *M. tuberculosis*, but extrapulmonary disease is uncommon except for the rapidly growing mycobacteria. **Treatment** of *M. kansasii* infections is similar to that for *M. tuberculosis*, but *M. avium-intracellulare* is usually resistant to chemotherapy, and four to six agents should be used concurrently for treatment.

J. **Septicemia**   Septicemia refers to a toxic state when the host's abilities to localize an infection are overwhelmed. The **sources** may be an infection in any site but most commonly the lungs, abdomen, urinary tract, surgical wounds, and sites of indwelling vascular catheters. The management of septicemia is directed to the original source of infection. If an obstruction, abscess, or infected foreign body is present, it is difficult to treat a septic episode effectively. Septicemia, if untreated, may progress to septic shock.

1. **Septic shock.** Septic shock is a hypotensive state that may occur during microbial, usually bacterial, infection. Once shock has developed, irreversible changes may occur that can be fatal. **Septic shock is a medical emergency.** Recognition that a patient is in septic shock should prompt the physician to institute a variety of diagnostic and therapeutic procedures as follows:

   a. **Fluid therapy.** Restore blood pressure to normal. Administering fluids to the patient in septic shock is by far the most important therapeutic maneuver. Sepsis, especially that resulting from gram-negative bacteria, causes increased capillary permeability and effective fluid volume loss that may be massive. On recognition of septic shock, a large-bore intravenous catheter should be inserted and fluids given rapidly. Since intravascular volume is depleted, normal saline or crystalloid are the most effective fluid sources. It is not uncommon for a patient in septic shock to require more than 4 liters normal saline within the first hour. **Titration of fluid therapy** must be based on peripheral blood pressure, perfusion of the microcirculation, and fluid status of the pulmonary vasculature. **Assessment of mental status and urine flow** can be used to monitor tissue perfusion at the capillary level. The most rapid and simple means to monitor for pulmonary venous overload are with a careful **chest examination** for rales and serial **arterial blood gas** determinations. On occasion, placement of a Swan-Ganz catheter is warranted, but for patients in shock the delay necessary may not be appropriate.

b. **Empiric broad-spectrum antibiotic coverage.** Determine and treat the source of infection. While administering fluids, quickly examine the patient and review the history. Empiric broad-spectrum antibiotic coverage should be instituted and should include agents for treatment of both gram-negative and gram-positive bacteria. In most situations, a **first-generation cephalosporin and an aminoglycoside** are appropriate therapy. However, if history or physical examination suggests a microbial agent that would not be covered by these antibiotics, additional empiric coverage is indicated. In patients already on broad-spectrum coverage, other antimicrobial (e.g., antipseudomonal, antifungal) agents may be added while awaiting culture results. During the interval between ordering antibiotics and their administration, obtain blood and other appropriate cultures.

c. **Corticosteroids.** Evidence for the efficacy of corticosteroids for treatment of septic shock is not firm. They appear to be of most benefit when given early in the course. Either dexamethasone 3 mg/kg or methylprednisolone 30 mg/kg, i.v., should be given as a single dose immediately, with a follow-up dose in 24 hr.

d. **Other treatment. Severe acidosis** (pH less than 7.1) should be treated with $NaHCO_3$ as necessary. Disseminated intravascular coagulation usually resolves without heparin therapy as the septic process is controlled.

2. **Sepsis in neutropenic patients.** Because infections in neutropenic patients (neutrophil count less than 1,000) can be rapidly fatal, empiric antibiotic therapy is indicated for any signs of sepsis. After initial evaluation, empiric therapy with bactericidal antibiotics should be given. The usual **treatment of choice** is an aminoglycoside and a semisynthetic penicillin, such as oxacillin, or a first-generation cephalosporin. If *P. aeruginosa* is suspected, carbenicillin or ticarcillin should be substituted for oxacillin or the cephalosporin. If cultures yield a likely pathogen, specific therapy for that agent should be instituted. If cultures do not yield a pathogen, and fever and neutropenia continue, empiric antibiotics should be continued. If the clinical picture worsens, additional new cultures are recommended. For patients remaining febrile and neutropenic after 7 days of empiric antibiotics, amphotericin B 0.5 mg/kg/day may be

added, but it is more important to **reassess the patient** than to give more drugs. When neutropenia resolves, patients usually defervesce spontaneously within 48 hr. If no focus for infection is discovered, antibiotics usually can be discontinued. For persistent fever after resolution of neutropenia, a diagnostic evaluation to determine the source of the infection is indicated.

3. **Sepsis of abdominal origin.** Fecal contamination may occur through trauma, surgery, or inflammation of the bowel wall (e.g., diverticulitis, appendicitis, colitis). The consequent infections are caused by **mixed bacterial flora**, which includes aerobic gram-negative rods and anaerobic organisms. After fecal spillage or sepsis of other abdominal origin, such as cholangitis or an infected pancreatic pseudocyst, empiric antimicrobial treatment should be instituted. **Therapy** should consist of an aminoglycoside and an agent active against anaerobes (such as metronidazole, clindamycin, or chloramphenicol). Isolation of agents from wound or blood cultures should determine definitive therapy. Hospitalized patients on long-term antimicrobial therapy for an abdominal abscess caused by fecal spillage also are at risk for developing disseminated fungal disease usually due to *Candida* or *Aspergillus* species.

4. **Community-acquired sepsis.** Persons who have not been hospitalized recently but who appear to be in a toxic condition may be ill for a variety of reasons. Careful history, physical examination, and screening laboratory tests will reveal the causes of most such problems, and the treatments for these have been indicated previously. The physician also should be aware of several other conditions that require rapid intervention:

   a. **Toxic-shock syndrome** (TSS) is caused by exotoxin-producing *S. aureus* strains and is primarily an intoxication. Most cases occur in young women and are associated with the use of tampons, but posttraumatic, postpartum, and postoperative cases also occur. **Treatment** consists of supporting blood pressure with fluids and adrenergic agents if necessary, eliminating the nidus of infection by removing foreign bodies (including tampons), and administering antistaphylococcal antibiotics, usually oxacillin or a first-generation cephalosporin.

   b. **Rocky Mountain spotted fever (RMSF)** is endemic in the areas surrounding the southern and central Appalachian Mountains, and/or Long Island, and less often in the Rocky Mountain region. Sporadic cases occur in most parts of the United States. RMSF is a tick-borne rickettsiosis that may be fatal unless treated early. **Diagnostic clues** are a history of tick exposure and a macular rash beginning on the extremities and progressing centrally; however, these may not be present and the diagnosis should be considered in any patient from an endemic area with unexplained fever and toxicity. **Treatment** is oral tetracycline 40 mg/kg/day or chloramphenicol 50 mg/kg/day in four divided doses, continued for 14 days.

   c. **Malaria must be considered in febrile persons who return from endemic areas. Diagnosis** is made by examination of a thick film of peripheral blood. For uncomplicated infection caused by organisms other than chloroquine-resistant *P. falciparum*, treatment is oral chloroquine phosphate 1 g followed by 500 mg in 6 hr, then 500 mg/day for 2 days. Chloroquine-resistant *P. falciparum* infection is treated with fansidar (500 mg sulfadoxine and 25 mg pyramethamine), 3 tablets stat. For seriously ill, obtunded patients, intravenous quinine may be obtained from the Centers for Disease Control.

d. Uncommon problems. Management of **typhoid fever** and septicemic *Salmonella* infections is discussed in section II. C. 3. For acutely ill patients living in rural parts of the southwestern United States, **plague** should be considered in the differential diagnosis. **Tularemia**, which may present as an acute toxic state, should be considered in rabbit hunters or those with tick exposures.

BIBLIOGRAPHY

Textbooks

Anderson, R. J. and Schrier, R. W., eds. (1981): *Clinical Use of Drugs in Patients with Kidney and Liver Disease*. W. B. Saunders, Philadelphia.
Kucers, A., and Bennett, N. McK. (1979): *The Use of Antibiotics: A Comprehensive Review with Clinical Emphasis*, 3d ed. William Heinermann Medical Books Ltd., London.

Articles on Specific Agents

Cockerill, F. R. III, and Edson, R. S. (1983): Trimethoprim-sulfamethoxazole. *Mayo Clin. Proc.*, 58:147–153.
Dhawan, V. K., and Thadepulli, H. (1982): Clindamycin: A review of fifteen years of experience. *Rev. Infect. Dis.*, 4:1133–1153.
Dolin, R., Reichman, R. C., Madore, H. P., Maynard, R., Linton, R. N., and Webber-Jones, (1982): A controlled trial of amantadine and rimantidine in the prophylaxis of influenza A infection. *N. Engl. J. Med.*, 307:580–584.
Edson, R. S., and Keys, T. F. (1983): The aminoglycosides: Streptomycin, kanamycin, gentamicin, tobramycin, amikacin, netilmicin, sisomicin. *Mayo Clin. Proc.*, 58:99–102.
Eliopoulos, G. E. and Moellering, R. C., Jr. (1982): Azlocillin, mezlocillin, and piperacillin: New broad-spectrum penicillins. *Am. Intern. Med.*, 97:755–760.
Erffmeyer, J. E. (1981): Adverse reactions to penicillin. *Ann. Allergy*, 47:288–300.
Farber, B. F., and Moellering, R. C., Jr. (1983): Retrospective study of the toxicity of preparations of vancomycin from 1974 to 1981. *Antimicrob. Agents Chemother.*, 58:138–141.
Goldman, P. (1980): Metronidazole. *N. Engl. J. Med.*, 303:1212–1218.
Medoff, G., and Kobayashi, G. S. (1980): Strategies in the treatment of systemic fungal infections. *N. Engl. J. Med.*, 302:145–155.
Moellering, R. C., Jr., Krogstad, D. J., and Greenblatt, D. J. (1981): Vancomycin therapy in patients with impaired renal function: A nomogran for dosage. *Ann. Intern. Med.*, 94:343–346.
National Institute of Allergy and Infectious Diseases Collaboratiave Antifungal Study. (1983): Treatment of systemic mycoses with ketoconazole: Emphasis on toxicity and clinical response in 52 patients. *Ann. Int. Med.*, 98:13–20.
Neu, H. C. (1982): The new beta-lactamase stable cephalosporins. *Ann. Intern. Med.*, 97:408–419.
Whitley, R. J., Soong, S. J., Hirsch, M. S., et al. (1981): Herpes simplex encephalitis: vidarabine therapy and diagnostic problems. *N. Engl. J. Med.*, 304:313–318.
Zaske, D. E., Irvine, P., Strand, L. M., Strate, R. G., Cipolle, R. J., and Rotschager, J. (1982): Wide interpatient variations in gentamicin dose requirements for geriatric patients. *J.A.M.A.*, 248:3122–3126.

Endocarditis

Dinubile, M. J. (1982): Surgery in active endocarditis. *Ann. Intern. Med.*, 96:650–659.
Geraci, J. E., and Wilson, W. R. (1982): Culture-negative endocarditis. *Mayo Clin. Proc.*, 57:149–154.

Wilson, W. R., Giulani, E. R., Danielson, G. K., and Geraci, J. E. (1982): General considerations in the diagnosis and treatment of infective endocarditis. *Mayo Clin. Proc.*, 57:81–85.

Gastroenteritis

Blaser, M. J., Wells, J. G., Feldman, R. A., et al. (1983): Campylobacter enteritis in the United States, a multicenter study. *Ann. Intern. Med.*, 98:360–365.

Jewkes, J., Larson, A. G., Price, A. B., et al. (1981): Aetiology of acute diarrhea in adults. *Gut*, 22:388–392.

Silva, J., Batts, D. H., Fekety, R., et al. (1981): Treatment of *Clostridium difficile* colitis and diarrhea with vancomycin. *Am. J. Med.*, 71:815–822.

Meningitis

Durack, D. T., and Spanos, A. (1982): End of treatment spinal tap in bacterial meningitis. Is it worthwhile? *J.A.M.A.*, 248:75–78.

Rahal, J. J., and Simberkoff, M. S. (1982): Host defense and antimicrobial therapy in adult gram-negative bacillary meningitis. *Ann. Intern. Med.*, 96:486–474.

Osteomyelitis

Meyers, B., Berson, B., Gilbert, M., et al. (1973): Clinical patterns of osteomyelitis due to gram-negative bacteria. *Arch. Intern. Med.*, 131:228–233.

Waldvogel, R., Medoff, G., and Swartz, M. (1970): Osteomyelitis: A review of clinical features, therapeutic considerations and unusual aspects. *N. Engl. J. Med.*, 282:198–206.

Pneumonia

Schwartz, J. S. (1982): Pneumococcal vaccine: Clinical efficacy and effectiveness. *Ann. Intern. Med.*, 96:208–220.

Tillotson, J. R., and Lerner, A. M. (1966): Pneumonias caused by gram-negative bacilli. *Medicine* (Baltimore), 45:65–76.

Yu, V., Kroboth, F. K., Shonard, J., et al. (1982): Legionnaires' disease: New clinical perspective from a prospective pneumonia study. *Am. J. Med.*, 73:357–361.

Sepsis

National Academy of Medicine (1982): The toxic-shock syndrome. *Ann. Intern. Med.*, 96:831–996.

Peters, W. P., Johnson, M. W., Friedman, P. A., and Mitch, W. E. (1981): Pressor effect of naloxone in septic shock. *Lancet*, 1:529–530.

Pizzo, P. A., Robichaud, K. J., Gill, F. A., and Whitebsky, F. G. (1982): Empiric antibiotic and antifungal therapy for cancer patients with prolonged fever and granulocytopenia. *Am. J. Med.*, 72:101–111.

Sexually Transmitted Diseases

Corey, L. (1982): The diagnosis and treatment of genital herpes. *J.A.M.A.*, 248:1041–1049.

Rothenberg, R. B., Simon, R., Chipperfield, M., et al. (1976): Efficacy of selected diagnostic tests for sexually transmitted diseases. *J.A.M.A.*, 235:49–51.

Urinary Tract Infections

Souney, P., and Polk, B. S. (1982): Single-dose antimicrobial therapy for urinary tract infections in women. *Rev. Infect. Dis.*, 4:29–34.

Stamm, W. E., Counts, G. W., Running, K. R., et al. (1982): Diagnosis of coliform infection in acutely dysuric women. *N. Engl. J. Med.*, 307:463–468.

11.

Gastrointestinal Diseases

John Goff

11.

Gastrointestinal Diseases

I. ESOPHAGEAL DISEASE

A. Reflux Esophagitis

1. **Pathophysiology and diagnosis.** The reflux of gastric (acidic) or duodenal (alkaline) juice into the esophageal lumen can cause damage to the squamous mucosa. Damage is dependent on the characteristics of the refluxed material, lower esophageal sphincter (LES) competence, and the duration of contact (speed of clearing). The **diagnosis** is made primarily on a historical basis (heartburn, pyrosis, regurgitation), but objective evidence of disease needs to be confirmed with endoscopy, motility studies, a Bernstein test, or an esophagram if the symptoms do not respond to initial treatment or if the patient develops dysphagia.

2. **Initial therapy includes:**

   a. **Head-of-bed elevation** with 6-inch blocks (not elevation of patient's head with pillows) to allow gravity to aid in esophageal clearance at night.

   b. **Dietary changes.** Patients should not lie down immediately after eating; they should avoid fatty foods, smoking, alcohol, and chocolate because they decrease LES pressure; and they should try to lose weight.

   c. **Drugs** that lower LES pressure (anticholinergics, theophylline, meperidine, estrogens) should be avoided if possible.

   d. **Antacids** are the primary treatment for reflux symptoms. The dose will vary from 30 ml orally at bedtime to hourly doses, but generally 30 ml, p.o., 1 and 3 hr p.c. and h.s. is most helpful. Algenic acid (Gaviscon®) forms a foam that floats on top of the gastric contents. Thus, when reflux occurs, the Gaviscon®, rather than gastric acid, is the refluxed material. Gaviscon® can be substituted for antacids or used in conjunction with antacids. The usual dosage is 15 to 30 ml, p.o., 1 to 2 hr p.c. and h.s., or 1 to 2 chewable tablets 1 to 2 hr p.c. and h.s.

3. **Second-line therapy** for patients unresponsive to initial treatment:

   a. **Cimetidine** (300 mg, p.o., q.i.d.) or other H_2-blocking agents; these will decrease acid production very effectively and will prevent esophageal irritation when reflux occurs.

   b. **Drugs that increase LES pressure** and improve reflux symptoms, such as bethanechol and metoclopramide. **Bethanechol** is a pure cholinergic drug. Its usual dose is 25 mg, p.o. 30 min a.c. and at h.s.; however, a single 25-mg dose p.o. at h.s. may be as effective without as many side

237

effects. **Metoclopramide** has several neurologic effects, including a cholinergic effect; 10 to 20 mg, p.o., q.i.d., will increase LES pressure and speed gastric emptying. These two agents can be used together in very selected patients.

4. **Third-line therapy. Surgery** to prevent reflux is reserved for patients not responding to medical management and those who have documented reflux with esophageal damage or complications of esophagitis, including severe stricture formation, bleeding, or pulmonary aspiration. Barrett's epithelium (gastric glands in the esophagus) may represent an indication for earlier surgical intervention.

5. **Complications of therapy** include

   a. **Diarrhea,** which can be caused by excessive use of magnesium-containing antacids. This can be reversed by alternating doses with a pure aluminum hydroxide antacid such as Amphogel®.

   b. **H₂ blockers** have several, though infrequent, side effects (see II. for enumeration).

   c. **Cholinergic agents** should be avoided in patients with asthma, hyperthyroidism, coronary artery disease, and peptic ulcer disease.

   d. **Metoclopramide** will produce mental changes or extrapyramidal reactions in up to 10% of patients. These symptoms are treated by stopping metoclopramide, plus diphenhydramine 50 mg, i.m., if the symptoms are severe.

B. Infectious Esophagitis

1. **Pathophysiology and diagnosis.** The two most common esophageal infections are candidiasis and herpes simplex. These usually occur in patients with malignancy, diabetes mellitus, or immune compromise but can occur in otherwise normal patients. Patients usually complain of dysphagia or odynophagia. The diagnosis is made from brushings and biopsies obtained at **endoscopy.**

2. **Treatment**

   a. **Analgesia** is best obtained by using a combination of antacid and a topical anesthetic every 1 to 2 hr (Oxaine M suspension).

   b. **Antifungal drugs** for candidiasis:

      (1) **Nystatin** suspension, 250,000 U, p.o., every 2 hr, or the patient can use nystatin suppositories or lozenges for 2 to 6 weeks.

      (2) **Flucytosine** (100 mg/kg, p.o.), **amphotericin B** (5 to 10 mg/day, i.v.), **miconazole** (250 mg, p.o., 3 to 6 times a day), and **ketoconazole** (200 to 400 mg, p.o., q.d.) for 2 to 6 weeks can be used as alternate therapies or for more severe cases.

   c. **Acyclovir** 5 mg/kg infused over 1 hr every 8 hr for 7 days may be useful for herpes esophagitis in the immune compromised host. The dose is less in renal insufficiency.

C. Diffuse Esophageal Spasm

1. **Pathophysiology and diagnosis.** A history of liquid and solid dysphagia with or without chest pain, plus an abnormal esophagram or esophageal scintigraphy

will strongly suggest the diagnosis of diffuse esophageal spasm (DES). The diagnosis is confirmed by esophageal manometry. The etiology and pathophysiology of DES are unknown. Drugs, acid, hot or cold liquids, and some foods may precipitate the syndrome.

2. **Treatment** in order of preference:

   a. **Antireflux** measures as outlined above may be useful if acid reflux is producing spasm.

   b. **Anticholinergic drugs** can decrease spasm. **Propantheline** is recommended in a dose of 15 to 30 mg, p.o., q.i.d.

   c. **Nitrates** will benefit some patients. An initial trial of sublingual nitroglycerine (NTG) 1/150 g p.r.n. is followed by long-acting nitrates (e.g., isosorbide dinitrate 10 to 40 mg, p.o., q.i.d.) if the NTG benefits the patient.

   d. **Calcium channel blockers** relax smooth muscle, and nifedipine 10 to 20 mg, p.o., q.i.d., or verapamil 80 to 160 mg, p.o., q.i.d., can improve symptoms in selected patients with DES.

   e. Balloon dilatation or surgical myotomy should be reserved for severely symptomatic patients who are resistant to medical treatment.

II. PEPTIC ULCER DISEASE

A. Duodenal and Gastric Ulcers

1. **Pathophysiology and diagnosis. Duodenal ulcers** (DU) are caused by the effects of acid and pepsin on the duodenal mucosa. A combination of increased duodenal acid and decreased mucosal resistance results in mucosal disruption. The cause of **gastric ulcers** (GU) is more complex and less well defined. Factors that influence the formation of GU include gastric acid and pepsin secretion, delayed gastric emptying, duodenogastric reflux, gastric blood flow, gastric mucus and bicarbonate secretion, drug ingestion (aspirin and other prostaglandin inhibitors), and psychological stress. A GU in the absence of acid should alert one to consider Crohn's disease, malignancy, or infection as the etiology.

   The **diagnosis** of an ulcer should be suspected when patients complain of upper abdominal pain. Food-relieved pain usually signals a DU, whereas food-increased pain is more common with GU. An upper gastrointestinal (UGI) series will diagnose most peptic ulcer disease (PUD), but since 10% or more can be missed, endoscopy must be performed if the X-rays are negative. Total healing of a GU must be documented to exclude the possibility of gastric cancer. DU healing does not need to be documented if symptoms resolve.

2. **Initial therapy** for both DU and GU includes the following.

   a. **Smoking** should be discontinued, especially in DU patients, because continuation has been shown to decrease the healing rate despite other treatment.

   b. **Dietary** changes are of no proved benefit or detriment; nevertheless, patients should avoid foods that increase their symptoms.

c. Antacids of high buffering capacity (see Table 1) given 7 times a day (30 ml, p.o., 1 and 3 hr p.c. and h.s.) have been shown to heal DU but are of questionable benefit in GU.

d. H$_2$ blockers (cimetidine 300 mg, p.o., q.i.d., or ranitidine 150 mg, p.o., b.i.d.) decrease acid secretion and make excellent substitutes for antacids because of equal or better effectiveness compared to antacids and increased patient compliance.

e. Sucralfate (Carafate®) promotes DU/GU healing by forming a protective coating over the ulcer. It is used in patients with intolerance for or unresponsiveness to H$_2$ blockers. The dosage is 1 g, p.o., 30 min a.c. and h.s.

3. **Second-line therapy** is for use in patients unresponsive to the individual use of the above drugs. **Cimetidine failures** need to have the Zollinger-Ellison syndrome excluded while trying alternate forms of therapy:

a. Add regular doses of antacid.

b. Switch to ranitidine.

c. Add anticholinergic (propantheline 15 mg, p.o., q.i.d.)

d. Increase dosage of cimetidine to 600 mg, p.o., q.i.d.

Drugs that have been effectively used in European trials to treat peptic ulcers and may soon be available in the United States include colloidal bismuth, carbenoxolone, trimipramine, prirenzepine, and prostaglandins.

4. **Third-line therapy. Surgical intervention** is indicated with ulcers unresponsive to medical management (nonhealing over 8 to 12 weeks), frequent ulcer recurrences, repeated or continued bleeding, gastric outlet obstruction, and perforation.

5. **Complications of therapy**

a. Antacids (see above under esophagitis).

b. Cimetidine side effects include gynecomastia, granulocytopenia, mental confusion (especially in the elderly or patients with renal or liver disease), interstitial nephritis, and rarely, increased liver enzymes. **Delayed metabolism** of propranolol, theophylline, warfarin, and benzodiazepines caused

TABLE 1. *Comparison of various liquid antacids*

Antacid	Dose required to neutralize 100 mEq acid (ml)	Na content per dose (mg)
Al (OH)$_3$		
Amphojel®	75	4.5
ALternaGEL®	40	0.8
Al (OH)$_3$ + Mg(OH)$_2$		
Maalox® TC	25	4.0
Maalox® Plus	45	11.7
Mylanta® II	30	6.8
Riopan® Plus	55	3.3
Gelusil® II	35	10.1

by cimetidine can lead to drug toxicities. In **renal failure** the dose of cimetidine must be decreased to 300 mg, p.o., b.i.d.

c. **Anticholinergic drugs** cause dryness of the mouth and should be avoided in patients with pulmonary disease, prostatism, delayed gastric emptying, or glaucoma.

6. **Complications of PUD and their treatment**

a. **Recurrent ulcers,** gastric or duodenal, are common occurrences. Generally treatment is the same as for primary ulcers. **Prevention** of recurrences with cimetidine 400 mg, p.o., either at h.s. or b.i.d. has been demonstrated in DU patients. Multiple, poorly controlled recurrences are an indication for surgery. **Noncompliance** must be remembered as a major reason for recurrences or poor ulcer healing.

b. **Hemorrhage** (see XII.).

c. **Gastric outlet obstruction** results from edema and scarring secondary to ulcers near the pylorus. A **nasogastric tube** is useful for making the diagnosis and **mandatory** for treatment. A positive saline load test, more than 400 ml still in stomach 30 min after instillation of 700 ml of normal saline, confirms the diagnosis. Suction should be maintained for a minimum of 72 hr. **Cimetidine** 300 mg, i.v., every 6 hr should be started. Volume depletion, hypokalemia, and hypochloremic alkalosis can be corrected with intravenous normal saline and KCl. **Surgery** is indicated if the patient has a history of chronic obstructive problems or if unable to reverse present episode of obstruction.

d. **Penetration and perforation** usually require surgical intervention because of poor response to routine medical treatment.

7. **Complications of surgery for PUD and their treatment**

a. **Alkaline (bile) reflux gastritis** occurs when duodenal contents reflux into the stomach after pylorus-destroying surgery and, in conjunction with a small amount of acid, produce gastric inflammation. Therapy is **acid reduction** with antacids or cimetidine [aluminum hydroxide antacids are best since they also bind bile acids (Amphojel®, ALternaGEL®)]; and **bile acid binding** with cholestyramine (4-g packs) or colestipol (5-g packs), 2 p.o. with breakfast and 1 p.o. with lunch and supper. Sucralfate 1 g, p.o., 30 min a.c. and h.s. also may be beneficial. **Improved gastric emptying** and decreased duodeno- or jejunogastric reflux can be obtained by using metoclopramide 10 to 20 mg, p.o., q.i.d. **Surgery** frequently is necessary because medical management often is not effective (creation of Roux-en Y).

b. **Dumping syndrome** is the term applied to a group of postvagotomy or partial-gastrectomy symptoms that include one or more of the following: postprandial pain, bloating, diarrhea, vomiting, nausea, and vasomotor symptoms. **Dietary changes** are most important for control of dumping. Patients should eat 6 or more small high-protein, low-carbohydrate meals per day and should drink liquids only between meals. Milk products usually need to be avoided. **Anticholinergic drugs** and **antidiarrheal agents** are of benefit in selected patients.

   c. **Poor gastric emptying** of solids with or without bezoar formation can occur after vagotomy or antrectomy. **Dietary** intake of nondigestible roughage must be discouraged. Patients need to chew their food very well or blenderize it if their dentition is poor. **Metoclopramide or bethanechol** will improve selected cases. **Enzyme preparations** containing cellulose such as Arco-Lase®, Ku-Zyme®, Kanulase®, and Celluzyme™ will help digest phytobezoars and prevent their recurrence.

   d. **Diarrhea** is a frequent symptom after gastric surgery. After excluding malabsorption as a cause (see weight loss, below), the treatment is as for any patient with chronic diarrhea (see VII.).

   e. **Weight loss** is common after gastric surgery. If the decrease is greater than 15 pounds, then an evaluation to exclude **malabsorption** from bacterial overgrowth, pancreatic insufficiency, and celiac sprue is indicated. Patients often develop **anemia** or metabolic **bone disease** from chronic mild malabsorption. The anemia is treated with iron, folate, or cobalamin as indicated by appropriate tests. Parenteral iron is frequently needed in these patients. Oral calcium and vitamin D will prevent or improve the bone disease.

B. Gastritis and Duodenitis   Gastritis and Duodenitis are diffuse superficial mucosal disruptions of the stomach and duodenum. Their etiology is similar to ulcer disease in the same location; thus, the initial therapy is identical. Gastritis is frequently associated with **drug ingestion** (especially prostaglandin inhibitors) and promptly responds to removal of the irritating agent.

C. Stress Ulcers   Stress ulcers develop in severely ill patients (sepsis, burns, CNS trauma, fulminant hepatic failure, etc.). **Treatment** must be aggressive because of the high mortality associated with bleeding in severely ill patients. A combination of intravenous cimetidine and oral antacids is recommended.

Preventive therapy is indicated in these patients. **Antacid** is the best agent for increasing gastric pH and preventing bleeding. It should be given by nasogastric tube (30 ml or more) every hour as needed to keep the gastric pH >4. **Cimetidine** 300 mg, p.o., every 6 hr, may be used, but available data suggest it is less effective than antacid.

D. Zollinger-Ellison Syndrome   This syndrome is caused by gastrin-secreting tumors, usually in the pancreas. The increased acid secretion causes the patient to have refractory or malignant duodenal ulcer disease. **Medical therapy** consists of high-dose H_2 blockers, often in combination with an anticholinergic drug. **Surgical exploration** to establish tumor resectability or perform a highly selective vagotomy is advisable. Patients refractory to medical management with unresectable tumors are treated with a **total gastrectomy.**

III. MALABSORPTION

   A. Pathophysiology and Diagnosis   Malabsorption is caused by inadequate amounts of bile and pancreatic juice, decreased small-bowel mucosal function, increased number of bacteria in the upper intestine, or a combination of these factors. Some **tests** of malabsorption require all phases of digestion and absorption to be intact to obtain normal results (triolein breath test, stool fat); other selectivity test isolated functions (pancreatic secretion test, hydrogen breath test, d-xylose absorption test, small-bowel biopsy). Once a specific diagnosis has been made, rational treatment can begin.

B. Treatment of Selected Malabsorptive Disorders

1. **Celiac sprue** is treated by total removal of gluten-containing grains from the diet (wheat, rye, barley, oats). The patient needs to be cautioned that gluten (wheat) is added to many products (ice cream, canned vegetables, candy, processed meats, etc.), thus label reading becomes very important. Milk should be avoided and vitamin/mineral supplements provided during the recovery phase.

2. **Bacterial overgrowth** in the upper small intestine develops when obstruction, diverticula, achlorhydria, or blind loops cause stagnation. The bacteria compete for nutrients, deconjugate bile salts, and damage the mucosal brush border. **Surgical correction** of the stagnation is the most effective therapy. **Antibiotics** will control symptoms in patients with nonsurgically correctable disorders (intestinal diverticulosis, scleroderma, diabetes mellitus, Crohn's disease). Control usually can be obtained and maintained by 2-weeks-on–2 weeks-off courses of tetracycline or metronidazole 250 mg, p.o., q.i.d. Occasionally, cycling several different antibiotics will be necessary.

3. **Short-bowel syndrome** occurs when the remaining functional surface area of jejunum or ileum is insufficient to absorb enough nutrients to sustain life.

   a. **Medical therapy. Cimetidine** 300 mg, p.o., q.i.d., will suppress the acid hypersection that occurs in about 50% of patients transiently after massive small-bowel resection. **Cholestyramine** (4-g pack, p.o., with water; 2 with breakfast and 1 with lunch and supper) or cholestipol (5-g packs) are used to prevent bile acid irritation of the colon and subsequent diarrhea in patients with ileal resections. Patients with more than 100 cm of ileum resected can have worsening of lipid absorption with these agents because they deplete the bile acid pool. **Antidiarrheal agents** will increase transit time and may facilitate absorption (see VII.).

   b. **Parenteral alimentation** often is necessary to correct nutritional deficiencies in poorly controlled patients. Some patients may require home total parenteral nutrition (TPN) because of insufficient absorptive surface and limited adaptive hyperplasia of the remaining intestinal mucosa.

   c. **Oral feedings** are necessary to prevent atrophy of the remaining intestinal mucosa. Feedings should begin with elemental diets (amino acids, simple sugars, and medium-chain triglycerides) and can be advanced to more complex foods as tolerated by the patient. Remember that commercial preparations are hypertonic and usually will need to be diluted, at least initially, to avoid an osmotic diarrhea. **Steatorrhea** can be decreased by maintaining patients on a 50- to 75-gm-fat diet with medium-chain-triglyceride supplementation, as needed, to supply an adequate caloric intake. The diet also should be low in oxalate to prevent the development of renal calculi. Milk usually must be avoided. (See Chapter 21 for details on these preparations).

   d. **Mineral and vitamin supplementation** is important, especially in patients relying totally on oral feedings. Table 2 lists common dosages of supple-

TABLE 2. *Supplements for patients with malabsorption or maldigestion*

Supplements	Dosage	Route
Vitamins		
A	5,000–50,000 U/day	p.o.
D_3	25,000–50,000 U/day	p.o.
D_2 (ergocalciferol)	50,000–400,000 U/day	p.o.
1,25-dihydroxychole-calciferol (calcitriol)	0.25–1.0 mEq/day	p.o.
K_1 (phytonadione)	5–10 mg/day	s.o. or i.m.
K (menadiol)	5–10 mg/day	p.o.
E	50–500 U/day	p.o.
Folic acid	1 mg/day	p.o.
B_{12} (cobalamin)	100–1000 μg/month	i.m.
B complex	1–2 tabs/day	p.o.
C	100–1000 mg/day	p.o.
Minerals		
Calcium (carbonate, lactate, gluconate)	1.5–3.0 g/day (elemental)	p.o.
Magnesium (oxide, sulfate, gluconate, citrate)	1–6 g/day	p.o. or i.m.
Iron (sulfate, gluconate, fumarate)	325 mg t.i.d.	p.o.
Imferon (iron dextran)	1–5 ml/wk	i.m.
Zinc	15–30 mg/day	p.o.
Other minerals (with multiple vitamins)	1–2 tab/day	p.o.

ments often required by patients with short-bowel syndrome and chronic malabsorption.

4. **Pancreatic insufficiency** is discussed in XI.B.

5. **Lactase deficiency** develops in up to 90% of adults from many ethnic and racial groups (blacks, Orientals, American Indians, Mexican-Americans). **Diagnosis** is primarily made by a history of pain, bloating, flatulence, or diarrhea after ingesting milk or milk products. Objective confirmation can be obtained by documenting a lack of increase in serum glucose or an increase in breath hydrogen after ingesting 12.5 to 50 g of lactose. **Treatment** consists of avoiding milk and milk products with high lactose contents. Aged cheeses have the least lactose content and may be tolerated by some patients. Yogurt usually is tolerated because of its intrinsic lactase content. Patients may purchase lactase as a powder to add to milk before they drink it (LactAid®). Patients who avoid milk should supplement their diets with 1 to 2 g calcium per day.

6. **Drugs** such as cholestyramine, cathartics, colchicine, neomycin, ethyl alcohol, and tetracycline may cause malabsorption.

IV. INFLAMMATORY BOWEL DISEASE

A. Ulcerative Colitis

1. **Pathophysiology and diagnosis.** The etiology of ulcerative colitis (UC) is unknown. The disease is characterized by superficial inflammation and ulceration of the colonic mucosa. It invariably involves the rectum and can extend continuously to involve the entire colon in many patients. The **diagnosis** is made by observing edematous, friable, rectosigmoid mucosa in the absence of identifiable pathogens. **Barium enemas and colonoscopy** help define the extent of disease and any associated complications (strictures, cancer) but are

usually done during a quiescent phase to avoid complications and exacerbations.

2. Initial therapy for mild exacerbations

a. **Sulfasalazine** (Azulfidine®) 500 mg, p.o., b.i.d. or q.i.d. may be given, with increasing doses every 2 to 4 days as tolerated to a maximum of 8 g/day. The slow increases in dose helps prevent excessive gastric upset. Enteric-coated tablets may decrease the nausea produced by stomach irritation from sulfasalazine.

b. **Corticosteroid enemas** or foam are very useful for patients with primary proctitis or severe rectal symptoms. Cortenema® or Proctofoam® are used per rectum twice daily. A mixture of 1.6 g hydrocortisone powder (alcohol hemisuccinate) per quart of safflower oil given as 2-oz enemas is cheaper than the commercial preparations and equally effective.

c. **Dietary changes** are of modest benefit in mild flares of UC. However, changing the diet to liquids or elemental foods will decrease the diarrhea and is advised in more severe cases.

d. **Anticholinergic and antidiarrheal drugs** are best avoided in patients with flares of UC because of their limited effectiveness and risk of producing toxic megacolon.

3. Second-line therapy is for patients not responding to the initial therapy or with more severe disease at the outset.

a. **Corticosteroids** orally (prednisone 30 to 60 mg, p.o., q.d. or b.i.d.) or intravenously in more severely ill patients (hydrocortisone 100 mg every 8 hr) are highly effective in producing remission. ACTH is not superior to prednisone or hydrocortisone. Patients who have responded to corticosteroids can be withdrawn from them over 4 to 12 weeks without immediate recurrence of colitis.

b. **Azathioprine** in doses up to 2.5 mg/kg/day, p.o., have not been shown to be of significant benefit. However, selected patients may respond, and patients who are not operative candidates often can be maintained on lower doses of corticosteroids if azathioprine is added to their treatment regimen.

c. **Parenteral alimentation** is indicated to reverse or prevent nutritional deficits, since UC patients with moderate to severe disease are unable to ingest enough to offset their increased losses and catabolic state. TPN does not alter the natural history of the colitis.

d. **ACTH** has a controversial role in the therapy for UC. Doses vary from 20 to 120 U/day, i.m. or i.v.

4. Third-line therapy is reserved for patients unresponsive to the regimens outlined above or for those with frequent recurrences. **Total colectomy** cures most patients, although a few will have persistent extracolonic manifestations (sclerosing cholangitis, arthritis).

5. Maintenance of remission by using **sulfasalazine** 2 g/day, p.o., has been proved experimentally. Corticosteroids should not be used for long-term maintenance because of the risks of major side effects. During remission, patients are still at risk for developing carcinoma. They need **annual colonoscopy** after 8 years from the time of diagnosis of UC to screen for cancer and dysplasia. Severe dysplasia or repeated finding of lesser degrees of dysplasia are indications for elective colectomy.

6. **Toxic megacolon** is a medical emergency. It is defined by a transverse colon diameter greater than 6 cm in association with systemic toxicity. If patients do not respond to treatment in 24 to 48 hr, they need an emergent colectomy. **Dehydration and hypokalemia** need to be vigorously corrected parenterally. Transfusion may be necessary, and TPN usually will be necessary. **Nasogastric suction** will help decompress the distended bowel.

   Antibiotics are indicated to prevent sepsis if perforation occurs or to treat it if it has already developed. Ampicillin 1 g, i.v., every 4 hr; tobramycin 2 mg/kg, i.v., followed by 1 mg/kg every 8 hr; and clindamycin 600 mg, i.v. every 6 hr (or their equivalents) are recommended. **Hydrocortisone,** 100 mg, i.v., every 8 hr is sufficient to prevent stress-induced adrenal insufficiency in patients who have recently been taking corticosteroids, and it is adequate for treatment of the toxic megacolon. Barium enema, colonoscopy (not a careful sigmoidoscopy), anticholinergics, and antidiarrheal agents must be avoided.

7. **Complications of therapy**

   a. **Sulfasalazine.** Dose-related side effects develop in 20% of patients receiving more than 4 g/day, p.o. Slow acetylators have increased frequency of toxic side effects, including nausea, vomiting, abdominal discomfort, and headache. These are treated by decreasing the dose.

   Idiosyncratic, possibly hypersensitivity reactions, include fever, skin rash, arthralgias, hepatitis, and rarely, anemia or aplastic anemia. These side effects usually develop in 1 to 4 weeks after starting sulfasalazine. Treatment consists of drug withdrawal. **Folate absorption** is decreased by sulfasalazine; thus, folic acid supplementation (1 mg, p.o., q.d.) is indicated in patients on long-term treatment.

   b. **Corticosteroids.** Side effects occurring during initial (acute) administration are edema or hypertension from sodium retention, hyperglycemia, psychosis, and rarely, hypokalemic alkalosis. Additional side effects from long-term use are an increased susceptibility to infection, osteoporosis, myopathy, cataracts, Cushingoid appearance, acne, hirsutism, and a very small increase in PUD.

   c. **Azathioprine** can cause bone marrow depression, increased susceptibility to infection, pancreatitis, fever, and rash.

B. **Crohn's Disease**

1. **Pathophysiology and diagnosis.** Crohn's disease is an idiopathic inflammatory process that involves all layers of the gut wall and may have noncaseating granulomas. The lesions are characterized by deep ulcerations that lead to fistula or abscess formation. Frequently "skip areas" are found (normal mucosa separating ulcerated areas). The **diagnosis** is made by a combination of history, physical examination, roentgenograms, endoscopic examination, and biopsy. As with UC, infectious causes must be excluded before the diagnosis can be made.

2. Initial therapy for patients with mild to moderate symptoms:

a. **Dietary changes,** depending on the severity of the disease. **Maintenance of nutrition** is extremely important, and parenteral feeding should be used if needed, although in milder exacerbations a regular diet with supplementation usually is adequate. Bulk should be avoided if obstruction is suspected. Lactose intolerance may coexist and can result in increased symptoms if milk intake is greatly increased as part of a liquid diet.

b. **Antidiarrheal agents** (diphenoxylate, loperimide, etc.) can be useful in controlling diarrhea but must be used with caution and avoided totally if perforation, obstruction, or toxic megacolon are suspected.

c. **Bed rest** is advisable, especially if symptoms are moderate to severe.

d. **Sulfasalazine** (2 to 8 g/day, p.o., in divided doses) will improve symptoms in some patients with Crohn's disease. However, it is least effective in those with small-bowel involvement only and most effective in those with colon involvement only. **Corticosteroids** very effectively control Crohn's disease. The usual dose is 40 to 60 mg, p.o., every morning in mild to moderate cases. It can be used in conjunction with sulfasalazine, but advantages of combined therapy have not been proved.

3. Second-line therapy is for more severely ill patients or those unresponsive to the initial regimen.

a. **Aggressive nutritional support is mandatory.** This may be accomplished orally but usually requires parenteral feeding during exacerbations because anorexia, pain, or vomiting prevent adequate oral intake.

b. **Intravenous corticosteroids** may be administered at dose equivalent to 300 mg hydrocortisone daily in 2 to 4 divided doses.

c. **Azathioprine** (2 to 3 mg/kg/day) or **6-mercaptopurine** (1.5 mg/kg/day) may be of benefit, although clinical trials using these agents have produced only marginally positive results. They can be combined with corticosteroids and will allow a dose reduction without a decrease in beneficial effects. **Metronidazole** (750 to 1,500 mg/day, p.o., in divided doses) has shown some benefit in uncontrolled trials. The most promising results have been noted in patients with perineal disease.

4. Third-line therapy is for patients unresponsive to the medical regimens outlined above or who develop abscesses, fistulas, or obstruction. These patients require **surgical resection** of the involved bowel.

5. Treatment during remission is different from that of patients with UC.

a. **Prednisone, sulfasalazine, and azathioprine** have not been shown to prolong remission. Therefore, the **ultimate goal** in most patients is to taper off these drugs gradually over 4 to 12 weeks once remission is achieved. Maintaining Crohn's patients on low-dose prednisone is acceptable if unable to sustain a remission without it.

b. The **diet** for most patients between flares is regular food with liquid supplements as needed to insure adequate calorie intake. Patients with residual ileal damage or after large ileal resections may need part of their fat intake replaced by medium-chain triglycerides (25%) to decrease stea-torrhea and increase calorie absorption. These people also often need monthly cobalamin (1,000 μg, i.m.).

c. **Colestipol** (5-g packets) or **cholestyramine** (4-g packets) are bile-salt-binding resins that will decrease bile-salt-induced diarrhea in patients with ileal disease or resection. The usual dose is 2 packs, p.o., with breakfast and 1 each with lunch and supper.

d. **Antibiotics** (tetracycline 250 mg, p.o., q.i.d., or metranidazole 250 mg, p.o., q.i.d. for 7 to 14 days) are indicated when bacterial overgrowth proximal to a small-bowel stricture is suspected or diagnosed.

e. **Antidiarrheal** agents are frequently necessary to control loose stools during clinical remissions (see VII.).

6. **Complications of therapy** for Crohn's disease may result from **sulfasalazine, azathioprine, and corticosteroids** (see IV.A.7.). **6-Mercaptopurine** is a metabolite of azathioprine; thus, the side effects are similar. **Metronidazole** in the large doses required for therapy of Crohn's disease frequently is not tolerated because of nausea, abdominal discomfort, headaches, a metallic taste, and peripheral neuropathy. Metronidazole also has an Antabuse®-like effect when taken with alcohol. **Colestipol and cholestyramine** can increase steatorrhea by decreasing the bile acid pool further in patients with large (usually greater than 100-cm) resections of ileum. Absorption of fat-soluble vitamins (A, D, E, and K) can be impaired as well. These agents also can produce significant constipation.

V. PSEUDOMEMBRANOUS COLITIS

A. **Pathophysiology and Diagnosis**   Pseudomembranous colitis (PMC) is caused by an overgrowth of toxin-producing *Clostridium difficile,* which usually occurs after antibiotic exposure. The toxin causes characteristic raised yellow plaques (pseudomembranes) to develop on the rectal and colonic mucosa. Patients develop systemic symptoms, including fever, abdominal pain, and diarrhea (often Hemoccult®-positive). The **diagnosis** is made by the history (antibiotic use), the physical findings at sigmoidoscopy, and measurement of the level of *Clostridium* toxin in the diarrheal stools.

B. **Therapy for PMC**

1. **Colestipol** (5-g packets) or **cholestyramine** (4-g packets) given orally 4 times a day has been variably successful. However, because its cost is low, it should be tried first in milder cases. These resins bind to the toxin, preventing it from causing further mucosal and systemic injury.

2. **Vancomycin** 125 mg to 500 mg, p.o., q.i.d. for 7 to 14 days, is the **drug of choice** for treating PMC. Approximately 15% to 20% of responders will relapse, requiring a second course or alternate therapy. The major disadvantage to its use is its extremely high cost. Vancomycin given orally is poorly absorbed.

3. **Bacitracin** 250,000 U, p.o., q.i.d., is a slightly less expensive, alternate form of therapy, but there is only limited clinical data supporting its usefulness.

4. Metronidazole 250 mg, p.o., q.i.d., also has been reported to be effective, but it has on rare occasion been reported to cause PMC.

VI. DIVERTICULAR DISEASE

A. Diverticulosis

1. **Pathophysiology and diagnosis.** Diverticulosis is an acquired condition in which portions of the mucosa and submucosa of the colon herniate through the muscle layers at the point where the nutrient artery penetrates the muscle. The etiology remains unclear, but epidemiologic evidence suggests that the highly refined Western diet promotes its development. The **diagnosis** is made by barium enema or colonoscopy. Less than 25% of people with diverticulosis develop symptoms or complications.

2. **Therapy** of uncomplicated symptomatic diverticulosis is similar to the treatment of irritable bowel syndrome (see below).

B. Bleeding   Bleeding from diverticula can occur. Its management is discussed under GI bleeding (XII.).

C. Diverticulitis

1. **Pathophysiology and diagnosis.** Diverticulitis results from inflammation of the diverticular wall, usually producing microperforations. These can progress to a large phlegmonous mass, abscess with fistula formation, or bowel obstruction. The **diagnosis** is made by history, physical exam (left lower quadrant tenderness or mass), sigmoidoscopy, and barium enema. Ultrasound or computed tomography (CT) scan can help define abscesses in diverticular disease.

2. **Initial therapy** for mild to moderate diverticulitis:

   a. **Nothing by mouth** and nasogastric suction if vomiting is present or the patient's abdomen is distended.

   b. **Intravenous hydration** and electrolyte replacement as needed.

   c. **Avoid analgesics** until serial examinations of the abdomen can be made to exclude a perforation with peritonitis.

   d. **Antibiotics** are indicated for most cases serious enough to be hospitalized. Milder cases can be treated with ampicillin or a cephalosporin; more severe cases require broader-spectrum coverage, including anaerobes (e.g., ampicillin, gentamicin, and clindamycin).

3. **Second-line therapy,** consisting of surgical intervention, is reserved for perforation with peritonitis, progressive abscess formation despite antibiotics, and bowel or urinary obstruction in acute cases. **Chronic complications** requiring surgical treatment include recurrent severe attacks, fistula formation, chronic partial bowel obstruction, and urinary tract involvement.

VII. DIARRHEA

A. Acute Diarrhea   Acute diarrhea is generally defined as more than 200 g of stool per day, usually associated with increased frequency of passage (>3/day) and of less than 3 weeks duration.

1. **Diagnosis** of the cause is made by taking a careful history, including travel, exposures, and ingestions (drugs); examining the stool for white blood cells,

parasites, and blood; culturing the stool for pathogens; and doing a sigmoidoscopy if blood or white blood cells are present in the stools.

2. **Treatment**

   a. **Hydration** orally with electrolyte-containing fluids (e.g., Gatorade) if tolerated or intravenously if necessary is the most important treatment.

   b. **Narcotic antidiarrheal agents** (see VII.B.2.) should be used cautiously or not at all initially. They may prolong the course of some infectious diarrheas and can induce toxic megacolon in UC patients.

   c. **Kaolin, pectin, bulk agents** (e.g., Metamucil®, Mitrolan®) are useful in decreasing the diarrheal episodes in mild, uncomplicated cases of acute diarrhea.

   d. **Pepto-Bismol®** (bismuth subsalicylate) in large doses (30 to 60 ml, p.o., every 30 min for eight doses) has been shown to be effective in decreasing the symptoms of acute traveler's diarrhea. It may be useful for other forms of mild to moderate diarrhea as well.

   e. **Antibiotics** are indicated only for severely ill patients with fever, leukocytosis, and bloody diarrhea. Empiric therapy for *Shigella* or *Campylobacter,* using ampicillin (or trimethoprim-sulfamethoxazole) or erythromycin, respectively, is appropriate, depending on local disease prevalence while culture results are pending. Antibiotics can result in the production of resistant strains of bacteria or pseudomembranous colitis; thus, their use must be limited to appropriately documented bacterial diarrheas.

   f. **Antiparasitic agents** are used only when a specific diagnosis is made by stool examination or rectal mucosal biopsy.

      (1) **Giardiasis** can cause acute or chronic diarrhea. Treatment is with metronidazole 250 mg, p.o., t.i.d., or quinacrine 100 mg, p.o., t.i.d., for 7 days. Patients with relapses or frequent recurrences need to be investigated for hypogammaglobulinemia.

      (2) **Amebiasis** can cause acute or chronic diarrhea. Asymptomatic infections are treated with diiodohydroxyquin 650 mg, p.o., t.i.d. for 20 days or diloxanide furoate 500 mg, p.o., t.i.d. for 10 days. Invasive disease (colitis, ameboma, hepatic abscess, etc.) requires treatment with metronidazole 750 mg, p.o. or i.v., t.i.d. for 5 to 10 days. In severe cases metronidazole should be combined with either diiodohydroxyquin or diloxanide. Chloroquine 250 mg p.o., q.i.d. for 30 days also can be used for invasive disease.

   g. Delete any drugs that could be a cause of diarrhea.

B. **Chronic Diarrhea**   Chronic diarrhea is defined as more than 200 g of stool daily for >3 weeks.

   1. **Pathophysiology and diagnosis.** The four major mechanisms of diarrhea are:

      a. **Osmotic** diarrhea is caused by the presence of poorly absorbed solutes (Mg^{+2} or SO_4^{-2} salts, sugars—lactose, fructose, sorbitol, mannitol, lactulose, etc.) in the intestine or colon, which are hypertonic and cause fluid secretion into the gut lumen. This form of diarrhea stops when the patient takes nothing by mouth. The stool osmolality is >twice the sum of stool Na^+ plus K^+ concentration by at least 50 mOsm.

b. **Secretory** diarrhea develops when the gut is stimulated to secrete excessively, there is inhibition of fluid and electrolyte absorption, or both to variable degrees. The causes include enterotoxins from bacteria, excessive hormone secretion (vasoactive intestinal peptide, calcitonin, prostaglandins, gastrin, and others), some laxatives, bile salts, and fatty acids. This form of diarrhea will persist during prolonged fasting. The stool osmolality equals twice the stool Na^+ plus K^+ concentration.

c. **Mucosal injury or exudative** diarrhea results when the mucosal integrity of the gut is disrupted. The diarrhea is primarily caused by decreased absorptive capacity but is also related to loss of fluid and protein from the mucosa into the gut lumen. Invasive infectious pathogens, inflammatory bowel disease, and celiac disease are the most common causes of exudative diarrhea.

d. **Altered motility** can cause diarrhea either by allowing bacterial overgrowth (stasis) or by moving contents along too fast to be properly processed and absorbed by the gut mucosa. Common causes of altered transit include diabetes mellitus, hyperthyroidism, vagotomy, gastrectomy, scleroderma, and irritable bowel syndrome.

2. **Therapy** of chronic diarrhea usually is directed first at treating the underlying disease. Listed below are some general considerations for patients with uncorrectable diseases or idiopathic chronic diarrhea.

a. **Drugs** should be systematically withdrawn from a patient's regimen if possible or medication changed to exclude their role in causing the diarrhea.

b. **Dietary changes** may help some patients. Removing all milk products should be tried. A detailed dietary history, looking for excessive intake of any food–particularly beans, caffeine, fresh fruits, raw vegetables, or any foods that seem to precipitate symptoms—should be taken. Removal of all wheat products (gluten-free diet) is rarely indicated in patients without abnormal small-bowel biopsies, but it may be helpful in a small group of patients who poorly absorb wheat, with resultant colonic fermentation of the malabsorbed carbohydrates that produces bloating and diarrhea.

c. **Bile-salt-binding agents** (colestipol and cholestyramine; see IV.B.) are constipating and particularly useful for bile-salt-related diarrheas.

d. **Antibiotic usage** for chronic diarrhea is appropriate only when a diagnosis of small-bowel bacterial overgrowth is suspected or diagnosed. Tetracycline or metronidazole 250 mg, p.o., q.i.d. for 2 weeks, with repeated courses as needed, are the **drugs of choice.**

e. **Narcotic antidiarrheal agents** are potent inhibitors of gut motility and to a lesser extent of secretion. There is a potential for patients to become addicted to all of these agents. They must be used with caution or avoided in patients with lung disease, bladder outlet obstruction, glaucoma, and severe advanced liver disease.

Lomotil® (diphenoxylate hydrochloride, 2.5 mg per tablet) is a congener of meperidine. The dosage is 1 to 2 tablets, p.o., every 4 to 6 hr up to a maximum of 8 tablets per day. **Imodium®** (loperimide hydrochloride, 2 mg per capsule) may control chronic diarrhea not improved by Lomotil®. The dosage is 1 to 2 capsules, p.o., every 4 to 6 hr up to a maximum of 8 capsules per day. **Paregoric** (camphorated tincture of opium) is useful in doses of 4 to 8 ml, p.o., every 4 to 6 hr. **Deodorized tincture of opium** can be given in doses of 0.5 to 1.5 ml, p.o., every 4 to 6 hr. **Belladonna alkaloids** will decrease gastrointestinal secretions and motility, but side effects of dry mouth, blurred vision, urinary retention, impotence, and mental changes limit their use. Common doses are atropine 0.5 mg, p.o., every 6 hr; scopolamine methyl bromide 2.5 mg, p.o., every 6 hr; propantheline 15 to 30 mg, p.o. every 6 hr; hyoscyamine 0.1 to 0.3 mg, p.o. every 6 hr; and belladonna tincture 0.6 ml, p.o., every 6 hr. **Codeine** 15 to 60 mg, p.o., every 4 to 6 hr, is very useful for controlling diarrhea, although its abuse potential is great.

VIII. CONSTIPATION   Passage of hard, small-volume stools less than 2 to 3 times a week, associated with subjective complaints (bloating, fullness, anorexia, etc.), is a reasonable definition of constipation, although many normal subjects have similar bowel-movement patterns.

A. Pathophysiology and Diagnosis   Constipation is caused by either slow transit through the colon or obstruction in the anorectal area. Drugs that decrease transit time include narcotic analgesics, anticholinergics, antidepressants, ganglionic blockers, and others. Metabolic conditions that can prolong colonic transit are diabetes mellitus, hypothyroidism, hypercalcemia, hypokalemia, and pregnancy. Many neurologic disorders involving the peripheral or central nervous system can produce constipation. Extra- or intraluminal tumors, benign or infection-related strictures, muscle disorders (scleroderma, dermatomyositis, myotonic dystrophy), and painful anorectal lesions (ulcers, fissures, prolapse) can produce constipation. In addition, there probably exists a condition known as psychogenic constipation.

B. Therapy   Therapy for constipation must be individualized. Patients with new onset of constipation from decreased activity, dietary changes, or drugs can usually be managed by reversal of the inciting event or removal of the drug, plus use of mild cathartics. Chronic constipation requires prolonged stepwise restraining of bowel function and if possible withdrawal from heavy laxative use. One must never treat a patient with suspected obstruction with strong laxatives.

    1. Bulk agents are the best products available for increasing stool volume and moisture without having any direct effect on the colonic mucosa. Increasing the dietary fiber to approximately 30 g/day with bran is a simple way to improve constipation. Similar results are attainable by using 1 to 4 tablespoons per day of a psyllium-seed preparation (Metamucil®, Konsyl®, Konsyl®-D, Perdiem®). A synthetic bulk agent (Mitrolan®) in tablet form is convenient but more expensive.

    2. Stool softeners or emollient laxatives that purportedly increase stool moisture because of their surface-active properties include Colace® (docusate sodium) 50 to 200 mg, p.o., q.d., and Surfak® (docusate calcium) 24 mg, p.o., q.d.

Mineral oil 15 to 45 ml, p.o., q.d. also is classified as an emollient laxative but never should be combined with a docusate compound because it will promote the intestinal absorption of the mineral oil. Mineral oil can prevent lipid-soluble vitamins from being absorbed.

3. **Saline cathartics** are moderately potent laxatives. These nonabsorbable or poorly absorbed agents cause increased colonic volume through their osmotic effects. Milk of magnesia (15 to 30 ml, p.o., q.d.), magnesium sulfate (5 to 10 g, p.o., q.d.), magnesium citrate (200 ml, p.o., q.d.), sodium phosphate (Fleet Phospho®-Soda 60 to 120 ml, p.o., q.d.) and lactulose (Cephulac® 20 to 30 g 1 to 4 times q.d.) are commonly used agents in this group.

4. **Stimulant cathartics** are generally the strongest oral agents and the most likely to produce colonic mucosal damage when used excessively. Some of the more common stimulant cathartics include castor oil (15 to 30 ml, p.o., q.d.), bisacodyl (Dulcolax® 10 to 30 mg, p.o., or a 10-mg suppository, p.r., q.d.), phenolphthalein (100 mg, p.o., q.d.), cascara sagrada (aromatic cascara fluid extract 5 ml, p.o., q.d.) and senna (Senokot® 2 to 4 tablets, p.o., q.d.).

5. **Enemas** are useful either to prepare the rectosigmoid for endoscopic examination or to relieve severe constipation. Many substances are used for enema solutions, and there are several recommended safe and effective preparations. **Tap-water or saline** enemas (1 to 2 liters at 100 to 105 °F, p.r.) are popular and effective. They are frequently ordered to be given until the rectal return is clear. Care must be exercised because tap-water enemas can lead to significant hypokalemia or water intoxication. Saline enemas are less of a problem if isotonic sodium chloride is used, but they can cause volume depletion if a hypertonic solution is used.

Soap-suds enemas (2/3 oz castile soap in 2 liters water at 100 to 150 °F, p.r.) produce results by distention and mucosa irritation. Occasionally, the irritant effect can produce a colitis.

Phosphate enemas (Fleet, 4½ oz, p.r.) work primarily by irritant and osmotic effects. The main side effect of their use is sodium retention.

Mineral oil retention enemas (3 to 6 oz, p.r.) are given to soften and lubricate impacted stool. This enema is meant to be retained for 1 to 8 hr before expulsion.

6. **Manual disempaction** may be necessary initially in patients with severe constipation.

IX. ANORECTAL DISORDERS

A. Hemorrhoids

1. **Pathophysiology and diagnosis.** Hemorrhoids or piles are caused by dilatation of the superior (internal) or inferior (external) hemorrhoidal venous plexus. Two major theories for their development exist. One holds that they are secondary to upright posture or straining to evacuate the rectum, and the other theory suggests that hemorrhoids possibly have arteriovenous communications resulting in increased pressure with dilatation and rupture. The diagnosis is made by direct examination.

2. **Treatment** of uncomplicated hemorrhoids includes the following:

   a. **Stool softeners** or bulk agents to help prevent straining.

   b. **Tucks®️ pads** (witch hazel) used as the last wipe after defecating to decrease local discomfort and help with hygiene.

   c. **Sitz baths** for decreasing symptoms and improving hygiene—the patient is instructed to sit in a warm tub of water 2 to 3 times a day.

   d. **Suppositories** containing anesthetics, astringents, steroids, and emollients (modest symptomatic benefit).

   e. **Surgery,** including injection, cryosurgery, rubber-band ligation, anal dilatation, hemorrhoidectomy, and lateral internal sphincterotomy, is recommended for severe or intractable cases.

3. **Thrombosed external hemorrhoids** are generally treated symptomatically. If seen early, an incision with clot removal will quickly relieve pain and shorten the time of healing. The external thrombosed hemorrhoid is covered with skin; it should not be confused with a thrombosed, prolapsed internal hemorrhoid that is mucosal-covered and may be treated differently. The latter requires surgical consultation, whereas the former usually does not.

B. Anorectal Abscesses

1. **Pathophysiology and diagnosis.** Anorectal abscesses are predominantly caused by anal crypt infections that track inward. They may dissect into many planes. The **diagnosis** is made by digital rectal examination in a patient with rectal pain. Fever may be present.

2. **Therapy** is surgical drainage. Antibiotics are reserved for patients with signs or symptoms of systemic toxicity.

C. Fissures

1. **Pathophysiology and diagnosis.** Fissures are longitudinal tears in the anal skin caused by trauma (hard stool, foreign body, intercourse). More than 90% of simple fissures are in the posterior midline. Chronic fissures are characterized by an enlarged anal papilla superiorly and a sentinel pile inferiorly.

2. **Therapy** consisting of the same symptomatic measures listed above under hemorrhoidal therapy will heal nearly half of these lesions in 2 to 8 weeks. More chronic lesions will require surgical intervention.

X. IRRITABLE BOWEL SYNDROME   Irritable bowel is defined as gasrointestinal symptoms (including bloating, flatulence, dyspepsia, abdominal cramping, nausea, vomiting, constipation, diarrhea, or a combination of these symptoms) that cannot be attributed to any other specific cause after an appropriate evaluation. The most common symptom complex is pain with diarrhea, constipation, or alternating diarrhea and constipation.

A. Pathophysiology and Diagnosis   Irritable bowel syndrome has no known cause at this time. The symptoms seem to be caused by an abnormal or exaggerated response of the gut to use stimuli such as cholecystokinin, food, gaseous distention, and stress. Many patients also have mild to moderate psychiatric disorders. As stated above, the **diagnosis is one of exclusion of other causes** for the patient's complaints.

B. Therapy   Therapy for irritable bowel is empiric. Treatment for each patient must be individualized. Time spent explaining the disorder, stressing to the patient that he is not crazy, and reassuring the patient that he does not have cancer will be of more benefit than any other single intervention.

1. **Increased bulk** in the diet is usually beneficial, although often patients will complain of more pain when bulk is increased. Patients with worse symptoms should be encouraged to persist for 3 to 4 weeks before abandoning this treatment, since many will improve after the initial deterioration. (See VIII.B. for dosages.)

2. **Anticholinergic drugs** that are of benefit to patients with pain and diarrhea include clidinium (Quarzan®) 2.5 to 5.0 mg, p.o., t.i.d., or q.i.d., dicyclomine (Bentyl®) 10 to 20 mg, p.o., t.i.d. or q.i.d., hyoscyamine (Levsin®) 0.125 to 0.25 mg, p.o., t.i.d. or q.i.d., or propantheline (Pro-Banthīne®) 15 to 30 mg, p.o., t.i.d. or q.i.d.

3. **Sedation** with low-dose benzodiazepines or phenobarbital can be very helpful especially in combination with the anticholinergics listed above. These should be avoided if the patient is depressed.

4. **Alterations in diet** may improve symptoms. Beneficial maneuvers include regularized eating habits, discontinue gum chewing, avoid gas-producing foods (sorbitol, legumes, cabbage), milk-free diet, gluten-free diet, and low-fat diet.

5. **Antidepressants** should be used if the patient is depressed, which many of them are.

6. **Psychiatric referral** may be necessary.

XI. PANCREATITIS

A. Acute Pancreatitis

1. **Pathophysiology and diagnosis.** Acute pancreatitis probably is caused by premature activation of enzymes in the pancreas leading to an autodigestive process. The initiating factors within the pancreas remain obscure. The **diagnosis** is made by a combination of history, physical examination, and laboratory studies. The patients often have a history of heavy alcohol intake or have cholelithiasis. They complain of upper abdominal pain with radiation to the back, nausea, and vomiting. An elevated serum or urine amylase in this setting strongly supports the diagnosis of acute pancreatic inflammation.

2. **Therapy** for mild to moderate severe pancreatitis is primarily designed to rest the pancreas (decrease pancreatic secretion). **Nothing by mouth** (NPO) should be continued until all vomiting, nausea, and pain are resolved.

    a. **Nasogastric suction**   (NG) is optional treatment in most patients. Persistent vomiting, an ileus on abdominal films, absent bowel sounds, or a history of a good response to NG suction previously are indications for its use.

    b. **Intravenous hydration** is extremely important. Patients are frequently third-spacing fluid and can require 6 or more liters of fluid in the first 24 hr.

    c. **Calcium replacement** usually is not necessary, but replacement with intravenous calcium gluconate should be initiated if the serum level falls to 7 mg/dl or less.

d. Analgesia is important. At present, meperidine is favored over morphine because it has less effect on the sphincter of Oddi. Dosage ranges from 50 to 150 mg, i.m., every 3 hr.

e. Antibiotics are not indicated unless there is a very strong indication that an associated infectious process is present.

f. Antacids or cimetidine may be used without fear of exacerbating the pancreatitis. They decrease acidification of the duodenum, which may help further decrease pancreatic stimulation. However, clinical trials have shown no additional benefits of cimetidine therapy over simple NPO.

g. Anticholinergics, Trasylol, glucagon, and somatostatin have not been shown to be beneficial. Any drugs that could potentially be contributing to the pancreatitis must be withdrawn (e.g., hydrochlorthiazide, furosemide, sulfonamides, estrogens, azathioprine).

h. Diet after resolution of symptoms: Initially, patients may resume a clear liquid diet, but this should be modified to a low-fat, low-protein liquid diet in more severe cases or in patients with a history of difficulty resuming oral intake. Dietary advancement must not be too rapid. In most cases patients will progress to a regular diet over 3 to 5 days.

3. **Therapy for severe pancreatitis** includes all of the above measures, plus:

a. Peritoneal lavage has been shown to improve the early mortality from severe (hemorrhagic) pancreatitis but has not been proved to improve overall survival. A balanced electrolyte solution with 15g/liter of dextrose (Dianeal) is usually used. Some authors also recommend adding 1,000 U of heparin, 8 mEq potassium, and 250 mg ampicillin to each liter. Two liters of fluid are instilled into the peritoneal cavity and left there for 30 min. This is then drained and repeated hourly for 48 to 96 hr.

b. Parenteral alimentation is indicated in any patient likely to be unable to take calories orally for more than 2 weeks.

c. Surgical intervention with stone removal, biliary drainage, partial pancreatectomy, or drain placement may be necessary in severe cases not responding to medical management.

B. **Chronic Pancreatitis**

1. **Definition and diagnosis.** Chronic pancreatitis is progressive pancreatitic damage despite removal of presumptive precipitating causes. It is manifested by pain, malabsorption, diabetes mellitus, and pancreatic calcifications in varying combinations.

2. **Therapy**

a. Pain relief is often difficult to achieve in these patients. **Narcotic analgesics** are useful but often lead to addiction. **Surgical therapy** (pancreatic duct drainage, celiac ganglionectomy, splanchnectomies, or total pancreatectomy) can be helpful in selected cases. **Pseudocyst drainage** (if one is present) may provide significant pain relief. **Pancreatic enzymes** have been reported to relieve pain even if clinical insufficiency is not present (see malabsorption).

b. Diabetes mellitus is treated with insulin. There is no role for other hypoglycemic agents.

c. Malabsorption is managed by replacing pancreatic enzymes orally. Viokase® (pancreatin) or Cotazym®(pancrelipase) 2 tablets before, during and after each meal; plus 2 to 4 tablets, p.o., with any snacks; or 2 tablets, p.o. every 2 hr while awake are standard and usually effective regimens. The dose of Pancrease® (enteric-coated pancrelipase) is one-half this amount. Occasionally, patients will require addition of sodium bicarbonate (1.3 g, a.c. and p.c., p.o.) or cimetidine (300 mg, p.o., q.i.d.) to prevent enzyme destruction by acid in the stomach or duodenum.

XII. GASTROINTESTINAL BLEEDING

A. Upper Gastrointestinal Bleeding

1. The **diagnosis** is obvious if a patient presents with hematemesis, but establishing the source of hemorrhage becomes more challenging when a patient presents with melena or hematochezia. Although a history of PUD, barrier-breaker ingestion, or upper abdominal pain are helpful, the diagnosis primarily is made by aspirating blood or Hemoccult®-positive coffee-ground material from the stomach. A negative NG aspirate can occur if a duodenal ulcer is bleeding with no duodenogastric reflux or if bleeding stopped long enough before intubation for all blood to have been emptied from the stomach.

The most accurate way (85% to 95%) to establish the exact bleeding source is with **endoscopy.** If a patient is bleeding too massively to be endoscoped, then arteriography can be helpful in locating the source; however, emergency surgery may be necessary before a diagnosis can be established when bleeding is massive and the patient cannot be adequately stabilized. The UGI series is used to establish a diagnosis electively in a stable patient with a minor to moderate-size bleed.

2. General therapy for **all** gastrointestinal bleeding

a. Assess the amount of blood loss by examining the patient. Look for signs of shock—hypotension, tachycardia, diaphoresis, and decreased urine output. **Orthostatic pulse changes** (>20/min increase) suggest a 500-ml deficit, whereas the addition of a fall in diastolic pressure (>10 mm Hg decrease) implies more than a 1,000-ml blood loss. The presence of shock implies 40% to 50% volume depletion. The hematocrit is the least sensitive indicator of acute blood loss, since it takes at least 24 hr to reequilibrate to a new stable level after an acute bleeding episode.

b. Establish venous access either peripherally with one or two large (14 to 18 g) intravenous catheters or, in the more seriously ill patient, start a central line. The latter also will be useful to measure central venous pressure, thus helping with fluid-management decisions. **Volume replacement** can begin immediately with normal saline—500 to 1,000 ml over the initial 30 min with repeats as necessary to keep the systolic blood pressure greater than 90 mm Hg until blood is available.

c. Blood transfusions are required for all patients who present in shock from bleeding. These patients and those who continue to actively bleed should be given fresh whole blood. Patients with less bleeding or those who have stopped bleeding may be given packed red cells. Transfusions are given to maintain the hematocrit at 30% (or 35% in patients with heart disease). A transfused unit of blood will increase the hematocrit 3 points if bleeding has stopped and no other volume expanders are being given simultaneously.

    d. **Fresh frozen plasma** (FFP) is indicated if fresh whole blood is not available and the patient requires >5 units of blood, or if the patient has a coagulopathy. At least 3, and often more, units of FFP are needed to produce an effect on the clotting times. **Platelet transfusions** are rarely needed unless massive or continued bleeding (>10 units of blood) has occurred or the patient has significant thrombocytopenia (<50,000 platelets).

3. **Initial therapy for upper gastrointestinal bleeding**

    a. **Gastric lavage** with saline or water to remove blood and establish if persistent bleeding is present. The use of iced saline has not been proved to stop bleeding. A 32 to 36F orogastric tube must be used to effectively remove clots. This also will clear the stomach so that endoscopy can be performed if indicated.

    b. **Esophagogastroduodenoscopy** is **not** a therapeutic modality and has not been shown to have any major effect on the ultimate outcome in bleeding patients. Presently, it may be beneficial to endoscope seriously ill patients, massive bleeders, alcoholics (especially if portal hypertension is suspected), and elderly (>60 years old) patients because the endoscopic findings will influence the type of treatment (i.e., early or delayed surgery, specific therapy for varices). The availability of therapeutic endoscopy (electrocoagulation, lasers, and sclerotherapy) may make early endoscopy more beneficial by providing effective treatment.

    c. **Cimetidine** (300 mg, i.v. every 6 hr) has not been shown to stop active bleeding. Cimetidine combined with **antacid** (30 ml, p.o. every 2 hr) has been proved to prevent recurrent bleeding. This is appropriate treatment for the first 48 hr in all types of upper gastrointestinal bleeding except perhaps varices.

4. **Specific therapy** for sources of upper GI bleeding

    a. **PUD.** For doses of **cimetidine** and **antacids,** see section 3. C. above. **Sucralfate** (Carafate®, 1 g, p.o., 30 min a.c. and h.s.) is an appropriate alternative to cimetidine and antacids or may be used in conjunction with them if given at different times. This drug is of no benefit if bleeding is persisting, since it will bind to the blood rather than the ulcer crater.

    Electrocoagulation (bipolar preferred over monopolar) or **laser phototherapy** are recommended for ulcers with visible vessels because of their high rebleeding rate (approximately 60%). Ulcers actively bleeding at endoscopy or rebleeding ulcers in poor-operative-risk patients also are indications. **Vasopressin** either intravenously or intra-arterially is of little or no benefit for PUD.

    Surgery is indicated for patients with uncontrollable massive bleeding, persistent bleeding requiring more than 5 units of blood in 24 hr or repeated transfusions over 48 to 72 hr, and for patients with recurrent bleeding, after stopping for 24 or more hr, despite appropriate medical therapy.

b. **Mallory-Weiss tear.** Vasopressin intravenously or intra-arterially may be useful (see below). **Electrocoagulation and laser phototherapy** are very useful for persistently bleeding tears. **Surgery** with oversewing of the bleeding site is necessary occasionally.

c. **Gastritis and stress ulcers. Prophylaxis** for prevention of stress ulcer is best achieved with antacids, although in some situations cimetidine has been shown to be beneficial. Either agent must be given with NG aspiration monitoring of the gastric contents. A pH maintained at greater than 4 will prevent hemorrhage.

Vasopressin intravenously or intra-arterially will control hemorrhage (see below). **Surgery** should be a last resort for gastritis because the recurrence rate after any operation, short of a total gastrectomy, approaches 50%.

d. **Aortoenteric** fistulas require surgery immediately when diagnosed.

e. **Angiodysplastic lesions** may be treated with electrocoagulation or laser phototherapy if available, otherwise surgery is indicated for isolated lesions.

f. **Variceal hemorrhage**

(1) **Vasopressin** is the initial therapy for actively bleeding varices. Intraarterial infusions offer little advantage over intravenous infusions. The preferred method of administration is a **continuous intravenous infusion.** The dose to start is 0.2 U/min with incremental increases to a maximum of 0.6 U/min over 2 to 3 hr as needed to control hemorrhage. Once bleeding has stopped, the rate should be kept constant for 12 to 24 hr and then decreased slowly over approximately 48 hr. The major **complications** of vasopressin are related to ischemia of the abdominal organs, extremities, and heart. Thus, it must be used with extreme caution in patients with atherosclerosis.

(2) **Balloon tamponade** with a Sengstaken-Blakemore tube should be added to the treatment regimen if bleeding persists in the face of vasopressin infusions. These balloons are highly effective in stopping bleeding at least temporarily but are dangerous. They should be used only by experienced clinicians.

There are several points to be emphasized in the use of the Sengstaken-Blakemore tube (S-B tube). If a 4-lumen tube is not available, an NG tube should be sewed or taped onto the S-B tube above the esophageal balloon and connected to intermittent suction to prevent pulmonary aspiration of saliva or blood. If time permits, the position of the gastric balloon should be confirmed radiographically after 25 ml of air has been insufflated before final inflation. Both balloons should be inflated simultaneously to gain control of the bleeding initially. The gastric balloon holds 200 ml of air, whereas the esophageal balloon is inflated so that it has 25 to 35 mm Hg pressure in it.

The gastric balloon is firmly pulled up against the gastroesophageal junction (2 to 4 lbs of traction) and secured at the nose with foam rubber and tape. Pulleys with weights should not be used, but a football helmet or baseball catcher's mask can be used for securing the tube and thus prevent alar necrosis. Scissors are to be placed conspicuously at the bedside so the tube can be quickly cut, deflating the balloons, if there is any upward migration with airway obstruction. A large hiatal hernia is a relative contraindication to placement of an S-B tube. The balloons ideally are deflated in about 24 hr to prevent esophageal necrosis. The esophageal balloon is deflated first, followed in 4 to 6 hr by the gastric balloon, with removal of the whole S-B tube 12 hr later if no further bleeding occurs.

(3) Endoscopic sclerotherapy can be undertaken either in an emergency under general anesthesia with a rigid endoscope or electively with mild sedation and a flexible endoscope. The **rigid instrument** is best used when active bleeding is persistent because of better suction and tamponade capabilities. Emergent sclerosis with sodium morrhuate or sodium tetradecyl sulfate has been effective in stopping bleeding. Long-term trials with repeated sclerosis have been less successful in preventing recurrent variceal hemorrhage.

(4) Propranolol given in doses sufficient to decrease the pulse by 25% has been shown to prevent recurrent variceal (and gastritis) hemorrhage in one study. This form of therapy should be limited to patients who have stopped bleeding and are not suitable candidates for shunt surgery.

(5) Portacaval shunts prevent rebleeding in 90% of patients who survive the surgery, however, the operative mortality is 25–80% and the frequency of life threatening encephalopathy or liver failure is nearly 20% after surgery. The Warren shunt (distal-splenorenal) has the lowest postoperative complications, but is technically very difficult to perform.

B. Lower Gastrointestinal Bleeding

1. **Diagnosis** is made by first excluding an upper gastrointestinal source. Then, the exact site in the lower gut can be established by use of sigmoidoscopy, colonoscopy, ^{99m}Tc-labeled red blood cells, angiography, or barium enema, depending on the rate of bleeding.

2. **Initial therapy** is as listed under gastrointestinal bleeding.

3. **Specific therapy** for lower gastrointestinal bleeding is more limited. **Angiography** is not only diagnostic but can be therapeutic if vasopressin is selectively infused into the bleeding artery or if autologous clot is injected.

Electrocoagulation (bipolar favored over monopolar) or **laser photocoagulation** have been effective in stopping bleeding from angiodysplastic lesions, ulcers, and tumors in uncontrolled reports. **Surgical resection** may be needed if bleeding persists or is not controllable with endoscopic therapy.

BIBLIOGRAPHY

Constipation

Agnew, J. (1980: *The Enema. A Textbook and Reference Manual.* Medical Academics Press, Colorado Springs, CO.

Cummings, J. H. (1974): Progress report. Laxative abuse. *Gut,* 15:758–766.

DeVroede, G. (1983): Constipation: Mechanisms and management. In: *Gastrointestinal Disease Pathophysiology, Diagnosis, Management,* edited by M. H. Sleisenger and J. S. Fordtran, pp. 288–308. W. B. Saunders Co., Philadelphia.

Diarrhea

Blaser, M. J., Berkowitz, I. E., LaForce, F. M., Cravens, J., Reller, L. B., and Wang, W. L. L. (1979): Campylobacter enteritis: Clinical and epidemiologic features. *Ann. Intern. Med.,* 91:179–184.

Netchvolodoff, C. V., and Hargrove, M. D. (1979): Recent advances in the treatment of diarrhea. *Arch. Intern. Med.,* 139:813–816.

Pickering, L. K., DuPont, H. L., Olarte, J., Conklin, R., and Ericsson, C. (1977): Fecal leukocytes in enteric infections. *Am. J. Clin. Pathol.,* 68:562–565.

Plotkin, G. R., Kluge, R. M., and Waldman, R. H. (1979): Gastroenteritis: Etiology, pathophysiology and clinical manifestations. *Medicine* (Baltimore), 58:95–114.

Raizman, R. E. (1976): Giardiasis: an overview for the clinician. *Dig. Dis. Sci.,* 21:1070–1074.

Read, N. W., Krejs, G. J., Read, M. G., SantaAnna, C. A., Morawski, S. G., and Fordtran, J. D. (1980): Chronic diarrhea of unknown origin. *Gastroenterology,* 78:264–271.

Wolfe, M. S. (1978): Giardiasis. *N. Engl. J. Med.,* 298:319–321.

Diffuse Esophageal Spasm

Castell, D. O. (1976): Achalasia and diffuse esophageal spasm. *Arch. Intern. Med.,* 136:571–579.

Diverticular Disease

Almy, T. P., and Howell, D. A. (1980): Diverticular disease of the colon. *N. Engl. J. Med.,* 302:324–331.

Cello, J. P. (1981): Diverticular disease of the colon—medical staff conference, University of California, San Francisco. *West. J. Med.,* 134:515–523.

Parks, T. G. (1975): Natural history of diverticular disease of the colon. *Clin. Gastroenterol,* 4:53–69.

Zollinger, R. W. (1968): The prognosis in diverticulitis of the colon. *Arch. Surg.,* 97:418–421.

Gastrointestinal Bleeding

Ayres, S. J., Goff, J. S., and Warren, G. H. (1983): Endoscopic sclerotherapy for bleeding esophageal varices: Effects and complications. *Ann. Intern. Med.,* 98:900–903.

Chojkier, M., and Conn, H. O. (1980): Esophageal tamponade in the treatment of bleeding varices. A decadal progress report. *Dig. Dis. Sci.,* 25:267–272.

Fogel, M. R., Knauer, M., Andres, L. L., Mahal, A. S., Stein, D. E. T., Kemeny, J., Rinkei, M. M., Walker, J. E., Siegmund, D., and Gregory, P. B. (1982): Continuous intravenous vasopressin in active upper gastrointestinal bleeding. *Ann. Intern. Med.,* 96:565–569.

Greenburg, A. G., Saik, R. P., Coyle, J. J., and Peskin, G. W. (1981): Mortality and gastrointestinal surgery in the aged. *Arch. Surg.,* 116:788–791.

Larsen, D. E., and Farnell, M. B. (1983): Upper gastrointestinal hemorrhage. *Mayo Clin. Proc.,* 58:371–387.

Lebrec, D., Poynard, T., Hillon, P., and Benhamou, J.-P. (1981): Propranolol for prevention of recurrent gastrointestinal bleeding in patients with cirrhosis. *N. Engl. J. Med.,* 305:1371–1374.

MacDougal, B. R. D., Theodossi, A., Westaby, D., Dawson, J. L., and Williams, R. (1982): Increased long term survival in variceal hemorrhage using injection sclerotherapy. *Lancet,* 1:124–127.

Malt, R. A. (1972): Control of massive upper gastrointestinal hemorrhage. *N. Engl. J. Med.,* 286:1043–1046.

Peterson, W. L., Barnett, C. C., Smith, H. J., Allen, M. H., and Corbet, D. B. (1981): Routine early endoscopy in upper gastrointestinal bleeding. *N. Engl. J. Med.,* 304:925–929.

Proceedings of the NIH and Consensus Workshop. (1981): *Dig. Dis. Sci.,* 27:1S–104S.

Ring, E. J., Oleaga, J. A., and Baum, S. (1980): Current status of angiographic techniques in the management of gastrointestinal bleeding. *J. Clin. Gastroenterol,* 2:99–103.

Swain, B. P., Storey, D. W., Northfield, T. C., Brown, S. G., Kirkham, J. S., and Salmon, P. R. (1981): Controlled trial of argon laser photocoagulation in bleeding peptic ulcers. *Lancet*, 2:1313–1316.

Terblanche, J., Northover, J. M. A., Bornman, P., Kahn, D., Barbezet, G. O., Sellars, S. L., and Saunders, S. J. (1979): A perspective evaluation of injection sclerotherapy in the treatment of acute bleeding from esophageal varices. *Surgery*, 85:239–245.

Vallon, A. G., Cotton, P. B., Laurence, B. H., Armengol Miro, J. R., and Salor Oses, J. C. (1981): Randomized trial of endoscopic argon laser photocoagulation in bleeding peptic ulcers. *Gut*, 22:228–233.

Inflammatory Bowel Disease

Kirsner, J. B., and Shorter, R. G., eds. (1980): *Inflammatory Bowel Disease*, 2d ed. Lea and Febiger, Philadelphia

National Cooperative Crohn's Disease Study. (1979): *Gastroenterology*, 77:825–944.

Irritable Bowel Syndrome

Alpers, D. H. (1983): Functional gastrointestinal disorders. *Hosp. Pract.*, April:139–153.

Burns, T. W. (1980): Colonic motility and the irritable bowel syndrome. *Arch. Intern. Med.*, 140:247–251.

Kirsner, J. B. (1981): The irritable bowel syndrome. A clinical review and ethical considerations. *Arch. Intern. Med.*, 141:635–639.

Lasser, R. B., Bond, J. H., and Levitt, M. D. (1975): The role of intestinal gas in functional abdominal pain. *N. Engl. J. Med.*, 293:524–526.

Lennard-Jones, J. E. (1983): Functional gastrointestinal disorders. *N. Engl. J. Med.*, 308:431–435.

Malabsorption

Green, P. H. R., and Tall, A. R. (1979): Drugs, alcohol and malabsorption. *Am. J. Med.*, 67:1066–1076.

Hofmann, A. F., and Poley, J. R. (1969): Cholestyramine treatment of diarrhea associated with ileal resection. *N. Engl. J. Med.*, 281:379–402.

Isaacs, P. E. T., and Kim, Y. S. (1979): The contaminated small bowel syndrome. *Am. J. Med.*, 67:1049–1057.

Longstreth, G. F., and Newcomer, L. A. D. (1975): Drug induced malabsorption. *Mayo Clin. Proc.*, 50:284–293.

Regan, P. T., and Dimagno, E. P. (1979): The medical management of malabsorption. *Mayo Clin. Proc.*, 54:267–274.

Sheldon, G. F. (1979): The role of parenteral nutrition in patients with short bowel syndrome. *Am. J. Med.*, 67:1021–1029.

Pancreatitis

DiMagno, E. P., Malagelada, J. R., Go, B. L. W., and Moertel, C. G. (1977): Fate of orally ingested enzymes in pancreatic insufficiency. *N. Engl. J. Med.*, 296:1318–1322.

Field, V. E., Hepner, G. W., Shabot, M. M., Schwartz, A. A., State, D., Worthen, N., and Wilson, R. (1979): Nasogastric suction in alcoholic pancreatitis. *Dig. Dis. Sci.*, 24:339–344.

Goff, J. S., Feinberg, L. E., and Brugge, W. R. (1982): A randomized trial comparing cimetidine to nasogastric suction in acute pancreatitis. *Dig. Dis. Sci.*, 27:1085–1088.

Graham, D. Y. (1977): Enzyme replacement therapy of exocrine pancreatic insufficiency in man. *N. Engl. J. Med.*, 296:1314–1317.

Graham, D. Y. (1979): An enteric coated pancreatic enzyme preparation that works. *Dig. Dis. Sci.*, 24:906–909.

Graham, D. Y. (1982): Pancreatic enzyme replacement. The effect of antacids or cimetidine. *Dig. Dis. Sci.*, 27:485–490.

Mallory, A., and Kern, F., Jr. (1980): Drug-induced pancreatitis: A critical review. *Gastroenterology*, 78:813–820.

Ranson, J. H. C., and Spencer, F. C. (1978): The role of peritoneal lavage in severe acute pancreatitis. *Ann. Surg.*, 187:565–573.

Ranson, J. H. C. (1980): Surgical treatment of acute pancreatitis. *Dig. Dis. Sci.,* 25:453–459.

Peptic Ulcer Disease

Ahmad, S. (1979): Side effects of cimetidine. *South Med. J.,* 72:509–513.

Christensen, E., Juhle, E., and Tygstrup, N. (1977): Treatment of duodenal ulcer. Randomized clinical trials of a decade. *Gastroenterology,* 73:1170–1178.

Drake, D., and Hollander, D. (1981): Neutralizing capacity and cost effectiveness of antacids. *Ann. Intern. Med.,* 94:215–217.

Fromm, D. (1977): *Complications of Gastric Surgery.* Wiley, New York.

Flesher, B., and Achkar, E. (1981): Aggressive approach to the medical management of peptic ulcer disease. *Arch. Intern. Med.,* 141:848–851.

Hanscom, D. H., and Buchman, E. (1971): The follow up period. Veterans Administration cooperative study on gastric ulcer. *Gastroenterology,* 61:585–591.

Isenberg, J. I., Peterson, O., Walter, L., Elashoff, J. D., Sandersfeld, M. A., Reedy, T. J., Ippoliti, A. F., VanDeventer, G. M., Frankel, H., Longstreth, G. F., and Anderson, D. S. (1983): Healing of benign gastric ulcer with low dose antacids or cimetidine: A double-blind randomized placebo controlled trial. *N. Engl. J. Med.,* 308:1319–1323.

Malagelada, J-R., and Cortot, A. (1978): H_2 receptor antagonist in perspective. *Mayo Clin. Proc.,* 53:184–190.

Morris, T., and Rhodes, J. (1979): Antacids and peptic ulcer–a reappraisal. *Gut,* 20:538–545.

Robert, A., and Kauffman, G. L. Jr. (1983): Stress ulcers in gastrointestinal disease. In: *Gastrointestinal Disease. Pathophysiology, Diagnosis, Management,* edited by M. H. Sleisenger and J. S. Fordtran, pp. 612–625. W. B. Saunders Co., Philadelphia.

Sun, D. C. H., and Stempien, S. J. (1971): Site and size of the ulcer as determinant of outcome. *Gastroenterology,* 61:576–584.

Pseudomembranous Colitis

Bartlett, J. G., Chang, T. W., Jurwith, M., Gorbach, S. L., and Onderdonk, A. B. (1978): Antibiotic associated pseudomembranous colitis due to toxin-producing clostridia. *N. Engl. J. Med.,* 298:531–534.

George, W. L., Rolfe, R. D., and Finegold, S. M. (1980): Treatment and prevention of antimicrobial agent induced colitis and diarrhea. *Gastroenterology,* 79:366–372.

Keeffe, E. B., Katon, R. M., Chan, T. S., Melnyk, C. S., and Benson, J. A. (1974): Pseudomembranous colitis. Resurgence related to newer antibiotic agents. *West. J. Med.,* 121:462 474.

Silva, J., Batts, D. H., Fekety, R., Ploufe, J. F., Rifkin, G. D., and Baird, I. (1981): Treatment of *Clostridium difficile* colitis and diarrhea with vancomycin. *Am. J. Med.,* 71:815–822.

Reflux Esophagitis

Bozymski, E. M., Herlihy, K. J., and Orlando, R. C. (1982): Barrett's esophagus. *Ann. Intern. Med.,* 97:103–107.

Cooper, J. D., and Jeejeebhoy, K. N. (1981): Gastroesophageal reflux: Medical and surgical management. *Ann. Thorac. Surg.,* 31:577–593.

Demeester, T. R., Johnson, L. F., and Kent, A. H. (1974): Evaluation of current operations for the prevention of gastroesophageal reflux. *Ann. Surg.,* 180:511–523.

Richter, J. E., and Castell, D. O. (1982): Gastroesophageal reflux. Pathogenesis, diagnosis and therapy. *Ann. Intern. Med.,* 97:93–103.

12.

Liver Diseases

Gregory T. Everson

12.

Liver Diseases

I. ACUTE HEPATITIS

A. Clinical Features Acute hepatitis is caused by viruses, drugs, alcohol, toxins, and disorders of metabolism. In most cases the history sugggests the etiology. In the absence of drug, alcohol, or toxin exposure, viral hepatitis is likely. **Drug-induced hepatitis** is the result of either the intrinsic hepatotoxicity of the drug (acetaminophen, CCl_4, isoniazid) or an idiosyncratic host response to the drug (Aldomet®, halothane, phenylbutazone). Fever, skin rash, and blood eosinophilia implicate host hypersensitivity to drug as the mechanism of hepatocellular injury. **Hepatitis A** (HA) is transmitted by the fecal-oral route and is the likely etiology of epidemic hepatitis occurring in crowded living conditions. **Hepatitis B** (HB) and **non-A, non-B hepatitis** (NANB) are parenterally transmitted. Sporadically acquired HB and NANB are probably the result of inapparent parenteral inoculation through minor mucosal breaks that occur with brushing teeth, eating meals, bowel movements, vaginal intercourse, and anorectal intercourse. **Subjects at greatest risk** for HB or NANB include spouses of patients with HB or NANB, male homosexuals, intravenous-drug abusers, workers exposed to blood or blood products, and patients requiring frequent transfusions of blood or blood products (hemophiliacs). On rare occasions, other viruses [Epstein-Barr (EB), cytomegalovirus (CMV), herpes, rubella] cause hepatitis in adults.

B. Viral Serology The proper classification of acute viral hepatitis depends on specific serologic tests: IgM antibody to HA (anti-HAV), HB_sA_g, anti-HB_c (IgG), and anti-HB_s. Table 1 shows the various permutations of these tests and their diagnostic interpretation. EB, CMV, herpes, or rubella hepatitis are diagnosed by a rise in antibody titer from acute to convalescent sera.

C. Therapeutic Measures

    1. General management. Indications for hospitalization include nausea and vomiting severe enough to result in dehydration, or severe impairment of liver function causing encephalopathy, ascites, gastrointestinal (GI) bleed, and rising prothrombin time in spite of parenteral vitamin K. All admitted patients should be placed on needle (HB, NANB) and stool (HA) precautions but not in isolation. Gloves should be worn when handling biological specimens, and specimens should be clearly labeled as coming from a patient with hepatitis. All used instruments should be autoclaved.

    2. Specific measures. No effective antiviral therapy exists for acute viral hepatitis, and **corticosteroids are contraindicated** as they may increase the risk of developing chronic hepatitis. Removal of the offending drug and/or alcohol

TABLE 1. *Interpretation of serologic tests in acute viral hepatitis*

Patient	HBₛAg	Anti-HBₛ	Anti-HB_c[a]	Anti-HAV	Interpretation
1	−	−	−	+	Acute HA
2	+	−	+	+	Acute HA and chronic HB carrier
3	+	−	+	−	Acute HB or chronic HB and acute NANB
4	−	−	−	−	Acute NANB
5	−	+	−	−	Acute NANB and late convalescent HB
6	−	+	+	+	Acute HA and convalescent HB
7	−	−	+	−	Early convalescent HB or chronic HB and acute NANB

[a]The present serologic test detects both IgG and IgM anti-HB_c. A recently developed radioimmunoassay specific for IgM anti-HB_c may resolve the question of acute versus chronic HB raised in patients 3 and 7. The IgM anti-HB_c is positive in high titer only in cases of acute HBV.

is the mainstay of therapy for drug-induced and alcoholic hepatitis, respectively.

3. **Immunoprophylaxis.** Adverse effects from **immune globulins** are rare. They should be given **intramuscularly**, and use, if necessary, is not contraindicated by pregnancy.

a. **Hepatitis A.** Postexposure **passive immunization** with immune serum globulin (ISG) is indicated only during the early incubation period. It must be given within 14 days of exposure. Preexposure prophylaxis of travellers to endemic areas may be deferred if only usual, well-traveled tourist routes are followed and residence is < 3 months. Table 2 lists the recommended use of ISG based on the type of HA exposure.

b. **Hepatitis B.** **Passive immunization** is effective in preventing postexposure clinical HB events. Since 1977 lots of ISG contain anti-HBₛ in titer of at least 1:100 by radioimmunoassay (RIA). HB immune globulin (HBIG) contains anti-HBₛ in titer of at least 1:100,000. The cost of HBIG is 20

TABLE 2. *Passive immunization in viral hepatitis*

Type	Exposure	Choice of immune globulin	Dose
A	Prior to travel to endemic area; projected residence of		
	<3 mo	ISG	0.02 ml/kg
	>3 mo	ISG	0.06 ml/kg initially and q 5 mo
	Household, sexual or close institutional contact	ISG	0.02 ml/kg
	Casual contact	None	—
	Common source	None	—
B	Parenteral[a]	HBIG	0.06 ml/kg initially and in 1 mo
	Vertical transmission (mother to newborn)	HBIG	0.5 ml within 24 hr of delivery and in 3.5 mo
	Sexual (exposed to patient with acute HB)	HBIG	0.06 ml/kg
NANB[b]	Parenteral	ISG	0.06 ml/kg

[a]Needle stick, transfusion, or mucus membrane exposure to HBₛAg-positive specimens.
[b]Efficacy of ISG in preventing posttransfusion clinical NANB hepatitis is suggested by recent studies. Use of ISG in cases of vertical transmission or sexual exposure has not been evaluated.

times that of ISG. Guidelines for use of these immune globulins after exposure to a patient with known or suspected acute HB are given in Tables 2 and 3. Concomitant administration of immune globulin and HB vaccine may be indicated if after initial exposure prolonged exposure to HB virus is likely (e.g., a neonate born to a chronic HB_sA_g-carrier mother).

c. **HB vaccine** has proved to be safe and efficacious. **Candidates for vaccination** are subjects who are or are likely to be anti-HB_s negative with a high probability of exposure to HB virus via either parenteral inoculation, vertical transmission, sexual contact, close personal contact, or work-related exposure to blood or blood products. Defined candidates include surgeons, dialysis staff and patients, blood bank personnel, emergency room staff, dentists, gastroenterologists, hematologists, neonates of mothers who are carriers of HB_sA_g, male homosexuals, and intravenous-drug abusers. Vaccine **dose** is 20 μg, i.m. Heptavax® initially and at 1 and 6 months (cost is approximately $100). Patients with renal failure should receive 40 μg instead of 20 μg.

Since the vaccine is derived from the blood of male homosexuals who are chronic carriers of HB_sA_g, there is concern that present batches of vaccine could potentially harbor the agent of acquired immune deficiency syndrome (AIDS). However, the method of preparing the vaccine kills all known infectious agents (including slow viruses) and the incidence of AIDS in the male homosexual population receiving vaccine in the New York study was decreased compared to the control population. Although absolute safety cannot be guaranteed, it is very unlikely that the agent of AIDS or other infectious agents could be transmitted via the vaccine.

d. **NANB hepatitis.** As no serologic markers are available for the agent(s) of NANB hepatitis, clear definition of efficacy of **passive immunization** awaits further investigation. The recommendations in Table 2 are based on the results of three studies of ISG in posttransfusion hepatitis and the relative safety of ISG.

TABLE 3. *Postexposure prophylaxis with immune globulins after parenteral inoculation[a], HB_sA_g status unknown*

Risk[b] of source being HB_sA_g⊕	Test for HB_sA_g	Prophylaxis
High	Yes	.06 ml/kg ISG immediately If HB_sA_g ⊖: nothing more If HB_sA_g ⊕: 0.06 ml/kg HBIG immediately and in 1 mo
Low	No	Nothing or 0.06 ml/kg ISG
Unknown[c]	No	Nothing or 0.06 ml/kg ISG

[a]Needle stick or direct mucus membrane exposure.
[b]High risk includes specimens from patients with acute viral hepatitis, patients from mental institutions, hemodialysis patients, male homosexuals, IV drug abusers, and persons of Asian origin. Low risk includes specimens from otherwise healthy people or average hospital patients.
[c]Source of specimen not known.

II. FULMINANT HEPATIC FAILURE

A. Clinical Features   Fulminant hepatic failure (FHF) is acute hepatocellular necrosis with hepatic encephalopathy that occurs within 8 weeks of the onset of symptoms. Evidence of preexisting hepatocellular disease must be absent. Two thousand cases of FHF occur in the United States each year: one-third viral, one-third drug-induced, and one-third miscellaneous (Wilson's disease, acute fatty liver of pregnancy, Reye's syndrome, jejunoileal bypass, ischemia, sepsis). FHF survival has increased from <10% in the 1940s to 20% to 25% at present because of improvements in the quality of nursing care and intensive care unit (ICU) monitoring.

B. Therapeutic Measures

1. **Corticosteroids.** Survival data from the only controlled trials of corticosteroids in FHF are shown in Table 4. On the basis of the results of these trails, **corticosteroids are not recommended in the routine management of FHF.** However, if FHF develops after withdrawal of corticosteroids used in treating another disease process, then reinstituting steroids may be indicated.

2. **Hepatic support systems.** The following methods have been used in FHF: exchange blood transfusion, plasmapheresis, cross-circulation with human and baboon donors, hemoperfusion through isolated human or animal liver, hemodialysis (conventional and polyacrylonitrate), and column hemoperfusion (microencapsulated charcoal, albumin-covered amberlite XAD-7 resin). Only exchange transfusion has been evaluated by controlled trial, and the mortality was greater in the treated group. As improvement in survival has not been shown by controlled trials with any of these methods, their use in FHF is not recommended (unless under protocol in a randomized controlled trial).

3. **Liver transplantation.** Only one patient with FHF who received a liver transplant has been reported. He did not survive. Thus, at present there is no established role for liver transplantation in FHF.

C. Management of Complications

1. **Upper GI bleeding.** Emergency endoscopy and identification of bleeding lesion is required. Management of bleeding lesion is described in Chapter 11, section XII.

2. **Encephalopathy. Restrict protein intake** (initially 0 g/day and increase only

TABLE 4. *Corticosteroid treatment of fulminant hepatic failure*

	Corticosteroids		Placebo	
Reference	No.	Survivors[a]	No.	Survivors[b]
Ware et al.	4	0	11	7
Redeker et al.	17	6	16	6
EASL	26	3	14	2
Rakela	37	9	20	5

[a]Overall survival, 21%.
[b]Overall survival, 33%.
EASL, European Association for the Study of the Liver.
No., refers to number of patients.

as encephalopathy improves); catharsis of GI tract, lactulose 30 ml every 4 hr initially, then adjust dose to achieve 2 to 4 loose stools per day. Treatment of cerebral edema with either dexamethasone 16 to 72 mg/day, hydrocortisone 600 mg/day, or glycerol 1.5 g/kg/day is ineffective in FHF. A recent study suggests that **mannitol** 1 g/kg, given intravenously as a 20% solution whenever intracranial pressure rises above 30 mm Hg for more than 5 min, may be effective in resolving cerebral edema and prolonging survival in FHF. If this therapy is undertaken, it necessitates placement of intracranial pressure transducers.

3. **Ascites.** A diagnostic paracentesis is indicated if excessive bleeding is **not** anticipated (excessively prolonged prothrombin time). In general, diuretics are contraindicated.

4. **Coagulopathy.** Vitamin K 10 mg/day, i.v., is recommended. Prophylactic infusions of clotting factors are not of proved benefit. **GI hemorrhage** should be treated with fresh whole blood, fresh frozen plasma, and fresh platelets (if needed). Disseminated intravascular coagulation is rare in FHF (except in acute fatty liver of pregnancy); heparin should not be given prophylactically.

5. **Sepsis.** Prophylactic antibiotics are not recommended. Blood, urine, and sputum should be cultured frequently (even in absence of fever or other signs of infection) and **antibiotic therapy** directed toward the specific organism.

6. **Renal failure. Hemodialysis** is reserved for patients with acute renal failure not caused by hepatorenal syndrome (HRS).

7. **Hypoglycemia.** Requirements of up to 2 kg glucose per day have been reported in FHF. Thus, frequent **blood glucose measurements** (every 6 hr or more often if levels are not stable) are necessary for adjusting intravenous glucose administration.

III. CHRONIC ACTIVE LIVER DISEASE

A. **Clinical Features** The Mayo Clinic treatment criteria for chronic active liver disease (CALD) include active hepatic inflammation continuing without improvement for >10 weeks (some authors recommend >6 months) documented by **liver biopsy** with SGOT >10× nl or SGOT >5× nl plus γ-globulin >2× nl. All studies of corticosteroid efficacy have been done in **symptomatic** patients with CALD. Major types of CALD include HB_sA_g-positive CALD, NANB CALD, and primary autoimmune CALD. Wilson's disease, hemochromatosis, alcoholic liver disease, alpha-1 antitrypsin deficiency and drug-induced liver injury (isoniazid, Aldomet®, nitrofurantoin, and oxyphenisatin) may present as CALD. Chronic persistent hepatitis and chronic lobular hepatitis are clinically benign conditions, histologically distinct from CALD, and should not be treated with corticosteroids.

B. **Therapeutic Measures**

1. **HB_sA_g-positive CALD.** In retrospective studies **corticosteroids** have been shown to be effective in this form of CALD, although less so than in primary autoimmune CALD. In addition, it has been shown that higher doses of steroid may be needed to achieve remission. However, in the only prospective controlled trial, survival in HB_sA_g-positive CALD was adversely affected by corticosteroids. In addition, induction of markers of viral replication occurs

during immunosuppressive therapy. Thus, it is impossible to make absolute therapeutic recommendations based on these data. Even so, the patient with marked biochemical and histologic activity who is clinically deteriorating probably should be given a trial of corticosteroid therapy (prednisone 30 to 60 mg/day for 2 months). If no beneficial response occurs, steroids should be rapidly tapered and discontinued. Limited trials of human leukocyte interferon and adenine arabinoside have shown no beneficial effect of either agent.

2. **Primary autoimmune CALD.** Three controlled trials have established the efficacy of **corticosteroids** (prednisone 15 to 30 mg/day) in this condition (Table 5). The initial favorable response persists up to 10 years, but few patients can be withdrawn from steroids without precipitating an exacerbation of the disease. In patients with steroid side effects, azathioprine (1 to 2 mg/kg/day) may be given in an attempt to reduce steroid dose but maintain clinical remission. Azathioprine alone is ineffective in CALD.

3. **NANB CALD.** Parenterally transmitted NANB hepatitis results in mild CALD with progression to cirrhosis in ≈10% of cases. No controlled trials of immunosuppressive therapy exist because of difficulty in defining etiology. A **limited therapeutic trial** of prednisone 15 to 30 mg/day for 6 months may be indicated in symptomatic patients with evidence of moderate to severe activity biochemically and histologically. If remission is induced, then steroids or steroids plus azathioprine should be reduced to the lowest dose necessary to maintain remission.

4. **Wilson's disease.** This diagnosis is confirmed by presence of Kayser-Fleischer rings, low serum ceruloplasmin (<200 mg/liter), elevated urinary copper excretion (>100 µg/24 hr), and elevated hepatic copper concentration (>250 µg/g dry liver). The disease should be suspected in patients < 35 years old with chronic liver disease (with or without neurologic symptoms or signs) or persistently elevated transaminases, alkaline phosphatase, and γ-glutamyl transferase, with no other clear etiology. Low-copper diet and D-penicillamine (1 to 2 g/day) is highly **effective therapy** for both the hepatic and neurologic sequelae of the disorder.

5. **Alcoholic hepatitis.** This diagnosis is usually evident from history, physical examination, and liver biopsy. The only effective therapy is **abstinence from alcohol**. According to data from controlled trials, **corticosteroids are not recommended**.

6. **Alpha-1-antitrypsin deficiency.** This form of liver disease is diagnosed by

TABLE 5. *Corticosteroids in chronic active hepatitis*

References[a]	Mortality (%)		Follow-up (yr)
	Corticosteroids	Placebo	
Cook et al.	14	56	4
Murray-Lyon et al.	5	28	2
Soloway et al.	6	35	3.5

[a]Although disease groups were heterogeneous, most had primary autoimmune chronic active liver disease.

absent alpha-1 antitrypsin in blood and PAS-positive globules in periportal hepatocytes on liver biopsy. No effective therapy exists, but **diagnosis is important for genetic counseling.**

7. **Drug-induced CALD.** In almost all instances drug-induced CALD will improve after withdrawal of the offending agent.

IV. CIRRHOSIS

A. **Clinical Features** Once the disease process has advanced to cirrhosis, specific therapy is of little benefit. The patient's subsequent clinical course is determined by **complications** resulting from cirrhosis including variceal hemorrhage, portosystemic encephalopathy, ascites, coagulopathy, poor nutritional status, and infection.

B. **Variceal Hemorrhage** Only 50% of upper GI bleeding in cirrhosis with varices is caused by varices. Therefore, since therapeutic decisions are affected by the cause of bleeding, **emergent endoscopy** should be performed. Management of variceal bleeding is outlined in Chapter 11.

C. **Portosystemic Encephalopathy**

1. **General.** A **precipitating event** usually can be identified: ingestion of a high-protein meal; drugs and medications (especially sedatives, narcotics, and tranquilizers); GI bleeding; sepsis; and, spontaneous bacterial peritonitis. Usual causes of acute change in mental status also must be excluded (see Chapter 23).

2. **Therapeutic measures**

a. **Treat precipitating cause** when possible.

b. **Diet. Restrict dietary protein** to 20 to 40 g/day. Some patients may be able to tolerate higher amounts of vegetable-base protein than animal-base protein. However, no adequate controlled trials comparing the two exist.

c. **Lactulose.** The goal is to induce two to three semiformed stools per day (usually 15 ml t.i.d.). **Severe diarrhea** may be induced by excessive doses of lactulose, which may lead to deterioration of a patient secondary to compromised serum electrolytes and intravascular volume. Several clinical trials have attested to the efficacy and safety of lactulose in both chronic and acutely ill patients with encephalopathy.

d. **Neomycin.** Studies comparing neomycin to lactulose have demonstrated similar efficacy. However, neomycin may be oto- and nephrotoxic after oral ingestion; it should not be used alone but **in combination** with lactulose. Trials comparing the combination of lactulose plus neomycin to either alone suggest that the combination is more efficacious. The suggested dose of neomycin is 1 to 2 g, p.o. or via nasogastric tube every 6 hr.

e. **Branched-chain amino acids.** One intravenous (Hepatamine), and two oral (Hepatic Aid; Travasorb Hepatic) preparations are available. Three controlled trials have given conflicting results. These preparations are expensive and their role in the treatment of either cirrhosis or hepatic encephalopathy has not been defined; therefore, their routine use is not recommended.

f. **Dopamine agonists.** L-DOPA is ineffective in acute hepatic encephalopathy complicating cirrhosis but has a short-lived beneficial effect in chronic hepatic encephalopathy. **Bromocriptine** in a dose of 2.5 to 15.0 mg/day, when added to lactulose and low-protein diet, was shown by controlled trial to be effective in chronic hepatic encephalopathy. **Neither** drug **is recommended for acute hepatic encephalopathy.** If a trial of these agents is undertaken in chronic hepatic encephalopathy, the patient should be monitored for evidence of orthostatic hypotension and constipation, complications of both drugs.

D. Ascites   Several factors contribute to the formation of ascitic fluid within the peritoneal cavity, including portal hypertension, increased hepatic lymph formation, altered Starling forces across the peritoneal capillary bed, and renal/humoral factors [including hyperaldosteronism, increased sympathetic tone, and excessive antidiuretic hormone (ADH) secretion, leading to renal sodium and water retention]. **Diagnostic paracentesis** is essential to exclude ascites from causes other than liver disease, particularly in febrile patients with abdominal pain. Diuretic therapy of ascites is **potentially dangerous**; it should be instituted only in the stable patient, with careful monitoring of electrolyte, acid-base, and hemodynamic status. Changes in therapy should be made gradually.

1. **Diagnostic paracentesis** (50 to 100 ml) is indicated in all patients with new-onset ascites, increasing ascites, ascites refractory to medical therapy, or ascites and clinical decompensation to rule out **spontaneous bacterial peritonitis** (SBP). An absolute PMN count >200/mm^3 is presumptive evidence of SBP. Low ascitic fluid pH has been described in SBP but only when PMN is >200/mm^3. Thus, the utility of ascitic fluid pH remains to be determined. The combination of ampicillin plus aminoglycoside is recommended initial therapy. This combination covers most organisms responsible for SBP including gram-negative bacilli, enterococcus, and *Streptococeus pneumoniae*. Antibiotic therapy is subsequently adjusted to the specific sensitivities of the cultured organism(s).

2. **Therapeutic measures**

a. **Hospitalization** is initially necessary to impose accurate dietary restrictions and monitor the effects of therapy. Daily monitoring of weight, fluid intake/output, and clinical exam are recommended. Serum electrolytes, BUN, and creatinine should be drawn every 1 to 2 days. The **goal of therapy** is uncomplicated weight reduction of 0.5 kg/day until ascites is gone.

b. **Initial regimen** is bed rest and restriction of <2 g **sodium** and 1,000 to 1,500 ml **water** per day. This includes any sodium or water administered with drugs or medications. Stricter sodium restriction (<500 mg/day) is advocated by some authors, but patient compliance with this regimen is poor. A recent study has shown that moderate sodium restriction (2 g/day) results in better patient compliance and few side effects. Water restriction also is indicated because of the diminished free-water clearance in cirrhosis with ascites.

c. **Diuretic therapy.** If weight loss is not achieved after 4 days, sodium and water restriction should be continued and **spironolactone** added, 100 mg, p.o., b.i.d. The dose should be increased to 200 mg, p.o., b.i.d., if the patient is not diuresing after 4 additional days. If spironolactone effect is observed (urine Na>K) but patient is not diuresing or if high-dose spironolactone (≥400 mg/day) is ineffective, then **furosemide** (40 mg/day) may be added. Start with a low dose and increase subsequent doses by 20 mg only as needed to obtain weight loss of 0.5 kg/day **safely**.

With close monitoring, diuretic therapy for ascites has been shown to be safe. If electrolyte imbalance (i.e., hyperkalemia from spironolactone), hypovolemia, or azotemia is induced during therapy, the dose of diuretic should be reduced. Severe complications, including hepatic encephalopathy, hepatorenal syndrome, and death, have all resulted from indiscriminate use of diuretics in cirrhotic patients.

3. **Hepatorenal syndrome** is functional renal failure occurring in the cirrhosis patient with ascites. This must be differentiated from prerenal azotemia secondary to hypovolemia and acute tubular necrosis. One must document normal intravascular volume, fractional urine excretion of sodium < 1, and unremarkable urine sediment to make the **diagnosis** of HRS. Numerous **therapies** for HRS have been tried without success, including dopamine, vasopressors, vasodilators, albumin infusions, and propranolol. The **peritoneovenous shunt** may reverse renal failure but is associated with numerous complications. Since efficacy is not defined, insertion is expensive, and complications are potentially life-threatening, use of the peritoneovenous shunt is not recommended outside of randomized controlled trials.

E. **Use of Drugs and Alcohol in Chronic Liver Disease**   Since many drugs depend on the liver for metabolism and excretion, modifications in dosage must be made in the patient with liver disease to avoid toxicity. On the basis of a recent review, the following approach to management of drug dosage is suggested.

High-risk drugs (e.g., meperidine, pentazocine, propranolol, lidocaine, and nitroglycerin) have high first-pass hepatic elimination (60%) and are essentially dependent on hepatic blood flow for removal from plasma. In the presence of either shunting of hepatic blood flow or markedly diminished hepatic extraction/excretion, blood levels of these drugs may become markedly elevated. In this setting **both initial and maintenance dosages of drug should be reduced**.

Limited-risk drugs (e.g., phenobarbital, diazepam, theophylline, rifampin, clindamycin, and chloramphenicol) have a low first-pass hepatic elimination (<30%) and depend on the metabolic capacity of the liver for removal from plasma. The peak drug level after an initial dose of a low-extraction drug is unaltered by liver disease. However, reduced liver metabolic capacity results in excessive accumulation and toxic levels of drug after repeated doses; **reduction in maintenance dosage of drug is therefore necessary**.

Low-risk drugs (e.g., naproxen, oxazepam, lorazepam, ampicillin, isoniazid, furosemide, spironolactone, digoxin, prednisone, and cimetidine) have essentially unaltered hepatic elimination even in the presence of severe liver disease. Therefore, dosage reduction is not necessary.

In spite of these guidelines individual variation is great, and one must realize that end-organ response may be altered in liver disease. In particular, nontoxic therapeutic blood levels of sedatives, narcotics, and tranquilizers may precipitate **hepatic coma** in a compensated patient with cirrhosis. Therefore, one should use these drugs sparingly in the cirrhotic patient.

Continued **alcohol intake** in a patient with Laennec's cirrhosis portends a poor prognosis. It is not known whether alcohol is especially toxic to patients with nonalcoholic chronic liver disease. Even so, in these patients it is probably wise to limit alcohol intake to <2 oz/week.

V. TREATMENT OF SPECIFIC LIVER DISEASES

A. Acetaminophen Overdosage   The major factor determining risk and severity of hepatotoxicity is the acetaminophen blood level (obtained >4 hr after drug ingestion) in relation to time of ingestion. Since **acetylcysteine** may be life-saving, the physician always should initiate therapy. The decision to continue or discontinue acetylcysteine is based on acetaminophen blood level.

Management includes

  a. Gastric lavage (do not give activated charcoal as it interferes with absorption of acetylcysteine).

  b. Acetylcysteine, orally or via nasogastric tube (loading dose, 140 mg/kg; maintenance dose, 70 mg/kg every 4 hr × 17 doses); follow SGOT, SGPT, alkaline phosphatase, and bilirubin.

B. Hemochromatosis   Hemochromatosis is an iron-storage disease inherited in an autosomal recessive pattern. The disease should be suspected in patients with chronic liver disease, transferrin saturation >60%, and/or ferritin >2× nl. **Diagnosis** is confirmed by quantitative liver iron >10 mg/g dry liver weight and/or no drop in hematocrit in spite of 1 U/week phlebotomy for 10 weeks or more. **Treatment** is removal of excess iron stores by phlebotomy to achieve and maintain mild anemia (hematocrit 36%). Asymptomatic family members homozygous for the hemochromatosis gene are discovered by **routine screening** (serum iron, total iron-binding capacity, and ferritin) of siblings and offspring of the patient with hemachromatosis.

C. Primary Biliary Cirrhosis   Specific therapy of primary biliary cirrhosis (PBC) is currently **experimental**. Patients have been treated with corticosteroids, azathioprine, chlorambucil, cyclosporin A, and D-penicillamine with limited or no success. Corticosteroids worsen metabolic bone disease in PBC and are contraindicated. D-penicillamine has been studied in three controlled trials, one showing increased survival, one showing decreased survival, and one showing no change in survival. Use of D-penicillamine in PBC therefore should be limited to controlled trials. Cholestyramine 2 to 5 g q.i.d. is useful in controlling **pruritus**. Multivitamins and calcium supplements are necessary to delay **osteopenia**. 25-OH vitamin D may be the preferred vitamin D analog in those patients documented to have **osteomalacia**.

D. Sclerosing Cholangitis   Steroids and immunosuppressive agents are probably ineffective in the treatment of this lesion. In patients with **inflammatory bowel disease** the activity of sclerosing cholangitis may or may not abate after colectomy. In fact, sclerosing cholangitis has occurred several years after colectomy. Thus, proctocolectomy is not recommended as standard therapy for sclerosing cholangitis occurring in inflammatory bowel disease.

BIBLIOGRAPHY

Acute Hepatitis

Centers for Disease Control (1982): Immune globulins for protection against viral hepatitis. *Ann. Intern. Med.*, 96:193–197.
Chau, K. H., Hargie, P., Decker, R. H., Mushahwar, I. K., and Overby, L. R. (1983): Serodiagnosis of recent hepatitis B infection by IgM class anti-HBc. *Hepatology*, 3:142–149.
Dienstag, J. L. (1983): Non-A, non-B hepatitis. *Gastroenterology*, 85:439–62, 743–768.
Favero, M. S., Maynard, J. E., Leger, R. T., Graham, D. R., and Dixon, R. E. (1979): Guidelines for the care of patients hospitalized with viral hepatitis. *Ann. Intern. Med.*, 91:872–876.
Mulley, A. G., Silverstein, M. D., and Dienstag, J. L. (1982): Indications for use of hepatitis B vaccine, based on cost-effectiveness analysis. *N. Engl. J. Med.*, 307:644–652.
Mushahwar, I. K., Dienstag, J. L., Polesky, H. F., McGrath, L. C., Decker, R. H., and Overby, L. R. (1981): Interpretation of various serological profiles of hepatitis B virus infection. *Am. J. Clin Pathol.*, 76:773–777.
Szmuness, W., Stevens, C. E., Zang, E. A., Harley, E. J., and Kellner, A. (1981): A controlled clinical trial of the efficacy of the hepatitis B vaccine (Heptavax B): a final report. *Hepatology*, 1:377–385.
Vyas, G. N., Cohen, S. N., and Schmid, R., eds. (1978): *Viral Hepatitis.* Franklin Institute Press, Philadelphia.

Chronic Active Liver Disease

Conn, H. O. (1978): Steroid treatment of alcoholic hepatitis. *Gastroenterology*, 74:319–322.
Conn, H. O., Maddrey, W. C., and Soloway, R. D. (1982): The detrimental effects of adrenocorticosteroid therapy in HBsAg-positive chronic active hepatitis: fact or artifact? *Hepatology*, 2:885–887.
Cook, G. C., Mulligan, R., and Sherlock, S. (1971): Controlled prospective trial of corticosteroid therapy in active chronic hepatitis. *Q. J. Med.*, N.S. 40:159–185.
Czaja, A. J., Ludwig, J., Baggenstoss, A. H., and Wolf, A. (1981): Corticosteroid-treated chronic active hepatitis in remission. *N. Engl. J. Med.*, 304:5–9.
Czaja, A. J., Davis, G. L., Ludwig, J., Baggenstoss, A. H., and Taswell, H. F. (1983): Autoimmune features as determinants of prognosis in steroid-treated chronic active hepatitis of uncertain etiology. *Gastroenterology*, 85:713–717.
Depew, W., Boyer, T., Omata, M., Redeker, A., and Reynolds, T. (1980): Double-blind controlled trial of prednisolone therapy in patients with severe acute alcoholic hepatitis and spontaneous encephalopathy. *Gastroenterology*, 78:524–529.
Dudley, F. J., Scheuer, P. J., and Sherlock, S. (1972): Natural history of hepatitis-associated antigen-positive chronic liver disease. *Lancet*, 2:1388–1393.
Kirk, A. P., Jain, S., Pocock, S., Thomas, H. C., and Sherlock, S. (1980): Late results of the Royal Free Hospital prospective controlled trial of prednisolone therapy in hepatitis B surface antigen negative chronic active hepatitis. *Gut*, 21:78–83.
Lam, K. C., Lai, C. L., Trepo, C., and Wu, P. C. (1981): Deleterious effect of prednisolone in HBsAg-positive chronic active hepatitis. *N. Engl. J. Med.*, 304:380–386.
Murray-Lyon, I. M., Stern, R. B., and Williams, R. (1973): Controlled trial of prednisone and azathioprine in active chronic hepatitis. *Lancet*, 1:735–737.
Schalm, S. W., Ammon, H. V., and Summerskill, W. H. J. (1976): Failure of customary treatment in chronic active liver disease: causes and management. *Ann. Clin. Res.*, 8:221–227.
Schalm, S. W., Summerskill, W. H. J., Gitnick, G. L., and Elveback, L. R. (1976): Contrasting features and responses to treatment of severe chronic active liver disease with and without hepatitis B antigen. *Gut*, 17:781–786.
Scullard, G. H., Robinson, W. S., Merigan, T. C., and Gregory, P. B. (1979): The effect of immunosuppressive therapy on hepatitis B viral infection in patients with chronic hepatitis. *Gastroenterology*, 77:A40.
Soloway, R. D., Summerskill, W. H. J., Baggenstoss, A. H., Geall, M. G., Gitnick, G. L., Elverback, L. R., and Schoenfield, L. J. (1972): Clinical, biochemical and histological remission

of severe chronic active liver disease: A controlled study of treatments and early prognosis. *Gastroenterology*, 63:820–833.

Wu, P. C., Lai, C. L., Lam, K. C., and Ho, J. (1982): Prednisolone in HBsAg-positive chronic active hepatitis: Histologic evaluation in a controlled prospective study. *Hepatology*, 2:777–783.

Cirrhosis

Ascites

Epstein, M. (1979): Deranged sodium homeostasis in cirrhosis. *Gastroenterology*, 76:622–635.

Epstein, M. (1981): The Leveen shunt for ascites and hepatorenal syndrome. *N. Engl. J. Med.*, 302:628–630.

Gitlin, N., Stauffer, J. L., and Silvestri, R. C. (1982): The pH of ascitic fluid in the diagnosis of spontaneous bacterial peritonitis in alcoholic cirrhosis. *Hepatology*, 2:408–411.

Gregory, P. B., Broekelschen, P. H., Hill, M. D., Lipton, A. B., Knauer, C. M., Egger, M., and Miller, R. (1977): Complications of diuresis in the alcoholic patient with ascites: a controlled trial. *Gastroenterology*, 73:534–538.

Hoefs, J. C., Canawati, H. N., Sapico, F. L., Hopkins, R. R., Weiner, J., and Montgomerie, J. Z. (1982): Spontaneous bacterial peritonitis. *Hepatology*, 2:399–407.

Reynolds, T. B., Lieberman, F. L., and Goodman, A. R. (1978): Advantages of treatment of ascites without sodium restriction and without complete removal of excess fluid. *Gut*, 19:549–553.

Sherlock, S., ed. (1981): Ascites. In: *Liver and Biliary System*, 6th ed., pp. 116–133. Blackwell Scientific Publication, London.

Drugs and alcohol in chronic liver disease

Bircher, J. (1983): Altered drug metabolism in liver disease—therapeutic implications. In: *Recent Advances in Hepatology I*, edited by H. C. Thomas and R. N. M. MacSween, pp. 101–113. Churchill Livingstone, Edinburgh.

Jurgen, L., and Axelsen, R. (1983): Drug effects on the liver. An updated tabular compilation of drugs and drug-related hepatic diseases. *Dig. Dis. Sci.*, 28:651–666.

Portosystemic encephalopathy

Atterbury, C. E., Maddrey, W. C., and Conn, H. O. (1976): Neomycin-sorbitol and lactulose in the treatment of acute portal-systemic encephalopathy. *Dig. Dis. Sci.*, 23:398–406.

Bircher, J., Haemmerly, U. P., Scollo-Lavizzari, G., and Hoffmann, K. (1971): Treatment of chronic portal-systemic encephalopathy with lactulose. *Am. J. Med.*, 51:148–159.

Conn, H. O., Leevy, C. M., Vlahcevic, Z. R., Rodgers, J. B., Maddrey, W. C., Seeff, L., and Levy, L. L. (1977): Comparision of lactulose and neomycin in the treatment of chronic portal-systemic encephalopathy. *Gastroenterology*, 72:573–583.

Greenberger, N. J., Carley, J., Schenker, S., Bettinger, I., Stammes, C., and Beyer, P. (1977): Effect of vegetable and animal protein diets in chronic hepatic encephalopathy. *Dig. Dis. Sci.*, 22:845–855.

Morgan, M. Y., Jakobovits, A. W., James, I. M., and Sherlock, S. (1980): Successful use of bromocriptine in the treatment of chronic hepatic encephalopathy. *Gastroenterology*, 78:663–670.

Wahren, J., Denis, J., Desurmont, P., Eriksson, L. S., Escoffier, J.-M., Gauthier, A. P., Hagenfeldt, L., Michel, H., Opolon, P., Paris, J.-C., and Veyrac, M. (1983): Is intravenous administration of branched chain amino acids effective in the treatment of hepatic encephalopathy? A multicenter study. *Hepatology*, 3:475–480.

Fulminant Hepatic Failure

European Association for the Study of the Liver. (1979): Randomized trial of steroid therapy in acute liver failure. *Gut*, 20:620–623.

Gregory, P. B., Knauer, C. M., Kempson, R. L., and Miller, R. (1976): Steroid therapy in severe viral hepatitis. *N. Engl. J. Med.*, 294:681–687.

Jones, A. E., and Schafer, D. F. (1982): Fulminant hepatic failure. In: *Hepatology*, edited by Zakim and Boyer, pp. 415–445. W. B. Saunders, Philadelphia.

Rakela, J., (1979): A double-blinded, randomized trial of hydrocortisone in acute hepatic failure. *Gastroenterology*, 76:1297.

Redeker, A. G., Schweitzer, I. L., and Yamashiro, H. S. (1976): Randomization of corticosteroid therapy in fulminant hepatitis. *N. Engl. J. Med.*, 294:728–729.

Ware, A. J., Jones, R. E., Shorey, J. W., and Combes, B. (1974): A controlled trial of steroid therapy in massive hepatic necrosis. *Am J. Gastroenterology*, 62:130–133.

Miscellaneous Liver Diseases

Black, M. (1980): Acetaminophen hepatotoxicity. *Gastroenterology*, 78:382-392.

Powell, L. W., Bassett, M. L., and Halliday, J. W. (1980): Hemochromatosis: 1980 update. *Gastroenterology*, 78:374–381.

Rumack, B. H., Peterson, R. C., Koch, G. G., and Amara, I. A. (1981): Acetaminophen overdose. *Arch. Intern. Med.*, 141:380–385.

Sherlock, S. (1981): Treatment and prognosis of primary biliary cirrhosis. *Sem. Liver Dis.*, 1:354–364.

13.

Hemorrhagic and Thrombotic Disorders

Ute Hasiba

13.

Hemorrhagic and Thrombotic Disorders

I. BLEEDING DISORDERS Management of persons who are actively bleeding or who are to undergo a hemostatic stress such as a surgical procedure can only be accomplished after hemostatic abnormalities have been defined or excluded. An adequate history, a physical examination, and the review and understanding of all underlying medical conditions will aid in selecting the appropriate laboratory tests.

A. History and Physical Examination An adequate **history** is particularly important if one is considering a congenital coagulopathy. The questions need to be specific, yet should not be leading; **present and past bleeding symptoms** need to be reviewed, as well as previous surgical procedures, regardless of whether they were associated with excessive bleeding or not. **Family history** should include asking for persons with diagnosed bleeding disorders as well as bleeding symptoms and surgical exposures in close relatives. A **drug history** is important not only to relate to bleeding symptoms, but also to interpret test result abnormalities; e.g., acetylsalicylic acid (ASA) and many other drugs may prolong the bleeding time in the absence of an underlying hemostatic defect. A history of delayed rebleeding with surgical procedures or unexplained swelling of joints following injury may suggest hemophilia. Excessive bleeding after ASA ingestion may be due to a mild platelet defect. Excessive bleeding from cuts, unexplained epistaxis, or even increased menstrual bleeding might be a clue to the diagnosis of von Willebrand's disease. A history of isolated instances of easy bruising is common and should only be pursued if there are other reasons to suggest a bleeding disorder. A review and understanding of all pathophysiologic events are very important in a person with active bleeding and will greatly help in the selection of the appropriate laboratory tests that can identify the hemostatic defect.

Petechiae observed during the **physical examination** suggest a platelet or vascular disorder. Deep hematomas imply a coagulation factor defect. Orthostatic blood pressure changes should alert one to look for a hidden source of blood loss such as the gastrointestinal (GI) tract or the retro- or intraperitoneal space.

B. Laboratory Studies

1. Platelet studies

　a. The **template bleeding time** is the best in vivo test to evaluate the platelet-vessel wall interaction. It is usually prolonged in the presence of thrombocytopenia or abnormal platelet function, but may also be slightly prolonged in the presence of certain vascular disorders. Each person with a platelet count over 100,000/μl and with a markedly prolonged bleeding time should be evaluated for abnormal platelet function.

   b. Platelet aggregation studies measure the interaction and clump formation of platelets when stimulated with various agents [adenosine diphosphate (ADP), collagen, epinephrine, arachidonic acid]. A photooptical instrument notes changes in light transmittance and records them graphically. Decreased responses to one or several aggregating agents will be obtained in the presence of congenital and acquired-platelet functional defects (for details see I.F.).

2. Coagulation tests. These tests **must** be interpreted according to each hospital's established normal ranges, since reagents and techniques influence normal values. Atraumatic venipunctures and blood drawn directly into the anticoagulant are most appropriate. Blood must be transported to the laboratory promptly, where the tests are performed immediately or the plasma is separated and frozen. The amount of anticoagulant must not vary; half-filled vacutainers will result in erroneous results. For patients with greatly increased or decreased hematocrits, blood should be collected into specially prepared tubes with adjusted amounts of anticoagulants.

   a. Prothrombin time (PT) measures a clot formation via the "extrinsic" system. The test is performed in citrated plasma, and the reagent consists of Ca^{2+} and thromboplastin. Results are best expressed in seconds and are compared with the results obtained with a normal standard. A prolonged PT indicates a deficiency in one or more of the clotting factors II, V, VII, X; a significant decrease in fibrinogen, or the presence of an inhibitor.

   b. Activated partial thromboplastin time (APTT) measures the fibrin formation via the "intrinsic system." The reagent consists of an agent capable of activating factor XII and a "partial thromboplastin," which provides phospholipids similar to those present in platelets (platelet factor 3); after an appropriate incubation time the citrated plasma is recalcified and the clotting time measured in seconds. Decrease of any clotting factor except factors VII and XIII will result in prolonged APTT. In addition, the APTT will be prolonged in the presence of a "lupus anticoagulant" or heparin. Mixtures of equal amounts of normal plasma and patient plasma will correct the APTT if it is due to clotting factor deficiencies but not if it is caused by an inhibitor or heparin.

   c. Thrombin time (TT) measures the time required for a standardized solution of thrombin to clot plasma. It is prolonged with hypofibrinogenemia or with an abnormal fibrinogen, and in the presence of certain anticoagulants [heparin, fibrin(ogen) degradation products].

   d. Reptilase® time. This commercially available purified venom from the snake, Bothrops Atrox is similar to thrombin in action; the Reptilase® time will be normal in the presence of heparin, but markedly prolonged with an abnormal fibrinogen.

   e. Fibrinogen is most commonly measured indirectly by comparing the thrombin time of the patient with that obtained with serial dilutions of plasma containing varying amounts of fibrinogen. Since the thrombin used in this assay is very strong and the patient's plasma is diluted, the measurement will not be affected by therapeutic levels of heparin or moderate amounts of inhibitory fibrin split products.

f. **Fibrin degradation products** are usually measured with various methods employing antisera developed against nonclottable fibrin(ogen) fragments. Blood samples must be collected in special tubes containing plasmin inhibitors to prevent in vitro fibrinolysis.

g. **Individual clotting factors** are most often measured as modified screening tests—APTT or PT. The tests are based on the ability of the patient's plasma to correct results obtained with a plasma known to be deficient in the factor to be measured.

h. **Factor XIII deficiency** will not prolong the APTT or PT, but the fibrin clot will dissolve after the addition of urea or monochloracetic acid.

3. **General approach to the diagnosis of hemorrhagic diatheses**

a. **Congenital bleeding disorders** are usually due to the deficiency of a single plasma coagulation factor. Prolonged screening test(s) (PT, APTT, TT, bleeding time) will help in choosing the appropriate specific coagulation factor assays, which will confirm the diagnosis. Occasionally, a very mild bleeding disorder will not result in a prolonged screening test; only a good history will allow us to select the appropriate further workup.

b. **Acquired coagulopathies** are usually associated with multiple hemostatic abnormalities. Patterns of abnormalities obtained with screening tests and adequate understanding of the pathophysiologic events occurring in the patient will allow us, in most cases, to classify the coagulopathy and to initiate the appropriate therapy. It is neither necessary nor useful to perform all coagulation factor assays or other tests that we expect to be abnormal. On the other hand, treating patients who have a prolonged PT or APTT with fresh, frozen plasma and without understanding why these tests are abnormal is inappropriate and a practice that should be strongly discouraged. A "lupus anticoagulant" is not associated with excessive bleeding, and an acquired antibody to factor VIII will not respond to fresh, frozen plasma (for other examples see I.D.).

C. **Congenital Coagulopathies**

1. **Hemophilia**

a. Clinical presentation. **Classic hemophilia (hemophilia A)** is a bleeding disorder characterized by decreased amounts of factor VIII:C [antihemophilic factor (AHF), antihemophilic globulin (AHG)]. **Hemophilia B or Christmas disease** is due to decreased amounts of factor IX [plasma thromboplastin component (PTC)]. Both disorders are X-linked, occurring almost exclusively in males. Hemophilia A affects 1 in 10,000 males, and hemophilia B, 1 in 50,000. The clinical presentations of hemophilia A and B are very similar and vary in proportion to the degree of factor deficiency. Patients with severe hemophilia (clotting factor assay <0.01 U/ml) have frequent spontaneous hemorrhages, especially into joints, whereas patients with mild hemophilia (clotting factor assay >0.05 U/ml) only experience excessive bleeding with trauma or surgery. Patients with moderately severe hemophilia (clotting factor assay between 0.01 U/ml and 0.05 U/ml) may have spontaneous hemorrhages, but rarely develop chronic arthropathy.

b. **Treatment for hemophilia A** consists of replacement with factor VIII-containing blood products; these include various pooled, lyophylized **factor VIII concentrates** and **cryoprecipitate.** The amounts to be infused vary, depending on the location of the hemorrhage (see Table 1). To achieve a specific in vivo level, the following formula should be employed:

Units of factor VIII = desired in vivo level in units $\times$ 100 $\times$ weight in kg $\times$ 0.5. The correction factor 0.5 derives from the plasma volume (blood volume $\times$ plasmacrit), assuming a normal hematocrit. One unit of factor is defined as the activity of the factor contained in 1 ml of normal plasma.

One bottle of factor VIII concentrate contains anywhere from 200 to 1,500 units of VIII:C. **Factor VIII concentrate** is usually administered by slow intravenous bolus at a rate of 5 to 10 ml/min.

Cryoprecipitate is prepared from individual blood units. One bag contains approximately 100 units of VIII:C in a volume of 15 to 30 ml; it should be administered by slow intravenous bolus or rapid infusion. The half-life of administered factor VIII:C in cryoprecipitate or concentrate is approximately 12 hr. Certain factor VIII concentrates are stable enough to be administered by continuous intravenous infusion. In patients undergoing **major surgery**, factor VIII:C levels should be maintained at >0.5 U/ml throughout the procedure and for 48 hr postoperatively; levels of 0.25 U/ml should be maintained for another 5 to 10 days, depending on the type of surgery.

c. **Treatment of hemophilia B** Major hemorrhages are treated with **factor IX concentrate** (prothrombin complex concentrate), which contains the clotting factors II, VII, IX, and X in highly purified form. Dosages calculated with the same formula as used for hemophilia A will result in lower levels of measurable factor IX:C, since the administered factor IX:C will be distributed equally between the intra- and extravascular space. Hemostatic control will, however, be comparable to that achieved in hemophilia A. Minor hemorrhages can be treated with **fresh, frozen plasma** (15 ml/kg will result in levels close to 0.2 U/ml). The half-life of administered factor IX in plasma or concentrate is approximately 18 hr.

TABLE 1. *Treatment of bleeding episodes in hemophiliacs*

Bleeding episode	Calculated dosage to reach level of	Repeat dosage
Early hemarthrosis	0.2 U/ml	None
Moderate hemarthrosis with slight swelling	0.4 U/ml	None
Massive hemarthrosis, muscle hemorrhage	0.4 U/ml	Every 8–12 hr for 2–4 days
Suspected or proven: CNS, retroperitoneal, GI, neck, or throat bleeding	1.0 U/ml	Maintain level between 0.5–1.0 U/ml for up to 2 weeks

d. **Complications of treatment**

(1) **Allergic reactions** due to factor VIII or IX concentrates are extremely rare, and routine pretreatment with diphenhydramine hydrochloride (Benadryl®) is not recommended. Frequent administration of cryoprecipitate and of fresh, frozen plasma may require prophylactic diphenhydramine hydrochloride, since hives or GI distress are often encountered.

(2) Transmission of **infectious agents.** Hepatitis (type B and type non-A, non-B), cytomegalic virus infection, and maybe agents involved in the pathogenesis of the acquired immune deficiency syndrome (AIDS) all may pose serious risks to frequently transfused patients with hemophilia. Because each lot of pooled, factor VIII or IX concentrate contains plasma from 5,000 to 20,000 donors, the risk of acquiring **hepatitis** is much higher with concentrate than with single-donor blood products—fresh, frozen plasma and cryoprecipitate. Therefore, infrequently transfused patients should receive single-donor products whenever feasible. Recently developed heat-treated concentrates may decrease the risk of viral transmission, but further studies are needed to confirm this possibility.

Desmopressin acetate (DDAVP®), a synthetic vasopressin, is capable of releasing stored factor VIII (VIIIR:RCo and VIII:C) from endothelium and produces a transient rise in factor VIII levels. Administering 0.3 μg/kg intravenously results in a four-to-sixfold increase of VIII:C and VIIIR:RCo and is the ideal agent to treat patients with mild hemophilia A and von Willebrand's disease.

(3) **Inhibitors.** 15% of all patients with hemophilia A develop an inhibitor (antibody to VIII:C). Inhibitors are extremely rare in hemophilia B. **Steroids** and/or immunosuppressive agents are ineffective in decreasing the inhibitor titer or in preventing an anamnestic response. The treatment of hemorrhagic episodes depends on the type of inhibitor, high or low antibody titer after exposure to factor VIII, antibody titer at the time of the bleeding episode, and type of hemorrhage (mild, severe, or life-threatening).

e. The following blood products may be used:

(1) **Prothrombin complex concentrates** (Konyne®, Proplex®) may control bleeding into muscles and joints in 25% to 40% of hemorrhagic episodes. A dose of 50 to 100 U/kg is usually administered and may be repeated in 4 to 8 hr. Response may vary with different lots of products; no laboratory tests are available to monitor the response.

(2) **Activated prothrombin complex concentrates** (Autoplex™, FEIBA®) should be reserved for **advanced** hemorrhages or for those not responding to nonactivated concentrates. They control bleeding into muscles and joints in approximately 60% of these hemorrhages. A dose of 50 to 100 correctional units may be repeated in 6 to 12 hr. No simple laboratory test is presently available to monitor the response. Activated and nonactivated prothrombin complex concentrates contain small amounts of VIIIC:Ag and may cause an anamnestic rise in the antibody titer.

(3) Factor VIII concentrate is the **product of choice** for patients who never develop high levels of antibodies despite frequent exposure to factor VIII. Factor VIII concentrate should also be used in patients with a history of high antibody levels in the past, but low levels (<20 Bethesda units) at the time they suffer a life-threatening hemorrhagic episode. In patients with antibody titers of >2 Bethesda units, **plasmapheresis** should precede the administration of factor VIII, since it will lower the antibody titer.

2. **von Willebrand's disease**

   a. **Clinical presentation and diagnosis.** Von Willebrand's disease is now recognized as a group of congenital bleeding disorders associated with qualitative or quantitative **abnormalities of the factor VIII molecular complex.** In classical von Willebrand's disease all measurable parameters associated with the factor VIII molecular complex are decreased. They include VIII coagulant activity (VIII:C), ristocetin cofactor activity (VIIIR:RCo), which measures the ability of the antibiotic ristocetin to induce binding of VIII vwf to platelets; and VIII-related antigen (VIIIR:Ag). The bleeding time is usually prolonged. In variants of von Willebrand's disease one or more of the VIII-associated parameters may be normal, yet the clinical syndrome is indistinguishable from classic von Willebrand's disease. Most patients with autosomal dominant von Willebrand's disease have clinically **mild** disease; they experience excessive bleeding with surgery, heavy menstrual periods, and mucous membrane bleeding (GI tract, epistaxis). **Severe** forms, inherited as an autosomal recessive trait, may also cause hemarthroses.

   b. **Treatment.** The blood product of choice is **cryoprecipitate**, since factor VIII concentrate does not correct the prolonged bleeding time. Administration of cryoprecipitate will result in a sustained rise of VIII:C lasting for 2 to 4 days, yet the bleeding time will remain normal for only 6 hr. In certain surgical procedures administration of cryoprecipitate every few days to maintain normal VIII:C levels will be adequate, whereas other procedures or massive GI bleeding will require more frequently administered cryoprecipitate to maintain a normal bleeding time. The usual dosage of cryoprecipitate is 1 bag of cryoprecipitate per 5 kg weight.

3. **Other congenital coagulopathies** are quite rare. Bleeding episodes require the administration of fresh, frozen plasma or other **blood products** rich in the deficient coagulation factor.

D. **Acquired Coagulopathies**

   1. **Disseminated intravascular coagulation (DIC)**

      a. **Etiology and clinical presentation.** DIC is a dynamic pathologic process triggered by the **activation of** the **hemostatic mechanism**; it usually results in lowered levels of clotting factors and in excessive fibrinolysis, both of which may lead to clinical bleeding. On the other hand, fibrin deposition may cause micro- or macrothrombosis and sometimes hemolytic anemia due to red cell fragmentation. DIC may be encountered in many clinical settings; **acute DIC** occurs with shock, sepsis, certain complications of pregnancy (amniotic fluid emboli and abruptiae placentae), hemolytic transfusion reactions, and massive tissue damage (burns, crush injury, and heat stroke). **Subacute or chronic DIC** may occur in leukemia, liver disease, or in patients with solid tumors and vasculitis.

The **clinical and laboratory manifestations** in a given patient **are extremely variable** and not only depend on the DIC but also on the underlying disorder. The intensity and duration of the activation of blood coagulation, the state of the fibrinolytic system, the rate of the blood flow, the state of the liver function, bone marrow, and the macrophage system will all influence the clinical and laboratory picture.

b. **Laboratory findings** in massive **acute** DIC will usually include thrombocytopenia, hypofibrinogenemia, increased fibrin split products, and variable decreases in clotting factors. **Subacute** or chronic DIC is much more difficult to diagnose, but soluble fibrin as measured by the **protamine gel test** will usually be present.

c. **Therapy. Prompt treatment of the underlying disease** and elimination of the trigger mechanism are the most important parts of therapy. Additional treatment must be individualized, and generalizations are difficult to make. A good understanding of the pathophysiology and of the natural history of the underlying disease contributes a great deal to logical and rational management of these patients. Frequently repeated clinical and laboratory evaluations are essential. If a patient is **actively bleeding** and has markedly decreased platelets, fibrinogen, and other clotting factors, **replacement therapy** is indicated with fresh, frozen plasma, platelets, and cryoprecipitate. Ten bags of cryoprecipitate provide 2 to 3 g of fibrinogen in relatively little volume and should therefore always be given in settings of profound hypofibrinogenemia. **Heparin** is seldom indicated but may be considered if adequate replacement therapy does not decrease the bleeding in acute DIC, if the patient has purpura fulminans or acral ischemia, and in patients with acute progranulocytic leukemia. Heparin should be administered by continuous intravenous infusion in the lowest doses that correct the process (usually 500–1,000 U/hr).

2. **Vitamin K deficiency**

a. **Etiology.** Vitamin K is a cofactor for the cocarboxylation of the coagulation proteins II, VII, IX, and X. Noncarboxylated proteins exhibit greatly decreased enzyme activity. Vitamin K deficiency is very **common**, especially in hospitalized patients. Conditions leading to vitamin K deficiency include obstructive liver disease; conditions that alter the patient's normal intestinal flora such as treatment with antibiotics; malabsorption syndromes; and nutritional deficiency, although the last is rarely the sole cause of significant vitamin K deficiency.

b. **Diagnosis.** Empirical administration of vitamin K for patients with a prolonged prothrombin time is an acceptable practice. Factor assays (II, VII, IX, and X) are rarely necessary to support the diagnosis.

c. **Treatment** of vitamin K deficiency always includes the **administration of vitamin K.** Dosage, route, and type of vitamin K depend on the clinical setting. Spontaneous bleeding is rare, unless the prothrombin time is more than 30 sec. Patients with significant bleeding should receive 10 to 20 mg of vitamin K_1, intravenously. This will correct the prothrombin time in 4 to 8 hr. Intravenous vitamin K_1 should be administered slowly (1 mg/min) to avoid hypotension. Serious hemorrhages will also require the administration of **fresh, frozen plasma** (15 ml/kg). In life-threatening situations, **prothrombin complex concentrate** (3–4 vials) will normalize hemostasis more rapidly and completely, but it carries a higher risk of hepatitis. In vitamin K-deficient persons without obvious bleeding or in those needing correction prior to surgery, 3 to 5 mg of vitamin K_1 should be given subcutaneously to correct the deficiency. Individuals who require chronic vitamin K replacement should receive the water-soluble vitamin K_3, which can be given orally.

3. Liver Disease

a. Clinical presentation. Since most proteins involved in hemostasis are produced in the liver, **severe liver damage** is usually associated with marked abnormalities in the hemostatic mechanism. Besides decreased production of clotting factors, formation of dysfunctional fibrinogen, activation of clotting mechanism leading to DIC, and enhanced fibrinolytic activity may aggravate the hemorrhagic diathesis. In addition, patients with certain types of liver disease are often thrombocytopenic and may have abnormal platelet function. These hemostatic derangements may cause spontaneous hemorrhage but more often aggravate bleeding from anatomical sites such as varices, or gastritis.

b. Treatment of significant bleeding should be attempted with **fresh, frozen plasma** (15–20 ml/kg). Prothrombin complex concentrates are **contraindicated** in most settings, since they may cause local thrombosis or frank DIC. This is partially because patients with liver disease have decreased levels of antithrombin III. Parenteral vitamin K_1 should also be given (5 mg subcutaneously for 3 days), although most patients will not respond.

4. Acquired anticoagulants. Acquired hemorrhagic diatheses due to specific depressants of clotting factors are relatively rare, but they may be associated with serious bleeding.

a. Antibodies that destroy factor VIII:C are clinically most important. They occur in postpartum women, after penicillin exposure, in patients with rheumatoid arthritis and systemic lupus erythematosus (SLE), as well as in otherwise healthy elderly persons. Some individuals may lose their inhibitor spontaneously; more than 50% will respond to steroids and/or immunosuppressive agents. Acute bleeding episodes are treated in similar fashion as those in hemophiliacs with inhibitors.

b. Acquired von Willebrand's disease is extremely rare; it occurs in patients with SLE, gammopathies, lymphomas, and solid tumors. Factor VIII:C and FVIII vW are both decreased, and antibodies to FVIII vW have been observed in some but not all patients. Treatment is that of the underlying disorder.

c. The **"lupus anticoagulant"** is **quite common**; it occurs in at least 10% of patients with **SLE**, in other autoimmune disorders, and with certain drugs, especially chlorpromazine and ampicillin. The anticoagulant is an antibody directed against certain phospholipids in platelets; it prolongs the APTT, but does not cause clinical bleeding. On the contrary, its presence in the blood is associated with an **increased thrombotic tendency**. Therapy should be directed at the underlying disorder. Surgery can be safely performed in the presence of the inhibitor, unless the patient also has a platelet functional defect.

E. Quantitative Platelet Disorders

1. **Thrombocytopenia** results from either decreased platelet production or increased peripheral utilization. **A bone marrow examination should always be performed** unless there is no doubt at all about the etiology of the thrombocytopenia. In a normal marrow, approximately 8 megakaryocytes are found per spicule; decreased numbers suggest decreased platelet production, whereas normal or increased numbers imply increased platelet consumption. One needs to keep in mind, however, that more than one factor may contribute to the patient's thrombocytopenia.

   a. Disorders causing thrombocytopenia primarily **by decreased platelet production** include aplastic anemia, drugs, and replacement of marrow by solid tumors. Indications for platelet transfusions will be discussed in section G.

   b. Thrombocytopenia with splenomegaly. Whereas a healthy spleen sequesters about 25% of all platelets released from the marow, massively enlarged spleens may pool up to 90% of the platelets. If marrow function is normal, this redistribution, however, seldom causes severe thrombocytopenia ($<50,000/\mu l$) or bleeding. Splenectomy should be reserved for those rare patients who have unmanageable bleeding.

   c. **Disorders causing thrombocytopenia primarily by increased peripheral destruction include:**

      (1) DIC (see D.1.)

      (2) **Idiopathic thrombocytopenic purpura (ITP).** ITP is an autoimmune disorder in which platelets react with an autoantibody, specific for the platelet membrane, and are destroyed by macrophages. The **diagnosis** of ITP is often **reached by excluding** other disorders of peripheral platelet utilization, such as thrombotic thrombocytopenic purpura (TTP), DIC, or a huge spleen. Documentation of platelet antibodies may be helpful, but these tests are still not universally available. ITP exists in two forms: The **acute self-limited form** following viral infections (e.g., measles) occurs most often in children; presumably it is due to absorption of viral antigen-antibody complexes onto platelets. The **chronic recurrent form** is primarily a disorder of young and middle-aged women, sometimes suffering from SLE. More than 25% of elderly persons with ITP have or will eventually develop lymphoproliferative malignancies.

Steroids are used to treat ITP. Adult patients should be treated with prednisone (1–2 mg/kg/day) until the platelet count reaches 100,000/μl, at which time it should be tapered slowly.

Splenectomy is indicated for those patients who do not respond to prednisone in 2 weeks, if prednisone cannot be decreased without recurrence of thrombocytopenia, or if the patient suffers a relapse within a few weeks. **Life-threatening bleeding at presentation**, although rare, requires immediate splenectomy. Platelets should be available at the time of surgery, but only administered if the patient still bleeds excessively after the splenic artery has been ligated.

Following splenectomy, 25% of patients will remain thrombocytopenic; steroids should be restarted, but if the platelet count cannot be maintained in the safe range with 10 mg of prednisone per day, **immunosuppressive agents** [cyclophosphamide (Cytoxan®) 2–3 mg/kg/day, or azathioprine 2–3 mg/kg/day] should be added. **Vinka alkaloids** (vincristine 0.025 mg/kg, vinblastine 0.125 mg/kg) every 7 to 10 days may improve the platelet count transiently but rarely result in long-lasting remissions.

Patients with chronic ITP and platelet counts exceeding 50,000/μl or patients with even lower platelets without bleeding should not be treated at all. Patients with refractory ITP who need to undergo surgery should be prepared with high doses of steroids, and those who never responded to steroids may achieve a transient rise in their platelet count with **intravenous gamma globulin** (0.4 g/kg daily for 5 days).

(3) Thrombocytopenia in sepsis. Thrombocytopenia is an early sign of bacterial sepsis. It may be due to DIC, aggregation of platelets by bacteria, or adhesion of platelets to damaged subendothelium. Bacteria-antibacteria immune complexes which attach to Fc receptors on platelets may contribute significantly to the thrombocytopenia. Treatment should be directed toward controlling the bacteremia, but platelet transfusions may be helpful in patients with significant bleeding, despite the fact that administered platelets are usually utilized within a few hours.

(4) Posttransfusion purpura is a very rare complication usually seen in multiparous PLA-1-negative women who have received blood containing PLA-1-positive platelets. Profound thrombocytopenia develops 7 to 10 days after the transfusion; the mechanism is not clear. Treatment is very difficult, since all platelets are incompatible.

(5) Drug-induced thrombocytopenia may be due to decreased platelet production but is more often immune-mediated. Drug-induced thrombocytopenia is relatively rare, but virtually any drug can been implicated. The drugs shown to have more than a rare association with thrombocytopenia include quinine, quinidine, heroin (cut with quinine), digitoxin, heparin, gold, penicillin, sulfamonides, and diuretics. **All drugs should be discontinued** in patients who develop sudden thrombocytopenia, unless another etiology for the thrombocytopenia has clearly been established. Drug-induced immune thrombocytopenia usually subsides within a few days but may persist for several weeks. Documentation of drug sensitivity in vitro is desirable but frequently difficult because available tests are either too insensitive, nonspecific, or difficult to perform. **Corticosteroids** do not lessen the duration of thrombocytopenia, but should be administered because of their capillary protective effect. Platelet transfusions should be reserved for those patients with life-threatening bleeding. Once recovery occurs, rechallenging with the suspected drug is not indicated, since the ensuing severe thrombocytopenia poses more risks than is gained from establishing a definitive diagnosis.

(6) **TTP** is a rare syndrome of uncertain etiology characterized by thrombocytopenia, microangiopathic hemolytic anemia, fluctuating neurologic symptoms, fever, and renal failure. The primary **histopathologic findings** are intravascular, hyaline microthrombi, but the pathophysiologic events leading to their development are not known. Most cases of TTP are fulminant, but chronic relapsing forms have also been recognized in recent years. Other conditions that have preceded or are associated with TTP include pregnancy, recent immunization, and viral diseases.

Appropriate therapy for TTP is still very **controversial.** Numerous treatment modalities have been used in various combinations; since controlled trials have never been performed, no regimen has been shown to be clearly superior. The fact that TTP may represent a syndrome of diverse etiologies adds to the difficulty in evaluating treatment modalities. **Steroids** alone are effective in less than 15% of the cases but are usually added to other treatment modalities; they may decrease vessel wall inflammation and may prolong platelet survival in TTP. **Antiaggregating agents**: Two small series of patients responding to aspirin and dipyridamole (Persantine®) alone have been reported, but most patients received antiaggregating agents in combination with other modes of therapy. The overall response rate was slightly more than 50%.

The best response rates, approaching 80%, have been obtained with **plasma exchange**, i.e., removing the patient's plasma and replacing it with fresh, frozen plasma. Frequency of exchanges and amounts to be exchanged have not been clearly determined, but most experts recommend daily exchanges of 3 to 5 liters. **Administration of fresh, frozen plasma** without removal of the patient's plasma has also been shown to be effective in approximately 50% of all patients; the reported series are small and most responders were women. Proponents of this therapy attribute its success to the replacement of an inhibitor of a platelet-aggregating substance felt to be missing in patients with TTP. Recently, **vincristine** has been shown to be effective in small groups of patients. This observation needs to be supported with further studies; the reason for the efficacy of vincristine in TTP is presently not known.

The role of **splenectomy** in TTP remains **controversial.** In combination with steroids and antiaggregating agents the overall response rate is approximately 50%. It has been suggested that the benefits of splenectomy may be because of intraoperative transfusions rather than to the removal of the spleen per se. In addition, patient selection may have influenced reported response rates, as severe neurologic impairment or fulminant clinical course may mitigate against an operative intervention. **Platelet transfusions** are contraindicated in any case of suspected TTP, since they may cause neurologic deterioration. Based on all available data, the therapeutic approach outlined in Table 2 is suggested.

2. **Increased platelets**

 a. **Reactive thrombocytosis** occurs commonly with solid tumors, inflammation, hemolysis, the postsplenectomy state, active bleeding, and iron deficiency. Even platelet counts exceeding 1,000,000/μl usually do not lead to bleeding or thrombosis.

 b. **Thrombocythemia.** Patients with myeloproliferative disorders often have strikingly increased platelet counts resulting from autonomous, increased production of megakaryocytes in the bone marrow; these platelets are abnormal and may cause thrombosis as well as bleeding. **Specific therapy** to lower platelet counts exceeding 500,000/μl should be initiated with hydroxyurea or ^{32}P. When the patient's platelet count exceeds 1 million, **antiaggregating agents** (aspirin 325 mg/day and dipyridamole 25 mg q.i.d.) may prevent thrombosis. Patients with diffuse hemorrhage should undergo emergency platelet pheresis.

F. **Qualitative Platelet Defects**

 1. **Congenital disorders.** In **Bernard Soulier syndrome**, platelet adhesion is decreased and platelets do not aggregate with **ristocetin**, despite normal plasma levels of factor VIII vWF. The platelets lack a receptor protein for factor VIII vWF, which appears to reside in the glycoprotein Ib fraction of the platelet membrane. In **Glanzmann's thrombasthenia** platelets do not aggregate at all with ADP, epinephrine, or collagen; glycoprotein fractions IIb and IIIa, which appear to be of importance in platelet-to-platelet interactions, are absent from platelet membranes. These rare, autosomal recessive disorders are often associated with severe bleeding episodes. On the other hand, **storage pool defects** are clinically mild. Platelets contain decreased amounts of ADP and serotonin in storage granules, secondary aggregation with ADP and epinephrine is absent, and response to collagen decreased. Persons with congenital platelet function defects may require **platelet transfusions** for significant bleeding and before surgical procedures. Five platelet concentrates/M² (or the

TABLE 2. *Treatment of TTP*

	Agent	Dose
At time of diagnosis:	Prednisone	1–2 mg/kg/day
	Aspirin	10 mg/kg/day
	Dipyridamole	25 mg q.i.d./day
	Plasma exchange	50 ml/kg/day
If no response in 5 days, add:	Vincristine	1.4 mg/M² q 7 days
If rapid deterioration, consider:	Splenectomy	—

number of platelets calculated to provide 80,000 platelets/µl) will usually correct the bleeding time.

2. **Acquired platelet functional defects.** An ever-increasing number of clinical disorders have been found to be associated with abnormal platelet functions. This may result in spontaneous bleeding, easy bruising, or excessive bleeding during surgery. Therefore, a template bleeding time should always be performed in patients with known underlying disorders who are to undergo major surgery or invasive procedures. **Uremia** causes serious bleeding, but the basic platelet defect is not well understood. Platelet factor 3 dysfunction has, however, been identified. Transient correction of the bleeding time has been observed after intravenous or intranasal desmopressin. Platelet function defects in **paraproteinemia** respond best to plasmapheresis. The **acquired storage pool disorder** has become a frequently recognized entity characterized by platelet functional abnormalities similar to those observed in congenital storage pool disorders. It has been postulated that a variety of substances, including antibodies and immune-complexes, can attach to platelets, initiate activation and the release reaction, and thus result in circulating platelets that are depleted in storage granule contents. This platelet functional defect is frequently observed in systemic lupus erythematosus and in chronic ITP. Therapy should be directed toward the underlying disorder.

3. **Drug-induced platelet function abnormalities.** ASA causes irreversible inhibition of cyclooxygenase, an enzyme required for prostaglandin formation. Thus, the platelet defect persists as long as the platelets circulate; the bleeding time may remain prolonged for up to 4 days. Certain emergency surgical procedures may require the administration of normal platelets. Other nonsteroidal anti-inflammatory agents reversibly inhibit the enzyme cyclooxygenase, and withdrawal of the drug results in immediate correction of the bleeding time. **Carbenicillin** causes significant platelet functional abnormalities and should therefore be **avoided** in patients with severe thrombocytopenia, since it may worsen their bleeding diathesis. Large doses of **penicillin G** and other penicillin derivatives, especially ticarcillin and piperacillin, may cause less severe platelet functional defects.

G. **Platelet Transfusions** Platelet counts in excess of 50,000/µl are usually not associated with significant bleeding, and severe spontaneous bleeding is rare in patients with platelets over 20,000/µl (in the absence of other hemostatic abnormalities). Patients with thrombocytopenia should be protected against trauma. In severe thrombocytopenia (<20,000/µl), intramuscular injections, enemas, and even toothbrushing may cause bleeding.

Random donor platelets are prepared in the blood bank from single units of blood. Each platelet concentrate contains 5.5 to 10×10^{10} platelets. Platelets may also be obtained by **pheresis of platelets** from appropriate donors. These platelets should be **reserved for** recipients who have developed potent antibodies to human lymphocyte antigens (HLA) or platelet-specific antigens and who have become refractory to random donor platelets.

1. **Indications for platelet transfusions** include: **significant bleeding**, with platelet counts of less than 50,000/µl; bleeding due to **certain types of abnormal**

platelet function (see I.F.); **major surgery** in patients with less than 80,000 platelets/µl; and, **prophylactic** platelet transfusions.

The use of platelets in **nonbleeding patients** undergoing induction and consolidation therapy for acute leukemia or other intensive chemotherapy remains **controversial**. Repeated exposure to random donor platelets leads to the development of alloantibodies (HLA and platelet specific) and renders patients refractory to random platelet transfusions when required for bleeding episodes later on. Initial use of HLA compatible platelets, however, remains **controversial**. Recent studies were unable to document the prevention of alloimmunization despite the sole use of HLA matched platelets, but more studies will be needed to support these findings. Advocates of prophylactic platelet transfusions point out that a hemorrhage, especially into the CNS, may be lethal before platelets can be administered. Available literature does not provide enough data on a safe level of platelets, since many factors other than the platelet count influence the risk of bleeding. Serious spontaneous bleeding is nonetheless rare, unless the platelet count is below 20,000/µl. We recommend prophylactic platelet support for thrombocytopenia below 20,000 µl/ml.

2. **Dosage.** One random donor platelet concentrate should increase the platelet count by 5,000 to 10,000/µl/M². The normal half-life of infused platelets should be 4 days; fever, infections, hepatosplenomegaly, vascular damage, and preformed platelet antibodies all shorten their survival.

3. **Monitoring.** A platelet count should be obtained 1 hr after the transfusion. An increment of less than 5,000 platelets/µl/M² body surface/platelet concentrate is considered poor and is usually due to potent preformed HLA antibodies (unless the patient has massive DIC or potent autoantibodies). Single-donor platelets from relatives or from an HLA donor pool should be considered if the patient has a poor increment with two consecutive random donor platelet transfusions.

4. **Complications** of platelet transfusions include fever and chills, usually due to leukoagglutinins and transmission of hepatitis.

H. **Vascular Purpura**   Vascular purpura comprises a heterogeneous group of conditions that are characterized by easy bruising and spontaneous bleeding, especially into skin and mucous membranes. **Hereditary abnormalities are rare**; they include hereditary hemorrhagic telangiectasia (Rendu-Osler-Weber) and inborn errors of collagen biosynthesis such as the Ehlers-Danlos (rubber man) syndrome. **Acquired vascular disorders** include conditions in which the basic structure of the vessel wall is altered by old age (senile purpura), by lack of ascorbic acid (scurvy), by steroids, or by amyloid deposition. The most frequently encountered vascular bleeding phenomena are associated with **infections**, either through the action of microbial toxins (e.g., meningococcemia) or through immunologically mediated processes. **Immunologic mechanisms** leading to vascular purpura include disorders associated with immune complex formation (SLE, essential mixed cryoglobulinemia), and those due to delayed hypersensitivity, sometimes referred to as allergic purpura seen with drugs and microbia (leukocytoclastic vasculitis). In addition, acquired vascular disorders may be caused by one of the so-called **"psychogenic purpuras,"** which include autoerythrocyte sensitization, autosensitization to DNA, as well as hysterical and factitious bleeding. There are no adequate in vitro tests to evaluate these disorders; the template bleeding time may be mildly abnormal, and additional platelet function tests may be required to differentiate between vascular and platelet functional defects. However, it is important to recognize the clinical settings that lead to vascular purpura so that unnecessary platelet functional testing can be avoided.

II. **THROMBOSIS**   Although great strides have been made in recent years to understand the pathophysiologic events that lead to thrombosis, simple, sensitive, and specific laboratory tools are still not available to establish the diagnosis of thrombosis, or help to identify those persons at increased risk of developing thrombosis (by some experts referred to as the "hypercoagulable state"). Accurate diagnosis of acute thrombotic episodes—frequently requiring invasive procedures—is, however, very important, since therapy is associated with significant morbidity.

A. **Diagnosis**

1. **Venous thrombosis.** Clinical signs of pain, edema, change in skin temperature, venous dilatation, and the Homans' sign are very unreliable and probably detect only half of the thromboses diagnosed by venography. **Venography** is considered to be the most accurate means of establishing the diagnosis of deep vein thrombosis (DVT), but cannot always determine the age of the thrombus. The major **side effect** of venography is thrombosis, but this occurs in less than 5% of patients with present imaging techniques. **Impedance plethysmography** is a sensitive and specific noninvasive diagnostic tool for proximal venous thrombosis in the thigh, but quite insensitive in the detection of calf vein thrombosis. False negative results may be encountered with nonobstructing thrombi or in the presence of collateral vessels. False positive results may be obtained in the presence of severe peripheral vascular disease and congestive failure. **Doppler ultrasound** is also sensitive and quite specific in experienced hands; false negative and positive results occur in similar settings as with plethysmography. **Fibrinogen leg scanning** is not very useful, since it is only sensitive in detecting calf vein thrombosis. The primary source of pulmonary emboli is probably from thigh rather than calf vein thrombi.

2. **Peripheral arterial occlusion.** Clinical methods such as peripheral pulses and flow assessments are inaccurate; yet plethysmography and Doppler ultrasound often provide enough information about the location and degree of occlusion to perform surgery without the need of angiography.

3. **Laboratory tests for thrombosis and prethrombotic states**

    a. No blood test, currently available, can support the diagnosis of active, local thrombosis. Sensitive methods measuring fibrin formation and proteolysis (such as radioimmunoassay for fragment E and fibrinopeptide A) have recently been developed. Although normal values help to exclude acute thrombosis, elevated levels are not specific for thrombosis.

    b. In persons with a **suspected congenital thrombotic** tendency, AT-III, plasminogen and protein C should be quantitated by chromogenic and immunologic methods. Abnormal fibrinogens are detected with the thrombin and Reptilase® time (see I. B.).

c. Elevated levels of PF_4 and βTG are observed when platelets undergo activation and release in the circulation and have been found in patients with **arterial thrombosis**; the sensitivity and specificity of these tests are still unknown. At present these tests do not help in the management of individual patients.

d. Certain clinical disorders are associated with **hemostatic abnormalities** that may predispose to thrombosis. Antilhrombin III (AT-III) levels may be low in patients with the nephrotic syndrome and in women taking birth control pills. AT-III and protein C are usually decreased in liver disease.

B. Congenital Thrombotic Diatheses   To date only a few congenital abnormalities in hemostatic parameters have been associated with a lifelong thrombotic tendency.

1. **AT-III deficiency** is an autosomal dominant disorder associated with recurrent venous and/or arterial thrombosis. AT-III is an α_2-globulin that inhibits the activated serine proteases IIa, Xa, IXa, and XIa by binding to the active serine residues, thus playing an important role in the prevention of excessive activation of the clotting sequences which may lead to thrombosis. This disorder may be due to decreased production of normal AT-III or a dysfunctional molecule. Ideally, the **diagnosis** should be established when the patient is not receiving anticoagulants nor is suffering from an acute thrombosis. Warfarin may raise AT-III levels, whereas active thrombosis and prolonged heparin therapy lower measurable plasma AT-III. All family members need to be tested to identify those with the deficiency before they develop a thrombotic episode. All affected persons need appropriate anticoagulants when other risk factors are present, e.g., pregnancy, the postoperative period, or prolonged bed rest. Once they develop a thrombotic episode, lifelong treatment with warfarin is probably indicated.

2. **Protein C deficiency.** Protein C is a vitamin K-dependent glycoprotein that inactivates the active forms of factors VIII:C and V; it also generates a potent fibrinolytic activity. Familial protein C deficiency is probably rare, but its incidence is not known, since few laboratories are currently able to measure protein C. Prophylactic anticoagulants are indicated for those persons who have a history of thrombotic episodes.

3. **Dysfunctional plasminogens and fibrinogens** resulting in inadequate fibrinolysis have recently been identified in several families suffering from frequent, recurrent venous thromboses. These disorders are probably rare, and the best management has not yet been established.

C. Treatment of Peripheral Thrombosis

1. **Superficial thrombophlebitis** is generally controlled with local heat, elevation, and anti-inflammatory agents such as indomethacin.

2. **DVT.** Although many specific clinical issues in the treatment of thromboembolism remain to be answered by further clinical trials, the following recommendations seem appropriate based on results obtained from recent clinical trials. **Proximal DVT** should be treated **with fibrinolytic agents**, especially in younger persons suffering their first thrombosis. All other persons should receive **heparin** for 10 days. Doses, routes of administration, and laboratory monitoring of heparin and the fibrinolytic agents are discussed in detail in

section III. **Calf vein thrombosis** should be treated with a course of heparin despite a low incidence of pulmonary emboli and postphlebitic syndrome, since extension of thrombosis into more proximal veins is frequently seen.

The initial episode of proximal DVT requires treatment with an anticoagulant for 6 months; 2 months' treatment appears to be sufficient for calf vein thrombosis. Warfarin remains the agent of choice. Recent studies suggest that less intense therapy resulting in prolongation of PT to 1.5 times the control may be as effective as more intensive therapy (PT 2.0–2.5 times the control), yet associated with less bleeding. Subcutaneous heparin in doses that result in prolongation of APTT to 1.5 times the control value should be used during pregnancy and in other persons where warfarin is contraindicated. Most persons who suffer a recurrent DVT while receiving adequate anticoagulants or shortly after discontinuation of therapy require long-term treatment with anticoagulants, at least for several years.

3. **Peripheral arterial thromboembolism.** Most peripheral arterial occlusive thrombi or emboli require either a **conventional surgical** procedure, a **transluminal embolectomy**, or an **angioplasty**. Low-dose fibrinolytic agents (5,000 units of streptokinase per hour) administered directly into the clot combined with transluminal angioplasty have shown promising preliminary results, but at present can be recommended only for centers with special interest in this therapeutic approach. Patients with peripheral arterial thromboembolism require long-term treatment with warfarin.

D. **Prevention of DVT** A number of clinical risk factors for the development of venous thrombosis have been identified; they include advanced age, previous thromboembolism, presence of malignancy, cardiac failure, prolonged immobility, obesity, varicose veins, hip fractures, and certain surgical procedures, especially orthopedic surgery of the lower limbs and extensive pelvic surgery.

1. **Low-dose heparin.** Low-dose heparin has been evaluated most extensively in **surgical settings**, where it appears to be effective in preventing DVT and pulmonary emboli in general and gynecological surgery, but not in hip or prostatic surgery. It should also be considered in **elderly** patients who are placed on bed rest, in those with congestive heart failure, and maybe in patients recovering from myocardial infarction.

Current **dosage** recommendations are 5,000 units subcutaneously every 8 to 12 hr. A highly concentrated form of heparin (20,000–40,000 U/ml) should be injected rapidly through a 25-gauge needle, and pressure should be applied at the injection site to minimize hematoma formation. **Laboratory** monitoring is not necessary, and major bleeding episodes are not encountered with this regimen.

2. **Dextran** appears to be as effective as low-dose heparin in general surgery and may also prevent DVT associated with hip fractures and orthopedic surgery in the lower extremities. Hypersensitivity and volume overload are the most serious **side effects**; clinically important bleeding is not encountered.

3. **Pneumatic leg compression** has shown to be of benefit in the prevention of DVT but has not been evaluated in the prevention of fatal pulmonary embolism. The major advantage resides in the lack of side effects.

   4. Antiplatelet agents have generally not been useful in the prevention of venous thrombosis. Beneficial effects from ASA in one large group of patients who underwent hip surgery need to be supported by further studies.

III. ANTICOAGULANTS

A. Heparin   Heparins are a nonhomogeneous group of sulfated mucopolysaccharides obtained from animal tissues. Heparin exerts its anticoagulant effect by potentiating the action of AT-III. The metabolic fate of heparin has not been fully elucidated, but removal from the circulation appears to occur primarily in the **reticular endothelial system**; enzymatic desulfation in the **liver** may also play some role. Severe renal disease affects elimination of heparin only slightly. Heparin **does not cross the placental** barrier.

Most **preparations** in clinical use are sodium salts obtained from porcine intestine, or bovine lung, containing 1,000, 5,000, 10,000, 20,000, or 40,000 USP U/ml. Calcium salts of heparin are also manufactured.

   1. Administration and laboratory control. In the treatment of acute, active thrombosis, heparin is best administered by **continuous intravenous infusion.** A loading dose of 5,000 to 10,000 units by bolus should be followed by 1,000 to 2,000 U/hr administered by mechanical infusion pump. The concentration of heparin should not exceed 20,000 U/liter of fluid, since mechanical pump failure during the infusion of a more concentrated solution can lead to massive overdose and serious bleeding. **Therapy should be monitored**; although a number of tests are available including the thrombin clotting time and activated clotting time, most hospitals use the APTT.

   Therapeutic levels of heparin (0.2–0.4 U/ml) usually result in APTTs between 1.5 to 2.0 times the control. Initially, the APTT should be **measured frequently** and the infusion rate adjusted accordingly; daily monitoring is advised once a steady dose has been established. In most patients, an adequate anticoagulant effect can be achieved with doses of between 20,000 and 30,000 U/24 hr. **Higher doses** of heparin may be needed in pulmonary embolism and possibly in patients with severe AT-III deficiency. For **long-term treatment** of venous thrombosis, heparin is administered s.c. every 12 hr in doses that prolong the PTT to 1.5 times the control value, measured 6 hr after a dose of heparin. This is the **treatment of choice for DVT during pregnancy.**

   2. Prevention and treatment of bleeding. Hemorrhage constitutes the primary toxicity of heparin. Factors **increasing the risk** of bleeding include age, other hemostatic abnormalities, and trauma. Patients on full-dose heparin should receive the minimum of invasive procedures, no intramuscular injections or drugs that interfere with platelet function. It is advisable to check hematocrits periodically and perform stool examinations for occult blood. When significant bleeding occurs, heparin should be stopped and the APTT checked. With therapeutic levels heparin no longer causes a prolongation of the APTT 4 hr after cessation of therapy, since it has a half-life of only 60 min.

   In rare occasions of life-threatening bleeding, **protamine sulfate** can be administered, which will neutralize heparin instantaneously. One mg of protamine sulfate will neutralize 100 units of heparin; the dose of protamine sulfate will depend on the amount of heparin in the circulation at that particular moment. Immediately after a bolus of 10,000 units, 100 mg of protamine is needed, but 60 min later 50 mg will be sufficient. If heparin is given as continuous intravenous infusion, one should consider that half of the amount given during the last hour needs to be neutralized (i.e., if the patient receives 1,000 U/hr, 5 mg of protamine is needed). Since protamine possesses anticoagulant properties itself, excessive dosages should never be given. Effective neutralization should be confirmed by performing an APTT. Protamine sulfate should be administered very slowly—50 mg over 10 min—to prevent hypotensive episodes.

3. **Side Effects. Severe thrombocytopenia** occurs in probably less than 2% of patients receiving porcine heparin, but is more frequently encountered with bovine heparin. **Thrombocytopenia may be associated with the development of new arterial or venous thrombi**, a complication associated with high mortality and morbidity. Periodic platelet counts should therefore be performed and heparin discontinued if the platelet count drops below 80,000/μl. The best management of such patients is not known, but warfarin and antiaggregating agents are presently recommended by most experts. **Prolonged administration** of heparin has been reported to cause osteoporosis and suppression of aldosterone secretion. Hypersensitivity reactions are rare.

B. **Oral Anticoagulants** Oral anticoagulants are a group of low molecular weight compounds that act in the **liver** by interfering with the vitamin K-dependent cocarboxylation of factors II, VII, IX, and X. The onset of action of the oral anticoagulants is delayed until the unaffected vitamin K-dependent factors are cleared from the circulation. Factor VII activity will be diminished in 8 to 12 hr, since it has the shortest half-life, but it will take 5 to 7 days until therapeutic anticoagulation has been reached, since the half-lives of factors II and X are greater than 48 hr.

Warfarin is the most commonly used oral anticoagulant. Tablets of 2 mg, 2½ mg, 5 mg, 7½ mg, and 10 mg, each in a different color, are available. Warfarin **therapy** is initiated with a dose of 10 mg/day for 3 to 5 days followed by a maintenance dose of 2 to 10 mg/day. The maintenance dose is determined by the patient's PT, which should be performed daily until it remains stable at about 2.0 times the normal control value.

1. **Indications**

a. In **proximal** DVT warfarin is started 5 to 7 days before heparin is discontinued and is given for 6 months. Two months may be sufficient to prevent recurrence in calf vein thrombosis. Pulmonary embolism requires treatment for 6 months. Recurrence of thrombosis or embolism shortly after warfarin has been discontinued or while on "therapeutic" dosage of warfarin requires long-term anticoagulation. Patients with congenital hemostatic abnormalities predisposing to thrombosis require lifelong anticoagulation therapy following their first thrombotic episode.

b. **Cerebrovascular disease.** Long-term oral anticoagulants may be indicated in patients with transient ischemic attacks.

c. **Cardiac embolism.** Oral anticoagulants reduce the incidence of systemic embolization in patients with valvular rheumatic heart disease and with prosthetic heart valves.

d. Peripheral arterial disease. Long-term oral anticoagulants are indicated after acute thromboembolic episodes.

2. **Contraindications.** Oral anticoagulants are contraindicated in **pregnancy**, since they cross the placental barrier and may cause serious fetal hemorrhage, and in **breast feeding women**, since they may enter the milk. They should be withheld in patients with uncontrolled **hypertension** or in patients who have had **recent CNS** or **eye surgery**; relative contraindications include other hemostatic defects, GI lesions such as varices or peptic ulcer. In addition, patients demonstrating inability or unwillingness to cooperate should not be placed on oral anticoagulants.

3. Factors adversely affecting the degree of anticoagulation may lead to either serious bleeding or subtherapeutic anticoagulation. **Changes** in liver function, excessive alcohol intake, a change in diet, and alterations in the normal bowel flora which lead to reduced absorption of vitamin K may all result in serious bleeding. **A variety of drugs may potentiate or inhibit the effect of warfarin** by causing changes in drug absorption, metabolism, or binding of the drug to albumin. The most important interactions are listed in Table 3. Effects of the same drug may vary from patient to patient, therefore, any drug change should be closely supervised by frequent PT determinations.

4. **Management of excessive coumadin effect and bleeding. Bleeding** may occur in the face of a PT in the therapeutic range; in this case a local source should be sought, especially if the bleeding is from the GI or genitourinary (GU) tract. Bleeding in the presence of a markedly prolonged PT generally does not warrant a search for an anatomical lesion. Besides the GI or GU tract, hemorrhage may occur into the retroperitoneal space, the adrenal, CNS, or the eye; intracranial hemorrhages may be fatal. **Potentially life-threatening bleeding** associated with a markedly prolonged PT is best managed by the

TABLE 3. *Drug interactions with warfarin*

Potentiate oral anticoagulants	Antagonize oral anticoagulants
Antibiotics	Barbiturates
Alcohol (acute abuse)	Estrogens
Anabolic steroids	Alcohol (chronic abuse)
Cimetidine	Griseofulvin
Clofibrate	Meprobamate
Phenytoin sodium (Dilantin®)	Haloperidol
Salicylates	Rifampin
All nonsteroidal anti-	
inflammatory agents	
Thyroxine	
Propylthiouracil	
Quinine	
Nortriptyline	
Allopurinol	
Ethacrynic acid	
Methyldopa	
Sulfonamides	

administration of prothrombin complex concentrate—one bottle per 10 kg weight can be administered in 15 to 30 min and will completely normalize the hemostatic defect. **Fresh, frozen plasma** carries less hepatitis risk, but a volume requiring several hours to infuse will only partially correct the PT.

If the PT is very much prolonged but bleeding is not life-threatening, 10 mg vitamin K, given intravenously or subcutaneously will correct hemostasis in 6 to 12 hr. Larger dosages are not advisable, since they render the patient refractory to further anticoagulation for up to 2 weeks. If the PT is only slightly outside the therapeutic range and bleeding is not life-threatening, the patient can be managed simply by omitting the next two or three warfarin doses. If the PT is greater than three times the control value, 1 to 2 mg of vitamin K should be administered subcutaneously, even if the patient is not actively bleeding.

5. **Management of patients needing surgery or invasive procedures.** Complete reversal of anticoagulation is often associated with recurrence of thrombotic events, but many surgical and dental procedures can safely be performed when the PT is 1.5 times the control value. If **surgery is elective**, partial normalization of hemostasis is best obtained by omitting one or two doses of warfarin; more rapid correction can be accomplished with very small doses of vitamin K (1–2 mg subcutaneously). **Emergency invasive** procedures are best covered by administering fresh, frozen plasma.

6. **Side effects.** Except for bleeding, toxic effects are rare. Anorexia, nausea, or diarrhea may occur; they are mild but may affect the level of anticoagulation because of changes in food intake and absorption. A hemorrhagic vasculitis is extremely rare, but can result in skin necrosis, especially over the breasts.

C. **Fibrinolytic Agents** Thrombolytic therapy has an advantage in the treatment of thrombotic disorders, since it is capable of **inducing the dissolution** of thrombi. Two plasminogen activators, **streptokinase (SK) and urokinase (UK)** are currently in clinical use. Besides allowing dissolution of thrombi and emboli, they also dissolve hemostatic plugs. In addition, they produce **profound changes** in the hemostatic mechanism caused by circulating plasmin—hypofibrinogenemia, inhibitory fibrin split products, and abnormal function of platelets. This "lytic state" may result in serious spontaneous bleeding.

1. **Indications.** Fibrinolytic agents are indicated for proximal (popliteal, femoral, iliac, axillary, and subclavian) venous thrombosis, massive or symptomatic pulmonary emboli, and arterial occlusions not amenable to surgical repair. The higher cost and greater bleeding risk with fibrinolytic agents compared with other anticoagulants appear to be justified in these clinical settings, since studies have shown that more complete and rapid lysis of clots decreases the incidence of the postphlebitic syndrome and may prevent pulmonary hypertension in patients who suffered pulmonary emboli. However, in **each patient the benefits to be gained must be weighed carefully against the risks**, especially in those considered at increased risk of developing serious bleeding complications.

2. **Contraindications.** The following are **absolute** contraindications: active internal bleeding; any cerebrovascular process, disease, or procedure within 2

months; bacterial endocarditis; and **pregnancy.** The following are considered **relative** contraindications: recent surgical procedures or trauma, major coagulation defects, history of GI lesions, severe hypertension, and remote cerebrovascular events.

3. **Dosage.** In the treatment of systemic thromboembolism, both agents should be initiated with an intravenous loading dose (250,000 units of SK over 30 min; 4,400 U/kg of UK over 10 min), followed by a continuous intravenous infusion (SK 100,000 U/hr; UK 4,400 U/kg/hr). In DVT fibrinolytic agents are administered for 48 to 72 hr; ideally, clinical improvement should be assessed every 24 hr by a noninvasive method such as plethysmography. Pulmonary emboli are treated for 24 hr. Fibrinolytic therapy is **always followed** with full-dose **heparin** for 7 to 10 days.

4. **Laboratory monitoring.** No available test measures what occurs within the clot directly. Laboratory tests are only used to document a lytic state, not to adjust the dosage. The most appropriate tests are **plasminogen** and **antiplasmin** levels. However, the most practical test, since it is readily available, is the TT. The TT should be no longer than 1½ times the control value before initiating therapy; values at least one-half to two times the control value indicate an adequate lytic state; after termination of therapy, values of less than two times the control value should be obtained before heparin is started.

5. **Complications. Bleeding is the only significant complication.** It can be **minimized** by avoiding all unnecessary handling of patients, all vessel punctures, and all agents that interfere with platelet function. Serious bleeding requiring transfusions occurs in less than 10% of patients.

6. **Management of bleeding.** Oozing from compressible puncture sites can be controlled by pressure dressings; more **severe bleeding** requires discontinuation of the lytic therapy, replacement of blood loss with red cells, and replenishing fibrinogen with cryoprecipitate. Antifibrinolytic therapy such as aminocaproic acid (Amicar®) is seldom needed because the half-life of the fibrinolytic agents is very short.

BIBLIOGRAPHY

Bowie, E. J. W., and Owen, C.A. (1980): The significance of abnormal preoperative hemostatic tests. In: *Progress in Hemostasis and Thrombosis*, Vol. 5, edited by E. B. Brown, pp. 179–209. Grune Stratton, New York.

Bukowski, R. M., Hewlett, J. D., Reimer, R. R., Groppe, C. W., Weick, J. K., and Livingston, R. B. (1981): Therapy of thrombotic thrombocytopenic purpura: An overview. *Semin. Thromb. Hemostas.*, 7:1–8.

Feinstein, D. I. (1982): Diagnosis and management of disseminated intravascular coagulation: The role of heparin therapy. *Blood*, 60:284–287.

Flute, P. T. (1979): Clotting abnormalities in liver disease. In: *Progress in Liver Diseases*, Vol. 6, edited by Fenton and Schaffner, pp. 301–312. Grune Stratton, New York.

Hull, R., and Hirsh, J. (1981): Advances and controversies in the diagnosis, prevention, and treatment of venous thromboembolism. In: *Progress in Hematology*, Vol. 7, edited by E. B. Brown, pp. 73–123. Grune Stratton, New York.

Kasper, C. K. (1981): Management of inhibitors to factor VIII. In: *Progress in Hematology*, Vol. 7, edited by E. B. Brown, pp. 143–165, Grune Stratton, New York.

Kelton, J. G., and Hirsh, J. (1980): Bleeding associated with antithrombotic therapy. *Semin. Hematol.*, 17:259–291.

Shapiro, S. S., and Thiagarajan, P. (1982): Lupus anticoagulants. In: *Progress in Hemostasis and Thrombosis*, Vol. 6, edited by T. H. Spaet, pp. 263–285. Grune Stratton, New York.

Sharma, G. V. R., Cella, G., Parisi, A. F., and Sasahara, A. A. (1982): Thrombolytic therapy. *N. Engl. J. Med.*, 306:1268–1276.

Slichter, S. J. (1980): Controversies in platelet transfusion therapy. *Annu. Rev. Med.*, 31:509–540.

Weiss, H. J. (1980): Congenital disorders of platelet function. *Semin. Hematol.*, 17:228–241.

14.

Treatment of Anemia

Thomas J. Meyer

14.

Treatment of Anemia

Anemia is a symptom or sign, not a diagnosis. As such, the treatment of anemia should be undertaken only after a thorough understanding of the underlying pathophysiology of the disease associated with the anemia. In many cases, the treatment of the underlying disease is necessary rather than the treatment of the anemia itself. Sometimes the underlying disease is very simple, as, for example, in the multiparous woman with a poor diet who becomes iron deficient. Sometimes it is very complex and not amenable to definitive treatment, as in the myelodysplastic syndrome. This chapter discusses the symptomatic treatment of anemias and assumes that the reader has thoroughly investigated the underlying condition and has arrived at a proper diagnosis. To emphasize the importance of these principles, when appropriate in each discussion a **warning** paragraph precedes the discussion of therapy. This serves as a checkpoint to remind the reader of pitfalls in the treatment of that form of anemia.

In addition, certain sections have a short paragraph on **monitoring therapy.** These sections point out common problems that develop during the course of therapy when treatment does not result in the expected improvement. The anemias can roughly be divided into anemias of decreased production and anemias of increased destruction (see Table 1).

I. ANEMIAS OF DECREASED PRODUCTION

A. Anemias Secondary to Systemic Disease

1. **Anemia of endocrine disease.** A variety of endocrine diseases are associated with anemia. These include pituitary deficiency, hypothyroidism, Addison's disease, and estrogen excess. The anemia resolves with treatment of the underlying endocrine disorder.

2. **Anemia of chronic disease**

   a. **Warning.** Exclude iron deficiency since this may mimic the anemia of chronic disease or may be associated with it.

   b. This very specific disorder, presumably from a reduced rate of erythropoietin production and/or impaired utilization of iron in a patient with chronic infectious, inflammatory, or malignant disease, is **not treatable** per se. Optimal management of the underlying disease is the only appropriate therapy.

   c. In anemia of chronic disease the **hematocrit** rarely falls below 30%; therefore, if a patient's anemia is lower, another contributing cause should be sought.

TABLE 1. *Classification of anemias*

Anemias of decreased production	Anemias of increased destruction
Systemic disease	Blood loss
Endocrine disorders	Intrinsic RBC abnormalities
Anemia of chronic disease	Membrane disorders
Anemia of renal failure	RBC metabolic and enzyme defects
Nutritional deficits	Hemoglobinopathies
Iron	Paroxysmal nocturnal hemoglobinuria
B$_{12}$	(PNH)
Folate	Extrinsic RBC abnormalities
Bone marrow failure	Antibody-mediated (drug related,
Aplastic anemia	autoimmune, cold agglutinins)
Pure red cell aplasia	RBC fragmentation syndromes
Myelodysplastic and myelophthisic	Bacterial infections, toxins, chemicals,
anemias	drugs
Thalassemia	Hypersplenism
Sideroblastic anemia	Hemolytic transfusion reactions

3. **Anemia of renal failure**

   a. **Warning**

   (1) Exclude **iron deficiency** since uremic patients often have occult gastrointestinal blood loss.

   (2) Exclude **folate deficiency** since hemodialysis removes folate.

   (3) Exclude **inadequate dialysis**, which can worsen anemia.

   b. When the abovementioned causes of anemia in patients with renal failure have been excluded, occasional patients remain symptomatic from anemia (e.g., angina, congestive heart failure, excessive fatigue). A trial of androgen nandrolone decanoate, 3 mg/kg i.m. every 2 weeks, may raise the hematocrit 5 to 6 percentage points.

   c. The **side effects** of this therapy (hirsutism, fluid retention, acne) must be weighed against the symptomatic improvement resulting from the modest increase in hematocrit. Patients who have had bilateral nephrectomies have, in general, lower hematocrits; thus **nephrectomy** should be avoided, if possible, in patients with end-stage renal disease (ESRD). **Androgens** will not raise the hematocrits of these patients. **Blood transfusion** in patients with ESRD should be avoided, since transfusions suppress residual erythropoiesis. Moreover, such transfusions are accompanied by risks (e.g., hepatitis) and unnecessary costs.

B. **Anemias of Decreased RBC Production Secondary to Nutritional Deficits**

   1. **Iron-deficiency** anemia

      a. **Warning**

      (1) Exclude blood loss from a malignancy of the GI tract.

      (2) Aspirin and nonsteroidal anti-inflammatory drugs are frequent causes of GI blood loss.

      (3) Is the patient taking antacids or drinking excessive milk or tea, which interfere with iron absorption?

      (4) Has thalassemia or sideroblastic anemia or lead poisoning been excluded?

(5) Keep iron preparations out of reach of children since iron ingestions may be fatal.

b. Two or three 300-mg tablets of ferrous sulfate, U.S.P. per day, preferably on an empty stomach, provide the maximum absorbed amount of iron (120–180 mg elemental iron). This is the least expensive form of iron therapy, and other salts or slow-release forms offer no advantage. If the patient cannot tolerate iron on an empty stomach, reduce the dose to one to two tablets per day. Although iron administration with food to avoid GI upset is tempting, only a very small percentage is absorbed in this setting. Orange juice with meals may increase food iron absorption, but probably doesn't promote ferrous iron absorption. Liquid iron preparations can be titrated to tolerance and gradually increased until the patient can take full doses of about 180 mg of elemental iron per day. Beware that liquid iron may stain teeth temporarily.

c. If the patient simply cannot (malabsorption, inflammatory bowel disease) or will **not tolerate** oral iron or the on-going iron loss occurs at a rate too rapid for oral iron replacement, **parenteral** iron may be administered. In a patient who can take oral iron and who is not having continued blood loss, parenteral iron confers no advantage over oral iron as to the rate of rise of hematocrit. Iron dextran (Imferon®) and iron sorbitex (Jectofer®) contain 50 mg iron/ml. Both can be administered i.m. but Imferon® can also be given intravenously. The i.m. administration of these drugs may cause skin staining and is uncomfortable; thus the **i.v. route is preferred.** A **test dose** of 0.5 ml diluted in 5 ml of saline and given slowly over 5 min is necessary because rare anaphylactoid reactions may occur. There is no evidence that the i.m. administration has a lower incidence of reactions than the i.v. form. Subsequent doses of 2 to 5 ml per day, given slowly over 5 min to prevent flushing reactions should be administered until the patient has received the total calculated dose. The **formula** for calculating the iron dose in grams is: [normal hemoglobin (15 g/dl) − patient's hemoglobin] × 0.255.

d. **Monitoring therapy**

(1) The **reticulocyte count** should rise in 7 to 10 days. If not, the diagnosis is suspect or the patient is not absorbing (or taking) the therapeutic iron.

(2) Patients may become **folate deficient** when iron is repleted, therefore a complete blood count should be repeated a month after therapy to be certain a megaloblastic anemia has not developed.

(3) Oral iron should be continued for 3 to 4 months after the **hematocrit** has returned to normal to replenish iron stores.

(4) It should be emphasized that some **maternal prenatal vitamins** that contain iron have been shown to have inappropriately low absorption of iron, presumably secondary to the interaction with other minerals contained in the compounds. Thus, mixed vitamin and mineral compounds cannot always be relied on to provide adequate amounts of iron for the deficient patient.

2. **B₁₂ (cobalamin) deficiency**

   a. **Warning**

      (1) Is the patient a strict **vegetarian**? In this setting, oral B_{12} supplementation is adequate.

      (2) Does the patient have blind loop syndrome with bacterial overgrowth or some other reversible malabsorption abnormality? These patients may respond to antibiotics or surgical correction of the blind loop.

      (3) Is the serum folate level normal? B_{12} deficiency can be secondary to malabsorption induced by folate deficiency.

   b. The **treatment** of B_{12} (cobalamin) deficiency requires **parenteral cobalamin** in the vast majority of cases. This is provided by 1,000 μg i.m. of cobalamin, either cyanocobalamin or hydroxocobalamin per day for 1 week on diagnosis, then once a week for a month, and then 1,000 μg per month for the life of the patient. **Hydroxocobalamin** can be used if the patient can only come in every 2 to 3 months, since it seems to be retained better than cyanocobalamin. It is slightly more expensive and not as available in the United States as in Europe. Since the major cost of B_{12} therapy is the cost of the i.m. injections, the slight increase in drug costs is not really significant. Patients should be supplied with medical alert bracelets and they and their families or friends should be carefully instructed in the nature of the patient's disease, since a surprising number of patients discontinue therapy or are lost to follow-up.

   c. **Monitoring therapy.** Reticulocytes peak at 5 to 10 days after the onset of therapy. If a full hematologic correction does not occur, the **diagnosis should be reconsidered.** Neuropsychiatric abnormalities will partially or fully correct although full benefit may not be seen until after 1 year of treatment. Some patients may have neuropsychiatric defects prior to the presence of anemia, which may respond to B_{12} replacement.

3. **Folate (folic acid, pteroylglutamic acid) deficiency**

   a. **Warning.** Has **vitamin B_{12}** deficiency been excluded? Folate replenishment may worsen or elicit CNS abnormalities if given to patients who are B_{12} deficient. For this reason, most multivitamin preparations do not contain folic acid.

   b. Normal diets contain adequate amounts of folic acid and most victims of folate deficiency are alcoholics, pregnant women, patients with malabsorption, patients on hemodialysis, or people who subsist on highly processed and cooked food. Rarely, patients on anticonvulsants (e.g., phenytoin) or other medications may become anemic from folate deficiency. When possible, the primary treatment is to **remove the underlying cause.** When this is not possible, oral replacement with folic acid is indicated.

   c. Since the daily requirement for folic acid is approximately 100 μg and the commercially available tablet contains 1 mg of folic acid, this is adequate to treat even most cases of malabsorption. Patients with **severe malabsorption** may require 5 mg by mouth per day. **Severely anemic patients** may be initially treated with i.m. folate (5 mg per day for 3 days). Body stores are replenished after 1 to 2 months of oral therapy. However, sustained replacement of 1 mg per day by mouth may be indicated in chronic alcoholism, hemodialysis, malabsorption, or unusual dietary habits.

d. Pregnant women should be prophylactically treated with folate-containing prenatal multivitamins.

e. Monitoring therapy. See comments under B_{12} deficiency regarding hematologic response.

C. Anemias of Bone Marrow Failure

1. Aplastic anemia

a. Warnings

(1) Exclude **environmental toxins** such as benzene or other solvents, cytotoxic agents, chloramphenicol, phenylbutazone, glue sniffing, insecticides, radiation exposure.

(2) Exclude **paroxysmal nocturnal hemoglobinuria** (PNH), which may mimic this disorder.

(3) Exclude **severe B_{12} folate deficiency** since the peripheral blood, but not the bone marrow, may mimic this disorder.

b. Aplastic anemia in a young person under 45 years of age with a histocompatible donor should be treated with **bone marrow transplantation.** Avoid blood products from relatives prior to this procedure, which may sensitize the patient to antigens that will interfere with the bone marrow graft. However, if transfusion is mandatory, packed RBCs or even frozen RBCs may minimize patient sensitization to antigens present in the blood. The actuarial survival for transplanted patients from the Seattle group is 75%, with a follow-up of 2 to 6 years. Patients who had not received blood transfusions before transplant did significantly better than those who had.

c. Patients who are not candidates for bone marrow transplant may be given a **trial of the synthetic androgen oxymetholone** at a dose of 2 to 4 mg/kg/day for several months. Occasional patients show a response, but the **side effects** of virilization, edema, acne, and liver toxicity may prevent prolonged therapy. A response should be evident within 2 to 3 months after the onset of androgen therapy.

d. Even more rarely, **corticosteroids** may give a partial response or may decrease the bleeding associated with the concurrent thrombocytopenia. Prednisone at 40 mg/m²/day may be tried for several months but should not be used longer without obvious benefit because of serious side effects. The **lowest dose** of steroid possible which still demonstrates benefit to the patient should be used. Generally, the only effect is on bleeding and 10 to 20 mg/day is adequate for the purpose of stabilizing microvasculature.

e. Several case reports suggest a response to **i.v. cyclophosphamide** (30 mg/kg/day for 4 days), but this should be considered experimental therapy.

f. Women with aplastic anemia may require **chronic suppression of menses** to prevent excessive blood loss from menorrhagia. This can be accomplished by **continuous** administration of Ovral® or a similar high-estrogen birth control pill.

g. RBC **transfusions**, occasional platelet transfusions, and very rarely white blood cell transfusions may be required. However, antibodies soon develop to all these blood components and reduce their effectiveness.

h. The patient who is not a candidate for bone marrow transplant has a mean survival of approximately 3 months, although there are some long-term survivors. Vigorous broad-spectrum antibiotic coverage immediately after appropriate cultures is indicated when patients with aplastic anemia become febrile.

2. **Pure red cell aplasia.** This rare disorder is associated with **thymic tumors** in 30% to 50% of adult patients. Antibodies against RBC precursors have been described, and thus immunologic manipulation might be expected to be effective. **Surgical excision** of the thymoma produces remission in approximately half the cases.

a. **Cyclophosphamide** at 2 mg/kg/day and titrated to produce a mild depression of the WBCs (3,000–4,000) has been reported to induce remission in another group of patients.

b. **Corticosteroids** and **splenectomy** have likewise been reported to benefit occasional patients.

c. **Plasmapheresis** was used in one patient with remarkable long-term resolution of the aplasia, but this approach should be considered experimental.

3. **Myelodysplastic and myelophthisic anemias.** The myelodysplastic anemias—variously called refractory anemia with excess blasts, preleukemia, dysmyelopoietic syndrome, or chronic erythremic myelosis—have in common a **primary abnormality of the bone marrow** with disordered maturation and the failure to produce adequate numbers of mature RBCs. The most difficult problem in many of these disorders is the **persistent anemia**.

a. RBC transfusion is the only reliable method of **treatment.** Washed RBCs may be used when the onset of sensitization to blood products results in transfusion reactions.

b. Steroids, androgens, cytotoxic agents, and vitamins have all been used with no consistent results.

c. The myelophthisic anemias have a similar problem with bone marrow failure except, of course, the normal bone marrow is replaced with tumor, infection, fibrous tissue, or another pathophysiologic disorder. **Supportive therapy** with RBCs, platelets, and rarely WBCs is the only **treatment** possible, except in the case of an infectious (e.g., tuberculosis) etiology in which treatment of the underlying disorder is effective.

4. **Thalassemia.** Thalassemias are a group of congenital disorders of hemoglobin synthesis. As such, they are **not amenable to definitive treatment.** Exciting experimental work involving genetic manipulation with 5-azacytidine and the transplantation of genetic material is underway and holds promise for the future.

All patients with thalassemia minor should be **warned against taking therapeutic iron** unless iron deficient, since this worsens the increased iron load that is already present from increased iron absorption.

a. Patients with **thalassemia major should avoid iron at all costs** since transfusion requirements supply excess iron. Most **children** with thalassemia major should be on a "hypertransfusion" program whereby they regularly receive RBCs to keep their hemoglobin above 10 g/dl. Preliminary trials with **hypertransfusion of "neocytes"** (young RBCs obtained from a cell separator) appear to show a decrease in transfusion requirements, in the rate of tissue iron accumulation, and in the incidence of symptomatic splenomegaly.

b. **Splenectomy** may be necessary if progressive splenomegaly is associated with decreasing RBC survival or abdominal discomfort. This procedure should be postponed as long as possible because of the danger of bacterial sepsis in asplenic children.

c. **Deferoxamine,** an iron chelator, has been used in an attempt to prevent morbidity and mortality from iron overload in thalassemia major patients. Chronic subcutaneous administration is possible but expensive, complicated, and dangerous in some patients. Although hepatic fibrosis seems to be improved, the major cause of death, cardiac hemosiderosis, has not been affected. The role of some of the technology mentioned above has not been clearly defined, and difficult decisions are required by patients, physicians, and health care systems.

5. **Sideroblastic anemia**

a. **Warnings**

(1) Exclude alcoholism, lead intoxication, antituberculosis, and antineoplastic medications.

(2) May be a **preleukemic** condition.

b. Sideroblastic anemia can be either hereditary or secondary to medications or to other underlying disease (neoplastic, primary bone marrow disorders, inflammatory disease). Thus, **treatment of any underlying disease**, if possible, is desirable. Withdrawal from alcohol results in resolution of the sideroblastic anemia associated with that condition.

c. **Pyridoxine,** 50 to 200 mg/day by mouth is **recommended** in other cases. This is most likely to be useful in the hereditary form but occasionally is helpful in the acquired form. In patients with tuberculosis who need to continue their medications, the anemia usually resolves when pyridoxine is added to the antituberculous drugs. Pyridoxal phosphate, the coenzyme form of the vitamin, has been reported to be beneficial when pyridoxine has been ineffective. However, it is not available in the United States, and the original studies showing a response have not been confirmed.

d. Many patients remain asymptomatic for years (median survival is 10 years for idiopathic form), and thus, if possible, **transfusions should be minimized** because of the danger of iron overload.

e. **Oxymetholone,** 100 mg/day, may be useful in some patients who require repeat transfusions (see **I. C. 1. for side effects** of this therapy).

II. ANEMIAS OF INCREASED DESTRUCTION

A. **Blood Loss** The **treatment** of blood-loss anemia is directed at prevention of continued bleeding. Transfusion may be required but should **only** be used **if absolutely necessary** to avoid the side effects of decreased blood volume. If the bleeding is chronic and the patient hemodynamically stable, the bone marrow can rapidly compensate for blood loss with a rate of about six to eight times baseline production. Occasionally a patient will develop iron deficiency in this setting and require iron replacement (see I. B. 1.).

B. **Intrinsic RBC Abnormalities**

1. **Membrane disorders of RBCs** (spherocytosis, elliptocytosis, stomatocytosis). In these hereditary disorders of the RBC membrane, **splenectomy** is the only definitive treatment. Indications for splenectomy in spherocytosis usually relate to biliary tract disease with pigmented stones rather than to complications of anemia from the hemolysis. Splenectomy should be undertaken after the patient is 13 years of age or older to prevent the septic episodes that occur in asplenic children. Membrane disorders other than spherocytosis tend to be milder and there is less experience with splenectomy.

2. **RBC enzymatic and metabolic disorders.** These defects occur in either the Embden-Meyerhof glycolytic pathway, e.g., pyruvate kinase deficiency, or the hexose monophosphate shunt, e.g., glucose-6-phosphate dehydrogenase (G-6-PD) deficiency.

a. The rare glycolytic disorders, which are associated with hemolytic anemia, gallstones, and splenomegaly, are generally treated with **splenectomy** when severely symptomatic. There is very little data available for definitive statements regarding therapy. Folic acid, 1 to 3 mg/day by mouth is indicated, and genetic counselling is appropriate.

b. **G-6-PD deficiency** is a sex-linked trait that occurs in 10% to 15% of American black males. In these patients, RBC survival is normal unless exposed to **oxidant stress** such as infections, ketoacidosis, and drugs. G-6-PD deficiency in other groups (e.g., orientals, Mediterranean peoples) tends to be less frequent but more severe. Table 2 lists agents that should be avoided in this condition.

3. **Hemoglobinopathies (sickle cell anemia)**

a. **Warning.** Patients with sickling diseases are as likely to develop other

TABLE 2. *Selected agents that commonly exacerbate hemolysis in G-6-PD deficiency*

Aspirin	Probenecid
Fava beans	Quinidine
Mothballs (naphthalene)	Quinine
Nitrofurans	Sulfonamides
Para-aminosalicylic acid	Sulfones
Phenacetin	Vitamin K (water-soluble analogs)
Primaquine	

conditions as is the general population. It should not be assumed that any painful episode in these patients is due to sickling, thus an adequate evaluation is important.

b. **Sickle cell anemia** is the most common inherited hematologic disease affecting mankind. There are hundreds of hemoglobinopathies, many asymptomatic, which cannot be discussed here; therefore, the management of sickle cell anemia will be used as a model for symptomatic therapy.

c. **Sickling crises** are initiated by infection, acidosis, fever, and hypoxia; therefore, these should be avoided whenever possible. Hydration, treatment of fever by acetaminophen (not aspirin which may cause acidosis), appropriate vaccinations for influenza and pneumococcal pneumonia, and folic acid, 1 mg/day, should be part of the care of these patients. Children who develop recurrent streptococcal or pneumococcal infections can be treated with prophylactic penicillin.

d. **Transfusion therapy** should be reserved for **symptomatic aplastic crises**, surgery, **pregnancy**, and progressive disease of the eyes, heart, lungs, genitourinary system, or CNS. Packed RBCs can be given at 3-week intervals to suppress the production of sickle cells. Chronic RBC transfusions, which result in iron overload, sensitization to transfused blood, and a heavy burden on blood donors, should be reserved for patients with severe disease.

e. **Painful crises** are best **treated** with i.v. fluids sufficient to produce 50 to 100 cc/hr urine output. Fever, vomiting, and diarrhea may increase the fluid and electrolyte loss, and thus careful attention must be paid to **fluid and electrolyte replacement. Sodium bicarbonate** should be administered to correct acidosis, since an acid pH exacerbates sickling and hemolysis. **Nasal O_2** is of questionable value but probably does no harm. **Narcotics** should be used liberally to control pain, and although addiction is a concern in these patients, data suggest adequate short-term pain relief will reduce the likelihood of this occurrence. **Meperidine** (Demerol®) should be avoided since it may precipitate seizures.

f. Abundant literature has been published about various antisickling agents such as cyanate, urea, and zinc. To date, no consistent benefit has been obtained from these agents. Molecular engineering involving gene transplantation and alteration in protein synthesis by 5-azacytadine are potential future approaches but are too preliminary to be clinically practical.

4. **Paroxysmal nocturnal hemoglobinuria (PNH)**

a. **Warnings**

(1) **Iron** replacement may worsen hemolysis.

(2) Blood **transfusion** can be dangerous and worsen hemolysis.

(3) **Heparin therapy** should be avoided because it may increase hemolysis.

b. This rare disease results from a population of RBCs whose membranes are unusually sensitive to lysis by complement. In addition, a hypercoagulable state exists, resulting in thromboses or embolic phenomena.

c. Because of the on-going hemolysis, iron is lost in the urine and **ferrous sulfate replacement** may be necessary. Paradoxically, replenishment of the iron may result in increased hemolysis because a new population of complement sensitive cells is produced. If this occurs, careful **transfusion prior to iron therapy** will allow the replenishment of iron without an increase in hemolysis.

d. Androgens (see I. C. 1.), corticosteroids (60 mg prednisone per day) and dextran (500–1,000 ml of a 6% solution) have all been used in difficult cases but without consistent success. **Warfarin** may be useful if recurrent thromboses or embolism becomes a problem. If blood **transfusions** are necessary, packed RBCs should be used. Frozen RBCs may also be used if other methods fail.

C. Extrinsic RBC Abnormalities

1. Idiopathic autoimmune hemolytic anemia

a. Warnings

(1) Exclude **lymphoma**, other tumors, ovarian cysts, collagen vascular disease, or drugs (methyldopa, penicillin, quinine).

(2) Exclude **hemolytic anemia** due to infectious agents (e.g., mycoplasma, clostridia), chemicals or other toxins (see II. C. 3.).

(3) Exclude **cold agglutinins** and paroxysmal cold hemoglobinuria, which will not respond to steroids or splenectomy. If cold agglutinin disease is present, administer blood slowly or through a blood warmer if transfusion is required.

b. The two approaches to **treatment** of autoimmune hemolytic anemia are:

(1) **Decrease clearance** of antibody-coated RBCs by the reticuloendothelial system (steroids, splenectomy). This effect will be seen in days.

(2) **Decrease antibody production** by immunosuppression (cytotoxic agents). This effect may take months.

c. Prednisone at a dose of 40 mg/m^2 should be started. If there is no effect in 3 to 4 days, the dose should be doubled. Most patients (70% to 90%) will respond to this treatment within a week. If a response occurs, the prednisone should be tapered at a rate of 2.5 to 5 mg every 3 days to the lowest dose that will prevent hemolysis. Alternate day steroids may be adequate and will reduce side effects.

d. Splenectomy is recommended for patients who are not controlled by prednisone in 2 to 3 weeks, or who relapse when prednisone is tapered. According to some authorities, splenectomy may be more likely to result in a good response if splenic sequestration is documented by radionucleide techniques prior to splenectomy. For those rare patients who fail steroids and splenectomy, **cytotoxic agents** can be used. A trial of cyclophosphamide, 2 mg/kg/day by mouth can be attempted as the prednisone is tapered. The white blood count must be followed closely to avoid depression below 3,000/microliter. If a response occurs, the cyclophosphamide can be tapered after 6 months. Controlled trials and large experience with cytotoxic agents do not exist, and their use must be carefully weighed in view of potentially serious side effects.

e. Cross matching for blood **transfusions** can be difficult because of the presence of the autoantibodies on the patient's RBCs. Dangerous alloantibodies also may be missed. Close interaction with the blood bank is required to successfully cross match and transfuse these patients. If transfusion is required for life-threatening anemia, the first 20 ml of blood can be given and then only saline for 30 min to observe for adverse effects before administering the remainder of the blood.

2. RBC fragmentation syndromes (microangiopathic hemolytic anemia). The following disorders result in RBC fragmentation:

a. Distorted cardiac valves or artificial valves. This may be so severe that it will require replacement of the valve.

b. Vasculitis.

c. Malignant hypertension.

d. Metastatic cancer.

e. Giant capillary hemangioma.

f. Disseminated intravascular coagulation, thrombotic thrombocytopenic purpura.

The appropriate **treatment** for these disorders is the removal of the underlying cause. Iron or folate deficiency may develop and should be replaced if the on-going hemolysis cannot be controlled. Hemolysis caused by defective cardiac valves in particular can result in massive losses of iron in the urine and require intravenous iron replacement (see I. B. 1.).

3. Hemolytic anemia due to infectious agents, chemicals, toxins, and drugs. Treatment of the **underlying condition** applies in: malaria; bartonellosis; clostridial sepsis; and, Borrelia recurrentis.

a. Common **chemicals and drugs** causing hemolytic anemia include: mothballs (naphthalene); nitrofurantoin; sulfasalazine; sulfonamides; methyldopa; penicillin; phenacetin; and, quinidine and quinine.

b. **Treatment of drug-induced hemolytic** anemias includes stopping the drug immediately and a short course of steroids at 40 mg/m^2/day until the drug has been cleared from the system.

4. Hypersplenism. The only treatment for this condition is **splenectomy.** However, much controversy exists as to the exact indication for this procedure. Splenectomy is rarely indicated for anemia alone, since the degree of anemia is generally not sufficient to require splenectomy. Hereditary spherocytosis (II. B. 1.) is the one condition where splenectomy is clearly indicated and cures the anemia. Continued bleeding from thrombocytopenia or infection from leukopenia seem the most common causes for recommending splenectomy in hypersplenism.

5. Hemolytic transfusion reactions

a. As soon as the transfusion reaction is suspected, the blood administration should be **terminated**, a check made for clerical errors (notify blood bank immediately if any are found), and the following tests performed:

(1) Plasma and urine hemoglobin (**note:** centrifuge a posttransfusion EDTA blood sample and the plasma will be a red or brown color if hemolysis has occurred).

(2) Direct Coombs' test. If this test is positive or if there is evidence of hemolysis, **complete retyping** of the patient and blood donor is indicated. The patient's serum should be screened for a red cell antibody.

(3) Smear and culture of donor blood.

b. Since the major morbidity and mortality come from **renal failure**, prevention of this complication should be as follows:

(1) Maintain **urine flow** utilizing normal saline at a rate to keep urine output at least 100 ml/hr.

(2) Administer **furosemide** 80 mg i.v. if necessary, to keep urine flow at 100 ml/hr when the i.v. fluids have assured a positive fluid balance. If there is no response in 2 hr, give 160 mg i.v. and double this dose at 2-hr intervals until 640 mg i.v. has been given. If there is no response to this, discontinue the administration of furosemide. **Vasopressors** should be **avoided** as much as possible, since this will only exacerbate the problem with renal ischemia.

(3) If the patient has a **fragile cardiopulmonary status**, it may be necessary to insert a Swan-Ganz catheter to monitor the pulmonary capillary wedge pressures to assure that adequate amounts of fluid have been administered.

(4) If the patient begins to bleed, consider disseminated intravascular coagulation (**DIC**), document this with laboratory tests, and treat appropriately (Chapter 13).

c. **Delayed hemolytic reactions** may occur from 3 to 14 days after transfusion. They are usually not as severe as acute reactions and are treated in the same way.

BIBLIOGRAPHY

Bentley, D. P., and Jacobs, A. (1975): Accumulation of storage iron in patients treated for iron-deficiency anemia. *Br. Med. J.*, 2:64–66.

Crosby, W. H. (1980): Improvisation revisited: Oral cyanocobalamin without intrinsic factor for pernicious anemia. *Arch. Int. Med.*, 140:1582.

Dean, J., and Schechter, A. N. (1978): Sickle-cell anemia: Molecular and cellular bases of therapeutic approaches. *NEJM*, 299:752–762, 804–810, 863–870.

Eichner, E. R. (1979): Splenic function: Normal, too much and too little. *Am. J. Med.*, 66:311–320.

Frank, M. M., Schreiber, A. D., Atkinson, J. P., et al. (1977): Pathophysiology of immune hemolytic anemia. *Ann. Intern. Med.*, 87:210–222.

Krantz, S. B. (1974): Pure red cell aplasia. *NEJM*, 291:345–350.

Kushner, J. P., Lee, G. R., Wintrobe, M. M., and Cartwright, G. E. (1971): Idiopathic refractory sideroblastic anemia. *Medicine*, 50:139–159.

Ley, T. J., DeSimone, J., Anagnou, N. P., et al. (1982): 5-Azacytidine selectively increases gamma-globin synthesis in a patient with B$^+$ thalassemia. *NEJM*, 307:1469–1475.

McCurdy, P. R. (1965): Oral and parenteral iron therapy. *JAMA*, 191:859–862.

Neff, M. S., Goldberg, J., Slifkin, R. F., et al. (1981): A comparison of androgens for anemia in patients on hemodialysis. *NEJM*, 304:871–875.

Oral Iron, (1978): *Med. Lett.*, 20:45.

Pineda, A. A., Brzica, S. M., and Taswell, H. F. (1978): Hemolytic transfusion reaction. *Mayo Clinic Proc.*, 53:378–390.

Propper, R. D., Cooper, B., Rufo, R. R., et al. (1977): Continuous subcutaneous administration of deferoxamine in patients with iron overload. *NEJM*, 297:418–423.

Rosse, W. F. (1980): Paroxysmal nocturnal hemoglobinuria—Present status and future prospects. *West J. Med.*, 132:219–228.

Seligman, P. A., Caskey, J. H., Frazier, J. L., et al. (1983): Measurements of iron absorption from prenatal multivitamin-mineral supplements. *Obstet. Gynecol.*, 61:356–362.

Storb, R., Thomas, E. D., Buckner, C. D., et al. (1980): Marrow transplantation in thirty untransfused patients with severe aplastic anemia. *Ann. Intern. Med.*, 92:30–36.

15.

Malignancies

Thomas J. Braun

15.

Malignancies

I. **GENERAL CONSIDERATIONS** The care and management of patients with cancer are often complex; however, certain fundamental principles should be followed. A **tissue diagnosis** must be obtained prior to initiating therapy. Second malignancies and nonmalignant complications or diseases are common; thus, when **diagnostic uncertainty** affects a therapeutic decision, the diagnosis should be ascertained with **additional tissue.** Appropriate therapy will depend on the **type of malignancy,** the **stage** of the tumor, the patient's overall **performance status,** the **intent** of therapy, and the presence of **other disease.**

The **goal** of therapy, cure or palliation, must be clearly in mind. Curative therapy may be directed at obvious disease or it may be adjuvant in an attempt to eradicate presumed microscopic disease. The best palliative approach may be identical to curative therapy. Objective parameters should be documented at the initiation of therapy and followed throughout the course as an indication of treatment efficacy. Before initiating a chemotherapeutic regimen, it should be asked if the goals of therapy could be better served by surgery or radiation therapy.

Drug efficacies, summarized by specific malignant disease, are presented in Table 1. An active drug should be used in its maximum tolerated dose. Optimal combinations contain **active** drugs with **different mechanisms of action** and **nonoverlapping toxicities.** Awareness of each drug's specific toxicity, mode of elimination, and possible drug interactions is important. The toxicity of one agent may impair the elimination or compound the toxicity of another agent in the combination. Performance status (Table 2) should always be documented at the initiation of therapy and followed through the course of treatment. For many tumors, performance status is the most important prognostic variable in predicting response to therapy. A complete blood count and laboratory studies reflecting the **integrity of the organ responsible for drug elimination** should also be evaluated prior to therapy.

Chemotherapy should be used only in the context of established, tried treatment schemes or as part of investigational protocols. This chapter should be used as an aid to the administration of well-designed treatment plans. The determination of an optimal treatment plan is well beyond the intent of this discussion.

II. **ANTINEOPLASTIC DRUGS**

    A. **Method of Administration**

        1. **Intravenous administration.** The sclerotic and phlebitic nature of many antineoplastic drugs mandates careful attention to detail during administration. The following points should be considered:

            (1) Areas of **compromised circulation** (superior vena caval syndrome,

TABLE 1. *General activity of chemotherapy in specific neoplasms*

Cancer type	Primary drugs	Alternative drugs
Diseases in which chemotherapy has major activity		
Trophoblastic tumors	Methotrexate, actinomycin D	Etoposide, cisplatin, vinblastine, bleomycin
Testicular carcinoma	Cisplatin, vinblastine, etoposide, bleomycin	Actinomycin D, mithramycin, doxorubicin, alkylating agents
Hodgkin's disease	Alkylating agents, vinca alkaloids, procarbazine, prednisone	Doxorubicin, etoposide, nitrosoureas
Acute lymphocytic leukemia	Vincristine, prednisone, anthracyclines, asparaginase, methotrexate, 6-mercaptopurine	Cyclophosphamide, cytarabine, etoposide
Lymphomas, histiocytic and lymphocytic	Alkylating agents, vinca alkaloids, doxorubicin, prednisone	Bleomycin, etoposide, procarbazine, nitrosoureas, methotrexate, etoposide
Embryonal rhabdomyosarcoma	Vincristine, actinomycin D, cyclophosphamide, doxorubicin	Methotrexate, cisplatin
Wilms' tumor	Alkylating agents, actinomycin D, vincristine	Doxorubicin
Ewing's sarcoma	Vincristine, actinomycin D, cyclophosphamide, doxorubicin	Cisplatin
Osteogenic sarcoma	Doxorubicin, vincristine, methotrexate, cyclophosphamide	Cisplatin, actinomycin D
Acute myeloid leukemia	Anthracyclines, cytarabine, thioguanine	Azacytidine, etoposide
Small cell carcinoma of the lung	Etoposide, doxorubicin, cyclophosphamide, vincristine	Methotrexate, procarbazine, nitrosoureas
Breast cancer	Tamoxifen, estrogens, doxorubicin, alkylating agents, methotrexate, fluorouracil	Aminoglutethimide, vinca alkaloids, mitomycin
Diseases in which chemotherapy has moderate activity		
Ovary carcinoma	Alkylating agents, doxorubicin, cisplatin	Fluorouracil
Chronic lymphocytic leukemia	Alkylating agents, prednisone	Vincristine
Myeloma	Alkylating agents, prednisone	Doxorubicin, nitrosoureas, vincristine
Adrenocortical carcinoma	Mitotane	Aminoglutethimide, doxorubicin
Gastric carcinoma	Doxorubicin, mitomycin	Fluorouracil, semustine
Bladder carcinoma	Cisplatin, doxorubicin	Cyclophosphamide, mitomycin
Endometrial carcinoma	Progestins, doxorubicin, cyclophosphamide	Cisplatin
Soft part sarcomas	Doxorubicin	Actinomycin D, cyclophosphamide
Islet cell carcinoma	Streptozocin, fluorouracil	Doxorubicin, cyclophosphamide
Nonsmall cell lung carcinoma	Cisplatin, vinca alkaloids	Mitomycin, cyclophosphamide
Head and neck squamous carcinoma	Cisplatin, methotrexate, bleomycin	Vinblastine, mitomycin

TABLE 1. *(Continued)*

Cancer type	Primary drugs	Alternative drugs
Diseases in which chemotherapy has minimal activity		
Prostatic carcinoma	Estrogens	Cyclophosphamide, doxorubicin, fluorouracil, cisplatin
Colorectal carcinoma	Fluorouracil	Nitrosoureas, mitomycin
Cervical carcinoma	Cisplatin, bleomycin	Mitomycin, methotrexate, cyclophosphamide
Pancreatic carcinoma	Fluorouracil, doxorubicin, mitomycin	Streptozocin
Melanoma	No good choice	Dacarbazine, nitrosoureas
Renal cell carcinoma	No good choice	Progestins, vinblastine

Adapted from *The Medical Letter*, 1983: vol 25, Jan 7.

superficial or deep vein thrombophlebitis, or surgical interruption of lymphatic or venous drainage) **should be avoided**. Proximal venous stasis will potentiate the phlebitic nature of many drugs.

(2) Small, distal, easily visible veins should be chosen.

(3) Because of their minimum patient discomfort, ease of insertion, and visibility, 23 or 25 gauge **scalp vein** needles are preferred.

(4) The needle **insertion site** should not be obscured with tape or dressings, and a major portion of the vein proximal to the insertion site should be well visualized.

(5) If possible, **avoid previously positioned catheters.** Their position, patency, and associated thrombosis may be uncertain.

(6) The catheter patency and proper venous position should always be confirmed prior to administration of the drug.

TABLE 2. *Performance status of cancer patients*

Zubrod scale	Rating		Karnofsky scale
		100	Normal activity, no evidence of disease
Normal activity	0	90	Normal activity, minimal symptoms
		80	Normal activity with effort
Symptomatic but ambulatory, cares for self	1	70	Cares for self, unable to carry on normal activity
Ambulatory more than 50% of time, occasionally needs assistance	2	60	Requires occasional assistance
		50	Requires considerable assistance and frequent medical care
Ambulatory less than 50% of time, nursing care needed	3	40	Disabled, requires special care
		30	Severely disabled, hospitalization indicated
Bedridden, hospitalization mandatory	4	20	Active supportive treatment necessary, very sick
		10	Imminent death
		0	Dead

(7) Optimally, the agent should be administered through a side port of a free-flowing i.v.

(8) **Do not** instill the drug under **force or impede the i.v. flow** during administration; this approach assures proper venous flow and minimizes drug concentration. The phlebitic and sclerotic potential is thus minimized.

(9) Always flush the catheter and vein with a substantial volume of i.v. solution after drug administration.

(10) Be aware of the sclerotic nature of any drug being given and give a potentially sclerosing agent as the last drug when used in combination with other antineoplastic agents.

2. **Management of extravasation.** Extravasation of a sclerosing agent may be painful prior to any obvious abnormality, or a silent extravasation may present as pain and necrosis days after the drug administration. There is **no good therapy** for the extravasation of sclerosing agents. Nevertheless, one commonly accepted scheme is listed in Table 3. Many points are debatable, and there is no firm documentation to support the efficacy of any particular approach. The prevention of an infiltration is far more important and of greater benefit than any therapy for extravasation.

3. **Intrathecal therapy. Methotrexate, cytarabine,** and **thiotepa** are the only neoplastic agents that can be instilled into the cerebrospinal fluid (CSF). Lumbar puncture may be used, but many prefer an **Ommaya reservoir** to repeated lumbar punctures because of its associated ease of drug administration and superior drug distribution. Important aspects of either method include strict sterile technique; use of sterile, nonbacteriostatic diluent (the bacteriostatic agent benzyl alcohol is neurotoxic); dilution of the drug solution with 2 to 5 ml of CSF; and flushing the needle or reservoir with CSF after drug administration to assure complete delivery.

Methotrexate (6–10 mg/m^2), cytarabine (20–60 mg/m^2), or thiotepa (1–10 mg/m^2) can be given twice weekly for leptomeningeal disease. Transient headache and nausea are common. Enough methotrexate can enter the systemic circulation to produce mild marrow toxicity and mucositis. Calcium leucovorin (folinic acid), 3 to 9 mg by mouth twice daily for 4 days, can be used to

---

TABLE 3. *Management of extravasations*

1. Terminate the infusion and aspirate as much as possible through the needle
2. Inject 50–100 mg hydrocortisone sodium succinate (Solu-Cortef®) through the retained needle and then remove it
3. Inject 50–100 mg hydrocortisone sodium succinate subcutaneously into the infiltrated area with a 25 gauge needle. Multiple sticks will be needed
4. If acutely painful, ethyl chloride topical spray will anesthetize the skin
5. Apply cold compresses for the first 24 hr
6. Apply 1% hydrocortisone cream to the infiltrated area twice daily for the duration of apparent inflammation
7. Specific antidotes such as sodium bicarbonate, hyaluronidase, vitamin E, or dimethyl sulfoxide are controversial
8. Adequate analgesia should be prescribed

minimize this usually mild systemic toxicity. Intrathecal thiotepa can also produce mild systemic effects. Intrathecal chemotherapy is obviously accompanied by a substantial risk of infection and chemical meningitis and should be performed only for a specific indication by an experienced physician.

B. **Classical Alkylating Agents**   Important toxicities, drug interactions, and dose modifications are listed in Tables 4 and 5.

1. **Busulfan's** cumulative and prolonged myelotoxicity requires particular attention. **Severe marrow toxicity** may occur with continuous daily therapy. Once blood counts begin to drop significantly, the nadir may not be reached for 30 days, and the bone marrow may take weeks to recover. Adrenal insufficiency or pulmonary fibrosis may appear with prolonged therapy.

2. **Chlorambucil and melphalan** doses can usually be titrated against blood counts without unacceptable or unique toxicity. The erratic absorption of oral melphalan may require dose escalation until marrow toxicity appears.

3. **Mechlorethamine,** nitrogen mustard, is a severe sclerosing and emetic agent. Generalized patient discomfort secondary to its immediate and generalized alkylating activity should be expected during drug administration and immediately thereafter. **Antiemetics** and occasionally sedation should accompany the treatment.

4. **Cyclophosphamide** is active both orally and intravenously. Patients receiving daily oral therapy should be watched carefully for the development of **asymptomatic hematuria**, representing the first signs of **hemorrhagic cystitis.** Large i.v. doses should also be accompanied by liberal hydration to avoid this complication. Frequent bladder emptying should be encouraged. The exact **dose reduction** required in the presence of **renal failure** is controversial. Fifteen percent of the urinary metabolites are active agents; however, some recommend as much as a 50% reduction in dose. Concurrent cyclophosphamide can potentiate doxorubicin cardiotoxicity. The influence of the hepatic microsomal oxidase system on cyclophosphamide activation and metabolism may account for differences in interpatient tolerance, but the effects in an individual patient are difficult to estimate.

5. **Thiotepa** is excreted as an active drug by the kidney, thus **dose reduction is required with renal failure.**

C. **Nonclassical Alkylating Agents**

1. **Nitrosoureas.** Carmustine (BCNU), lomustine (CCNU), and semustine (MeCCNU) all require special attention because of their **prolonged white cell and platelet nadirs.** Because these nadirs occur at 4 to 6 weeks, these drugs are usually given no more often than every **6 weeks.** In addition, the **pulmonary** and **renal toxicity** seen with **cumulative doses greater than 1 g/m²** with BCNU and MeCCNU requires determination of the total cumulative dose. The **neurotoxicity** seen with **BCNU** is often difficult to diagnose because of the other associated neurologic abnormalities in the patients usually receiving this drug. **Ataxia** may be the first sign of neurotoxicity.

2. **Streptozocin** is similar to the nitrosoureas in structure; however, it has its own unique clinical characteristics. **Renal failure** is the dose-limiting toxicity,

TABLE 4. *Chemotherapy administration and toxicity*

Class/name	Dose[a] administration	Acute toxicity	Chronic toxicity
Classical alkylating agents			
Busulfan (Myleran®)	2–12 mg p.o. daily	None	Marrow toxicity, skin pigmentation, pulmonary fibrosis, sterility, Addisonian syndrome
Chlorambucil (Leukeran®)	4–6 mg/m² p.o. daily	None	Bone marrow depression
Cyclophosphamide (Cytoxan®)	750–1,000 mg/m² i.v. q 3–4 wk: 100 mg/m² p.o. daily	Nausea and vomiting, cardiotoxicity at high dose	Marrow toxicity, alopecia, hemorrhagic cystitis, sterility, pulmonary fibrosis, impaired renal water with hyponatremia
Mechlorethamine (Nitrogen mustard)	15 mg/m² i.v. q 4 wk	Nausea and vomiting, local vesicant and phlebitis, infrequent anaphylaxis	Marrow toxicity, sterility, alopecia
Melphalan (Phenylalanine mustard)	10 mg/m² p.o. daily × 4 q 6 wk	Mild nausea	Marrow toxicity, sterility
Thiotepa	20 mg/m² i.v. q 1–4 wk	None	Marrow toxicity
Nonclassical alkylating agents			
Dacarbazine (DTIC)	800 mg/m² i.v. q 4 wk	Severe nausea and vomiting, phlebitis, pain with injection	Marrow toxicity, myalgias, arthralgia, alopecia, photosensitivity
Carmustine (BCNU)	200 mg/m² i.v. q 6–8 wk	Nausea and vomiting, phlebitis, pain with injection	Delayed marrow toxicity, pulmonary fibrosis, renal failure, ataxia as CNS toxicity
Lomustine (CCNU)	100 mg/m² p.o. q 6–8 wk	Nausea and vomiting	Delayed marrow toxicity, pulmonary fibrosis
Semustine (MeCCNU)	150–200 mg/m² i.v. q 6 wk	Nausea and vomiting	Delayed marrow toxicity, pulmonary fibrosis, renal failure
Cisplatin	50–120 mg/m² i.v. q 3 wk	Severe nausea and vomiting, anaphylatic reaction, diarrhea	Renal damage, ototoxicity, neurotoxicity, renal tubular damage with magnesium wasting, hemolysis, marrow toxicity at high doses
Estramustine phosphate	300 mg/m² p.o. daily	Nausea and vomiting, diarrhea	Gynecomastia, increased thromboembolic disease
Procarbazine	50–100 mg/m² p.o. daily, not continuously	Nausea and vomiting, disulfiram-like effect, CNS depression, monoamine oxidase inhibitor, hypersensitivity reactions	Marrow toxicity, peripheral neuropathy, stomatitis, sterility

TABLE 4. *(Continued)*

Class/name	Dose[a] administration	Acute toxicity	Chronic toxicity
Streptozocin	1.0–1.5 g/m² i.v. q 4 wk	Severe nausea and vomiting, insulin shock, severe local vesicant	Tubular renal damage, hepatotoxicity, mild marrow toxicity
Antibiotics Actinomycin D	0.5 mg/m² i.v. daily × 5 days q 3–4 wk	Nausea and vomiting, local vesicant and phlebitis, radiation recall (see text)	Marrow toxicity, oral and gastrointestinal ulceration, alopecia, acneiform eruptions
Bleomycin	10–20 U/m² i.v. weekly	Fever, anaphylactoid reactions	Acute pneumonitis, pulmonary fibrosis, stomatitis, alopecia, accentuated pulmonary oxygen toxicity, Raynaud's phenomenon, hyperpigmentation
Daunorubicin (Daunomycin)	60 mg/m² i.v. daily × 3 days	Nausea and vomiting, diarrhea, local vesicant and phlebitis, cardiotoxicity, red urine, radiation recall	Marrow toxicity, cardiotoxicity, alopecia, stomatitis, anorexia
Doxorubicin (Adriamycin™)	60 mg/m² i.v. q 3 wk	Nausea and vomiting, diarrhea, local vesicant and phlebitis, cardiotoxicity, red urine, radiation recall	Marrow toxicity, stomatitis, alopecia, cardiotoxicity, anorexia
Mithramycin	25–50 μg/kg i.v. q 4–7 days	Nausea and vomiting, fever, local vesicant	Thrombocytopenia, hemorrhagic diathesis, hepatotoxicity, nephrotoxicity, hypocalcemia, mucositis
Mitomycin	5–15 mg/m² i.v. q 4 wk	Nausea and vomiting, local vesicant and phlebitis	Delayed cumulative marrow toxicity, alopecia, stomatitis, pulmonary fibrosis, renal toxicity
Antimetabolites Methotrexate	40–60 mg/m² i.v. weekly: 2.5–10.0 mg p.o. daily	Mild nausea and diarrhea	Marrow toxicity, oral and gastrointestinal ulcerations, nephrotoxicity, hepatotoxicity, interstitial pneumonitis
Fluorouracil (5-FU)	600 mg/m² i.v. weekly	Nausea and vomiting, diarrhea	Oral and gastrointestinal ulceration, marrow toxicity, alopecia, chemical conjunctivitis, cerebellar dysfunction, increased pigmentation

TABLE 4. *(Continued)*

Class/name	Dose[a] administration	Acute toxicity	Chronic toxicity
Floxuridine (FUDR)	0.1–0.6 mg/kg i.a. daily: 0.5–1.0 mg/kg i.v. daily	Same as 5-FU	Same as 5-FU
Cytarabine (Ara-C)	100–200 mg/m² i.v. daily × 5	Nausea and vomiting, diarrhea	Marrow toxicity, oral ulceration, hepatotoxicity, conjunctivitis, pulmonary edema
Azacytidine	150–400 mg/m² i.v. daily × 5	Nausea and vomiting, diarrhea, fever	Marrow toxicity, hepatotoxicity, rhabdomyolysis
Mercaptopurine (6-MP)	80–100 mg/m² p.o. daily	Nausea and vomiting	Marrow toxicity, oral and gastrointestinal ulceration, hepatotoxicity, cholestasis
Azathioprine (Imuran®)	1–5 mg/kg p.o. daily	Nausea and vomiting	Marrow toxicity, oral and gastrointestinal ulcerations, hepatotoxicity, cholestasis, pancreatitis
Thioguanine (6-TG)	50–100 mg/m² p.o. daily	Nausea and vomiting	Marrow toxicity, stomatitis, hepatotoxicity
Hydroxyurea (HU)	50–75 mg/kg p.o. daily	Nausea and vomiting	Marrow toxicity, stomatitis, dermatologic reactions, alopecia
Epipodophyllotoxin Etoposide (VP 16-213)	100–400 mg/m² i.v. q 3–5 wk	Hypotension, nausea and vomiting, local phlebitis, anaphylaxis, fever	Marrow toxicity, peripheral neuropathy, alopecia, allergic reactions
Teniposide (VM-26)	100 mg/m² i.v. q wk	Nausea and vomiting, local phlebitis, hypotension	Marrow toxicity, alopecia, peripheral neuropathy
Hormonal therapy Aminoglutethimide	750–1,500 mg p.o. daily	Lethargy, dizziness, nausea, rash	Rash, fever, hypotension
Androgens Fluoxymesterone (Halotestin®)	10–30 mg p.o. daily	None	Masculinization, fluid retention, cholestatic jaundice, hypercalcemia
Testosterone propionate	50–100 mg i.m. 3 times weekly	None	Masculinization, fluid retention, hypercalcemia
Dromostanolone propionate	100 mg i.m. 3 times weekly	None	Masculinization, fluid retention, hypercalcemia
Testolactone (Teslac®)	250 mg p.o. qid	None	Hypercalcemia, minimal masculinization

TABLE 4. *(Continued)*

Class/name	Dose[a] administration	Acute toxicity	Chronic toxicity
Estrogens			
Diethylstilbestrol (DES)	1–3 mg p.o. daily	Nausea and vomiting, rare breast tumor stimulation	Fluid retention, uterine bleeding, thromboembolic disease, hypercalcemia, stress incontinence and urinary frequency in females, feminization in males
Ethinyl estradiol	1.5 mg p.o. 3 times weekly	Same as DES	Same as DES
Antiestrogens			
Tamoxifen	10–40 mg p.o. daily	Minimal nausea and vomiting, transient tumor pain	Hot flashes, transient and mild thrombocytopenia and leukopenia, vaginal bleeding, skin rashes, retinopathy and corneal opacities with high-dose therapy
Progestins			
Medroxyprogesterone acetate (Provera®)	400–800 mg i.m. or p.o. twice weekly	Local pain at injection site	Fluid retention
Hydroxyprogesterone caproate (Decalutin)	2–5 g i.m. weekly	Local pain at injection site	Cholestatic jaundice, fluid retention
Megestrol acetate (Megace®)	40 mg p.o. q.i.d.	None	Fluid retention
Vinca alkaloids			
Vincristine	1.4 mg/m² i.v. weekly 2.0 mg total dose	Local vesicant	Peripheral neuropathy, alopecia, constipation, adynamic ileus, neuritic pain, inappropriate ADH[b] secretion
Vinblastine	4–10 mg/m² i.v. weekly	Local vesicant, nausea, and vomiting	Marrow toxicity, alopecia, stomatitis, peripheral neuropathy
Vindesine	3 mg/m² i.v. weekly	Local vesicant, nausea, and vomiting	Marrow toxicity, alopecia, peripheral neuropathy
Miscellaneous			
Asparaginase	1,000 U/kg i.v. daily × 10 days	Nausea and vomiting, fever, anaphylaxis	Hepatotoxicity, pancreatitis, hyperglycemia, coagulation defects, CNS depression
Mitotane (O, P′-DDD)	2–16 g p.o. daily	Nausea and vomiting, diarrhea	CNS toxicity with depression, lethargy, dizziness, and visual disturbances, adrenal suppression, rash disturbances, adrenal

TABLE 4. *(Continued)*

Class/name	Dose[a] administration	Acute toxicity	Chronic toxicity
Hexamethylmelamine (HMM)	200–300 mg/m² p.o. daily	Nausea and vomiting	Marrow toxicity, CNS depression, peripheral neuritis
Amsacrine (AMSA)	60–200 mg/m² i.v. daily × 3–5 days	Nausea and vomiting local phlebitis, orange urine	Marrow toxicity, stomatitis, hepatic injury, alopecia

[a]Most antineoplastic agents can be given in various doses. The method, frequency, and site of administration, as well as the addition of other agents, all affect the dosage. The doses listed in this table should be considered only as a general guide. Specific protocols should be addressed for the exact dose in a particular situation.
[b]ADH, antidiuretic hormone.

and patients should be routinely monitored for **glomerular** and **tubular** abnormalities. Renal insufficiency requires dose modification. **Streptozocin** does not have the typical, prolonged marrow toxicity seen with the standard nitrosoureas. Patients should be warned of the **severe nausea** likely to develop 4 to 6 hr after drug administration.

3. **Cisplatin.** Conventional doses of cisplatin should not be given to a patient with a **creatinine clearance less than 50 ml/min.** Adequate hydration is essential and high doses (90–120 mg/m²) require **vigorous hydration and induced diuresis.** **Mannitol** is used to maintain a minimum urine flow of 200 ml/hr for the 4 hr following high-dose cisplatin, but **furosemide** may work as well; both require replacement of urinary **electrolyte losses.** Occasional **anaphylactic reactions** are seen. The **peripheral neuropathy** is potentiated by underlying neuropathy or other concurrent neurotoxins. Careful attention to **ototoxicity** manifested as high-frequency hearing loss is required in the older patient receiving multiple courses of cisplatin. The emetic stimulus is severe and dose dependent. Emesis usually begins 4 hr after therapy. **Adequate antiemetic premedication is essential.**

4. **Procarbazine** requires **dose modification** in the presence of significant **renal** or **hepatic** insufficiency; however, exact recommendations cannot be offered. A **disulfiram** effect occasionally occurs, and patients should be forewarned to avoid alcohol during therapy. Originally developed as a **monoamine oxidase inhibitor**, procarbazine can interact with tyramine-rich diets, sympathomimetics, or antidepressants and cause severe **hypertension.** The significant **nausea** associated with procarbazine can be attenuated by a divided dose schedule with the largest fraction given in the evening.

5. **Dacarbazine,** like cisplatin and streptozocin, can induce severe **nausea** and **vomiting** responsive to dopamine antagonists such as metoclopramide. No exact guidelines can be given for the empiric dose reduction required with renal failure. Local **pain** with injection is common and can be minimized by a slow, 20 to 30 min, injection rate.

6. **Estramustine phosphate** manifests usual **estrogenic** effects in men. No specific precautions are required.

D. Antibiotics

1. **Actinomycin D.** The cumulative toxicity and multiple ways in which it can be given require close attention to protocol. Like the anthracyclines, it may act as a **radiation** potentiator or exhibit radiation recall when given after radiation therapy. Thus, **unexpected** and severe **inflammation of skin or mucous membranes** may appear in previous or current radiation fields.

2. **Bleomycin** is excreted as an active drug by the **kidney**. Because of its short half-life (30 min), it is often given by continuous infusion, and attention must be paid to subtle changes in renal function. **Mucositis** is usually the initial sign of toxicity. The occurrence of **anaphylactic reactions**, reported primarily in patients with **lymphoma**, has led to the practice of administering a one-unit i.m. **test dose** the day prior to therapy. Although controversial, a routine test dose is often not used in patients with nonlymphomatous malignancy. The **fever** associated with bleomycin is usually less than 38°C and without fluctuation. High, spiking fever should not be attributed to bleomycin or any other chemotherapeutic agent. The incidence of **pulmonary fibrosis** increases at doses greater than 250 mg/m². The fibrosis is not steroid responsive; however, the acute pneumonitis seen after a single dose of bleomycin often responds to steroids. Patients with **underlying lung disease** are predisposed to the chronic toxicity. High, inspired oxygen concentrations should be avoided in patients who have recently received bleomycin. Attention must be paid to **oxygen concentration** in the patient with testicular or head and neck cancer who received bleomycin therapy prior to definitive surgery.

3. **Daunorubicin and doxorubicin.** Both anthracyclines are **sclerosing agents, cardiotoxic**, and **emesis inducers**. They also act as **radiation potentiators**, thus radiation mucositis and dermatitis must be anticipated with concurrent radiation therapy. Radiation recall is also seen (i.e., inflammation in area of previous radiation). **Stomatitis** is a problem with frequent low-dose doxorubicin but uncommon with large single doses. **Underyling heart disease, concurrent cyclophosphamide**, or previous **mediastinal radiation** are known to potentiate the **cardiotoxic** effects of these two agents. Acute ventricular or atrial **arrhythmias** can be seen with any cumulative dose; however, the more common cardiomyopathy is usually dose dependent. **Doxorubicin should be limited** to a cumulative dose of 550 mg/m². Above this level the incidence of cardiotoxicity increases substantially. Many physicians limit cumulative doxorubicin to 450 mg/m² and proceed only with specific attention to documented cardiac function and alternative therapeutic possibilities. A falling left ventricular ejection fraction or an ejection fraction less than 50% strongly suggests that the drug should be discontinued. Cardiomyopathy may develop months after the termination of doxorubicin, thus one cannot rely entirely on the present cardiac status. The incidence of cardiotoxicity in those patients with underlying risk factors increases at an approximately 100 mg/m² smaller cumulative dose. **Hepatic dysfunction requires dose modification.** There is no good theoretical basis to guide dose modification, thus the guidelines listed in Table 6 should be used only as general recommendations. The **alopecia** seen with these agents, although total, is reversible once the drugs have been stopped.

TABLE 5. *Chemotherapy drug interactions and dose modifications*

Class/name	Drug interaction[a]	Elimination	Dose modification for organ dysfunction	
			Organ dysfunction	Dose reduction
Classical alkylating agents				
Busulfan	None common	Metabolic inactivation and renal excretion	None	None
Chlorambucil	None common	Hydrolysis, metabolic inactivation, and renal excretion	None	None
Cyclophosphamide	Phenobarbital (increased activation)	Metabolic inactivation and renal excretion	Renal: creatinine clearance < 25 ml/min	15%–50% reduction
Mechlorethamine	Pentobarbital (synergistic toxicity)	Spontaneous hydrolysis	None	None
Melphalan	None common	Hydrolysis, metabolic inactivation, and renal excretion	None	None
Thiotepa	Pentobarbital (synergistic toxicity)	Renal excretion	Renal	In proportion to creatinine clearance
Nonclassical alkylating agents				
Dacarbazine	Phenytoin, phenobarbital (increased metabolism)	Metabolic inactivation and renal excretion	Renal	Empiric reduction with consecutive doses
Carmustine	None common	Metabolic inactivation and renal excretion	None	None
Lomustine	None common	Metabolic inactivation and renal excretion	None	None
Semustine	None common	Hepatic metabolism and renal excretion	Hepatic	None
Cisplatin	None common	Renal excretion	Renal	Empiric reduction in proportion to creatinine clearance
Estramustine phosphate	Estrogens (competitive inhibition)	Hepatic metabolism and excretion	None	None
Procarbazine	Ethanol, antidepressants, sympathomimetics, CNS stimulants	Hepatic metabolism and renal excretion	Renal, hepatic	Empiric reduction in proportion to hepatic and renal dysfunction
Streptozocin	Phenytoin (antagonizes cytostatic effect)	Metabolic inactivation and renal excretion	Renal: creatinine clearance < 25 ml/min	50%–75% reduction
Antibiotics				
Actinomycin D	None common	Hepatic metabolism and renal excretion	Hepatic, renal	Empiric reduction in proportion to creatinine clearance[b]
Bleomycin	None common	Renal excretion	Renal	

Drug	Interactions	Metabolism/excretion	Organ	Dose adjustment
Daunorubicin	None common	Hepatic metabolism and excretion	Hepatic	Empiric reduction
Doxorubicin	None common	Hepatic metabolism and excretion	Hepatic	Empiric reduction
Mithramycin	None common	Renal excretion	Renal	In proportion to creatinine clearance[b]
Mitomycin	None common	Hepatic metabolism	None	None
Antimetabolites				
Methotrexate	Salicylates, sulfonamides, phenytoin, probenecid, coumadin (increased toxicity)	Renal filtration and secretion	Renal	In proportion to creatinine clearance[b]
Fluorouracil	None common	Hepatic metabolism and renal excretion	Hepatic	Empiric reduction
Floxuridine	None common	Hepatic metabolism	Hepatic	Empiric reduction
Cytarabine	None common	Metabolic inactivation	None	None
Azacytidine	None common	Renal excretion	Renal	Empiric reduction
Mercaptopurine	Allopurinol (increased toxicity)	Hepatic metabolism and renal excretion	Hepatic, renal	Empiric reduction
Azathioprine	Allopurinol (increased toxicity)	Hepatic metabolism and renal excretion	Renal, hepatic	In proportion to creatinine clearance, empiric reduction
Thioguanine	None common	Hepatic metabolism and renal excretion	Renal, hepatic	Empiric reduction
Hydroxyurea	None common	Hepatic metabolism and renal excretion	Hepatic	Empiric reduction
Epipodophyllotoxin				
Etoposide	Dextrose (precipitation)	Hepatic metabolism and renal excretion	Hepatic, renal	Empiric reduction[c]
Teniposide	None common	Hepatic metabolism and excretion and renal excretion	Hepatic	Empiric reduction[c]
Hormonal therapy				
Aminoglutethimide	Dexamethasone (increased metabolism)	Hepatic metabolism	None	None
Androgens				
Fluoxymesterone	None common	Hepatic metabolism and excretion	Hepatic	Empiric reduction
Testosterone propionate	None common	Hepatic metabolism and excretion	Hepatic	Empiric reduction
Dromostanolone propionate	None common	Hepatic metabolism and excretion	Hepatic	Empiric reduction
Testolactone	None common	Hepatic metabolism and excretion	Hepatic	Empiric reduction
Estrogens				
DES	None common	Hepatic metabolism and excretion	Hepatic	Empiric reduction
Ethinyl estradiol	None common	Hepatic metabolism and excretion	Hepatic	Empiric reduction
Antiestrogens				
Tamoxifen	None common	Hepatic metabolism and excretion	None	None

TABLE 5. *(Continued)*

Class/name	Drug interaction[a]	Elimination	Dose modification for organ dysfunction	
			Organ dysfunction	Dose reduction
Progestins				
Medroxyprogesterone acetate	None common	Hepatic metabolism and excretion	Hepatic	Empiric reduction
Hydroxyprogesterone caproate	None common	Hepatic metabolism and excretion	Hepatic	Empiric reduction
Megestrol acetate	None common	Hepatic metabolism and excretion	Hepatic	Empiric reduction
Vinca alkaloids				
Vincristine	Other neurotoxins	Hepatic metabolism and excretion	Hepatic	Empiric reduction[c]
Vinblastine	Other neurotoxins	Hepatic metabolism and excretion	Hepatic	Empiric reduction[c]
Vindesine	Other neurotoxins	Hepatic metabolism and excretion	Hepatic	Empiric reduction[c]
Miscellaneous				
Asparaginase	None common	Metabolic inactivation	None	None
Mitotane	Barbituates, coumadin, phenytoin (stimulates microsomal oxidases)	Metabolic inactivation and hepatic excretion	Hepatic	Empiric reduction
Hexamethylmelamine	None common	Hepatic metabolism	Hepatic	Empiric reduction
Amsacrine	None common	Hepatic metabolism and excretion	Hepatic	Empiric reduction

[a]Only relatively common drug interactions with drugs other than chemotherapeutic agents are listed.
[b]Minimal to no removal by dialysis.
[c]A general recommendation is to reduce the dose by 50% for a bilirubin >1.5 mg% and by 75% for a bilirubin >3.0 mg%.

TABLE 6. *Treatment of hypercalcemia of malignancy*

Agent	Dose and administration	Onset	Contraindications	Complications
Saline, furosemide		Immediate	Impaired cardiac or renal function	Fluid overload, hypovolemia, hypokalemia, hypomagnesemia
Salmon calcitonin	2–8 MRCU/kg i.m. s.q. q 8–24 hr	2–6 hr	Allergy	Allergic reactions
Phosphates	1–1.5 g daily	24 hr	Hyperphosphatemia, impaired renal function	Diarrhea, soft-tissue calcification
Neutra-Phos®	250 mg p.o. qid[a]			
Neutra-Phos-K®	250 mg p.o. qid[a]			
Fleet Phospho-soda	3 ml p.o. bid[a]			
Mithramycin	25 µg/kg i.v. q 3–7 days	24–48 hr	Renal failure, thrombocytopenia	See Table 4
Corticosteroids	26–60 mg p.o. daily	48–120 hr	None	CNS reactions, hyperglycemia, hypokalemia

[a]Dose calculated to supply 1,000 mg inorganic phosphate daily. Dilute Phosphosoda 1:100 to minimize diarrhea. Neutra-Phos can be diluted to 250 ml.
MRCU, Medical Research Council units; p.o., by mouth.

4. **Mithramycin** is used in the treatment of hypercalcemia and recurrent testicular carcinomas. **Thrombocytopenia** is the most sensitive indication of toxicity. When used in the treatment of **hypercalcemia**, the usual dose is **25 μg/ kg i.v.** The osteoclast-mediated, hypocalcemic effect usually lasts 4 to 7 days. The drug is not dialyzed and is entirely dependent on **renal excretion. Do not** confuse a mitomycin order with a mithramycin order or a milligram dose for a microgram dose.

5. **Mitomycin.** The insidious, **cumulative marrow toxicity** of mitomycin often appears after three to four doses. Patients treated for a prolonged period occasionally develop **renal** insufficiency, active urinary sediment, thrombocytopenia, and a microangiopathic hemolytic anemia; thus, the peripheral blood smear, urinalysis, and serum creatinine should be followed.

E. **Antimetabolites**

1. **Methotrexate.** The patterns of drug interaction and toxicity vary with the dose given. Like other cycle-specific antimetabolites, the **period of exposure** is as important as the size of the dose. Patients with underlying **folate deficiency** are particularly sensitive to methotrexate. Organic anions such as **aspirin** and **probenecid** interfere with the renal tubular secretion of methotrexate and may increase the toxicity of chronic, low-dose therapy. Early toxicity may be missed. Drugs that interfere with the **albumin binding** of methotrexate such as **sulfonamides** and **coumadin** increase free drug level and toxicity. Methotrexate is very insoluble in acid, thus **renal methotrexate precipitation** may occur with higher doses. Doses greater than 100 mg/m² require a urinary pH above 7 and adequate urine flow. **Abnormal renal function requires dose modification.** Patients receiving prolonged, low-dose methotrexate may develop **interstitial pneumonitis** or **hepatotoxicity.** Methotrexate may accumulate in pleural and ascitic fluids and then slowly reenter the systemic circulation, producing severe and unexpected toxicity. Massive doses of methotrexate (8 g/m²) can be given when followed by calcium leucovorin rescue. One should not attempt high-dose methotrexate therapy without access to readily available methotrexate serum levels. A discussion of the details of high-dose methotrexate therapy is beyond the scope of this chapter.

   Calcium leucovorin bypasses the metabolic site of action of methotrexate and is used to minimize its toxicity. Three to 6 mg can be given i.v. four times per day. Oral tablets (5 mg, 25 mg) are also available. Duration of leucovorin therapy depends on the nature of the toxicity and, optimally, on the serum methotrexate level.

2. **Fluorouracil and floxuridine** (5-FU and FUDR) have similar patterns of activity and toxicity. They differ primarily in degree of hepatic metabolism and dose. Like methotrexate, the pattern of toxicity varies with the dose given. **Oral 5-FU** is erratically absorbed and **should be avoided** if possible. Dose modification for hepatic failure is controversial. Since both drugs are extensively **metabolized by the liver and then excreted by the kidney**, dose modification is suggested when there is significant impairment of either organ. However, usual doses of 5-FU are often given despite significant hepatic dysfunction without untoward toxicity.

3. **Cytarabine. Ara C** is usually given as a continuous infusion of 100 to 200 mg/m² for 3 to 5 days. Larger doses (3 g/m²) are also given as an i.v. bolus twice daily for 3 to 5 days. The higher dose is associated with a **CNS toxicity** not seen at the lower dose. Cytosine arabinoside may also be given as a small subcutaneous dose. All three dose schedules are currently used in the treatment of acute leukemia.

4. **Azathioprine** and its metabolite, **mercaptopurine**, are metabolized by xanthine oxidase. **Concurrent allopurinol requires a 50% to 75% reduction in mercaptopurine or azathioprine dose.** An empiric dose reduction based on the degree of marrow toxicity is required with hepatic dysfunction.

5. **Thioguanine** is given orally and has little unique toxicity. Although a purine analog like azathioprine and mercaptopurine, it is not metabolized by xanthine oxidase, and concurrent allopurinol does not necessitate a dose modification.

6. **Hydroxyurea.** Conventional doses (1–2 g daily) are not usually associated with symptomatic toxicity. Significant **nausea** or a maculopapular **rash** usually precludes therapy with more than 4 to 5 g/day. A divided daily dose will minimize GI toxicity. As white cell counts may fall precipitously, they should be checked frequently when initiating therapy or when using doses higher than 1.5 g/day.

F. **Epipodophyllotoxins   Etoposide (VP-16) and teniposide (VM-26).** Both drugs can cause severe **hypotension** if administered rapidly and **should be infused slowly over 30 min. Anaphylactic reactions** occasionally occur with each drug. VP-16 also comes in an oral preparation; however, wide variability in absorption has limited its use. **Hepatic dysfunction** will impair the elimination of both drugs. A modification schedule similar to that used with doxorubicin is suggested. There are no adequate guidelines for dose modification with **renal dysfunction**, although the kidney is involved in the elimination of both drugs.

G. **Hormonal Therapy**

1. **Aminoglutethimide.** Approximately 50% of people receiving aminoglutethimide experience some **acute toxicity** and should be warned. The **acute effects** of lethargy, drowsiness, ataxia, and transient rash usually resolve within 4 to 6 weeks and are minimized by small initial doses of the drug and the concurrent use of an increased hydrocortisone dose. The recommended initial aminoglutethimide dose is 500 mg/day for 2 weeks with a subsequent increase to 1,000 mg (250 mg p.o. q.i.d.). **Hydrocortisone** is begun at 100 mg/day for 2 to 3 weeks and then reduced to 40 mg daily. Given aminoglutethimide's ability to increase dexamethasone metabolism, **other steroids should not be substituted for hydrocortisone.** When aminoglutethimide is discontinued, it is not necessary to taper the steroid dose as the adrenal gland returns to a normal state of secretion and response to stress within a few days after the withdrawal of aminoglutethimide and hydrocortisone.

2. **Androgens.** All androgens require **dose reduction with significant liver disease.** Transaminase values and serum bilirubin levels should be routinely followed. The virilizing effects of androgens are part of the desired physiologic effect and should not be considered as toxicity. **Female patients need to be warned** of a gradual increase in facial hair, acne, voice deepening, and

increased libido. Because of their adequate absorption, oral preparations such as **fluoxymesterone** and **oxymethalone** are preferred. For refractory anemias, oxymethalone is usually started at 1 mg/kg/day and increased to a maximum of 5 mg/kg/day. Testolactone has a minimal virilizing effect and may not be as efficacious as the other androgen preparations.

3. **Estrogens.** The demonstrated increased **cardiovascular toxicity with diethylstilbestrol** (DES) in daily doses of 5 mg or greater is the basis for the recommended DES dose in prostatic cancer of **1 to 3 mg daily.** There is no clear evidence that a 3-mg daily dose is more toxic or efficacious than 1 mg daily. In those men who have not had complete suppression of testosterone production with the 1-mg dose, an increase to 3 mg is logical. The recommended dose for the treatment of breast cancer is 5 mg three times daily. Breast cancer patients with **metastatic bone disease** are at risk of **hypercalcemia** when placed on estrogen therapy. Occasionally (5% to 10% of patients), flares of disease will be induced with estrogen administration. Thus, patients should be examined and serum calcium levels checked 2 to 3 weeks after beginning DES. **Urinary stress incontinence** is often the most troublesome toxicity in older women.

4. **Antiestrogens.** The recommended dose of tamoxifen is 10 mg b.i.d. by mouth but many recommend 20 mg b.i.d. in premenopausal patients. Large loading doses are being investigated but cannot be considered standard therapy. Significant toxicity is uncommon, but an occasional patient will have to stop therapy because of unacceptable lethargy and nausea. As with the estrogens, hypercalcemia and, rarely, tumor flare can occur. Some tumor flares will be followed by an objective response with continuation of therapy; however, others may represent continuing tumor stimulation. Careful observation and clinical judgment are required to make the differentiation between these two responses. **Retinal toxicity** has been observed at much higher doses and is not a significant problem at currently recommended doses.

5. **Progestins. Abscess formation** may occur with intramuscular progestin therapy. The more commonly used oral agents are associated with minimal toxicity. **Mild fluid retention** and occasional **vaginal spotting** are the most common toxicities. The standard dose of megestrol acetate is 40 mg q.i.d. by mouth. The use of a 1- to 1.5-g/day dose is advocated by some but remains controversial.

H. **Vinca Alkaloids**

1. **Vincristine.** A single injection is usually limited to 2 mg. The **neurotoxicity** is **cumulative** and often requires a dose reduction after 4 to 5 weeks of therapy. The **neuritic pain** associated with all three vinca alkaloids may present as **jaw** or **deep muscle pain. Constipation** is often the limiting toxicity, although toxicity of any peripheral or cranial nerve is possible.

2. **Vinblastine.** The chemical structure differs minimally from vincristine, but the pattern of toxicity and disease activity is substantially different. **Marrow suppression, primarily of neutrophils**, is the limiting toxicity to a single dose. With prolonged, regular therapy **neurotoxicity** becomes prominent. **Vindesine**, the first metabolite of vinblastine, has somewhat less marrow

suppression but is also limited by **neurotoxicity** when given regularly. All three vinca alkaloids require **dose modification** in the presence of **hepatic dysfunction** and must be respected as severe **local vesicants.**

I. **Miscellaneous**

1. **Asparaginase.** The frequency of **hypersensitivity reactions** requires skin testing prior to asparaginase administration. The standard stock solution is diluted 1:100 and used as a **test solution.** If a positive skin test occurs, one must decide between a desensitization schedule or the administration of *Erwinia asparaginase* instead of the standard *Escherichia coli* preparation. The drug must be given slowly (not less than 30 min), and the patient watched for a possible anaphylactic reaction. The chance of an anaphylactic reaction increases with the number of previous treatments.

2. **Mitotane.** The gastrointestinal and CNS toxicities can be minimized by starting at 1 or 2 g/day. Doses are then escalated as tolerated. Given the resultant inhibition of adrenocortical function, adequate **glucocorticoid and mineralocorticoid replacement is required.**

3. **Hexamethylmelamine. Neurotoxicity** may manifest as agitation, hallucinations, or a parkinsonian-like syndrome. **Gastrointestinal toxicity** is usually dose limiting.

III. **THERAPY OF SPECIFIC PROBLEMS**

A. **Neurologic Complications**

1. Patients with **intracerebral neoplasms** require supportive medical therapy while receiving primary radiation or surgery. Patients with apparent brain metastases without an obvious primary site should be considered for prompt biopsy and subsequent radiation. The delay associated with a search for the primary site may be detrimental. **Dexamethasone** is the steroid most commonly used to minimize cerebral edema because of its minimal mineralocorticoid effect and its relatively prolonged biologic activity, although other glucocorticoids may work as well. Symptomatic patients should receive **10 mg dexamethasone followed by 4 mg q.i.d.** Occasional patients may require up to 100 mg for adequate control of edema. If symptoms allow, dexamethasone should be **tapered slowly** after the completion of radiation therapy.

Phenytoin and phenobarbital should be used to control **symptomatic seizures.** The use of phenytoin in the seizure-free patient with brain metastasis is controversial. Because of **phenytoin's ability to increase dexamethasone metabolism** by hepatic microsomes, many treat seizure-free patients with steroids without prophylactic antiepileptics.

2. **Carcinomatous leptomeningitis** represents a difficult therapeutic problem. **Symptomatic tumor deposits** are treated with **radiation therapy,** but radiation to the entire neuroaxis is very myelotoxic. Intrathecal therapy is indicated when the tumor type is responsive to methotrexate, cytarabine, or thiotepa. **Dexamethasone** may minimize local edema around tumor deposits. Effective systemic therapy should be started if possible.

3. **Epidural metastases. Prompt diagnosis** and the initiation of radiation therapy are the **most important** elements in the treatment of extradural or extrame-

dullary, intradural disease. The extradural mass in the patient without known malignancy should be approached **surgically** to allow rapid decompression and **diagnosis. Dexamethasone** in the schedule noted above should be started at diagnosis.

B. Metabolic Complications

1. **Hyperuricemia and the tumor lysis syndrome.** Patients presenting with **elevated uric acid concentrations** and **bulky, rapidly growing, therapy-sensitive** tumors are at risk of developing **renal urate crystal precipitation. A 600 to 900 mg loading dose of allopurinol** should be given for 2 days followed by a dose of 300 mg/day. Large, initial doses of allopurinol are occasionally complicated by a maculopapular rash that resolves with a decreased dose. All patients at risk should be **well hydrated** (urine output >2 liters/day). Patients with elevated uric acid concentrations or urinary urate crystals should receive sodium bicarbonate supplementation to their intravenous fluid (50 mEq/liter) to keep their urinary pH greater than 7.0. Acetazolamide (Diamox®), 250 mg i.v. q 6 hr, can be used in patients who cannot tolerate large alkaline volume administration. **Alkalinization should be discontinued once uric acid concentrations normalize** to avoid possible renal phosphate precipitation. If adequate urine output cannot be maintained, an **osmotic diuresis** with 12.5 g mannitol in a 20% solution should be attempted. Hemodialysis may be required if these measures are not effective. Management of the **hyperkalemia, hypocalcemia**, and **hyperphosphatemia** associated with renal insufficiency and tumor lysis does not differ from the standard approach to these problems. The risk of tumor lysis and uric acid precipitation in the kidney diminishes 4 to 5 days after chemotherapy treatment and maximal cell lysis has passed.

2. **Hypercalcemia.** The severity of hypercalcemic symptoms and the presence of cardiovascular or renal disease will determine the appropriate treatment (Table 6). Furosemide-induced saline diuresis of at least 100 ml/hr must be accompanied by **adequate volume replacement** to avoid a rise in calcium with diuretic-induced dehydration. Thiazide diuretics are contraindicated because of their hypercalcemic effect. The degree of symptoms and level of hypercalcemia will determine the rate of diuresis necessary. **Total volume status, cardiac function**, and serum **potassium** must be watched carefully.

Glucocorticoids are particularly effective in the hypercalcemia associated with **B cell neoplasms** and **breast cancer**. They should be started early in the treatment because of their delayed hypocalcemic effect.

Salmon calcitonin rapidly lowers serum calcium but the **duration of action is short** (< 12 hr). Repeated administration is associated with **tachyphylaxis** and the development of antibodies. A pause in calcitonin therapy may diminish the tachyphylaxis. Consequently, calcitonin is ideal for the symptomatic patient with renal or cardiac disease prohibiting vigorous saline diuresis but is of limited value in the chronic management of malignancy-associated hypercalcemia.

Inorganic phosphate, 1 to 2 g/day, as oral phosphate can be used to control chronic hypercalcemia. Serum **phosphorous levels** and **renal function** must be followed carefully to avoid a calcium-phosphorous concentration product above 65 and soft-tissue calcium precipitation. Intravenous phosphate with its risk of tissue calcium precipitation has **no role** in the routine care of the hypercalcemic patient.

Mithramycin, 25 μg/kg, can be given every 48 hr but therapy **no more frequently** than **twice weekly** is **much safer** (see II. D.). The hypocalcemic effect often lasts 4 to 7 days. The **renal clearance, broad toxicity** pattern, and ability to cause local tissue **sclerosis** must be understood to use the drug effectively.

Treatment of the primary malignancy determines what other measures are required to keep the patient asymptomatic, usually requiring a serum calcium level below 12 mg/dl. Contributing factors such as immobilization and increased dietary calcium should be minimized. Often a combination of steroids, maximal sodium intake, and oral phosphates will have to be used.

C. **Pain Control**   A systematic approach to the patient with cancer and pain is required. Local, correctable causes of pain must be sought. **Obstruction** of a hollow viscus or local **tissue infiltration** by tumor or infection requires specific therapy. Minor pain is best treated with **acetaminophen. Aspirin** and **nonsteroidal anti-inflammatory agents** must be used with caution when drug- or disease-induced **thrombocytopenia** is present. Renal insufficiency secondary to nonsteroidal anti-inflammatory drugs is also a concern in the often dehydrated, hypercalcemic patient with malignancy. **Tolerance does not develop to acetaminophen** or **aspirin**, and they may be continued when stronger analgesics are added. Codeine (30–60 mg q 4 hr), with its high oral potency and lack of tolerance development is the next drug added. Pain refractory to codeine can be treated with **hydromorphone** or **oxycodone**. Inadequate pain control with these two drugs requires **methadone** or **levorphanol**. An **elixir of morphine** (10 mg/5 ml) given as 20 to 60 mg every 2 to 4 hr or oxymorphone suppositories can be used when the patient is unable to swallow tablets.

Certain principles should be followed when using **narcotics** in a cancer patient. The pharmacologic properties listed in Table 7 should be exploited to the patient's benefit. Narcotics are best ordered on a **fixed schedule**, with the patient given the right to refuse the medication if he desires. Untoward effects such as **constipation, nausea**, or **sedation** should be anticipated and not allowed to interfere with adequate analgesia administration. The sedation and nausea abate within a few days, and standard antiemetics can be used to control the initial nausea. Constipation is universal, and therapy with adequate doses of a cathartic such as milk of magnesia, 30 to 90 ml/day, will preclude a major problem. The degree of pain control 1 to 2 hr after oral ingestion determines if the **dose was adequate. One should avoid undue concern for narcotic drug addiction** in this patient population. It is very uncommon. **Drug tolerance should be expected.** Dose escalation may be required after 2 to 4 weeks at a particular dose. The **dose increment required to overcome tolerance increases geometrically** as the tolerant dose increases. Cross tolerance between narcotics is not complete. When switching to another narcotic because of tolerance, one-half the equianalgesic dose should be used as the starting dose. The long half-lives of levorphanol, methadone, and their sedating metabolites require attention to possible **excessive sedation in the first**

TABLE 7. *Narcotic analgesics*

Name	Dose[a] and administration	Peak[b] (min)	Duration[b] (hr)	Oral/parenteral potency ratio	Plasma half-life (hr)
Morphine	10 mg i.m.	30–60	4–6	0.17	2–3.5
	60 mg p.o.	90–120	4–6		
Hydromorphone	2 mg i.m., i.v.	30–60	3–4	0.20	2–3
(Dilaudid®)	8 mg p.o.	60–90			
Codeine	120 mg i.m.	30–60	4–6	0.65	3
	200 mg p.o.	90–120			
Oxycodone	30 mg p.o.	60	3–4	0.50	2–4
(in Percocet®)					
Levorphanol[c]	2 mg i.m.	30–60	6–8	0.50	12-16
(LevoDromoran®)	4 mg p.o.	90–120			
Methadone[c]	10 mg i.m.	30–60	6–8	0.50	15-30
(Dolophine®)	20 mg p.o.	90–120			
Meperidine	75 mg i.m.	60–90	4–5	0.25	3–4
(Demerol®)	300 mg p.o.	90–120			
Oxymorphone	1 mg i.m.	30–60	3–6	0.17	2–4
(Numorphan®)	6 mg p.o.	90–120			
Pentazocine[d]	60 mg i.m.	30–60	3	0.30	2–3
(Talwin®)	180 mg p.o.	90–120			

[a]Recommended starting dose equianalgesic to 10 mg i.m. morphine sulfate.
[b]Based on analgesic effect not plasma concentrations.
[c]Drug and active metabolites may accumulate with repetitive dosing causing excessive sedation.
[d]Antagonist properties may precipitate withdrawal in narcotic-dependent patients, relatively high incidence of CNS toxicity.

weeks of therapy. With careful observation these two drugs can be titrated to a single dose size of 60 mg if needed.

D. **Antiemetic Therapy**   The severity of the emetic stimulus should be **anticipated.** Patients are advised to have an **empty stomach** and to refrain from a full diet for 12 hr after drug administration. The appropriate antiemetic from Table 8 should be administered on a regular schedule and started prior to the chemotherapy. The control of once established nausea and vomiting is much more difficult than its prevention. **Phenothiazines** may be used for **minimal** emetic stimuli or for the nausea and anorexia that may persist for days after the administration of strongly emetic agents. **Cannabinol derivatives**, nabilone and tetrahydrocannabinol, have moderate antiemetic effects. The associated disorientation, dizziness, and euphoria are much more common and disturbing in older patients and limit their utility.

Major emetic stimuli such as **cisplatin, dacarbazine**, and **doxorubicin** are not effectively treated with phenothiazines. **Metoclopramide**, 2 mg/kg i.v., can be given 30 min before cisplatin and every 2 hr thereafter for a total of five doses. Five doses of 7.5 mg droperidol can also be given intravenously by the same schedule when administering cisplatin. Older patients experience a 1% to 3% incidence of **extrapyramidal manifestations** with these two regimens. However, younger patients will experience this toxicity more frequently (>25%) and severely. Diphenhydramine, 25 mg i.v., will abolish the extrapyramidal reactions. **Younger patients should receive prophylactic diphenhydramine. Dexamethasone**, 20 to 60 mg i.v. 30 min prior to chemotherapy, is also helpful. Metoclo-

TABLE 8. *Antiemetic agents*

Class/name	Dose and administration	Efficacy	Toxicity
Phenothiazines			
Prochlorperazine (Compazine®)	10 mg p.o. q6hr 25 mg p.r. q8hr*a*	+	Extrapyramidal effects, sedation
Thiethyperazine (Torecan®)	10 mg p.o. q8hr 10 mg p.r. q8hr*a*	+	Extrapyramidal effects, hypotension
Chlorpromazine (Thorazine®)	25 mg p.o. q6hr 100 mg p.r. q6hr*a*	+	Extrapyramidal effects, hypotension
Butyrophenones			
Droperidol (Inapsine®)	0.5–7.5 mg i.v., i.m. q 2–4 hr	+ +	Hypotension, extrapyramidal effects, sedation, contraindicated in parkinsonian patients
Haloperidol (Haldol®)	0.5–2.5 mg i.v., i.m. q 1–4 hr	+ +	Same as droperidol
Others			
Metoclopramide (Reglan®)	2 mg/kg i.v. q2hr	+ + +	Extrapyramidal effects, sedation, diarrhea, contraindicated in parkinsonian patients
Tetrahydrocannabinol (THC)	5–10 mg/m² p.o. q4hr	+ +	Euphoria, dizziness, sedation, postural hypotension
Dexamethasone	10–20 mg i.v. prior to chemotherapy	+ +	No specific acute toxicity
Benzquinamide (Emete-con®)	25 mg i.v. q4hr*b* 50 mg i.m. q4hr	+ +	Sedation, hypotension

*a*Phenothiazines administered by rectum are erratically absorbed.
*b*Contraindicated in patients with cardiovascular disease.
p.o., by mouth; p.r., per rectum.

pramide, diphenhydramine, and dexamethasone in combination are often required with high-dose cisplatin or dacarbazine.

E. Infections The treatment of infectious diseases is discussed in Chapter 10, but special considerations are required in the often neutropenic patient with malignancy. The effects of therapy and the basic disease process predisposing the patient to infection and requiring special consideration include: abnormalities in **cell-mediated immunity** often seen in patients with lymphoid neoplasms receiving lymphoid radiation or glucocorticoids; **transient neutropenias** (<7 days) frequently seen in patients with solid tumors receiving cytotoxic therapy; **prolonged neutropenia** related to marrow ablative therapy for acute leukemia; and, abnormalities of **immunoglobulin quantity** and **function** seen with chronic B cell malignancies such as chronic lymphocytic leukemia and multiple myeloma. Understanding these predisposing factors allows one to anticipate specific infectious problems and to modify the diagnostic and therapeutic approach.

1. Prophylactic therapy in the neutropenic patient. Patients with absolute neutrophil counts below 1,000/mm³, and particularly those below **500/mm³**, are at great risk of bacterial infections and fever. The anticipated duration of neutropenia determines the type of prophylactic intervention. Patients with expected **transient neutropenia**, <500/mm³ for <7 days, require instruction about the importance of fever and careful analysis of all symptoms; however, **prophylactic antibiotics, hospitalization**, or **isolation** are **not required.**

Invasive procedures should be kept to an absolute minimum. Many recommend prophylactic antibiotics when an invasive procedure is required.

Expected **prolonged neutropenia** requires a different approach. Protective isolation with a laminar air flow room and mask and gown, daily bathing with hexachlorophene or povidone-iodine soap, nonabsorbable oral antibiotics, and sterilization of all food are protective when available and need to be used simultaneously. To use only a few of these interventions is not useful. A practical approach available in most hospitals includes a private room, careful hand washing, only essential invasive procedures, and no fresh fruits or vegetables. **Prophylactic trimethoprim-sulfamethoxazole**, 320 mg and 1,600 mg, respectively (two tablets twice daily), is recommended by many but remains controversial as trimethoprim-sulfamethoxazole **resistant infections** begin to appear in patients receiving prophylactic therapy.

2. **Fever and neutropenia.** Temperature greater than 38.3°C in a neutropenic patient requires a careful physical examination, chest X-ray, and cultures of blood, urine, sputum, throat, and any suspicious skin lesion. Without adequate neutrophils, typical inflammatory signs on physical examination, X-rays, or tissue analysis may not be present. The physical examination should be repeated frequently during the first few days of fever if a source is not found. Once cultures have been obtained, broad-spectrum antibiotics should be started. An **aminoglycoside** combined with a **semisynthetic penicillin** active against *Pseudomonas* or a **cephalosporin** in the penicillin-allergic patient (gentamicin and ticarcillin or cephazolin) is the usual recommendation, but the exact antibiotic choice depends on the **characteristics of infection in the particular hospital.** A significant prevalence of *Staphylococcus* requires the addition of bactericidal gram-positive (oxacillin or cephalosporin) coverage. The hospital's antibiotic-resistance pattern will determine the choice of aminoglycoside. A positive culture allows the optimal antibiotic and dose to be chosen. Despite the identification of a gram-positive source, broad-spectrum antibiotics should be continued to minimize the incidence of gram-negative secondary infection. If positive cultures are obtained, antibiotics are continued for the usual duration and until the neutropenia has resolved. Staphylococcal bacteremia with clear evidence of tissue infiltration should be treated for 4 to 6 weeks. Staphylococcal infection without tissue infiltration is adequately treated with 14 days of proper therapy, assuming the neutropenia has resolved. Duration of therapy in the patient who has responded to appropriate treatment of customary duration but remains neutropenic is controversial. If the fever resolves without the identification of a source, antibiotics are continued for the duration of the neutropenia.

3. **Persistent fever and neutropenia.** Persistent fever requires repeated examination and review of the antibiotic regimen. Antibiotic levels are indicated. After 3 to 4 days of fever, the addition of another antibiotic to provide coverage of all hospital-resident anaerobic or gram-positive organisms should be considered. Although controversial, many recommend temporarily stopping all antibiotics for 24 to 48 hr and reculturing. **Amphotericin** should be strongly considered after 4 to 7 days of fever unresponsive to a multidrug antibiotic

program, particularly with a history of previous fungal infection or colonization.

F. Transfusion Therapy

1. Prophylactic **white cell transfusions** are not indicated in the neutropenic patient. They are indicated in the patient with culture-documented **gram-negative** infection and neutropenia of less than 500/mm³ who remains febrile on appropriate antibiotics with sufficient serum concentration levels for at least 48 hr. Some authors further demand that the expected duration of neutropenia be greater than 7 days. The white cells should be ABO compatible and optimally human leukocyte antigen (HLA) compatible or from an ABO compatible family member. Once started, the WBC transfusions are repeated daily. Leukoagglutinin reactions are common and range from fever to life-threatening pulmonary infiltratates. **Simultaneous amphotericin** may exacerbate the pulmonary complications of WBC transfusions and should be avoided.

2. **Red cell transfusions** are discussed in Chapter 14. Radiation of red cells is not necessary in all patients with malignancy, but those patients with profound abnormalities of cell-mediated immunity, advanced Hodgkin's disease, or total lymphoid radiation should receive only **radiated blood products** to eliminate the risk of graft versus host reactions.

3. Prophylactic **platelet transfusions** are controversial, as discussed in Chapter 13. The patient's overall prognosis, duration of expected thrombocytopenia, and previous blood product exposure need to be considered when deciding on the use of prophylactic platelets. **Lumbar puncture**, thoracentesis, and surgical procedures all require a platelet level greater than **50,000/mm³**. Intracranial surgery requires greater than 100,000/mm³.

G. Malignant Pleural Effusions

Malignant pleural effusions are best treated with effective **systemic therapy.** A central pulmonary mass with a cytology negative chylous effusion may benefit from mediastinal radiation in an attempt to relieve proximal lymphatic obstruction. More commonly, pleural seeding with tumor accounts for the effusion, and local therapy is needed for palliation. Repeated thoracenteses are impractical because of the usual recurrence of fluid within 1 or 2 weeks. Obliteration of the pleural space requires a fully expanded lung and removal of all fluid. Chest tube drainage alone may induce pleural symphysis, but instillation of a sclerosing agent may improve the chance of sclerosis. Tetracycline, 500 mg in 30 ml water; nitrogen mustard, 10 to 40 mg; or thiotepa, 30 to 45 mg, can be used. Tetracycline is preferred by many because it has no associated marrow toxicity, but no agent has proven superior in inducing sclerosis. All are accompanied by severe chest pain and fever. Mild nausea and vomiting are seen with nitrogen mustard.

H. Superior Vena Caval Obstruction

Patients presenting with superior vena caval obstruction and no history of malignancy require a **tissue diagnosis** because of the variations in effective therapy for some of the malignant possibilities (the various lymphomas, thymomas, germ cell tumors, oat cell). If tissue cannot be obtained with an acceptable risk of bleeding, a **thoracotomy** with biopsy under direct visualization and controlled hemostasis may be required.

Relief of vena caval compression with radiation or chemotherapy is the essence of therapy, and other medical therapies are of unproven and questionable value. **Steroids** are often prescribed, but the minimal inflammation accompanying the syndrome is evidence against their value unless the primary tumor is steroid-sensitive. Although intraluminal thrombosis is often present at autopsy, **fibrinolytic therapy and heparinization** are usually not used because of their risk with concurrent increased intracranial venous pressure. Anticoagulation may have a role in the uncommon patient with the acute onset of symptoms and apparent minimal external compression. **Diuretics** may occasionally produce transient symptomatic improvement at the expense of a further decrease in cardiac filling and systemic hypovolemia. The routine use of a diuretic is, however, **discouraged.**

I. **Other Problems**

1. **Cardiac tamponade** of malignant etiology is acutely treated like the tamponade of nonmalignant etiology. Subsequent therapy requires effective primary treatment of the malignancy and often a drainage procedure or pericardial sclerosis. Specific therapy depends on the patient's overall clinical presentation and his physician's preference and experience.

2. **Leukostasis syndromes** with **CNS** and **pulmonary** manifestations may be seen with greater than 50,000 myeloblasts/mm³. Mature myeloid cells and lymphoblasts seldom produce this syndrome. A cytarabine continuous infusion, 200 mg/m²/day, or 3 to 4 g of hydroxyurea daily are the fastest ways to lower the circulating blast count.

3. **Acute promyelocytic leukemia** complicated by disseminated intravascular coagulation is discussed in Chapter 13. As heparinization during induction is effective and important, the possibility should be considered in all new leukemics.

BIBLIOGRAPHY

Chabner, B. A., editor (1982): *Pharmacologic Principles of Cancer Treatment.* W. B. Saunders, Philadelphia.

Cohen, L. F., Balow, J. E., Magrath, I. T., Poplack, D. G., and Ziegler, J. L. (1980): Acute tumor lysis syndrome: A review of 37 patients with Burkitt's lymphoma. *Am. J. Med.*, 68:486–491.

Dorr, R. T., and Fritz, W. L. (1980): *Cancer Chemotherapy Handbook.* Elsevier Science Publishing, New York.

Foley, K. M. (1982): The practical use of narcotic analgesics. *Med. Clin. North Am.*, 66:(5)1091–1104.

Gilbert, R. W., Kim, J. H., and Posner, J. B. (1978): Epidural spinal cord compression from metastatic tumor: Diagnosis and treatment. *Ann. Neurol.*, 3:40–51.

Higby, D. J., and Burnett, D. (1980): Granulocyte transfusions: Current status. *Blood*, pp. 2–8.

Mazzaferri, E. L., O'Dorisio, T. M., and LoBuglio, A. F. (1978): Treatment of hypercalcemia associated with malignancy. *Semin. Oncol.*, 5:(2)141–153.

Posner, J. B. (1977): Management of central nervous system metastases. *Semin. Oncol.*, 4:(1)81–91.

Seigel, L. J., and Longo, D. L. (1981): The control of chemotherapy-induced emesis. *Ann. Intern. Med.*, 95:352–359.

16.

Musculoskeletal Diseases

James C. Steigerwald

16.

Musculoskeletal Diseases

In patients with joint disease, arthrocentesis and synovial fluid analysis should be considered an essential part of the diagnostic workup. It is impossible, for example, to diagnose pseudogout or gout accurately without demonstrating calcium pyrophosphate dihydrate or uric acid crystals in synovial fluid. Likewise, septic arthritis can only be confirmed by proper examination and culture of the synovial fluid. Thus, a knowledge of proper technique for arthrocentesis and subsequent synovial fluid analysis is necessary before appropriate therapy can be begun.

I. **ARTHROCENTESIS**

A. **Indications**

　1. An unexplained synovial effusion.

　2. As part of the treatment of septic arthritis.

B. **Techniques**

　1. General

　　a. Mark area where needle is to be inserted with your fingernail.

　　b. Clean skin thoroughly with pHisoHex®, iodine, and/or alcohol.

　　c. Gloves, drapes, and masks are not necessary if the area to be aspirated is not touched after cleansing.

　　d. Anesthetize skin with ethyl chloride spray or use a 25-gauge needle to raise a skin wheal and then infiltrate down to, but not into, the joint capsule with 1% lidocaine.

　　e. Use a 21-gauge needle for entering the joint unless infection or hemarthrosis is suspected, then use an 18-gauge needle.

　　f. Once in a joint always remove as much fluid as possible.

　2. Specific joints

　　a. **Knee.** With the patient supine and the knee extended, insert the needle medially or laterally about 2 cm posterior and inferior to the superior tip of the patella. With the patient sitting and the knee flexed at a 90 degree angle, insert the needle medial to the patellar tendon just underneath the patella. If the suprapatellar bursa is distended, it may be aspirated directly.

　　b. **Ankle.** With the patient supine and the leg-foot angle at 90 degrees, insert the needle vertically just medial to the extensor hallucis tendon and lateral to the medial malleolus.

　　c. **Subtalar joint.** With the patient supine and the leg-foot angle at 90 degrees, insert the needle perpendicular to the skin just below or posterior to the lateral malleolus.

d. **Shoulder.** With the patient seated and the arm resting comfortably on the lap, the needle is inserted just medial to the head of the humerus and below the tip of the coracoid process. The needle is directed superiorly and laterally, being careful not to hit the humerus.

e. **Elbow.** With the patient seated and the elbow flexed to 90 degrees, the needle is inserted perpendicularly to the skin just below the lateral epicondyle.

f. **Wrist.** With the hand and wrist placed palmar surface down, the needle is inserted perpendicularly to the skin, just distal to the radius and ulnar to the anatomic snuff box. In a normal wrist you can generally see an indentation at this area. Because of the multiple bones in the area, however, the needle should be inserted slowly and if contact is made with bone it should be redirected without withdrawing it from the skin.

g. **Small joints of hands and feet.** A 25-gauge needle should be used and "teased" in dorsally under the extensor tendons. It is frequently helpful to have someone pull on the finger to achieve maximum extension and to open up the joint space.

h. **Hip.** Because of the difficulty of aspirating this joint, it should only be done by an experienced physician—preferably under fluoroscopic guidance.

i. **Prepatellar bursa.** This bursa does not communicate with the knee. If there is swelling below the knee, with the leg extended the needle should be inserted parallel to the bursa to prevent insertion of the needle into the knee joint. In an infectious bursitis this may prevent introducing the infection into the joint space.

j. **Olecranon bursa.** This bursa does not normally communicate with the elbow. The arm should be fully extended and the bursa entered parallel to the arm. This prevents insertion of the needle into the elbow joint.

II. SYNOVIAL FLUID ANALYSIS

Place some fluid in appropriate **culture tubes.** If gonococcal infection is suggested, chocolate agar or Thayer-Martin media should be used.

Place a drop of fluid on a microscope slide for Gram stain.

Place fluid in **heparinized tubes** for white blood cell count and differential as well as crystal analysis. For the **white blood cell count** the synovial fluid should be diluted with normal saline. If the usual acidic white blood cell diluting fluid is used it will clot the protein in synovial fluid, thus giving an inaccurate cell count.

Other tests, including synovial fluid glucose levels, are rarely helpful and are not done routinely.

If no fluid or only **blood** appears to be aspirated, try and express a drop or two from the syringe for culture, Gram stain, and crystal analysis.

III. INFECTIOUS ARTHRITIS
Infectious arthritis can be a devastating disease if there are delays in diagnosis or appropriate treatment.

A. Predisposing Factors

1. Concurrent extraarticular illness.
2. Serious chronic illness.
3. Prior arthritis in the affected joint.
4. Concurrent or recent immunosuppressive therapy.
5. Concurrent or recent antibiotics.
6. Previous joint surgery—especially total joint replacement.

B. Principles of Management

1. **Hospitalization.** Since treatment requires close observation and frequent aspiration of the joint, the patient should be hospitalized.

2. Even after initial joint fluid aspirations with Gram stain, culture and white blood cell counts with differential, repeat aspirations are indicated as often as **fluid is reaccumulating.** This could entail 2 to 3 aspirations per day in the first days of treatment. All fluids should be **cultured** until negative cultures are returned, and synovial fluid white blood cell counts should be monitored to see that they are decreasing.

3. **Intravenous antibiotics** (for details see below).

4. **Surgical drainage** is indicated for:

   a. Septic hips.

   b. Inability to adequately remove fluid because of **tissue debris** or loculation of fluid.

   c. **Persistent elevation of synovial fluid white blood cell count** ($>30,000$ cells/cc) and rapid reaccumulation of fluid (>20 cc) after 7 to 10 days of needle drainage and appropriate antibiotic therapy.

5. **Physical therapy.** As soon as acute swelling and pain have diminished, range-of-motion exercises should be instituted to prevent permanent loss of motion in the joint.

C. Specific Joint Infections

1. **Predominant organism in relationship to age**

   a. Less than 2 yr—*Hemophilus influenzae*

   b. 2 to 15 yr—*Staphylococcus aureus*

   c. 15 to 30 yr—*Gonococcus*

   d. Over 30 yr—*Staphylococcus aureus*

2. **Gonococcal arthritis** is a complication of disseminated gonococcal infection **characterized by** fever, typical skin lesions, migratory polyarthritis, and tenosynovitis. Within a few days the arthritis will usually **localize** in one or more joints.

   Treatment includes:

   a. Needle aspiration of the affected joint(s).

   b. Ten to 12 million units of i.v. **penicillin G** per day until there is a good response (usually 1–3 days) and then 2 g/day of ampicillin for 10 to 14 days.

   c. Patients **allergic to penicillin** can receive 1.5 g of oral tetracycline initially and then 2.0 g/day for 10 days.

   d. Pregnant women who are also **penicillin-allergic** can be treated with erythromycin 500 mg every 6 hr i.v. for 3 days, follwed by 2 g/day by mouth for an additional 7 days.

   e. Infection due to penicillinase-producing *Neisseria gonorrhoea* can be treated with cephalothin 2 to 4 g/day for 10 to 14 days.

3. *S aureus*, if untreated, can destroy a joint in 10 to 14 days. **Treatment** includes:

   a. Frequent needle aspirations.

   b. Intravenous nafcillin 8 to 12 g/day for 2 to 4 weeks.

   c. In nafcillin-allergic patients, cephalothin 6 to 8 g/day, clindamycin 1 to 3 g/day, or vancomycin 2 g/day—all for 2 to 4 weeks—can be used.

4. Streptococcal infection

Treatment includes:

   a. Frequent needle aspirations.

   b. Intravenous penicillin G 10 to 12 million U/day for 2 to 3 weeks.

   c. In penicillin-allergic patients, erythromycin 2 to 4 g/day for 2 to 3 weeks.

5. Gram-negative infections (*Escherichia coli, Proteus* species, and *Pseudomonas aerugenosa*) have increased in frequency in the past 20 years. *Pseudomonas* infection is especially common in i.v. drug abusers.

Treatment includes:

   a. Frequent needle aspirations.

   b. Gentamycin 4.5 to 6 mg/kg/day plus carbenicillin 30 g/day for 4 + weeks.

6. Antibiotics following initial Gram stain and culture but before culture results are available: (Dosages given below are for patients with normal renal and hepatic function.)

Organism suspected	Antibiotic	Dosage
Gram-positive cocci	Penicillinase-resistant penicillin	Oxacillin 8 g/day or nafcillin 8–12 g/day or methicillin 12 g/day
Gram-negative cocci	Penicillin G	10–12 million U/day
Gram-negative bacilli	Gentamycin Carbenicillin	4.5–6 mg/kg/day 30 g/day
No organism on Gram stain	Gentamycin + Nafcillin	4.5–6 mg/kg/day 8–12 g/day

7. Viral infections commonly present with arthralgias/arthritis. The most common are hepatitis, infectious mononucleosis, and rubella. They are self-limited. **Treatment** includes salicylate or nonsteroidal anti-inflammatory agents (NSAIDs).

8. **Mycobacteria/fungal arthritis** present as a chronic mono or pauciaiticular arthritis. A positive culture or tissue diagnosis should be made before committing patient to therapy.

D. **Infectious Bursitis** Most commonly seen in the **prepatellar bursa** or the **olecranon bursa**; generally associated with local trauma.

1. **Principles of management**

a. **Aspiration** of bursa for Gram stain, culture, and cell count. **Do not** insert needle into joint since neither of these two bursae communicates with elbow (olecranon bursa) or knee (prepatellar bursa).

b. **Hospitalization is usually not necessary** in an otherwise healthy patient if the patient can return to the physician on a daily basis until infection responds to treatment.

c. *S aureus* is the major cause of infectious bursitis. In the absence of Gram-stain evidence to the contrary, institute treatment with dicloxacillin 2.0 g/day for 7 to 10 days.

IV. **BACK PAIN** Back pain, especially of the low back, is second only to respiratory infection as a cause of absence from work in the United States. Although the differential diagnosis of back pain is quite broad and includes many serious and potentially remediable disorders, only a small percentage of patients have infectious, neoplastic, inflammatory, or metabolic disease as a cause of their pain. **Most patients** have back pain as a result of either structural weakness of the back or direct spinal nerve compression.

A. **Cervical Spine** Cervical pain may be caused by mechanical compression of surrounding structures, by inflammatory processes involving the joints, muscles, fascia, or by compromise of the vascular tissue. Some of the more **common causes** of pain are reviewed.

1. **Osteoarthritis**

a. Osteoarthritis in the cervical spine is **characterized** (as elsewhere in the body) **by degeneration** of cartilage. It may be associated with:

(1) Disc degeneration and decreased joint spaces.

(2) Marginal spur formation: Anterior spurs are rarely symptomatic. Posterior spurs are frequently symptomatic. Apophyseal spurring and sclerosis are frequently symptomatic.

b. **Treatment** is directed toward specific symptoms and includes:

(1) **Rest**

(2) Control aggravating factors such as occupational stress.

(3) Moist **heat** for 20 to 30 min two to three times per day is especially useful for muscle spasm.

(4) **Salicylates** or other NSAIDs. These are given primarily for their **analgesic** effect and secondarily for anti-inflammatory purposes. Therefore, lower doses are frequently sufficient.

(5) **Cervical collar** may help stabilize the cervical spine and relieve nerve root irritation.

(6) **Cervical traction.** If the above measures have failed, the patient should be **instructed** on the use of cervical traction.

(7) **Surgery** is rarely needed and only for neurologic complications.

2. **Rheumatoid arthritis.** The **cervical spine** is involved in more than 75% of patients with rheumatoid arthritis. Because of erosion of the transverse membrane, the atlantoaxial joint is prone to subluxation in several directions with spinal cord compression symptoms in severe cases. Cervical **pain radiating to the occiput** is, however, the most common complaint. The diagnosis is confirmed by obtaining lateral radiographic views of the cervical spine with the neck flexed and then extended. There should be no more than 3.5-mm separation between the odontoid and the anterior arch of the axis on either of these views.

Treatment includes:

a. **Awareness of the condition** so that the neck is not forciably flexed for any medical or surgical procedure. It is not unreasonable to send a patient with this problem to any procedure in a cervical collar.

b. **Aggressive anti-inflammatory medications** (see Chapter 17).

c. **Cervical collar.** If condition is present it should be used when symptomatic or when riding in a car even if the patient is asymptomatic.

d. **Surgical decompression** if neurologic signs develop.

3. **Axial arthropathies.** The cervical spine is not uncommonly involved in patients with an axial arthropathy. The disease involves primarily the apophyseal joints, but eventually there may be calcification of the anterior longitudinal ligaments with resulting fusion of the vertebrae and a stiff or immobile neck.

Treatment includes:

a. **Aggressive anti-inflammatory medication** (see Chapter 17).

b. **Physical therapy.** If fusion seems inevitable, try to have the patient fused in an optimal position, not with the chin resting on the chest.

4. **Fibrositis.** **Widespread** chronic complaints of pain with local tenderness in many areas, disturbed sleep pattern, and absence of any laboratory evidence of inflammation characterizes the patient with fibrositis. Among the most common areas of pain and tenderness are the **cervical spine and paravertebral areas.** This condition may exist as a primary fibrositis or in association with other connective tissue diseases including rheumatoid arthritis.

Treatment includes:

a. **Reassurance** that the disease is not physically crippling.

b. **Local measures** including massage or injections of 1 to 2 cc of 1% lidocaine into most bothersome trigger points.

c. **Tricyclic antidepressants** to reduce alpha wave sleep pattern and to allow for improvement in the quality of sleep. Dosage is quite variable, but low dosage should be utilized when beginning therapy (i.e., 10 mg of amitriptyline).

d. Analgesics—salicylates or NSAIDs can be tried but are generally without much benefit.

e. Narcotics should **not** be used.

5. Polymyalgia rheumatica (see Chapter 17). Characterized by **aching and muscle stiffness** in the proximal muscle groups, including the neck, and generally associated with an elevated Westergren sedimentation rate exceeding 50 mm/hr. In **treatment** corticosteroids are used (see Chapter 17).

6. Vertebrobasilar insufficiency may be caused by impingement of vessels in cervical spondylosis. A multiplicity of signs and symptoms relate to compression but should definitely be thought of if **turning the head** to one side or another causes vertigo, oculovisual changes, or sudden weakness in legs with or without fainting.

Treatment is directed to relief of impingement by: **conservative measures** (see Treatment of Osteoarthritis of the Neck); and, if persistant or progressive neurologic signs are present, **decompressive surgery** is indicated.

B. Thoracic Spine   Pain in the thoracic spine area is less common than in either the cervical or lumbosacral areas. Thoracic spine involvement is rare in rheumatoid arthritis and uncommon with the axial arthropathies, except in very severe cases. Degenerative changes of the spine may occasionally cause nerve compression, which most often responds to conservative management. Other more serious **causes** of thoracic back pain are **pathologic fractures, tumors, and infections.**

1. Pathologic fractures. Pain occurs weeks before fracture is seen on radiographs.

a. Metabolic. Senile, postmenopause, or steroid-induced diseases.

b. Tumors

(1) Primary such as **multiple myeloma.**

(2) Metastasic—breast, kidney, thyroid, prostate, and lung are most common.

2. Infection

a. Bacterial. Most common in senior citizens and i.v. drug users. Infection usually begins in disc space and spreads to bone. Diagnosis is made via culture of disc space. **Treatment** includes rest and suitable antibiotic therapy.

b. Tuberculosis. Pain is generally present for months before radiographic evidence of disease is seen either as a soft-tissue abscess or as disc space narrowing and bone destruction. **Tomograms** are helpful. Diagnosis is made by needle aspiration. **Treatment** is with antituberculous drugs alone unless progressive neurologic signs have developed.

C. Lumbosacral Spine   **Low back pain** is one of the major causes of long-term disability and loss of earnings in all societies. Eighty percent (80%) of adults will experience it sometime during their lifetime. It results in more than 1,400 lost work days annually per 1,000 workers in the United States. More importantly, less than 50% of patients with low back pain of more than 6 months' duration ever return to full gainful employment. The most common causes of low back pain are discussed here.

1. **Lumbosacral strain/sprain**
   a. **Clinical: Acute,** often traumatic; **chronic,** often atraumatic; **aggravated by motion,** relieved by rest; deep musculoskeletal pain; poorly localized and aching; wide radiation not dermatomal; no change with valsalva; characterized by muscle spasm, tenderness, and decreased range of motion; no neurologic deficit.
   b. **Predisposing factors:** Spondylolisthesis—a forward displacement of one vertebrae on another; trauma; hyperlordosis (disc degeneration, obesity, protuberant abdomen, muscle spasm).

2. **Degenerative disc disease** with nerve root compression (Table 1).

   Clinical: Most common in third to fourth decade; history of previous back pain; direct nerve pressure causes sharp laciniating pain; increased pain with valsalva, coughing; dermatomal radiation; sensory and/or motor findings with loss of deep tendon reflexes.

3. **Spondylolisthesis.** Indicates a forward displacement of one vertebra on another that involves the anterior body (and hence in association with spondylosis) or the entire segment (therefore an intact pars). **Congenital:** L5 on S1 most common. **Degenerative:** L4 on L5. Mild degrees are generally asymptomatic. With severe spondylolisthesis, backache is more severe with activity.

4. **Spinal stenosis** is most commonly seen in elderly patients with severe degenerative disc disease. It is characterized by the syndrome of lumbar pseudoclaudication. With **ambulation** there is increasing pain, numbness, and weakness in one or both legs which is lessened or relieved by rest.

   Spinal stenosis is **diagnosed** by **transverse axial tomography** and **computerized axial tomography** (CAT), which are at least as sensitive as myelography and are thus the procedures of choice for diagnosis.

   Differential diagnosis of back symptoms of mechanical and inflammatory disease are shown in Tables 2 and 3.

5. **Treatment of low back pain**
   a. **Lumbosacral sprain syndrome:**
      (1) May resolve spontaneously.
      (2) Local heat.

TABLE 1. *Clinical presentation of nerve root compression*

Nerve root compression			Two major syndromes		
Root	Disc	Pain radiation	Sensory deficit	Motor deficit	Deep tendon reflexes
L5	L4-5	Back to dorsum of foot, great toe	Lateral leg, mediodorsal foot	Foot, great toe extensors	Normal
S1	L5-S1	Back to sole and heel	Heel, lateral foot	Plantar flexors	Absent ankle jerk

TABLE 2. *Differential history of back symptoms of mechanical and inflammatory type*

History	Mechanical	Inflammatory
Past history	±	+ +
Family history	−	+
Onset	Acute	Insidious
Age (yr)	15–90	<40
Sleep disturbance	±	+ +
Morning stiffness	+	+ + +
Involvement of other systems	−	+
Effect of exercise	Worse	Better
Effect of rest	Better	Worse
Radiation of pain	Anatomical (S1, L5)	Diffuse (thoracic, buttock)
Sensory symptoms	+	−
Motor symptoms	+	−

(3) Mild analgesics and/or anti-inflammatories.

(4) Sedation/muscle relaxants (diazepam).

(5) Bedrest with bedboard.

(6) Exercise to strengthen the back, decrease lordosis.

b. **Nerve root compression:**

(1) Bedrest (1 or more weeks).

(2) Analgesics.

(3) Sedation.

(4) Exercise.

(5) Surgery (laminectomy). Indications for laminectomy are: **Absolute:** Cauda equina syndrome (pressure on the sacral roots causing bladder and bowel dysfunction and inability to walk); marked muscular weakness; and, progressive neurologic deficit. **Relative:** Intolerable pain in an emotionally stable individual; pain unrelieved by complete bedrest; recurrent incapacitating sciatica pain.

c. **Spondylolisthesis. Conservative therapy** as for lumbosacral spasm is generally effective. **Surgery** is indicated for uncontrolled pain or progressive neurologic signs.

TABLE 3. *Differential findings on examination between back pain of mechanical and inflammatory type*

Findings	Mechanical	Inflammatory
Scoliosis	+	−
Range of movement: decreased	Asymmetrically	Symmetrically
Local tenderness	Local	Diffuse
Muscle spasm	Local	Diffuse
Straight leg raising	Decreased	Normal
Sciatic nerve stretch	Positive	Absent
Hip involvement	−	+
Neurodeficit	+	−
Other systems	−	+

   d. Spinal stenosis. Surgery is indicated for all patients with severe symptoms.

   e. Compression fractures. Treatment depends on underlying cause.

   f. Inflammatory disease of low back. See Chapter 17.

V. ENTRAPMENT NEUROPATHIES Peripheral nerves may be compressed at specific anatomical sites causing characteristic clinical features. The more common entrapment neuropathies are discussed.

A. Median Nerve The median nerve arises from nerve root fibers C6, C7, C8, and T1. Entrapment occurs most commonly at the carpal tunnel, although occasionally cervical osteoarthritis (spondylosis) may cause median nerve compression.

   1. Carpal tunnel syndrome

     a. Sensory symptoms occur weeks to months before motor involvement and are characterized by: Numbness/paresthesias of the thumb, index, long, and one-half of the ring finger. Symptoms are frequently bilateral. Treatment at this stage is over 90% successful.

     b. Motor symptoms. Weakness and atrophy of the thenar muscles.

     c. Diagnosis

       (1) Tinel sign: Paresthesias are caused by percussion of the nerve at the volar aspect of the wrist.

       (2) Phalen maneuver: Reproduction of symptoms occurs by flexion of the wrist for more than 1 min.

       (3) Nerve conduction studies demonstrate a delayed sensory latency across the wrist. Later a motor latency can also be shown.

       (4) Electromyogram (EMG) is generally abnormal.

     d. Treatment depends on cause.

       (1) Wrist splints are most useful at night.

       (2) Medication—Anti-inflammatory drugs are recommended for rheumatoid arthritis; thyroid replacement in case of hypothyroidism.

       (3) Local injection of the carpal tunnel with ½ cc of 1% lidocaine and ½ cc of a long acting corticosteroid preparation may be efficacious.

       (4) Surgical release is always indicated if muscle weakness and thenar atrophy are present.

   2. Cervical osteoarthritis (spondylosis) generally coexists with the carpal tunnel syndrome.

     a. Sensory and motor symptoms—are similar to those for carpal tunnel. In addition, patients frequently have complaints of pain in cervical area.

     b. Diagnosis

       (1) See carpal tunnel.

       (2) Roentgenogram of cervical and upper thoracic spine.

       (3) Nerve conduction studies from supraclavicular region to the hand.

       (4) EMG, proximal as well as distal arm muscles.

  c. **Treatment** See treatment for carpal tunnel and for cervical spine osteo-arthritis (IV. A. 1.).

B. **Ulnar Nerve** The ulnar nerve arises from nerve root fibers C8 and T1. Entrapment can occur at the elbow (most commonly), the wrist, or secondary to osteoarthritis of the cervical spine.

  1. **Elbow** (cubital fossa syndrome)

   a. **Sensory symptoms:** Numbness/paresthesias occur on the palmar and dorsal surface of the fifth finger, ulnar half of the ring finger, and ulnar side of the hand.

   b. **Motor symptoms** are characterized by weakness of: Flexion and weakness of abduction of the wrist; flexion of the ring and fifth finger; abduction and opposition of the fifth finger; abduction of the thumb; adduction of the thumb; and, adduction and abduction of the fingers.

   c. **Diagnosis**

    (1) Sensory and motor changes in distribution of ulnar nerve.

    (2) Nerve conduction studies.

    (3) EMG.

   d. **Treatment**

    (1) **Nonsteroidal anti-inflammatory medications** should be used if the cause of the problem is **rheumatoid arthritis.**

    (2) **Surgery** is indicated when the motor branch of the nerve is involved.

  2. **Wrist:** Caused by ganglion, trauma, inflammatory arthritis.

   a. **Sensory symptoms** include: Numbness and paresthesias confined to the **palmar** surfaces of the fifth finger, the ulnar half of the ring finger, and the ulnar side of the hand. The dorsum of the hand has normal sensation.

   b. **Motor symptoms** are the same as for the elbow except that flexion of the wrist, fourth, and fifth fingers is intact.

   c. **Diagnosis**

    (1) Sensory and motor changes as described.

    (2) Nerve conduction studies show latencies of ulnar nerve in the hand but not the forearm.

   d. **Treatment**

    (1) NSAIDs for inflammatory arthritis.

    (2) Splinting of wrist.

    (3) Surgery when motor branch of nerve is involved.

  3. **Cervical osteoarthritis**

   a. **Sensory symptoms** are the same as for the elbow. In addition, there frequently is cervical spine pain.

   b. **Motor symptoms.** See elbow.

   c. **Diagnosis**

(1) See elbow.

(2) Roentgenograms of cervical and upper thoracic spine.

(3) Nerve conduction studies from Erb's point to hand.

(4) EMG.

d. Treatment. See treatment for the elbow and cervical spine osteoarthritis (IV. A. 1.).

C. Radial Nerve   The radial nerve arises from the posterior trunk of the brachial plexus and nerve root fibers C5, C6, C7, and C8. Entrapment occurs predominantly at the axilla.

Axilla   (Saturday night palsy) is often seen in people who fall asleep with their arm hung over the back of a chair or other similar object. It can also be seen secondary to pressure from crutches in the axilla.

1. Sensory symptoms include numbness and paresthesias of the posterior radial surface of the thumb and the metacarpal area of the thumb, index, and long fingers.

2. Motor symptoms include weakness of: Extension of the forearm, wrist, and fingers (wrist drop); supination of the forearm; and, triceps.

3. Diagnosis

a. History of trauma.

b. Clinical findings.

c. Nerve conduction studies.

d. EMG.

e. Roentgenograms to rule out fracture.

4. Treatment. Early recognition is important in order to institute treatment appropriate to cause.

D. Common Peroneal Nerve   The common peroneal nerve is a branch of the sciatic nerve which is most frequently entrapped where it divides into the deep and superficial peroneal nerves (in the popliteal area where it winds around the neck of the fibula).

1. Sensory symptoms include decrease or loss of sensation over the lateral leg and dorsum of the foot.

2. Motor symptoms include weakness of extension of foot and ankle.

3. Diagnosis

a. Clinical findings.

b. Arthrogram if popliteal cyst is present.

c. Nerve conduction studies.

d. EMG.

4. Treatment

a. Corticosteroid injections to the knee to decrease size of popliteal cyst.

b. Surgery if injections are not successful or if a cyst is not the cause.

E. Posterior Tibial Nerve The posterior tibial nerve is a branch of the tibial nerve. It can be entrapped in the tarsal tunnel in a flexor retinaculum along the medial malleolus of the ankle.

1. **Sensory symptoms** are worse at night and include paresthesias on the sole of the foot and dorsum of the toes.

2. **Motor symptoms** include weakness of intrinsic muscles of the foot.

3. **Diagnosis**

   a. Clinical findings, especially if there is active synovitis in the area of entrapment.

   b. Nerve conduction studies.

   c. EMG.

   d. Roentgenograms, especially with history of trauma.

4. **Treatment**

   a. Corticosteroid injection into the tarsal tunnel.

   b. Surgery if injections are not helpful.

F. Lateral Femoral Cutaneous Nerve The lateral femoral cutaneous nerve arises from lumbar nerve roots L2 and L3. It may be entrapped at the anterior superior ilial spine where it passes through a tunnel in the inguinal ligament. This is seen in people with one shortened lower extremity (adduction of the hip opposite the shortened extremity stretches the fascia and nerve against the entrapment point), marked obesity (especially if a girdle is worn), and systemic diseases such as diabetes.

1. **Sensory symptoms**

   a. Burning pain and parenthesias in the lateral thigh.

   b. Decreased sensation in areas of pain.

2. There are no **motor** symptoms.

3. **Diagnosis**

   a. Clinical findings.

   b. Sensory nerve conduction studies.

4. **Treatment**

   a. Correction of shortened leg length.

   b. Weight loss and/or removal of girdle.

   c. Surgery to decompress nerve.

VI. METABOLIC BONE DISEASE The regulation of bone metabolism is dependent on a number of factors including: adequate mechanical stress to the musculoskeletal system; sufficient mineral intake (especially calcium) to allow calcium homeostasis without bone resorption; normal levels of biologically active vitamins; and, appropriate hormonal interactions—specifically parathyroid hormone, calcitonin, and gonadal hormones. If any of these regulating mechanisms fail, the calcium homeostatic system is maintained by utilizing the major source of calcium in the body-bone.

Osteopenia is a reduction in bone mass below normal levels. It does not indicate the nature of the underlying abnormality of bone metabolism. Osteopenia may take one (or a combination) of three forms: osteoporosis, osteomalacia, and osteitis fibrosa.

A. Osteoporosis   Osteoporosis is an absolute decrease in bone mass with a parallel loss of protein matrix and bone mineral. It is the most common metabolic bone disease and affects one of four white women by the age of 65 years. These patients have suffered one or more fractures in osteoporotic bones. As such it is indirectly responsible for more than 1 billion dollars of hospital expenses per year.

Predisposing factors include: Small or lighter bones at the time of skeletal maturity (age 35 ± years). Dietary deficiencies in calcium and/or protein. Gastrointestinal absorption of calcium decreases with age; therefore, the amount of calcium in the diet should increase. Prolonged immobilization. Premature menopause. Long-term corticosteroid therapy, i.e., 5 mg or more of prednisone (or its equivalent) for at least 6 months.

1. Diagnosis

    a. Generalized malignancy should be excluded.

    b. Serum calcium, inorganic phosphate, and alkaline phosphatase levels should be normal.

    c. Thyroxine and cortisol levels are normal in idiopathic osteoporosis.

    d. Osteoporosis can occur, however, in hyperthyroidism and Cushing's syndrome.

    e. Serum and urine protein electrophoresis will allow diagnosis of multiple myeloma and light-chain disease.

    f. A 24-hr urine collection for calcium, and phosphorus should be obtained.

    g. A bone biopsy, preferably with tetracycline labeling, will confirm the diagnosis but is rarely necessary.

2. Treatment

    a. Adequate exercise or mobilization after illness.

    b. Dietary calcium supplementation (1–2 g calcium/day) is enough to ensure a 24-hr urine calcium level of > 100 mg/24 hr; levels over 300 mg/24 hr predispose to stones and should be avoided. If this treatment is unsuccessful in preventing progression of disease, then **vitamin D$_3$, 50,000 IU**, one to three times per week may be added. The dosage is adjusted to keep the 24-hr urine calcium between 100–300 mg. The serum calcium levels should also be periodically monitored. If symptoms or signs persist, the following regimen may be used.

    c. Estrogens can be administered to postmenopausal women. They are most effective when given within the first 1 to 2 yr following menopause but may be of some benefit even later. Their effect persists only while they are being given. They are used in cyclic fashion in as low a dosage as possible, i.e., 0.625 mg 21 days/month. The major risk of therapy is uterine bleeding, with a slightly increased possibility of endometrial cancer.

    d. In men a combination of 1 to 1.5 g **calcium**/day plus **vitamin D$_3$**, 50,000

IU, one to three time per week, plus **sodium fluoride** 40–60 mg/day may be of benefit. Sodium fluoride should always be used in conjunction with supplemental calcium to prevent actual bone weakness. Side effects occur in about one-third of patients receiving fluoride and consist primarily of gastrointestinal upset and synovitis.

   e. In the most refractory cases in women, the best regimen appears to be **calcium** (1.0–1.5 g/day), **sodium fluoride** (40–60 mg/day), and **cyclic estrogens** (0.625–2.5 mg/day).

   f. Corticosteroid-induced osteoporosis is caused by direct inhibition of bone formation and decreased calcium absorption from the gastrointestinal tract. Treatment includes: Adequate physical activity; as low a dose as possible of corticosteroids; **calcium 750 to 1,000 mg/day** plus **vitamin D₃** as 50,000 IU one to three times a week. Twenty-four hour urine calcium should be monitored for therapeutic effect or for signs of potential toxicity.

B. Osteomalacia   Deficient mineralization of bone matrix is due to inadequate concentration and/or utilization of calcium and phosphorus. The absolute bone mass may be normal, increased, or decreased.

   1. Predisposing factors

   a. Vitamin D deficiency: Inadequate intake of vitamin D in diet (rare in the United States) or reduced sunlight exposure (rare). Vitamin D malabsorption occurs secondary to impaired gastrointestinal function, pancreatic insufficiency, or insufficient bile salts. Abnormal vitamin D metabolism may occur in severe liver or renal disease, systemic acidosis, and with the anticonvulsant drugs, e.g., phenobarbital and phenytoin.

   b. Phosphate wasting syndrome: Acquired renal tubular defects with isolated phosphate loss, combined renal tubular defects (Fanconi syndrome), renal tubular acidosis, and use of phosphate binding antacids may cause osteomalacia.

   2. Diagnosis

   a. Serum calcium and phosphate levels may be normal or decreased and the alkaline phosphatase level may be normal or increased.

   b. Gastrointestinal studies can confirm a malabsorption syndrome, e.g., 72-hr stool fat.

   c. Tubular reabsorption of phosphate is decreased in phosphate-wasting syndromes.

   d. A bone biopsy with tetracycline labeling can confirm the diagnosis of osteomalacia, as can a reduced serum level of 25-hydroxyvitamin D.

   3. Treatment

   a. With inadequate dietary intake, vitamin D supplements should be given (15,000 IU of vitamin D for 4–6 weeks followed by 400 IU/day.) The diet should also contain at least 750 to 1,000 mg of calcium per day.

   b. With malabsorption syndromes, the primary defect should be corrected when possible (e.g., gluten-free diet with sprue) and calcium 1,000 to

2,000 mg/day plus vitamin D, 50,000 IU one to seven times per week is required.

c. **With severe liver or renal disease or with the use of anticonvulsant medication,** vitamin D supplementation with 50,000 IU/day and 1.0 or more g of calcium are required to restore normal balance. Monitor by checking serum calcium and phosphate levels, 24-hr urine collection for calcium and phosphorus along with measurements of serum levels of 25-hydroxyvitamin D. After normal levels are achieved, usually 2 to 6 months, supplemental vitamin D (1,600 IU/day) should be provided to maintain them.

d. **With phosphate-wasting syndromes** the aim of therapy is to maintain serum phosphate levels between 3 and 4 mg/dl. This requires

(1) 1.5 to 5.0 g phosphate/day. One teaspoonful of Fleet's Phospho®-Soda contains 129 mg of phosphorus. Higher dosages may be required in children.

(2) Vitamin D, 50,000 IU/day is also required.

C. **Osteitis Fibrosa**   Osteitis fibrosa is increased parathyroid hormone-mediated osteoclastic bone resorption with replacement of normal bone with fibrous tissue. Chronic renal disease is a **predisposing factor.**

1. **Diagnosis**

a. In **primary** hyperparathyroidism, serum calcium levels are usually elevated and phosphorus levels are decreased.

b. In **secondary** hyperparathyroidism (e.g., renal disease) serum calcium levels are usually normal or decreased and phosphorus levels are normal or increased.

c. Serum levels of parathyroid hormone are increased in both primary and secondary hyperparathyroidism.

2. **Treatment**

a. **Primary hyperparathyroidism** requires surgery in most cases.

b. **Secondary hyperparathyroidism.** The use of 1, 25-dihydroxyvitamin D works best in patients with low or normal serum calcium levels. The **goal** of therapy is to maintain a 24-hr urine calcium level between 100 and 300 mg. In severe cases with high serum calcium levels, pretreatment partial parathyroidectomy may be necessary.

VII. **LOCALIZED DISORDERS OF BONE: PAGET'S DISEASE**   Paget's disease of bone is a localized disorder involving one or many bones and characterized by increased osteoclastic activity resulting in localized osteolytic lesions. Over several years there is an evolution such that large numbers of osteoblasts are found forming bone at sites of previous osteoclastic lesions. This eventually results in progressive skeletal deformity.

A. **Symptoms**

1. **Pain.** Generally worse on weight bearing and most prominent in the hips. Pain results from periarticular bone involvement. Nerve root pain may occur secondary to bony abnormalities of the vertebrae with nerve root compression.

2. Bony deformities occur, including bowing of the tibia and/or the femur.

3. Increased skin temperature occurs over affected bones.

4. Loss of hearing, secondary to narrowing of cranial ostea and compression of the auditory nerve, may occur.

5. High output cardiac failure may occur secondary to increased blood flow through affected bones.

B. **Diagnosis**

1. Clinical signs and symptoms noted above.

2. Elevation of the serum alkaline phosphatase.

3. Elevation of urinary hydroxyproline levels.

4. Typical findings on roentgenograms.

5. Technetium 99 bone scan is usually abnormal only when disease is active in a particular area.

C. **Treatment** Patients symptomatic with pain will often respond to **salicylates** or any of the other **NSAIDs**. Since most patients with Paget's disease are over 60 years of age, these drugs should be used carefully to prevent any decline in renal function secondary to prostaglandin inhibition.

Criteria for specific treatment include: Disabling pain not relieved by salicylates NSAIDs; progression of skeletal deformity; neurologic complications; increasing deafness; and, high output cardiac failure. Immobilization hypercalcemia/hypercalcuria, especially before and after major surgery is also an indication for therapy.

Three agents have been successful: calcitonin, diphosphonates, and mithramycin.

1. **Calcitonin** inhibits osteoclastic activity. **Salmon calcitonin is the drug of choice** and is 30 to 50 times more potent than human calcitonin.

   The dosage schedule, after a **test dose** of 1 Medical Research Council (MRC) unit is given subcutaneously without adverse reaction, is 50 MRC units three times/week up to 100 MRC units/day, depending on the severity of the symptoms.

   During treatment clinical and biochemical data are followed. If no response occurs after 6 months of 100 MRC units/day, the drug is discontinued. If a good response occurs, the dosage may be lowered and eventually stopped. If symptoms recur, another course of therapy is indicated.

   Side effects immediately following injection include nausea, vomiting, diarrhea, fever, flushing, and taste abnormalities. Antibody resistance to calcitonin occurs in 10% of cases. The escape from therapeutic effect of calcitonin may be due in part to the occurrences of antibodies.

2. **Diphosphonates** bind to hydroxyapatite crystals and block their growth and dissolution. They also inhibit osteoclastic bone resorption.

   The dosage schedule for etidronate disodium diphosphonate is 5 mg/kg/day for 6 months given as a single oral daily dose. This is successful in about 80% of patients.

   Clinical and biochemical parameters should be followed. If there is an inadequate response to 5 mg/kg/day, the patient may be retreated after a 6 to 12 month interlude with 10 mg/kg/day for 6 months or 20 mg/kg/day for 1 to 3 months. There is, however, a definite **increase of osteomalacic bone disease in these higher dose treatment groups.** If the patient's initial response is good but he eventually suffers a relapse, retreatment at 5 mg/kg/day for 6 months is indicated.

Side effects of diphosphonates include: increased bone pain; fractures in areas of osteomalacia; and, diarrhea.

  3. **Mithramycin** inhibits RNA biosynthesis, and osteoclastic proliferation is selectively inhibited.

Dosage schedule for treatment of Paget's disease is 15 to 50 μg/kg/day for 10 days or weekly for 10 weeks. The drug should be given by slow i.v. infusion over 6 to 12 hr.

Clinical and biochemical parameters should be followed during treatment. Remissions may last several years. If the initial response is good, retreatment may be useful with recurrent symptoms.

Side effects of mithramycin include a reversible rise in hepatic enzymes and serum creatinine; decreased platelet counts, which may lead to hemorrhage, nausea, vomiting, and malaise; and potentially unknown effects on RNA synthesis.

VIII. OSTEOARTHRITIS   Osteoarthritis or degenerative joint disease in its primary form effects peripheral and central articulation and is characterized by degeneration of cartilage, subchondral bone thickening, eburnation or marbling of bone, marginal spur formation, and subarticular bone cysts. A **heritable primary form** involving Heberden's nodes and multiple joints occurring around menopause has been reported. Inflammatory erosive forms, primarily involving the hands, have also been seen.

The term **secondary osteoarthritis** is used if there are known direct causes of the arthritis. Included in this category are the osteoarthritic problems secondary to previous inflammatory joint disease, metabolic or endocrine diseases, previous trauma to the joint, and those joints with developmental abnormalities and subsequent biomechanical dysfunction.

The most commonly involved joints include:

  1. Distal interphalangeal (DIP), Heberden's nodes.

  2. Proximal interphalangeal (PIP), Bouchard's nodes.

  3. First carpometacarpal joints.

  4. Hips, 65% to 75% associated with a previous underlying abnormality.

  5. Knees, especially if valgus or varus deformities are present.

  6. First metatarsophalangeal (MTP), bunion joint.

  7. Cervical spine (C4–C6 region) with muscle spasm and radicular pain.

  8. Lumbar spine (L3–S1 region) with muscle spasm and radicular pain.

A. Symptoms

  1. A local disorder usually involving one or a few joints and without systemic manifestations.

2. Pain is described as deep and aching, occurring with weight bearing and/or activity and relieved by rest.

3. Morning stiffness is localized and of brief durations (5–30 min).

B. Signs

1. Local joint tenderness.

2. Crepitus with palpable osteophytes is sometimes present.

3. Synovitis is absent or mild and effusions are infrequent except for knees.

4. Even with joint deformity there is good preservation of function until late in the disease.

C. Treatment   Objectives are to relieve pain, minimize disability, and delay the progression of the disease.

1. General considerations

a. Correction of factors producing excessive joint strain; e.g., obesity, or difference in leg length (corrective shoes).

b. Physical therapy: Hot packs, massage, and ultrasound are helpful in relieving muscle spasm. Exercise helps maintain range of motion.

c. Supportive devices including a cane or crutch for lower extremity problems or soft cervical collars for radicular neck pain.

2. Drug therapy

a. Analgesics. Mechanical causes of pain without much secondary inflammation may respond well to analgesics alone as follows:

(1) Acetaminophen 300-mg or 500-mg. Take one or two capsules four/day.

(2) Propoxyphene hydrochloride 65 mg every 4 to 6 hr as needed for pain.

(3) Use narcotic medications such as codeine very sparingly. They may be most helpful at bedtime to allow patient to rest.

b. Salicylates and NSAIDs. There is good evidence of mild inflammation in most patients, with up to 30% of them having calcium pyrophosphate dihydrate or hydroxyapatite crystals in the synovial fluid or in the surrounding soft tissues. Therefore, anti-inflammatory therapy may be quite beneficial (Table 4).

c. The following **precautions** for the use of NSAIDs **in the elderly** are:

(1) Renal elimination is decreased so gastrointestinal elimination is increased, therefore overall gastrointestinal toxicity is increased.

(2) Start all NSAIDs at 50% of usual dosage and recheck patient within 2 to 4 weeks for signs of toxicity and therapeutic benefit.

(3) After 1 month of therapy at low dosage without side effects or benefits, increase dosage cautiously.

(4) Any drug must eventually be used at full dosage (if tolerated) for 2 to 3 weeks before considering the patient a nonresponder.

3. Intraarticular corticosteroid injections. Intraarticular corticosteroid injections may be used two or three times per year in any one joint. This should give

TABLE 4. *NSAIDs*

Drug	Daily dose	Frequency/day
Salicylates	1.8 g–3.6 g/day	3–6×
Indomethacin (Indocin®)	50–100 mg/day	2–4×
Ibuprofen (Motrin®)	1,200–3,600 mg/day	3–4×
Naproxen (Naprosyn®)	250–750 mg/day	2×
Sulindac (Clinoril®)	200–400 mg/day	2×
Meclofenamate sodium (Meclomen®)	300–400 mg/day	2×
Piroxicam (Feldene®)	10–20 mg/day	1×

substantial relief for at least 3 to 4 weeks to be judged successful and worth repeating and is most useful for:

a. **Knee.** See V. D. 4. Inject 2 cc of long-acting corticosteroid along with 1 cc of local anesthetic.

b. **Cystic Heberden's node.** Inject ¼ cc of long-acting corticosteroid directly into cyst.

4. **Surgical therapy.** If severe pain or disability persists despite optimal medical therapy and roentgenograms show progression of disease, surgery should be considered. Three procedures are most often utilized:

a. **Debridement.** Use of the arthroscope to remove loose bodies, etc., from the knee or shoulder.

b. **Realignment** procedures. Osteotomy is most helpful for the knee.

c. Total joint **replacements**. Hip and knee replacements are most successful.

IX. **SPORTS MEDICINE: THE MUSCULOSKELETAL SYSTEM**   More than 130 million Americans exercise or are engaged in some form of sports activity. Twenty-five million of them are runners. Because of the increasing number of participants, many of whom are newly converted sports or running enthusiasts, sports-related injuries now account for many physician visits.

A. **Shoulder Injuries**   Very few injuries other than those occurring in contact sports involve acute trauma to the shoulder. Most shoulder injuries result from repetitious use of the upper extremity. The musculotendinous unit of the shoulder is the structure that is most subjected to overuse. In addition, ligaments, joint capsule, and limbus may sustain injury from overuse.

To best diagnose the cause of the patient's shoulder problem, the location of discomfort and the exact structures involved must be determined. Identifying the structure may be difficult because of the deep-lying position as well as the close proximity of these structures.

The **differential diagnosis** of the more common shoulder problems is best considered by separating those with symptoms and findings in the anterior part of the shoulder from those located posteriorly.

1. **Anterior shoulder problems** include:

   a. **Impingement syndrome.** An overuse tendinitis of the rotator cuff and subacromial bursitis. Invariably in its chronic form there is some degeneration and partial tearing of the rotator cuff, specifically, the supraspinatus portion. Impingement occurs in the subacromial area and beneath the coracoacromial ligament.

   Treatment of the impingement syndrome consists of: Rest and avoiding any activity that causes pain; pendulum exercises; alternating heat and ice; and NSAIDs. Local steriod injection in association with other measures. Surgery may be necessary for refractory cases.

   b. **Anterior shoulder instability** may be frank recurrent dislocations or, more commonly, subluxations, giving symptoms of the shoulder "slipping in and out" with the arm externally rotated and abducted. Physical finding may include apprehension with passive stress in external rotation and abduction. Anterior inferior glenoid tears of the limbus may be associated with this problem. **Treatment** of anterior shoulder instability should initially involve muscle strengthening of the internal rotators through an active exercise program. **Surgery** may be necessary if symptoms persist and interfere with activity.

   c. **Bicipital tendinitis** is commonly confused with the impingement syndrome. It may present as an acute tendinitis but more commonly develops from **chronic irritation**. The **findings** are those of a very localized palpable tender area directly over the bicipital tendon as it passes through the bicipital groove of the humeral head. The pain experienced by the patient is also located anteriorly and aggravated by shoulder motion. **Treatment** is conservative and the same as for impingement syndrome.

   d. **Anterior glenoid (limbus) tears.** See anterior shoulder instability.

   e. **Acromioclavicular (AC) joint degeneration** presents as anterior shoulder pain that can be localized with careful palpation to the AC joint. A history of an injury may be recalled; however, considerable time may have elapsed between the injury and the symptoms.

2. **Posterior shoulder problems** include:

   a. **Posterior subluxation** of the shoulder may be essentially asymptomatic, that is, without pain, with only a sensation of subluxation. Painful subluxation may have associated posterior glenoid traction osteophytes.

   Patients with symptoms of recurrent posterior subluxation of the shoulder are frequently "loose-jointed" individuals and should be carefully examined to see if certain movements easily cause subluxation. Treatment should be conservative with restriction of aggravating activities. Only rarely does surgery play a role in the treatment of this condition.

   b. **Posterior glenoid tears** occur as a result of posterior subluxation. Generally, these are related to a specific injury with repetitive action such as throwing. Symptoms are those of crepitation and pain. Tenderness is well localized posteriorly and crepitation palpable with certain motions. The diagnosis is confirmed by **arthroscopy.**

    c. Compression injury to nerves about the shoulder most commonly involve the **suprascapular nerve** as it passes beneath the transverse scapular ligament in the suprascapular notch and the **axilliary nerve** as it exits through the quadrilateral space. Both nerves may be injured acutely or by repetitive stress. **Treatment** is conservative, with restriction of activity and observation.

  3. Reflex sympathetic dystrophy. Pathogenesis of reflex sympathetic dystrophy involves **excessive stimulation** of the sympathetic nervous system. It frequently follows: Soft-tissue injury, (40%); fractures, (25%); surgery, (20%); myocardial infarction, (12%); and, cerebral vascular accidents (3%).

Classical signs and **symptoms** of reflex sympathetic dystrophy are generally associated with a **precipitating event** and include:

  a. Pain and swelling in an extremity.

  b. Trophic skin changes in the same extremity.

    (1) Skin atrophy or pigmentary changes.

    (2) Hypertrichosis.

    (3) Hyperhidrosis.

    (4) Nail changes.

  c. Signs and symptoms of vasomotor instability.

  d. Pain and/or limited motion of the ipsilateral shoulder.

Treatment of reflex sympathetic dystrophy is as follows:

  a. Trigger point and/or joint injections with corticosteroids.

  b. Physical therapy.

  c. High-dose prednisone, 60 to 80 mg/day in divided doses for 4 to 14 weeks.

  d. Stellate ganglion blocks at 2- to 4-day intervals for 2 to 6 weeks.

  e. Sympathectomy, if disease is progressive and patient has a positive response to sympathetic nerve blocks.

B. Elbow Injuries Lateral epicondylitis (i.e., **tennis elbow**) generally occurs in beginning or less experienced players. It is caused most often by improper technique when using the backhand stroke.

This injury is generally due to an acute inflammatory process with or without partial rupture of the tendon at the tendon periosteal junction, secondary to repetitive supination of the wrist against resistance, as in extension of the wrist with the hand pronated in tennis, or by repetitive use of a screwdriver. **Predisposing factors** include inadequate forearm, wrist or metacarpal-phalangeal (MCP) extensor power and flexibility.

Treatment of acute lateral epicondylitis includes: Rest; ice within first 48 hr and then moist heat is preferable; NSAIDs; local injection using a mixture of ½ to ¾ cc **lidocaine** and ½ to ¾ cc injectable **steroid** (it is necessary to inject down to the periosteum for a successful result). Dimethylsulfoxide **(DMSO)** is not approved as yet but studies are ongoing.

TABLE 5. *Classification of runners*

Level I	Jogger	Novice or recreational runner averaging 2–18 miles per week (mpw) at 8–16 min/mile
Level II	Sports runner	20–40 mpw at 8–10 min/mile pace
Level III	Long distance runner	40–70 mpw at 7–8 min/mile pace (most marathon runners)
Level IV	Elite	70–170 mpw at 5–7 min/mile pace (world class)

TABLE 6. *Overuse syndromes in runners: relationship between distance run and incidence of injuries*

Miles/week	% Injured runners	Miles/week	% Injured runners
0–20	48	60–80	5
20–40	32	80+	2
40–60	13		

From Pagliano and Jackson, *Runner's World*, pp. 42–50, Nov. 1980, with permission.

Prevention of epicondylitis includes avoiding activities that cause stress to tendons. In tennis make sure: Racket grip is correct size; technique is appropriate, especially for backhand (don't hit with wrists flexed); proper warm-up before strenuous exercise; use of a 4-in strap around forearm just distal to elbow.

C. **Running Injuries: The Knee** Tables 5, 6, and 7 present the classification of runners, and the incidence and etiology of runners' injuries.

The knee is extremely vulnerable to many stresses applied to the lower extremity. Because of its anatomic location, an abnormality proximally in the hip, distally in the ankle or foot, or malalignment of all or part of the leg may be the source of

TABLE 7. *Etiology of running injuries*

Training errors (60%)
    Excessive mileage
    Intensive workouts
    Rapid change in routine
    Terrain (hills, hard surfaces, sand, sloped, or
      banked surfaces)
    Interval training—multiple runs of short duration
      with little rest between bursts
Anatomic factors (20%)
    Pronated foot
    Cavus foot
    Leg length difference
Shoes (20%)
    Soft heels increase force on heel
    Wide heels allow hyperpronation
    Inflexible soles increase muscle stress
    Flat soles give poor traction in mud and snow
      so should be studded
    Irregular wear of heel or sole causes increased muscle
      stress

the problem encountered at the knee. To fully evaluate a knee problem, the entire lower back, hip, and lower extremity needs to be examined.

To best determine the cause of the patient's knee problem, a thorough history must be elicited, followed by localization of the discomfort and identification of the structure involved. Basic understanding of the anatomy is obviously very important.

A **differential diagnosis** can be developed by considering problems that arise from extraarticular structures and from those that are related to intraarticular structures.

1. **Extraarticular** problems

   a. **Iliotibial band syndrome** is an inflammation of the tissue between the iliotibial band and the lateral femoral condyle caused by repeated rubbing as the knee is flexed and extended. Characteristically, this is seen in long-distance runners who have dramatically increased their mileage.

   Treatment includes: Decreasing running distance; ice for 20 min after exercise; stretching exercises; NSAIDs; steroid injection; and, correction of footwear, if necessary.

   b. **Pes anserinus bursitis** is seen most commonly in runners. The hamstrings act as knee flexors and internal rotators of the tibia. The bursa located between the tibial insertion of the medial collateral ligament and the three tendons as they cross to attach to the proximal medial tibia is locally tender with swelling.

   Treatment includes: Limitation of activity (running); ice after exercise; NSAIDs; steroid injection; and, shoe orthotics to correct foot deformity, if present.

   c. **Patellar tendinitis,** or jumper's knee, is an inflammation to the lower pole of the patella. It is particularly common in basketball players, certain track athletes, and, occasionally, runners.

   Treatment includes: Decreased activity; ice after exercise; NSAIDs; and, neopreme patellar stabilizer. **Do not** give steroid injection, and surgery rarely indicated.

   d. **Joint laxity** as an inherited trait or ligamentous laxity secondary to an old ligament tear may be a source of knee pain after a running or jumping activity. Usually, there is a small effusion and rather vague discomfort without good localization.

   Treatment should be directed toward muscle rehabilitation, bracing, if necessary, and adjustment of activity.

   e. **Popliteal tendinitis** is usually associated with running downhill and in conditions causing hyperpronation, such as running on banked surfaces. There will be localized tenderness just anterior to the fibular collateral ligament attachment to the femur.

   Treatment is the same as for the iliotibial band syndrome.

   f. **Medial collateral ligament (MCL) bursitis** is an uncommon condition that may be related to chronic overuse, a direct contusion, or a mild to moderate MCL sprain. A local injection of an anesthetic may help make the diagnosis.

Treatment consists of: Ice; decreased activity; NSAIDs; and, local steroid injection.

g. **Extensor mechanism malalignment** is no more than a tracking abnormality of the patellofemoral joint. It has been called "runner's knee," lateral compression syndrome, chondromalacia of the patella, and patellar subluxation.

The most obvious malalignment problem involves the **entire lower extremity**, often called "malicious malalignment syndrome." It is characterized by femoral anteversion producing internal femoral torsion, genu valgum, external tibial torsion, a Q angle (the angle formed by drawing lines from the anterior superior iliac spine and the tibial tubercle through the midpoint of the patella) over 20°, and general joint laxity, causing a hypermobile patella and pronated (flat) feet.

Not all patients with anterior (patella) knee pain fit this picture. In some, the lateral retinaculum is contracted with tightness of the vastus lateralis combined with weakness of the vastus medialis, producing lateral displacement of the patella. Hamstring tightness is also a common finding.

Patella tracking problems cause a rather vague pain located anteriorly around the patella. Running, knee bends, stairs, and hill climbing aggravate this pain.

Treatment consists of: Eliminating any activity that causes pain; isometric exercises until pain subsides; short arc extension exercises (30°); NSAIDs; hamstring stretching; and, patella-stabilizing braces; it also may require change of exercise and sport activity. Realignment procedures may be necessary in some cases.

2. **Intraarticular** problems

   a. **Meniscal tears,** either those from an acute injury or from degenerative tears, produce **typical symptoms** of "popping," "locking," and "giving way." Joint effusion is commonly present with local joint line tenderness over the menisucus. Quadricep atrophy is usually very prominent and full knee extension may be blocked. **Diagnosis** is confirmed by arthroscopy.

   Treatment consisting of meniscal trimming and a muscle rehabilitation program should be completed before returning to sports activity involving running and jumping.

   b. **Synovial plicae** are normal synovial folds that may become injured by direct contusion or by repetitive overstress. The most common plica involved is the **medial** plica, which gives symptoms of pain and clicking over the medial femoral condyle when the knee is moved. **Diagnosis** is confirmed by arthroscopy.

   Treatment consists of: Ice; decreased activity; NSAIDs; local steroid injection; and, rarely, synovial resection may be necessary.

   c. **Old trauma,** such as ligamentous injuries, previous meniscectomy, or osteochondritic defect, causes symptoms of knee pain, effusion, and crepitance, all aggravated by activity. **Synovitis** may be a prominent part of the symptom complex. The findings will depend on the "old injury." **Diagnosis** of the intraarticular pathology can be confirmed and graded by arthroscopy.

Treatment consists of: Decreased activity; changes of activity to cycling and swimming; NSAIDs; muscle-strengthening program; and, arthroscopic debridement.

    d. Chondromalacia of patella is not a clinical diagnosis but rather a **pathologic process**. The condition is poorly understood but best considered as part of the malalignment syndromes. Treatment specifically for this pathologic process is the same as outlined for malalignment problems. **Mechanical shaving** of the lesion should be considered in refractory cases.

D. Foot and Lower Leg Injuries

    1. Shin splints. Pathogenesis includes overuse of underdeveloped or untrained muscles, particularly the posterior tibial muscle. Small tears at the origin, belly, or musculotendinous junction of the involved muscle may occur with herniation of the muscle through the fascia. Shin splints may be associated with a periostitis, especially if the runner tries to run through the initial injury.

    Treatment: Rule out ischemic compartment syndromes or stress fractures; rest; stretching exercises prior to running; proper footwear (may need orthotics to prevent hyperpronation); and, avoid running on hard surfaces.

    2. Plantar fasciitis. Generally follows excessive walking or running on a pronated foot, especially if there is a loose, poorly fitted heel counter in the shoe. This puts undue tension on the plantar fascia. Seen more commonly in people with a flattened longitudinal arch (flat feet). **Spur formation** results from traction of the plantar fascia on the periosteum of calcaneus.

    Treatment. Raising the heel ¼ in removes tension placed on the calcaneus by the Achilles tendon, and releases tension of the fascia by plantar flexing the foot. Additional measures include: heel cup; local injection (may require two to three injections for relief); and, **surgery** to release plantar fascia.

X. ENDOCRINE DISORDERS
Musculoskeletal problems associated with endocrine disorders are not uncommon. The more prevalent associations are listed below.

A. Adrenal Gland

    1. Osteonecrosis (aseptic necrosis of bone). This may occur in endogenous Cushing's disease but is more common in patients receiving high-dose long-term corticosteroid therapy for another illness. Patients receiving corticosteroids with systemic lupus erythematosus and patients post renal transplant appear to be most at risk.

        a. Symptoms and signs. The most common area for osteonecrosis to develop is the femoral head where pain is the first symptom. In other areas (femoral condyles, humeral head, ankle, carpal, or tarsal bones), pain and swelling may be present. Symptoms usually precede any radiologic changes by two to three months.

b. **Diagnosis** necessitates evaluation of clinical symptoms and roentgenograms of affected area. Technetium 99 bone scan may be positive before there are any changes on roentgenograms. A positive scan shows no isotope in the affected section of bone.

c. **Treatment:** Reduce dosage of corticosteroid as much as possible. Non- or partial weight bearing should be followed if involved bone is in the lower extremities. Decompression of involved area by removing core of bone has been reasonably successful for femoral head. Total joint replacement may be necessary for very symptomatic cases.

2. **Corticosteroid withdrawal syndrome** is caused by too rapid a taper of corticosteroids in patients who have been on long-term, high-dose therapy. Patients complain of weakness, fatigue, myalgias, arthralgias, and may develop a low-grade fever. Physical examination demonstrates tender muscles and periarticular structures but no synovitis.

Treatment: Although symptoms will resolve spontaneously, a temporary halt or slowing of corticosteroid taper is beneficial.

B. Diabetes Mellitus

1. **Neuropathic/Charcot joints** occurs predominantly in the **lower extremities** and appears to be a consequence of severe long-standing peripheral neuropathy. It is most common in the tarsal and tarsometatarsal joints but is also seen in the metatarsophalangeal joints, ankles, and knees.

Clinical presentation involves painless soft-tissue swelling and deformity. **Diagnosis** includes awareness of clinical condition and physical findings. Roentgenograms show typical changes.

Treatment: Non-weight bearing may prevent progression of disease. Orthotic devices may also be helpful to prevent deformities.

2. **Diabetic osteopathy** is one of the more unusual complications of diabetes mellitus. This presents as patchy or generalized osteopenia involving the bones of the forefoot (osteolysis of the forefoot). There may also be some erosive changes in the involved bones. Pain is the overriding **symptom**. Roentgenogram showing typical feature confirms diagnosis.

No treatment appears to be effective, although the process may improve spontaneously.

3. **Periarthritis of shoulder** is more common in diabetics than in a control population. The condition should be treated aggressively to prevent the development of a frozen shoulder.

4. **Carpal tunnel syndrome** is increased in patients with diabetes mellitus. See section on carpal tunnel for treatment (V. A. 1.).

5. **Dupuytren's contracture and finger joint contractures.** The latter are prominent in diabetic children. If severe contracture develops and is not responsive to physical therapy, **surgical** release may be necessary.

C. Hypothyroidism/Myxedema   Musculoskeletal complaints are among the most common presenting complaints of myxedematous patients.

1. Clinical features

    a. Muscle stiffness and pain originate from a mild myopathy and are associated with elevated muscle enzymes, especially the creatinine phosphokinase (CPK).

    b. Arthropathy may be related to the myxedema itself with thick viscous synovial fluid or may contain calcium pyrophosphate dihydrate crystals, e.g., pseudogout.

    c. Carpal tunnel syndrome also may occur.

2. Diagnosis. Clinical findings and appropriate laboratory evaluation including a CPK and thyroid function studies and nerve conduction studies are indicated.

3. Treatment. Thyroid replacement.

BIBLIOGRAPHY

Kelley, W. N., Harris, E. D. Jr., Ruddy, S., and Sledge, C. B, (1981): *Textbook of Rheumatology.* W. B. Saunders, Philadelphia.

McCarthy, D. J. (1979): *Arthritis and Allied Conditions.* (1979): Lea and Febiger, Philadelphia.

Specific

Bland, J. H., Merrit, J. A., and Boushey, D. R. (1977): The painful shoulder. *Semin. Arthritis Rheum.*, 7:21–47.

Brody, D. M. (1980): Running injuries. *Clinical Symposia*, 32(4):2–36.

Goldberg, D. L., and Cohen, A. S. (1976): Acute infectious arthritis. A review of patients with nongonococcal joint infections. *Am. J. Med.*, 60:369.

Handsfield, H. N., Wiesner, P. J., and Holmes, K. K. (1976): Treatment of the gonococcal arthritis-dermatitis syndrome. *Ann. Intern. Med.*, 84:661.

Jayson, M. (1976): *The Lumbar Spine and Back Pain.* Sector Publishing Ltd., London.

Kopell, H. D., and Thompson, W. A. L. (1963): *Peripheral Entrapment Neuropathies.* Williams and Wilkens Co., Baltimore.

Riggs, B. L., Seeman, E., Hodgson, S. F., et al. (1982): Effect of the fluoride/calcium regimen on vertebral fracture occurrence in postmenopausal osteoporosis. *NEJM*, pp. 446–450.

Singer, F. R. (1977): *Paget's Disease of Bone.* Plenum Medical Book Company, New York.

17.

Rheumatic Diseases

Brian L. Kotzin

17.

Rheumatic Diseases

I. RHEUMATOID ARTHRITIS

A. General Considerations Important for Management Rheumatoid arthritis (RA) is a chronic inflammatory systemic disease of unknown etiology. Although the joints bear the brunt of the inflammatory destruction, other organs are frequently involved. The arthritis tends to be symmetrical and can vary in intensity and extent from self-limited, intermittent involvement of a few joints to a progressive destructive arthritis of almost every peripheral joint. Especially early in the course of disease, it is extremely difficult to prognosticate for an individual patient. Later, one must frequently rely on the pace of disease in the past to attempt to predict the future. It should be emphasized that the time course of disease, as well as efficacy of therapy, is usually measured in months to years. Joint disease per se is rarely fatal but complications of the articular and extraarticular process may be.

Although there is no cure, significant advances in management have considerably lessened the disability. General principles regarding treatment exist, but because of disease and patient variability, therapy must be designed on an individual basis. The goals of management include relief of pain, especially by controlling inflammation; the prevention of joint destruction and deformity; and, the maintenance or restoration of joint and patient function. **Optimal management of RA requires the combined efforts of multiple members of a health care team.** In this chapter, drug therapy is emphasized, and although it has a central role, it represents only one of several important treatment modalities. Supportive measures include **patient education**, the judicial use of **systemic and local joint rest, exercise and physical therapy**, and **occupational therapy**. Physical therapy is frequently important to preserve joint range of motion and to strengthen muscles, while occupational therapy can review and provide assistive devices for activities of daily living as well as helping in joint protection. **For many patients, surgery (either prophylactic or reconstructive) is an important part of optimal management.**

Assessing the activity of joint disease and the efficacy of treatment can be difficult. Important **variables to evaluate** include the extent of systemic symptoms (i.e., fatigue), duration of morning stiffness, signs and symptoms of joint inflammation (i.e., pain, tenderness, swelling, etc.), progression of joint deformity, changes in joint and patient function (i.e., by reviewing activities of daily living and employment), and radiographic progression of joint destruction.

B. Drug Therapy Figure 1 shows a general scheme for the management of rheumatoid arthritis.

    1. Salicylates and nonsteroidal anti-inflammatory drugs (NSAIDs)

        a. General considerations. Salicylates, usually in the form of aspirin, are

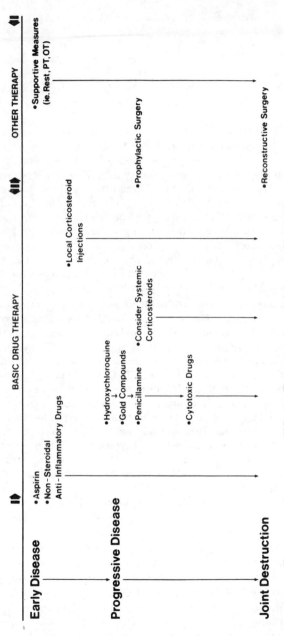

FIG. 1. The management of rheumatoid arthritis.

the cornerstone of drug treatment in RA. The major advantages of regular aspirin over other NSAIDs include low cost (10 to 30 times less expensive) and years of experience with a low incidence of serious complications. There is also no evidence that the other NSAIDs are more efficacious than aspirin in the treatment of RA. The newer nonsalicylate NSAIDs have a lower incidence of gastrointestinal (GI) intolerance and are easier to administer compared with aspirin (see below). The major **advantages** of the nonacetylated salicylates are lack of GI toxicity and absence of platelet function inhibition. Whether the nonacetylated salicylates are as effective as aspirin in RA remains unclear. The different NSAID preparations and adult dosages are shown in Table 1. All the drugs have antipyretic and analgesic effects in addition to their effect on inflammation.

b. **GI toxicity.** A major problem with the use of aspirin and other nonsalicylate NSAIDs is GI toxicity. This may present as: symptomatic **intolerance** (i.e., dyspepsia, heartburn, epigastric pain, and nausea), which is the major reason for noncompliance; an increase in **occult GI blood loss**, which occurs in most patients taking aspirin and is not usually clinically significant; and, major **upper GI hemorrhage**, which is a rare event (probably less than one episode per 1,000 users). It is important to realize that these forms of GI toxicity may not be correlated. For example, the asymptomatic patient may be equally likely to have major upper GI hemorrhage. Aspirin results in symptomatic intolerance more often than other NSAIDs. Indomethacin and phenylbutazone may result in more GI symptomatic toxicity than the other nonsalicylate preparations. Interestingly, **symptomatic intolerance to one NSAID does not necessarily predict intolerance to another**. The risk for major upper GI hemorrhage may be nearly equal for all the different drugs except for the nonacetylated salicylates, which result in almost no GI toxicity.

Local gastric damage from aspirin is immediate after ingestion. The systemic inhibition of prostaglandin synthesis and antiplatelet effect of the NSAIDs may, however, contribute to gastric toxicity and bleeding. Much of the local damage from aspirin can be prevented by adequate buffering **with nonabsorbable antacids** when the aspirin is ingested. The amount of buffering required cannot be accomplished in combination tablets that contain both antacid and buffer. Preparations of "buffered aspirin" are also much more expensive than regular aspirin.

Patients should be warned about the synergistic GI toxicity when both NSAIDs (especially aspirin) and ethanol are consumed.

c. **Interference with hemostasis. The ingestion of aspirin results in a pronounced irreversible inhibition of platelet function.** Less than one tablet can adversely affect nearly all the platelets in the body, although paradoxically, less inhibition of hemostasis may be seen at higher aspirin doses. Aspirin is thus contraindicated for patients on warfarin, patients with a bleeding diathesis, or for patients where hemostasis is critical. The other nonsalicylate NSAIDs have a variable and reversible effect on platelet function. The platelets remain defective only while significant drug levels

TABLE 1. *NSAIDs commonly used in the treatment of rheumatic diseases[a]*

Drug	Tablet/capsule size (mg)	Starting dose	Maximum daily dose (mg)
Aspirin:	325	650–975 mg q.i.d	Variable[b]
Enteric-coated aspirin (i.e., Ecotrin®, Easprin®)	325, 500, 975	650–975 mg q.i.d.	Variable[b]
Nonacetylated salicylates:			
Salsalate (Disalcid®)	500	1,000 mg t.i.d.	Variable[b]
Choline magnesium trisalicylate (Trilisate®)	500, 750	1,000 mg t.i.d.	Variable[b]
Choline salicylate (Arthropan®)	1 tsp = 650	1,300 mg q.i.d	Variable[b]
Magnesium salicylate	600, 545	1,000–1,200 mg t.i.d.	Variable[b]
Indomethacin (Indocin®)	25,50,75SR	25 mg t.i.d.	200
Ibuprofen (Motrin®)	400,600	400 mg q.i.d.	2,400
Naproxen (Naprosyn®)	250,375,500	250–375 mg b.i.d.	1,000
Fenoprofen calcium (Nalfon®)	200,300,600	300–600 mg q.i.d	3,200
Tolmetin sodium (Tolectin®)	200,400	400 mg t.i.d.	2,000
Sulindac (Clinoril®)	150,200	150–200 mg b.i.d.	400
Piroxicam (Feldene®)	20	20 mg q.d.	20
Meclofenamate sodium (Meclomen®)	50,100	50 mg t.i.d.	400
Phenylbutazone (Butazolidin®)	100	100 mg t.i.d.	400
Oxyphenbutazone (Tandearil®)	100	100 mg t.i.d.	400

[a]Not all possible drug preparations are included.
[b]Therapeutic dose and maximal daily dose are highly variable and depend on salicylate level.

are present. If possible, these drugs should be avoided in patients receiving anticoagulants, or used with extreme caution. The nonacetylated salicylates result in negligible platelet inhibition. **However, all salicylates interfere with vitamin K-dependent clotting factor synthesis and can markedly prolong the prothrombin time in patients on warfarin.** If salicylates are administered to such a patient, the prothrombin time must be followed carefully while therapeutic salicylate levels are being achieved. **In addition to its antiplatelet effect, phenylbutazone also has a marked interaction** with warfarin and greatly potentiates its action. Ethanol potentiates and prolongs the antiplatelet effect of aspirin.

d. **Effect on renal function.** NSAIDs may result in **reversible acute renal insufficiency secondary to vasoconstriction**, probably mediated by an effect on prostaglandin synthesis. If recognized early, and the drug discontinued, this complication is totally reversible. Diseases that result in decreased renal blood flow place the patient at increased risk. Thus, NSAIDs should be **used with caution in patients with** hypovolemia of any cause, congestive heart failure, cirrhosis, or the nephrotic syndrome. In addition, patients with preexisting renal disease (i.e., glomerulonephritis) are at increased risk. Decreasing renal function secondary to NSAIDs can be a great source of confusion in patients with lupus nephritis.

Increased **salt and water retention** has been reported with nearly all NSAIDs, perhaps related to their effect on renal hemodynamics. Rare reports of other forms of renal toxicity include the nephrotic syndrome and acute interstitial nephritis.

e. **Other toxicities**

(1) **Aspirin** and other **salicylates** have a number of important **drug interactions** in addition to the warfarin interaction mentioned above. For example, salicylates interfere with the action of uricosuric drugs (probenecid and sulfinpyrazone) and of spironolactone, and with the renal excretion of methotrexate.

(2) A syndrome of **aspirin hypersensitivity** includes nasal polyps, asthma, and occasionally serious anaphylactic-like reactions. It does not appear to be a true allergic reaction. Cross-reactivity with other nonsalicylate NSAIDs has been observed whereas the administration of nonacetylated salicylates has been tolerated.

(3) **Serious bone marrow toxicity** has been described with the use of **phenylbutazone and oxyphenbutazone.** Agranulocytosis can occur relatively early (weeks) after starting the drug, and patients usually recover if they can be supported through the acute episode. A much more serious problem is irreversible bone marrow aplasia, which is usually observed in patients on chronic therapy. The elderly patient appears to be at greater risk. Patients on these drugs should be monitored for bone marrow toxicity, although it is not clear that this complication can be prevented. **Chronic therapy with these drugs, especially in the elderly population, should be avoided.**

(4) Therapeutic doses of **some NSAIDs, especially indomethacin**, have been associated with **CNS side effects**, including confusion, drowsiness, decreased concentration, headache, depression, and psychosis. These side effects are more likely to occur in elderly patients.

(5) Therapeutic doses of **meclofenamate** sodium have resulted in **diarrhea** in a significant percentage of patients.

(6) **Liver enzyme elevations** have been frequently observed with the use

of aspirin and other NSAIDs, especially in patients with systemic lupus and juvenile rheumatoid arthritis. This has not been a problem in patients with adult RA.

(7) Many CNS and metabolic complications may occur with **severe salicylate intoxication** and are not discussed here.

(8) Treatment with nonsalicylate NSAIDs is generally **not recommended during pregnancy**. Aspirin therapy has been associated with both prolonged gestation and labor and should be avoided if possible in the third trimester.

f. Administration of aspirin. Figure 2 presents a scheme for the administration of aspirin in RA. The **goal** of therapy is to achieve a serum salicylate level of 15 to 30 mg%. A difficult problem in the administration of aspirin relates to the marked individual variability of the serum level that results from a given dose. Thus 8 to 36 tablets (325 mg per tablet) may be required to achieve a therapeutic salicylate level in different patients, and it is impossible to predict the therapeutic dose prior to administration. Because of this variability and the danger of salicylate intoxication (especially in elderly patients), it is important to **monitor salicylate levels** either clinically or by laboratory methods. The development of tinnitus indicates that the level is greater than 20 mg%. Unfortunately, **children and many elderly patients may not note tinnitus** (elderly patients may just manifest increased hearing loss). **In these patients, serum salicylate levels should be periodically obtained.**

One should start with a relatively low aspirin dose (2 to 3 tablets q.i.d.) and slowly increase the dosage at weekly intervals. As one achieves higher serum salicylate levels, metabolic pathways are saturated and the serum half-life increases. Thus, at high serum levels, a small increase in dosage can result in a relatively large increase in serum level. In addition, at high serum levels, urinary excretion becomes a major route of salicylate elimination, and small changes in urine pH may drastically change serum salicylate levels. **Absorbable antacids should be avoided** in the patient taking chronic salicylate therapy; the resulting increased urine pH can greatly increase renal excretion of salicylate and decrease serum levels. Similarly, a continuously lowered urine pH can decrease excretion and result in salicylate intoxication.

g. Use and efficacy of other NSAIDs. There is no evidence that one NSAID is more efficacious than another in the treatment of RA. Furthermore, there is no easy way to predict which drug will result in the best response in an individual patient.

All nonsalicylate NSAIDs should be administered with food initially. These drugs are definitely easier to administer than salicylates. A **2- to 3-week trial** is necessary before concluding that a drug is not efficacious.

Although aspirin does interact with other NSAIDs, this does not preclude combination therapy. Thus, indomethacin at bedtime might add significant benefit to a chronic aspirin regimen. Other combinations are possible,

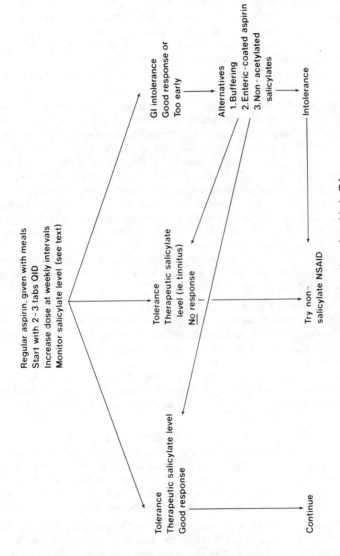

Regular aspirin, given with meals
Start with 2–3 tabs QID
Increase dose at weekly intervals
Monitor salicylate level (see text)

Tolerance
Therapeutic salicylate level
Good response

Continue

Tolerance
Therapeutic salicylate
level (ie. tinnitus)
No response

Try non-
salicylate NSAID

GI intolerance
Good response or
Too early

Alternatives
1. Buffering
2. Enteric-coated aspirin
3. Non-acetylated
salicylates

Intolerance

FIG. 2. Administration of aspirin in RA.

although the maximal benefit from a single drug should be assessed first. The GI toxicity for combinations is additive.

h. Use of NSAIDs in elderly patients. As discussed above, it is more difficult to assess salicylate levels in elderly patients clinically. Furthermore, salicylate intoxication in these patients may result in more neurologic, metabolic, and cardiovascular complications. Elderly patients may be at greater risk for GI and renal complications of NSAIDs, the neurologic toxicity observed with indomethacin, and the bone marrow suppression associated with phenylbutazone.

2. **Remittive drugs.** Unlike NSAIDs, remittive drugs may be capable of **reversing the progression of the underlying disease** and inducing a remission. They also may have the capability to decrease the radiographic progression of erosive disease. Unfortunately, the potential toxicity of these drugs is greater than that of the NSAIDs. The **decision to use these drugs** is based on severity of disease, prior response to conservative measures and to NSAIDs, and the effect of the disease on patient function. The trend has been to use these drugs earlier in disease, before patients have evidence of irreversible structural damage. They should not be viewed as measures of last resort. A common situation for the use of these drugs is in a patient with several months of progressive disease despite prior maximal therapy with conservative measures and NSAIDs. Patients should be advised that improvement with remittive drugs may not be apparent for months. **None** of the remittive drugs **are recommended during pregnancy.**

a. **Antimalarials.** The most commonly used drugs in this group include hydroxychloroquine (Plaquenil®) and chloroquine, with **hydroxychloroquine as the drug of choice**. Although the list of potential toxic effects is large, they are generally uncommon and reversible. Indeed, at the doses recommended, the antimalarials are remarkably well tolerated. They are clearly less toxic than other remittive agents and are easier to administer (i.e., routine laboratory testing is not required, see below). Thus, especially in relatively early disease, hydroxychloroquine is probably the remittive drug of choice.

Hydroxychloroquine should be started at 200 mg by mouth (p.o.) per day, and if well tolerated, can be increased to 400 mg/day, which is the maximum recommended dose. A beneficial effect is generally not seen before 6 weeks of treatment, and the drug should be continued at least 3 to 4 months before a decision regarding efficacy is made. If a good response is achieved, the maintenance dose can be decreased to 200 mg/day in some patients.

The complication of major concern is visual impairment due to retinal toxicity. This toxicity is related to the rate of administration and to the total cumulative dose, and at the doses recommended, it is rarely seen. Patients should be examined by an ophthalmologist every 6 months while on treatment. This exam should include a careful fundoscopic exam and studies of visual acuity, visual fields, and color vision. At the first sign of any abnormality, the drug must be stopped immediately.

b. **Gold compounds.** Numerous studies have documented the efficacy of gold compounds in rheumatoid arthritis. The most frequently used preparations are gold sodium thiomalate (Myochrysine®) and aurothioglucose (Solganal®). The former is an aqueous solution and the latter is prepared as an oil suspension. Doses and the expected clinical efficacy for both drugs are the same. Preliminary studies suggest that aurothioglucose, which is somewhat more difficult to administer, may be less toxic than gold sodium thiomalate. These studies need to be confirmed.

(1) Administration. Gold compounds are difficult to administer because they require repeated injections and close clinical and laboratory follow-up to monitor for toxicity. The drugs are given by deep intramuscular injection. **Test doses** of 10 mg and 25 mg are given 1 week apart, followed by 50 mg at weekly intervals. This dose is continued until maximum clinical improvement or until 1 g total dosage if no response is seen. Improvement is generally not seen before 500-mg cumulative dose. When a clinical response is obtained, maintenance therapy is necessary for continued improvement; the dosing interval is gradually increased to 50 mg every 2 to 4 weeks. At the first sign of relapse, the frequency of injections is increased. Prior to each injection, patients should undergo a **symptom review** for toxicity, complete blood count (including platelet count), and dipstick test for proteinuria (see below).

(2) Toxicity. Gold compounds should not be given to patients who have had a previous serious gold reaction. The drug should be cautiously used in patients with renal, hepatic, hematopoietic, or dermatologic disorders. However, gold is not contraindicated in Felty's syndrome (see below). **Adverse reactions to gold are frequent** (occurring in up to 50% of patients) and can occur at any time during therapy. Fortunately most reactions are mild. **Hematologic toxicity**, including agranulocytosis, thrombocytopenia, and aplastic anemia, is the most serious complication of gold therapy. **Frequent hematologic monitoring** is mandatory.

Nephropathy with gold therapy is usually manifested by proteinuria. A membranous glomerulopathy has been observed on kidney biopsies. Rarely, patients will progress to the nephrotic syndrome. Kidney toxicity is almost always reversible, and progression to renal failure is extremely rare. Treatment can be temporarily interrupted and cautiously restarted in patients with mild amounts of proteinuria. Gold should not be reinstituted in patients who have manifested severe proteinuria.

The most common side effects are mucocutaneous reactions. Rashes are frequently preceded by pruritus, and can resemble other dermatologic conditions (i.e., pityriasis rosea or lichen planus). **Stomatitis** may accompany the rash or may occur alone. In patients with mild mucocutaneous reactions, the drug should be stopped initially. After the reaction has cleared, the drug can be cautiously reinstituted at a lower dose.

Nitritoid reactions resemble the pharmacologic effects of nitrites and include facial flushing, light-headedness, and even syncope. This complication is usually seen shortly after injection with gold sodium thiomalate and can be eliminated by switching to aurothioglucose.

Other less frequent complications have been described with gold therapy, of which the administering physician should be aware. These include enterocolitis, cholestatic jaundice, peripheral neuropathy, and acute pulmonary toxicity.

(3) Oral gold. An oral gold preparation (Auranofin®) has been developed and is now being tested in clinical trials. Diarrhea and abdominal cramps are common **side effects** not seen with injectable gold. However, overall, complications appear to be less frequent and less severe than those due to parenteral gold. It is likely that oral gold will be approved shortly for use in RA.

c. Penicillamine. Penicillamine (Cuprimine®, Depen®) is another effective remittive agent used in the treatment of RA. It is a potent chelating agent and has been used in the past for the treatment of patients with Wilson's disease. The mechanism of action in RA remains unclear. Most trials suggest that the efficacy of penicillamine is equivalent to gold. Because of potential toxicity similar to that of gold, penicillamine must be administered with great care.

(1) Administration. The basic principle of administration is to introduce the drug gradually, with slow increments, until a clinical response is achieved. The initial dose is 250 mg given orally in a single dose at least 1.5 hr after a meal and not with other medications. The dose can be increased by 125 to 250 mg every 2 months until a clinical response or a maximal dose of 750 mg is achieved. Eight to 12 weeks of therapy are generally required before the earliest clinical response is apparent. Penicillamine treatment requires frequent clinical and laboratory monitoring (see below). To ensure patient follow-up, refill prescriptions should **not** be given. A complete blood count (including platelet count) and dipstick test for proteinuria should be performed at 2-week intervals for the first 6 months of therapy and then at least monthly after a maintenance dose is reached.

(2) Toxicity. Toxic reactions are common and may be severe. Hematologic toxicity is the most serious and includes leukopenia, thrombocytopenia, agranulocytosis, and aplastic anemia. The drug must be discontinued when there is evidence of a decreasing trend and certainly with platelet counts less than $100,000/mm^3$ or WBC less than $3,000/mm^3$.

Proteinuria, secondary to an immune-complex glomerulonephritis, can occur in up to 20% of patients. In most patients, low-grade proteinuria will resolve despite continued therapy. The drug should be discontinued if sustained proteinuria exceeds 1.0 to 2.0 g/day, if there is associated hematuria, or if renal function decreases (rare). It may take many months for the nephrotic syndrome to clear after discontinuation of the drug.

Skin rash is the most common side effect and frequently is accompanied by pruritus. **Stomatitis**, similar to that in gold therapy, is also seen. **Taste loss** is very frequent but may resolve with continued therapy. A rare complication is **the development of another autoimmune disease** such as Goodpasture's syndrome, myasthenia gravis, polymyositis, systemic lupus, vasculitis, or pemphigus.

3. **Cytotoxic drugs.** Cytotoxic drugs are used for patients who are refractory to more conventional therapy (~5%–15% of all RA patients), either because of lack of efficacy or unacceptable side effects. Because of their potential toxicity, these drugs are reserved for patients with severe disease, and careful follow-up is mandatory.

Azathioprine and **cyclophosphamide** have been studied the most extensively in the treatment of RA. With these drugs, complete remissions are rare, but response rates have been reported as high as 60% to 80%. The mechanism of action is probably related to their suppressive effects on the immune system. Although cyclophosphamide is the more immunosuppressive, there is **no** evidence that it is clinically more efficacious than azathioprine. Cyclophosphamide is more toxic and a more difficult drug to administer than azathioprine. For example, **side effects not seen with azathioprine** include alopecia, bladder toxicity, and profound gonadal toxicity. Furthermore, cyclophosphamide appears to have a greater oncogenic potential. **Therefore, at this time, azathioprine is the cytotoxic drug of first choice in RA.**

a. **Azathioprine** Azathioprine (Imuran®) is rapidly converted to 6-mercaptopurine after absorption. It should be initiated at 1.0 to 1.25 mg/kg/day, given as a single oral dose. If tolerated, this dose should be continued for 2 to 4 months. Maximum clinical benefit is usually not observed for 4 to 6 months. If the clinical response is unsatisfactory, the dose can be slowly increased (0.5 mg/kg/day at approximately monthly intervals) to a maximal dose of 3.0 mg/kg/day.

The most **serious** toxicity during therapy is **bone marrow suppression**, primarily leukopenia. Complete blood counts (including platelet count) should be followed weekly during initiation of therapy and during dosage increases, and at 2-week intervals after a stable dose is achieved. It should be emphasized that the nadir WBC may not be reached for 2 to 4 weeks after the last dose. Therefore, the physician must follow trends as well as the absolute WBC. Patients receiving azathioprine are at increased risk for infection, especially with the development of leukopenia. GI intolerance is common but can be decreased by giving the dose at bedtime. Some patients develop elevated liver enzymes early in therapy, which usually resolves during continued therapy. Chronic liver damage (i.e., cirrhosis) has not been a problem with the use of azathioprine in RA. The major long-term risk of azathioprine therapy is the **development of malignancy**, including lymphoma. However, this risk appears to be less in RA patients than renal transplant patients. The dose of azathioprine should be decreased to 25% of the recommended dose in patients taking **allopurinol**. The dose should also be decreased in patients with **renal insufficiency**.

b. **Cyclophosphamide.** Cyclophosphamide (Cytoxan®) should be initiated at a dose of 1.0 to 1.25 mg/kg/day, given as a single oral dose. The initial dose is continued for at least 2 months. If well tolerated and the clinical response suboptimal, the dose can be increased by 0.5 mg/kg/day increments at approximately monthly intervals to a maximal dose of 2.5 mg/kg/day. Cyclophosphamide can be an **extremely toxic** drug and is further discussed in section II of this chapter and in Chapter 15.

c. **Methotrexate.** Thus far, the clinical efficacy of methotrexate in RA has only been suggested in uncontrolled studies, and controlled studies are in progress. The experience with the use of this drug has been more extensive in other rheumatic diseases (i.e., psoriatic arthritis and inflammatory myositis) and in psoriasis. Methotrexate appears to be less toxic than drugs such as azathioprine and cyclophosphamide, and this probably accounts for its early popularity in the treatment of RA.

Methotrexate is initiated at 7.5 mg/week, given as 2.5 mg p.o. q 12 hr × 3 doses, as a single oral dose, or as a single intramuscular (i.m.) dose. If well tolerated and little or no improvement is noted, the dose can be increased by 2.5 mg increments every 2 weeks, to a maximum dose of 30 to 40 mg/week.

Patients given methotrexate should have blood counts checked prior to each dose initially and then at 2-week intervals after a maintenance dose is achieved. **Stomatitis and GI intolerance are frequent.** Stomatitis appears to be dose-related, and if mild, the drug can be stopped and then reinstituted at a lower dosage. Unlike that for cyclophosphamide and azathioprine, the long-term oncogenic potential of methotrexate appears to be minimal. **The major long-term complication is chronic liver damage, including cirrhosis.** Liver enzyme elevations may not predict which patients will develop cirrhosis, and periodic liver biopsies are recommended at cumulative dose intervals of 1.0 to 1.5 g, depending on other risk factors. Chronic alcohol ingestion, obesity, and diabetes appear to increase the risk of cirrhosis in patients treated with methotrexate. The drug should probably be avoided in alcoholic patients. The guidelines for use of methotrexate in RA are similar to those in psoriasis (see Chapter 22). As noted above, salicylates interfere with the renal excretion of methotrexate and may increase the toxicity at a particular dose.

4. **Systemic corticosteroids.** The use and toxicity of these drugs are discussed in greater detail in section II. Corticosteroid therapy does not appear to alter the natural history of RA (not remittive). However, these drugs have potent **anti-inflammatory effects** and can be extremely valuable in maintaining patient function during periods of active disease. They are also especially valuable for patients with associated incapacitating systemic symptoms (fatigue, anorexia, weight loss, etc.). **Chronic use** results in considerable toxicity, however, and these drugs must be used judiciously. Unfortunately, on too many occasions, corticosteroids are used inappropriately, in excessive dosages, and for unjustifiably prolonged periods of time.

Corticosteroids should be **reserved** for a subgroup of patients who have continued active disease despite conservative measures and NSAIDs. They are sometimes introduced to maintain patient function (hopefully, as a temporary measure) while remittive therapy is introduced. If a good response is obtained, corticosteroids can be tapered. Unfortunately, once started, it is difficult to taper patients off therapy. Patients refractory to conventional therapy frequently require chronic corticosteroid treatment.

Prednisone is almost always the oral preparation used and is initiated at a dose of 5 to 10 mg/day (higher doses are not recommended). The dose should be tapered slowly to the lowest possible dose that maintains the desired benefit. Occasionally, patients can be tapered to every other day therapy.

5. **Intraarticular corticosteroids.** Intraarticular administration of corticosteroids is frequently useful as a temporary measure in RA and has limited toxicity when used judiciously. Injections are best employed when only one or a few joints are active, but **one must be absolutely certain that arthritis is not secondary to infection.** If infection is a possibility, synovial fluid should be removed and analyzed prior to injection. Corticosteroids should also not be injected into grossly unstable joints. There is evidence that repeated intraarticular injections may damage cartilage. The duration of benefit after injection is highly variable, but frequently is reproducible for a particular patient. The preparations and techniques used are discussed in Chapter 16.

6. **Experimental therapy.** At this time, pulse megadose corticosteroid therapy, lymphoplasmapheresis, total lymphoid irradiation, and levamisole are experimental therapies for the treatment of RA. Their use should be limited to the study situation with informed consent under the approval of a human subjects committee.

C. **Extraarticular Manifestations of RA** Some selected extraarticular complications of RA that affect management decisions are discussed briefly.

1. **Rheumatoid nodules** do not usually require any special therapy. Peripheral nodules may occasionally impair function and when subjected to repeated pressure, may ulcerate and become infected. This should be prevented if possible by conservative measures. Occasionally, surgical removal is necessary.

2. **Ocular complications** in RA may take several forms. **Sjögren's syndrome** with keratoconjunctivitis sicca is the most common and is discussed in section V. **Episcleritis**, which usually presents as a red eye with or without ocular discomfort and without visual changes, generally requires no specific therapy. In contrast, **scleritis** is a much more serious problem, is frequently accompanied by severe pain, and can result in scleromalacia perforans and vision loss. Necrotizing scleritis requires skilled management that is coordinated with an ophthalmologist. Topical steroids alone are often ineffective in arresting the disease and frequently must be supplemented with high-dose systemic steroids or even cytotoxic drugs.

3. **Felty's syndrome** is a rare complication of RA, almost always occurring in the setting of long-term rheumatoid factor positive disease. The syndrome includes **splenomegaly and neutropenia** (WBC $< 2,000/\text{mm}^3$), although some patients do not have splenomegaly by exam. These patients frequently have other extraarticular manifestations. **Leg ulcers**, probably related to vasculitis, are common. The major complication of Felty's syndrome is **recurrent infec-**

tion, but the degree of neutropenia correlates poorly with the number and severity of infections. In most cases, bone marrow exam reveals myeloid hyperplasia presumably reflecting increased peripheral destruction. Treatment includes therapy directed at the underlying disease (i.e., remittive drugs). Other therapy may be necessary in patients experiencing frequent or severe infections. Splenectomy may result in a good short-term response. Unfortunately, long-term success is variable, and many patients will have recurrent infections. Lithium salts have been used successfully to raise the neutrophil count, but their ability to prevent infection remains unclear.

4. **Neurologic complications are frequent in RA. Entrapment** or compressive neuropathies (e.g., carpal tunnel syndrome) are common (discussed in Chapter 16). **Peripheral neuropathy** may also be a result of the systemic RA process. A mild sensory peripheral neuropathy may correlate with articular disease activity and usually requires no special therapy. Much more serious is a **fulminant symmetrical sensory-motor neuropathy or mononeuritis multiplex**; both are associated with a high mortality rate. These reflect severe vasculitis and require aggressive therapy (i.e., cyclophosphamide and high-dose corticosteroids, see VI.). **Cervical subluxation** can be very serious, resulting in compression of the cervical cord. C1-C2 subluxation is the most common but subluxation can also occur at lower levels (C3-C5) of the cervical spine. C1-C2 subluxation can also be associated with posterior compression of the occipital nerve (with severe occipital pain) and compression of the vertebral arteries. Therapy is generally designed to prevent abrupt cervical motion that might occur during anesthesia or during falls or whiplash injuries. More aggressive intervention with surgery is indicated for patients with **progressive** neurologic defects or intractable pain.

5. **Vasculitis** may develop in the patient with rheumatoid factor positive disease, particularly with high titers. Vasculitis is usually of the **small vessel** variety (see VI.), characterized by nailfold infarcts or palpable purpuric lesions. Without visceral involvement or severe peripheral limb ischemia, therapy is directed at the underlying disease. Rarely, patients develop a fulminant systemic necrotizing vasculitis with mononeuritis multiplex and visceral involvement. These patients require aggressive therapy (i.e., cyclophosphamide and high-dose steroids; see VI.).

D. **Infectious Arthritis in the Setting of RA**   It may be extremely difficult to diagnose infectious arthritis in a patient with RA. This difficulty in diagnosis frequently leads to a delay in therapy, which results in a poor outcome. Clues to the diagnosis include: one or a few joints disproportionately active compared with the others; fever or other systemic signs of infection; and, changes in a prosthetic joint (i.e., increased pain, increased swelling, or loosening). The management of infectious arthritis is discussed in Chapter 16.

II. SYSTEMIC LUPUS ERYTHEMATOSUS

A. **General Considerations Important for Management**   Systemic lupus erythematosus (SLE) is an autoimmune disease of unknown etiology, characterized by multisystem involvement and protean manifestations. Women of childbearing age are primarily affected. A hallmark of the disease is the presence of serum autoantibodies, especially antinuclear antibodies. The clinical presentation and course of SLE are extremely variable. Some patients have spontaneous remissions, others respond favorably to conservative measures and NSAIDs, and a few die from a multisystem disease unresponsive to high-dose corticosteroids and cytotoxic drugs. Treatment depends on the organ systems involved and must be tailored to the individual patient. The **goal** of therapy is to suppress disease manifestations while minimizing the cumulative toxicity of therapy, especially corticosteroids. Outcome has been steadily improving, with present 5-year survival rates greater than 90% even in patients with severe disease. Overaggressive treatment in the past, especially with corticosteroids, has probably resulted in an increased number of infectious deaths. As emphasized below, many of the disease manifestations can be treated with mild forms of therapy. Physicians have also become aware that infection may mimic manifestations of the disease as well as result in disease flares. **Thus, infection must always be ruled out prior to aggressive therapy.**

Drug therapy is emphasized in the sections below. **As in RA, conservative measures such as patient education, systematic rest, exercise, and physical therapy are also important in the management of SLE.**

B. **Systemic (Constitutional) Symptoms** Fatigue, malaise, anorexia, weight loss, and fever are common in SLE. Fever is usually low grade, but occasional patients have high spiking temperatures. Therapy usually depends on other organ involvement. Symptoms usually respond to conservative measures and antipyretic therapy (especially as part of NSAID treatment). Rarely, patients with debilitating systemic symptoms will require corticosteroids (prednisone, $\leq$ 0.5 mg/kg/day, see below).

C. **Arthralgia/Arthritis** The arthritis is almost always nondestructive and is rarely deforming. Therapy includes **salicylates** and/or other **NSAIDs**. (See I. for discussion of NSAIDs.) Elevation of liver enzymes with salicylates or NSAIDs is more common in SLE compared with RA, but is usually not clinically important. In addition, NSAIDs may result in reversible renal dysfunction, especially in the patient with preexisting lupus nephritis (see I.).

Some patients will have marked improvement in their arthritis after instituting **hydroxychloroquine** therapy. The administration of this drug in SLE is similar to that in RA (see above). Other remittive drugs used in RA (i.e., gold compounds and penicillamine) are usually **not** indicated for the treatment of arthritis in SLE.

D. **Dermatologic Manifestations** Cutaneous disease in SLE frequently includes the classic malar ("butterfly") rash, localized maculopapular eruptions, discoid lesions, photosensitive skin eruptions, and alopecia. Localized, self-limited disease can be treated with topical corticosteroid preparations (see Chapter 22). More extensive disease may respond to **hydroxychloroquine** (administration and toxicity are similar to that for RA, see I.). Rarely, severe generalized skin disease may require more aggressive treatment with systemic corticosteroids. Patients with demonstrated **photosensitivity** should be instructed to avoid sun exposure and to use potent sunscreens (i.e., those that contain para-aminobenzoic acid and have a sunscreen rating of 15).

E. **Serositis** Pleuritis and pericarditis are common in SLE, but complications such as tamponade are rare. Patients frequently report benefit after treatment with

NSAIDs (e.g., indomethacin). Occasional patients may require moderate-dose corticosteroid treatment (prednisone ≤ 0.5 mg/kg/day).

F. Renal Disease

1. **General considerations.** The most important determinant of prognosis in SLE is the presence and degree of kidney involvement. Clinical evidence of lupus nephritis is present in more than 50% of patients, but the extent of damage varies considerably. Many aspects of the management of lupus nephritis, in addition to drug therapy, are controversial, such as clinical value of the renal biopsy and use of serologic correlates of disease activity.

   Not all patients with lupus nephritis need to be treated aggressively with corticosteroids and/or cytotoxic drugs. Therapy should be tailored to the clinical severity of the glomerular involvement. Patients with mild clinical lupus nephritis (i.e., slight proteinuria, urinary sediment abnormalities, and normal, stable renal function) may not need aggressive therapy directed at the kidney involvement. In some patients, the histologic extent of renal involvement may be helpful information. Frequently, treatment in these patients may need to be directed at extrarenal manifestations. Patients with **late-stage lupus nephropathy** may have slowly progressed to chronic renal insufficiency (serum creatinine frequently >4 mg%), with renal biopsy showing extensive glomerular sclerosis. In these patients, corticosteroids and cytotoxic drugs have little effect on the progression to end-stage renal failure, but do increase the likelihood of infection.

   Hypertension is a relatively common and an underappreciated feature of severe lupus nephritis. It may also be exacerbated by corticosteroid treatment. **Good control of hypertension (see Chapter 4) is critically important for a successful outcome in lupus nephritis.**

2. **Corticosteroid therapy. Patients with active lupus nephritis and severe clinical manifestations (decreasing renal function and/or high-grade proteinuria) should be treated vigorously with high-dose corticosteroids as the first line therapy.**

   a. **Preparations.** Although many different corticosteroid preparations are available, only a few are used in the treatment of rheumatic diseases. **Prednisone** is the most commonly used oral preparation and has about four times the anti-inflammatory potency of hydrocortisone, with little mineralocorticoid activity. **Prednisolone** has similar activities as prednisone, but does not require activation by the liver. **Methylprednisolone** (Solu-Medrol®) is frequently used for parenteral administration. This drug has approximately 20% greater anti-inflammatory potency per weight, compared with prednisone. **Parenteral hydrocortisone** (Solu-Cortef®) frequently is used to cover patients during acute situations such as anesthesia. All of these preparations are relatively short-acting steroids. There appears to be little need for more potent systemic steroid preparations (i.e., dexamethasone) in the treatment of rheumatic diseases.

   b. **Initial dose.** An attempt should be made to control the disease quickly. The initial dose should be approximately 1 mg/kg/day (~60 mg/day) in three divided doses. Although not well studied, divided doses are probably more effective and more toxic than a single daily dose. It may take several weeks (4 to 8 weeks) to achieve control of active nephritis.

c. **Tapering.** The rate at which the steroid dose can be decreased is extremely empirical. Initial reductions can be relatively large (i.e., 10 mg every 1–2 weeks) to a daily dose of 40 mg/day. The drug should then be decreased at smaller decrements, for example, 5-mg decrements every 1 to 2 weeks until 20 mg/day, then 2.5-mg decrements every 1 to 2 weeks to maintenance dose. **The goal is to achieve the lowest daily dose that maintains the clinical benefit.** Some patients can be tapered to alternate-day treatment.

Problems that can arise as a result of steroid tapering include: **flare of the underlying disease; hypoadrenalism** (see below); and, the **steroid withdrawal syndrome.** The steroid withdrawal syndrome may include malaise, anorexia, low-grade fevers, arthralgias, myalgias, and postural hypotension. This syndrome must **not** be confused as a flare of the underlying disease and does not necessarily require a change in the tapering schedule.

d. **Toxicity. The toxicity of continuous high-dose corticosteroid therapy is overwhelming,** and includes the following:

(1) **Increased susceptibility to severe infections** secondary to immune suppression. Opportunistic infections are similar to those that occur in patients with cellular immune deficiency diseases.

(2) **Suppression of the hypothalamic–pituitary–adrenal axis with adrenal insufficiency.** Patients who have been on suppressive doses of corticosteroids within the preceding year should carry or wear identification to alert medical personnel that adrenal insufficiency may develop in emergency situations. Patients at risk for adrenal insufficiency should be "covered" with large doses of corticosteroids during anesthesia (100 mg hydrocortisone intravenously 2–4 hr prior to anesthesia and then 100 mg every 6–8 hr during surgery and the first 24 hr). Patients should also be covered during periods of **extreme** stress (e.g., severe infection).

(3) **Endocrine and metabolic complications are** numerous. These include a change in body habitus (i.e., truncal obesity, moon facies), acne hirsutism, menstrual irregularities, impotence, catabolic state with negative nitrogen balance, hyperglycemia, and hyperlipidemia. Suppression of growth in children can also be a serious complication.

(4) **Fluid and electrolyte abnormalities** include sodium and water retention and rarely hypokalemia. **Hypertension** can develop or be exacerbated.

(5) Steroid-induced **osteopenia** can result in a markedly increased incidence of bone fractures. Prophylactic treatment with calcium (1,000 mg/day) and vitamin D (50,000 units, 2 × per week) has been recommended to decrease the rate of bone loss in patients on corticosteroids. This may be especially important for high-risk patients—i.e., white females, (especially postmenopausal and those of small stature). Therapy with calcium and high-dose vitamin D should be introduced slowly,

and urinary calcium excretion should be monitored to prevent possible induction of urolithiasis.

(6) **Psychological problems** can develop and range from anxiety and insomnia to frank psychosis.

(7) **Myopathy** is manifested by proximal muscle weakness, especially prominent in the lower extremities (see III.).

(8) **Avascular necrosis,** especially of the femoral head, can be a severe complication of high-dose corticosteroid therapy and can clinically present years after therapy.

(9) **Ophthalmologic complications** include increased intraocular pressures and the development of posterior subcapsular cataracts.

(10) Other complications include pancreatitis, peptic ulcer disease, and pseudotumor cerebri.

e. **Alternate-day corticosteroid therapy** has been shown to be associated with less toxicity than daily administration. Unfortunately, alternate-day therapy is **usually not successful in suppressing disease activity** (this is true for most rheumatic diseases). However, some patients can be tapered to alternate-day therapy as a maintenance regimen.

f. **Pulse "megadose" corticosteroid therapy** (1 g methylprednisolone i.v./ day for 3 days) has been used to treat lupus nephritis. It was originally believed that this form of therapy might obviate the need for continuous high-dose corticosteroid treatment. It may be effective in a subgroup of patients. Early transient decreases in renal function have been described prior to improvement. The long-term benefit from this therapy remains unclear. At this time, until more studies are completed, pulse therapy should be regarded as investigational.

3. **Cytotoxic drugs.** The most commonly studied cytotoxic (or immunosuppressive) drugs have been **azathioprine and cyclophosphamide.** The use of these drugs has received enthusiastic support from many anecdotal clinical reports. However, although these drugs are frequently used in the treatment of lupus nephritis, controlled studies have failed to demonstrate that they are either efficacious or effective in sparing the dose of steroids.

At this time, these drugs should be reserved for patients who are corticosteroid-treatment failures. These patients fall into three groups: patients who continue to show renal deterioration despite an adequate trial of high-dose steroids; patients who respond to steroids but who require an unacceptably high maintenance dose to maintain a response; and, patients who have unacceptable side effects from steroids. Patients should be provided with complete informed consent, considering the unknown benefits and known toxicities of these drugs.

For reasons outlined above for RA, azathioprine is the cytotoxic drug of first choice because of its lower potential toxicity. The usual doses recommended for both azathioprine and cyclophosphamide are 1.5 to 3.0 mg/kg/day. Responses are generally not seen for several weeks. For a more complete discussion of these drugs, see sections I. and VI.

4. **Experimental therapy.** Alternate dosage schedules for cytotoxic drugs (i.e.,

intermittent bolus therapy), plasmapheresis, and total lymphoid irradiation should be limited to the study situation with appropriate human subjects committee approval.

G. **Central Nervous System Involvement** CNS involvement in SLE may result in markedly different clinical presentations, and therapy should be individualized. **It is always important to rule out other causes (especially infection) of a CNS problem in the setting of SLE.** The most common CNS problems are psychological, including **psychosis.** In the patient who is already on corticosteroids, one must differentiate steroid-induced psychosis from that secondary to SLE. Treatment of SLE-related psychosis includes antipsychotic drugs (see Chapter 25) and, frequently, high-dose steroids (~ 1 mg/kg/day). **Headaches** are also common and may include migraine-like features. Therapy may range from simple analgesia to the use of corticosteroids. A simple, uncomplicated **seizure** in the setting of active SLE may require no change in therapy or just antiseizure medications (see Chapter 23). **Multiple seizures** or status epilepticus are more serious and should be treated with both antiseizure medications and high-dose corticosteroids.

More serious CNS problems include **aseptic meningitis, hemiparesis** and other focal neurologic events, **organic brain syndrome** and **dementia,** and **coma.** These problems should prompt aggressive therapy with high-dose corticosteroids after other etiologies (i.e., infection) have been excluded. If a response to 1 mg/kg/day (in divided doses) is not immediately apparent, the dose should be increased in an attempt to gain control. Occasionally, doses greater than 100 mg/day appear to be required. After control is obtained, tapering from very high doses should be relatively rapid (i.e., to 60 mg/day in 1–2 weeks), if possible. Although they are frequently used, there is little evidence that cytotoxic drugs are effective in the treatment of CNS disease.

H. **Pneumonitis** In addition to pleural involvement (see above), patients with SLE may develop parenchymal lung disease. **Other causes (especially infection) of lung involvement should be excluded.** Patients with severe acute disease should be treated with **high-dose corticosteroid therapy.**

I. **Hematologic Involvement** The **anemia** in patients with SLE is usually the result of chronic disease and is usually not severe (hematocrit $\sim 30\%$). The hematocrit reflects the activity of the underlying disease, and treatment should be directed at other manifestations of disease. Some patients also have a positive Coombs' test, but they do not necessarily have a hemolytic anemia. Occasionally, patients will develop a Coombs' positive autoimmune hemolytic anemia, and they should be treated with high-dose prednisone (1 mg/kg/day). Patients who fail to respond or who require unacceptably high maintenance doses should be considered for splenectomy.

Thrombocytopenia in patients with SLE is very frequent, but is usually mild and requires no specific therapy. Occasional patients develop severe thrombocytopenia, secondary to peripheral destruction, and they should be treated with high-dose prednisone (1 mg/kg/day). Patients who fail to respond or who require unacceptably high maintenance doses should be considered for splenectomy.

Leukopenia in patients with SLE is also frequent and reflects both lymphopenia and neutropenia. It is rarely clinically important and does not require specific therapy.

A **circulating anticoagulant** can be demonstrated in 10% to 15% of patients with SLE, usually initially detected by an increased partial thromboplastin time (PTT). When present alone, it rarely results in a clinical bleeding diathesis, but may add to another hemostatic defect (e.g., thrombocytopenia, aspirin therapy). Rarely, a patient will require corticosteroid therapy for this problem.

III. **POLYMYOSITIS/DERMATOMYOSITIS**   Polymyositis is a disease of unknown etiology in which **muscles are damaged** by a chronic inflammatory process. In dermatomyositis there is an associated rash. The clinical hallmark of these inflammatory myopathies is **proximal muscle weakness**. The lower extremities are frequently involved first, and patients initially have difficulty arising from a low chair or toilet and climbing stairs. Involvement of the shoulder girdle may be manifested by difficulty reaching above the head or combing the hair. Neck muscles are also frequently involved. In severe cases, pharyngeal and upper esophageal musculature may become clinically involved, resulting in dysphagia and aspiration, and rarely progressive involvement of the respiratory muscles will develop. In the adult, these diseases may occur alone or in association with manifestations of other rheumatic diseases as part of an overlap syndrome. Occasionally, inflammatory myopathy may be associated with malignancy, which should be considered if the patient is over 50 years old. Criteria for **diagnosis** include a characteristic history and physical exam, the exclusion of other diseases, and documentation of muscle inflammation and damage by elevated serum muscle enzymes, electromyography, and muscle biopsy. Disease activity and response to therapy are usually followed by serial assessment of muscle strength and serum muscle enzyme (i.e., creatine phosphokinase) determinations.

A. **Corticosteroids**   The initial dose of prednisone is approximately 1 mg/kg/day in three divided doses. Therapy may need to be continued for 2 to 4 months before a maximum response is obtained. Suppression of muscle enzyme elevations usually precedes improvement in muscle strength. The dose is then slowly and carefully tapered (see II.) to a maintenance dose. Only rarely can patients be tapered off prednisone totally. After patients have been on corticosteroids chronically, the physician must carefully assess the contribution of steroid-induced myopathy to the muscle weakness.

B. **Cytotoxic Drugs**   Cytotoxic drugs are used in patients who respond to corticosteroid treatment incompletely or who require unacceptably high maintenance doses to suppress disease. **Methotrexate** has been used successfully, usually given parenterally (i.v. or i.m.). An initial dose of 10 mg/week is then followed by 10-mg increments at weekly intervals to a maximum dose of 50 mg/week. **Azathioprine** has also been recommended for the treatment of refractory myositis. (See I. regarding administration and toxicity of methotrexate and azathioprine.)

IV. **PROGRESSIVE SYSTEMIC SCLEROSIS (SCLERODERMA)**   Progressive systemic sclerosis (PSS) is a multisystem disease of unknown etiology, characterized by **fibrosis of the skin and visceral organs** as well as widespread vascular lesions. There is considerable individual variability in the extent and severity of involvement. In most cases, the **initial symptom** is Raynaud's phenomena. Although skin involvement is the hallmark of the disease, the extent of visceral organ involvement determines prognosis.

No treatment has proved effective in modifying the natural course of PSS. Drugs such as penicillamine may eventually be shown to be mildly effective, but at this time they remain investigational. **The routine use of corticosteroids and/or cytotoxic drugs is not warranted.**

However, treatment directed at different complications can decrease morbidity and mortality as well as improve the quality of life.

A. **Raynaud's Phenomenon** Supportive measures such as ensuring warmth (e.g., down mittens) and avoiding cigarettes can be helpful. Oral drugs that block sympathetic vasoconstriction may be helpful in individual patients. **Reserpine** (0.25–0.50 mg/day), **methyldopa** (750–1,000 mg in three to four divided doses), **guanethidine** (10–40 mg/day), and **phenoxybenzamine** (10 mg/day–10 mg q.i.d.) have been effective occasionally. Recently, the calcium channel blocker **nifedipine** has been shown to be beneficial in some patients. Nifedipine is initiated at 10 mg p.o. t.i.d. and can be slowly increased to a maximal dose of 40 mg p.o. t.i.d. Intraarterial reserpine has occasionally been given for acute relief of severe vasospasm. Surgical **sympathectomy** may help relieve severe vasoconstriction and help heal ischemic lesions but has little if any long-term benefit.

B. **Skin Involvement** No effective therapy has been demonstrated to decrease the progression of skin involvement. Skin ulcers require careful management including removal of nonviable tissue, treatment of infection, and measures to promote blood flow and healing.

C. **Esophageal Dysfunction** The goal of therapy is to decrease symptoms of dysphagia and reflux esophagitis and to prevent the progression of lower esophageal damage to stricture formation. Conservative measures such as elevating the head of the bed, not lying down after eating, and avoiding cigarettes and alcohol can be helpful. Antacids should be used optimally to decrease symptoms. Patients with persistent reflux symptoms should be treated with **cimetidine**, which decreases both symptoms and esophageal damage (see Chapter 11). Cholinergic agents such as bethanechol are rarely required and are rarely useful late in the course of esophageal disease. Esophageal dilation is required for patients with dysphagia secondary to stricture formation.

D. **Small-Bowel Involvement** Small-bowel dysmotility with secondary bacterial overgrowth is common. Patients with diarrhea or malabsorption should be treated with intermittent 2-week courses of a broad-spectrum antibiotic (e.g., tetracycline). Metoclopramide has **not** been shown to be of much help in promoting small-bowel motility. Episodes of adynamic ileus should be managed by intubation and decompression, without surgical intervention if possible.

E. **Myositis** Acute myositis should be treated with corticosteroids (see above). Chronic indolent myopathy, with little evidence of inflammation, responds poorly to corticosteroids.

F. **Arthralgia/Arthritis** Joint complaints can benefit from NSAIDs. These drugs should be avoided in patients at high risk to develop renal disease.

G. **Cardiopulmonary Involvement** **Early inflammatory interstitial lung** disease can be treated with a relatively short course ($\leq$3 months) of high-dose cortico-steroids (prednisone 40–60 mg/day). Although short-term improvement has been noted, the long-term effect of this treatment on the natural history of pulmonary disease remains unclear. Established parenchymal disease does **not** respond to corticosteroids and should be treated supportively (see Chapter 9). **Congestive heart failure** should be treated with standard therapy (see Chapter 6). Diuretics should be used cautiously in the patient at high risk to develop renal disease.

H. Renal Involvement Renal involvement is a major cause of death in PSS. Patients are usually hypertensive during a renal crisis, which strongly resembles malignant hypertension. Early recognition of impending renal crisis is extremely important. The development of elevated blood pressure, proteinuria, azotemia, microangio-pathic hemolytic blood smear, or pericardial effusion suggests impending renal crisis. Because of the potential important role of hyperreninemia, therapies that may increase renin levels (e.g., diuretics) perhaps should be avoided.

The major goal of therapy is blood pressure control. Recently, the introduction of **captopril** (Capoten®), an oral angiotensin-converting enzyme inhibitor, appears to have facilitated the treatment of this difficult problem. Captopril is initiated at a dose of 25 mg p.o. q.i.d. The dose can be increased to a maximum of 150 mg t.i.d. If control is still not adequate, another agent should be added. Side effects of captopril include leukopenia and agranulocytosis, proteinuria, rash, oral ulcers, hyperkalemia, and loss of taste. Combination antihypertensive regimens, especially using combinations that contain propranolol, parenteral nitrates, minoxidil, and clonidine have also been successful in individual patients (see Chapter 4). The progression to renal failure is not uncommon, and dialysis should be instituted as necessary. Bilateral nephrectomy should be considered as a measure of last resort in patients who exhibit life-threatening uncontrolled malignant hypertension.

V. SJÖGREN'S SYNDROME Sjögren's syndrome (SS) is a chronic inflammatory disease characterized by lymphocytic infiltration and destruction of the exocrine glands. Involvement of the lacrimal glands and salivary glands results in the most common clinical manifestations—keratoconjunctivitis sicca (dry eyes) and xerostomia (dry mouth). Sjögren's syndrome may occur alone (primary) or in association with another rheumatic disease (most commonly rheumatoid arthritis but also SLE and PSS). In its severe form, SS is a multisystem disease with involvement of multiple organ systems. Lymphoproliferation may extend beyond the exocrine glands and result in lymphadenopathy and parenchymal lung, kidney, and other organ damage (pseu-dolymphoma). Lymphoproliferation may also evolve into a true malignant lymphoma.

Treatment of the **dry eyes** is designed to provide symptomatic relief as well as prevent the major complications, including exposure keratitis and corneal ulceration. Therapy and follow-up should be coordinated with an ophthalmologist. Mild cases respond well to the repeated instillation of artificial tears (i.e., methylcellulose eye drops every 2 to 4 hr). Some patients are further improved by mucolytic agents. More severe cases may require closure of the nasolacrimal ducts, or even more extensive surgery to help provide continuous moisture.

Treatment of **xerostomia** may be extremely difficult and unsatisfactory. Lubricants often adhere to the mucous membranes and make symptoms worse. Increasing oral fluids and frequent rinsing may be helpful. In addition, supervision by a dentist is important to help control the rampant dental caries that may develop.

Occasional patients with extensive extraglandular lymphoproliferation may require treatment with high-dose corticosteroids and/or cytotoxic drugs (i.e., cyclophosphamide). Treatment of an associated rheumatic disease is essentially the same as that described for the disease alone.

VI. **VASCULITIS** Vasculitis is a pathologic process characterized by inflammation and necrosis of blood vessels, which results in a broad spectrum of clinical syndromes. There has been great difficulty and confusion attempting to categorize the different diseases. A clinically useful classification is important, especially to separate those diseases that respond to different treatment schedules. The classification outlined below uses vessel size as the major differentiating feature and in addition, syndromes with distinct clinicopathologic features (i.e., Wegener's granulomatosis) have also been separated. It is important in the management of vasculitic diseases to exclude an underlying infectious process.

A. **Vasculitis Involving Medium and Small Muscular Arteries: Polyarteritis Nodosa Group** Systemic necrotizing vasculitis involving medium and small arteries is usually a severe **progressive disease involving multiple organ systems.** If untreated, the 5-year mortality rate approaches 90%. Although studies thus far have been uncontrolled and retrospective, involving relatively few patients, patients with severe disease should be treated as outlined below for Wegener's granulomatosis, using **cyclophosphamide and corticosteroids.** Some patients with less severe disease may be initially managed with high-dose corticosteroids. However, cyclophosphamide should be immediately added if there is evidence of progression.

B. **Wegener's Granulomatosis** The clinical and pathologic features of Wegener's granulomatosis are distinctive and include **granulomatous vasculitis of the upper and lower respiratory tract** and a necrotizing glomerulonephritis. Untreated Wegener's granulomatosis usually pursues a rapidly fatal course represented by a 2-year mortality rate greater than 90%. The use of **cyclophosphamide** (Cytoxan®) has greatly improved the prognosis of this disease.

Patients with active disease and a relatively stable course should be started on oral **cyclophosphamide** 1 to 2 mg/kg/day. Most patients also require corticosteroids (prednisone 0.5–1.0 mg/kg/day) in divided doses. **Indications** for steroids include eye involvement, severe skin involvement, severe serosal inflammation, and severe systemic symptoms. The dose of cyclophosphamide should be increased by 25 mg every 2 weeks until a clinical response is obtained. It has been recommended that the lowest dose that maintains the response should be continued for 1 year after the disappearance of all disease activity. After the initial clinical response, prednisone should be tapered (see II.) to an alternate-day schedule, if possible.

Patients with rapidly progressive disease (i.e., rapidly progressive renal failure, severe pulmonary involvement, progressive peripheral neuropathy, or cerebral vasculitis) should be started on higher initial doses of cyclophosphamide (i.v. or p.o.)—4 mg/kg/day for 3 days, then tapered to 2 mg/kg/day over 3 days. Further treatment with cyclophosphamide is as described above. Patients should also be started on **prednisone** (1 mg/kg/day in divided doses). Tapering is as described above.

Cyclophosphamide can be associated with significant toxicity. The most serious toxicity during therapy is **bone marrow suppression, primarily leukopenia.**

Complete blood counts (including platelet count) should be performed weekly during initiation of therapy and then at 2-week intervals after a stable dose is achieved. Every attempt should be made to maintain the neutrophil count greater than 1,000/mm³ (preferably > 1,500/mm³). The nadir WBC will generally occur 2 weeks after the last dose. Thus, trends for decreasing counts must be followed carefully. Even after months of stability on a constant dose, the neutrophil count may begin decreasing, emphasizing the need for continued careful monitoring as long as the drug is given. Other **toxicities** include acute and chronic bladder damage (i.e., hemorrhagic cystitis), ovary or testicular damage (amenorrhea or azospermia), and alopecia. The major **long-term risk** is the induction of malignancy, including acute leukemia and non-Hodgkin's lymphoma.

Cyclophosphamide is **both activated and metabolized in the liver**. Drugs such as barbiturates may increase toxicity by increasing activation, whereas other drugs such as phenothiazines may increase toxicity by decreasing metabolism of the active drug. Corticosteroids may decrease the activity of cyclophosphamide; thus during corticosteroid tapering, the dose of cyclophosphamide may have to be decreased.

Some patients cannot be continued on cyclophosphamide or will not accept certain toxicities, and azathioprine can be used as an alternative agent. However, azathioprine does not appear to be as effective as cyclophosphamide, and it should not be used routinely as the first drug. Another secondary alternative to cyclophosphamide is chlorambucil, another alkylating agent.

C. **Small-Vessel Vasculitis**   Vasculitis involving small blood vessels (i.e., capillaries and venules) has also been termed **leukocytoclastic vasculitis** or the **hypersensitivity vasculitis** group, and includes a large group of different diseases, e.g., hypersensitivity vasculitis, serum sickness, Henoch-Schönlein purpura, essential mixed cryoglobulinemia, and others. In this group of diseases, the skin is almost always involved (i.e., palpable purpura, urticaria, vesicles, etc.) and is frequently the predominant organ involved. Other organ systems commonly involved include the joints, GI tract, and kidneys.

Treatment should be tailored to the **severity of visceral involvement**. If a precipitating agent (i.e., drug, chemical, microorganism, other disease) can be identified, it should be removed if possible. There is little evidence that corticosteroids and/ or cytotoxic drugs are effective, although they are frequently used. Plasmapheresis can be effective therapy in some patients with essential mixed cryoglobulinemia.

D. **Large-Artery Vasculitis: Giant Cell Arteritis and Associated Polymyalgia Rheumatica**   Giant cell arteritis (GCA) (also called temporal arteritis) is a disease of the elderly (90% of patients are over 60 years old). Characteristic features include systemic symptoms, cranial arteritis with visual loss, headache, and jaw claudication, and, less commonly, aortic arch or peripheral large-artery involvement. The most important complication is **visual loss**.

Whereas GCA implies a pathologic diagnosis, **polymyalgia rheumatica (PMR)** is a clinical syndrome also involving elderly patients characterized by proximal pain and stiffness (shoulders, hips, thighs, and neck), prominent morning stiffness, and no evidence of myositis or weakness. **GCA and PMR are closely related.** Of those patients with GCA 30% to 60% will manifest PMR, and 20% to 40% of patients with only PMR clinically will have pathologic evidence of GCA. The **sedimentation rate is almost always elevated in both GCA and PMR** and is consistently a valuable indicator of disease activity.

GCA responds dramatically to corticosteroid treatment. Frequently, therapy should be instituted prior to diagnostic tests such as temporal artery biopsy, especially in patients who report visual symptoms. **Prednisone is initiated at 1 mg/kg/day in divided doses,** and this dose is continued until all disease manifestations are suppressed and the sedimentation rate has reached base line. The dose is then gradually tapered (see II.) to a maintenance dose of 7.5 to 10 mg/day. The patient should be carefully followed clinically as well as with repeated sedimentation rates. Most patients should be treated for at least 2 years.

The symptoms of PMR almost always respond to low doses of prednisone (7.5–15.0 mg/day). Some patients with mild disease will respond well to NSAIDs. The patient on these regimens remains at risk to develop complications of GCA. However, such a patient can be instructed to report symptoms and can be followed carefully. If symptoms or signs of GCA develop, the patient can be treated successfully with high-dose corticosteroids. It is extremely rare for visual loss to be the presenting feature of GCA in this situation.

VII. **AXIAL ARTHROPATHIES (SERONEGATIVE SPONDYLOARTHROPA- THIES)** This group of diseases includes ankylosing spondylitis, Reiter's syndrome, psoriatic arthritis, and the arthritis associated with inflammatory bowel disease. Patients are almost always **rheumatoid factor negative** and do not have subcutaneous nodules. These diseases, especially when there is involvement of the axial skeleton, have a strong association with the major histocompatibility antigen HLA-B27.

A. **Ankylosing Spondylitis** Patients are usually 20- to 40-year old males **with inflammatory back pain.** The characteristics of inflammatory back pain (vs mechanical back pain) are important to recognize and include: insidious onset of low back pain without a precipitating event, lasting at least several months; associated morning stiffness; improvement with exercise; and, no associated neurologic signs or symptoms. Nearly all patients have radiologic evidence of bilateral sacroiliitis. Progression of disease results in calcification and fusion of the axial skeleton. Late complications of the spinal disease may include the cauda equina syndrome, spinal fractures, and cervical spine dislocation. One-third of patients also have peripheral joint involvement (especially hips, shoulders, and knees). Other extraarticular features that may require therapy include acute anterior uveitis and aortitis with aortic regurgitation.

Progression of the spinal disease cannot be prevented by current therapy. Goals of therapy include: relief of pain and discomfort, especially by decreasing inflammation; preservation of range of motion; and, maintenance of a good functional position (prevention of flexion deformities of the spine). Patients should be instructed regarding correct posture and sleeping habits. **Exercise and physical therapy are critical** and include daily extension exercises and activities such as swimming. **NSAIDs** can be extremely beneficial (see I.). Salicylates appear to be less effective than other NSAIDs, and indomethacin may be particularly effective. Phenylbutazone is sometimes beneficial in patients who do not respond to other NSAIDs (see toxicity in I.).

Although corticosteroids are occasionally beneficial, they should rarely be used. Other therapies (i.e., cytotoxic drugs and radiation) should be regarded as investigational and only used with appropriate human subjects committee approval.

B. Reiter's Syndrome   The classic syndrome affects young adult males and includes **arthritis, eye involvement** (usually conjunctivitis or iritis), **nonspecific urethritis (cervicitis** in females), and characteristic **mucocutaneous lesions** (painless oral ulcers, keratoderma blennorrhagica, circinate balanitis, and nail abnormalities). **However, most patients have an incomplete syndrome, frequently with only a characteristic arthritis.** The arthritis tends to be asymmetric, oligoarticular, and predominantly of the lower extremity. Heel pain is common. The arthritis may be intermittent and resolve without sequelae, but many patients have a chronic arthritis with functional disability. One-third of patients have chronic sacroiliitis.

The management of the arthritis is similar to that in ankylosing spondylitis. **Thus, conservative measures (exercise and physical therapy) and NSAIDs are central.** The judicious use of intraarticular corticosteroid injections is helpful (see I. and Chapter 16). Systemic corticosteroids are rarely indicated. In severe cases with destructive arthritis refractory to the above treatment, cytotoxic drugs such as methotrexate or azathioprine have been recommended (I.).

C. Psoriatic Arthritis   Approximately 7% of patients with psoriasis have arthritis. Skin involvement usually precedes the arthritis, but in approximately 10%, the reverse occurs. In some patients, flares of the skin disease and arthritis appear to correlate. Most patients have only a peripheral arthritis, which varies greatly in clinical presentation and severity. A minority have an associated spondylitis or spondylitis alone.

The treatment is similar to that recommended for RA in regard to conservative measures, NSAIDs, and intraarticular corticosteroid injections (see I.). Salicylates may be less effective than other NSAIDs. The arthritis may occasionally correlate with skin disease, which should be treated as described in Chapter 22. In some patients with persistent peripheral arthritis, **gold compounds** appear to be effective and are administered as recommended for RA.

Cytotoxic drugs such as **methotrexate** and azathioprine may be beneficial in severe cases refractory to the above measures (see I.). The greatest experience has been with methotrexate, which may be particularly helpful in patients with both refractory arthritis and skin disease. Systemic corticosteroids are rarely indicated in the treatment of psoriatic arthritis.

D. Arthritis Associated with Inflammatory Bowel Disease   There are two different forms of arthritis associated with inflammatory bowel diseases, ulcerative colitis and Crohn's disease. Some patients develop an **axial arthropathy**, remarkably similar to ankylosing spondylitis. This spondylitis can precede clinical bowel disease and shows no correlation with bowel disease activity. **Treatment is similar to that recommended for ankylosing spondylitis.**

A **peripheral arthritis** occurs in 10% to 20% of patients with inflammatory bowel disease. The arthritis usually involves a few joints of the lower extremity and is characteristically acute, self-limited, and nondestructive. It correlates strongly with bowel disease activity. **NSAIDs** (especially nonsalicylate preparations) may be extremely beneficial. **Major therapy is directed at the underlying bowel disease.**

VIII. CRYSTAL DISEASE

A. Gout

1. **General considerations important for management.** Gout is a term used for a group of heterogeneous diseases characterized by **hyperuricemia and: a characteristic arthritis** in which monosodium urate crystals are demonstrable within neutrophils in joint fluid; aggregated deposits of monosodium urate crystals **(tophi)** in the tissues, especially in and around joints; **uric acid urolithiasis**; and, nephropathy related to renal urate deposition. The development of gout requires prolonged accumulation of monosodium urate, usually requiring 10 to 20 years of sustained hyperuricemia. **Asymptomatic hyperuricemia is not gout.** The above disease manifestations may occur in different combinations. The arthritis is frequently first to appear, and tophi (if they develop) usually appear after the arthritis is clinically manifest.

Gouty arthritis is characterized by intermittent painful attacks involving one or a few joints. If untreated, a chronic arthritis phase may eventually develop. Approximately 50% of the initial attacks involve the metatarsophalangeal joint of the great toe (podagra), and 75% to 90% of patients with gout have podagra at some time. Attacks are frequently precipitated by severe medical or surgical stress. **The diagnosis of gouty arthritis is made by demonstration of monosodium urate crystals within neutrophils in the joint fluid**, generally requiring examination of the fluid by compensated polarized light microscopy. The serum uric acid level may be in the normal range at the time of an acute attack and thus be diagnostically misleading.

Optimal management also requires consideration of possible secondary causes of gout in a particular patient. Most patients (>90%) have idiopathic primary gout. Clues that suggest a patient may have secondary gout include diagnosing gout in a young individual (<35 years old) or a premenopausal female (90% of gouty patients are males). Secondary gout may be related to increased production (i.e., secondary to myeloproliferative diseases or various complete enzyme deficiencies), or related to decreased renal excretion of uric acid (i.e., secondary to chronic diuretic use, lead toxicity, etc.). It is also important to consider the contribution of ethanol abuse both as a precipitant of acute attacks and as a cause of sustained hyperuricemia secondary to increased production.

In the management of patients with gout, **it is extremely important to separate treatment of the acute inflammatory arthritis from treatment of the hyperuricemia.** One should not attempt to lower the uric acid level at the time of an acute attack. If a uric acid lowering agent has already been started prior to an acute attack, it should be continued.

2. **Management of acute inflammatory arthritis**

a. **NSAIDs. NSAIDs (nonsalicylate preparations) are the oral drugs of choice for the treatment of acute gouty arthritis.** Salicylates are **not** effective therapy. The largest experience has been with **indomethacin**, initiated at 50 mg t.i.d. (see I.). After an initial response, the drug is tapered to approximately 25 mg t.i.d. and continued until all signs and symptoms have resolved. **Phenylbutazone** has also been used frequently, usually started at 600 mg/day in three divided doses and then tapered to 300 to 400 mg/day. Other NSAIDs (including sulindac, naproxen, ibuprofen, and fenoprofen) can be used, beginning at maximal recommended dosages (see I.).

b. **Colchicine.** Although oral colchicine has been recommended for the treatment of acute gouty arthritis, at the doses required it is frequently associated with GI toxicity (abdominal pain, nausea, vomiting, and diarrhea) and is no more effective than NSAIDs. **Oral colchicine is therefore not recommended.**

In contrast, i.v. colchicine is extremely effective and well tolerated and is the drug of choice for patients who cannot take oral medications or who cannot tolerate NSAIDs. Initially, 1 to 2 mg is given, and this can be followed by 1 mg every 6 to 12 hr ($\times 2$ doses). **No more than 4 mg should** be administered to treat an acute attack. The drug dose is dissolved in approximately 25 ml of saline and slowly infused intravenously. **Great care must be taken to ensure that the drug does not extravasate from the vein**, since this may cause tissue necrosis. Patients with poor i.v. access should probably not receive this drug.

c. **Intraarticular corticosteroids.** Occasional patients may be treated locally with aspiration and then injection of the affected joint with corticosteroids (see Chapter 16).

d. **Systemic corticosteroids.** Rarely, patients who are refractory to conventional therapy or in whom conventional therapy cannot be instituted can be treated with systemic corticosteroids. Unfortunately, rebound attacks are not uncommon. Prednisone 40 to 60 mg/day in divided doses (or parenteral equivalent) is administered until clinical response, and then the drug is rapidly tapered over a few days.

3. **Management of hyperuricemia.** After the acute attack is controlled, consideration is given to control of the hyperuricemia. Some physicians recommend antihyperuricemic therapy after the first arthritis attack, whereas others suggest that this therapy be instituted after two or more attacks. Other factors such as serum uric acid level and 24-hr urinary uric acid excretion influence this decision. The goal of therapy is to lower the serum level to below saturation [saturation occurs at 7.0–7.5 mg% as determined by the autoanalyzer (colorimetric) method]. Thus, a good serum level on therapy will be less than 6 mg%. Antihyperuricemic therapy should be continued indefinitely.

Diet therapy (i.e., restriction of purine intake) is unlikely to lower the serum level by greater than 1mg%, although in certain individuals it may have a significant effect on 24-hr urinary excretion quantities. In a few obese individuals, **weight reduction** may lower the serum uric acid level into the normal range. **The role of ethanol abuse should not be overlooked**, both as a precipitant of acute attacks and as a cause of sustained hyperuricemia secondary to increased production.

Antihyperuricemic drugs may precipitate acute arthritis attacks in 10% to 20% of patients. Therefore, prior to their administration, **patients should**

be prophylactically treated with oral colchicine 0.5 to 0.6 mg b.i.d. Occasional patients who will not tolerate this low dose can be treated with nonsalicylate NSAIDs (e.g., indomethacin 25 mg t.i.d.). If no attacks have occurred after 6 months of good control of the serum level or after 6 months from the time all tophi have resolved, this prophylaxis can be discontinued.

a. **Uricosuric drugs.** These drugs increase the renal excretion of uric acid. **Complications include precipitation of urinary tract calculi**, which can be decreased by starting the drug slowly and maintaining good hydration, especially during initiation of therapy. **Probenecid** (Benemid®) has been shown to be an effective uricosuric drug. The initial dose is 250 mg p.o. b.i.d., which is increased to 500 mg b.i.d. after 3 to 4 days. The serum uric acid level should be checked every 2 weeks, increasing the daily dose by 500 mg until satisfactory control is achieved. The average effective dose is 1,000 to 1,500 mg/day (in two to three divided doses), and the maximum dose is 3,000 mg/day. Serious side effects with probenecid are rare. GI intolerance may be seen in up to 10% of patients. Probenecid influences the renal excretion and metabolism of a number of drugs. For example, indomethacin should be used at lower doses in patients taking probenecid. **Sulfinpyrazone** (Anturane®), another commonly used uricosuric drug, is initiated at 50 mg p.o. b.i.d. and then increased to 100 mg b.i.d. after 3 to 4 days. The average effective dose is 300 to 400 mg/day in three to four divided doses. The toxicity of sulfinpyrazone is similar to probenecid. **Salicylates markedly antagonize the action of both probenecid and sulfinpyrazone.**

Uricosuric drugs should not be used in patients with a history of uric acid urolithiasis, uric acid hyperexcretion (>800 mg/24 hr), and renal insufficiency (creatinine clearance less than 30 cc/min). They should also not be the primary drug in patients with extensive tophaceous disease.

b. **Inhibitors of urate production.** Allopurinol (Zyloprim®) is an inhibitor of xanthine oxidase and decreases urate production. Although it has a relatively short half-life, it is rapidly converted to the active metabolite oxipurinol, which has a half-life of 18 to 28 hr. The drug can be given as a single daily oral dose, usually beginning at 300 mg/day. It is unusual for patients to require more than 300 mg/day, although doses as high as 600 mg may rarely be necessary. The serum level is checked every 2 to 4 weeks until the appropriate dose is achieved. Allopurinol may not result in normalization of the serum level in some patients with tophaceous disease. Rather than continuing to increase the dose of allopurinol, the addition of a uricosuric agent is indicated. **Hypersensitivity reactions are the most common side effect of allopurinol and occur more frequently in the setting of renal insufficiency.** Care must be taken to use the lowest effective dose in this situation. Some reactions (including hypersensitivity vasculitis) may be serious. **Allopurinol markedly decreases the metabolism of 6-mercaptopurine and azathioprine**, and the dosage of these cytotoxic drugs should be reduced by 75%. Although the mechanism is less clear, allopurinol may also increase the toxicity of cyclophosphamide.

B. Calcium Pyrophosphate Disease ("Pseudogout")   It has been shown in recent years that calcium pyrophosphate dihydrate (CPPD) deposition can present in multiple ways and can mimic many of the common rheumatic syndromes. **Thus, CPPD deposition can mimic gout ("pseudogout")**, but also rheumatoid arthritis, osteoarthritis, traumatic arthritis, and neuropathic joint disease. CPPD disease is common and is especially frequent in the elderly. An important aspect of management is the consideration of associated diseases. Although many diseases have been associated, important ones to exclude in the typical patient include hyperparathyroidism, hemochromatosis, hypothyroidism, and gout.

1. Pseudogout. Pseudogout is characterized by acute intermittent attacks of **inflammatory arthritis**, most commonly affecting the knee. As in gout, attacks are commonly precipitated by severe medical or surgical stresses. The diagnosis is confirmed by demonstrating CPPD crystals within joint fluid leukocytes (by compensated polarizing light microscopy). Acute inflammation from other causes, such as infectious arthritis, can result in CPPD crystals being released into the joint fluid. Thus, in the setting of acute inflammatory arthritis, the presence of joint fluid CPPD crystals does not exclude infection.

The treatment of pseudogout is similar to that for acute gouty arthritis. Thus **NSAIDs (nonsalicylate)** are the oral drugs of choice (see above for dosage, etc.). **Joint fluid aspiration and intraarticular injection with corticosteroids** (see Chapter 16) can be very effective. Oral colchicine is **not** indicated, but occasionally i.v. colchicine may be effectively used. Rarely, patients who are refractory or who cannot tolerate the above therapy can be treated with systemic corticosteroids as outlined for gouty arthritis.

2. Chronic calcium pyrophosphate disease. Patients with CPPD disease may present as a chronic symmetric **polyarthritis** ("pseudorheumatoid"), as chronic osteoarthritis (with or without superimposed acute pseudogout attacks), and with extensive joint destruction, resembling neuropathic joint disease. **Joint radiographs** are very helpful in making the diagnosis.

Therapy is similar to that for osteoarthritis (see Chapter 16) and includes NSAIDs, analgesia, judicious use of intraarticular corticosteroids, and conservative measures such as exercise and physical therapy. There is no effective therapy designed to decrease the underlying CPPD deposition.

BIBLIOGRAPHY

Bohan, A., Peter, J. B., Bowman, R. L., and Pearson, C. M. (1977): A computer-assisted analysis of 153 patients with polymyositis and dermatomyositis. *Medicine*, 56:255.

Carette, S., Klippel, J. H., Decker, J. L., Austin, H. A., Plotz, P. H., Steinberg, A. D., and Balow, J. E., (1983): Controlled studies of oral immunosuppressive drugs in lupus nephritis. *Ann. Intern. Med.*, 99:1.

Champion, G. D., Day, R. O., Graham, G. G., and Paul, P. D. (1975): Salicylates in rheumatoid arthritis. *Clin. Rheum. Dis.*, 1:245.

Cupps, T. R., and Fauci, A. S. (1981): *The Vasculitides.* W. B. Saunders Co., Philadelphia.

Decker, J. L., Steinberg, A. D., Reinertsen, J. L., Plotz, P. H., Balow, J. E., and Klippel, J. H. (1979): Systemic lupus erythematosus: evolving concepts. *Ann. Intern. Med.*, 91:587.

Dinant, H. J., Decker, J. L., Klippel, J. H., Balow, J. E., Plotz, P. H., and Steinberg, A. D. (1982): Alternative modes of cyclophosphamide and azathioprine therapy in lupus nephritis. *Ann. Intern. Med.*, 96:728.

Dromgoole, S. H., Furst, D. E., and Paulus, II. E. (1981): Rational approaches to the use of salicylates in the treatment of rheumatoid arthritis. *Semin. Arthritis Rheum.*, 11:257.

Hughes, G. R., (editor) (1982): *Systemic Lupus Erythematosus. Clinics in Rheum. Dis.*, Vol. 8, W. B. Saunders Co., London.

Kelley, W. N., Harris, E. D., Ruddy, S., and Sledge, C. B. (editors) (1981): *Textbook of Rheumatology*, W. B. Saunders Co., Philadelphia.

Kelley, W. N. (editor) (1977): *Crystal-Induced Arthropathies. Clinics in Rheum. Dis.*, Vol. 3., W. B. Saunders Co., London.

McCarty, D. J. (editor) (1979): *Arthritis and Allied Conditions: A Textbook of Rheumatology*, 9th ed., Lea and Febiger, Philadelphia.

Whiting-O'Keefe, Q., Henke, J. E., Shearn, M. A., Hopper, J., Biava, C. G., and Epstein, W. V. (1982): The information content from renal biopsy in systemic lupus erythematosus. *Ann. Intern. Med.*, 96:718.

18.

Immunologic and Hypersensitivity Disorders

Alan L. Schocket

18.

Immunologic and Hypersensitivity Disorders

I. ANAPHYLACTIC/ANAPHYLACTOID REACTIONS These are systemic reactions resulting from the release of mediators such as histamine, prostaglandins, and leukotrienes from mast cells and basophils. These cause vasodilatation, increased capillary permeability, smooth-muscle contraction including bronchial and gastrointestinal, arrythmias, and exocrine hypersecretion.

A. Clinical Presentation The most serious **clinical manifestations** include vascular collapse with shock and upper airway obstruction due to laryngeal edema, either of which can be rapidly fatal. Patients having either of these manifestations have the highest incidence of death. Other symptoms and signs include urticaria (hives); angioedema; rhinorrhea and sneezing; itching, watery eyes; wheezing; abdominal cramps and diarrhea; and occasionally cardiac arrythmias. The **onset** of reaction following exposure may be seconds to minutes; orally it may be minutes to hours (usually less than 2 hr).

B. Causes

    1. Anaphylactic reactions refer to reactions mediated by the presence of specific IgE directed at an antigen to which the patient is exposed. Specific causes include:

        a. Drugs. The most common drug is **penicillin**, but any medication can cause a reaction, including horse serum, hormones, and so on.

        b. Ingestants. Foods are the most common cause, especially seafood and peanuts. Reactions to other additives have been described, including food coloring and preservatives.

        c. Insect stings. The most common stings include those of bees, wasps, and hornets. The danger is greatest when the sensitive individual is stung in the wilderness with little accessibility to medical care.

        d. Physical agents include exercise and cold exposure in sensitive individuals.

        e. Gamma globulin in IgA-deficient patients. Occurs secondary to exposure via gamma globulin injections or blood transfusions.

    2. Anaphylactoid reactions are initiated by mechanisms other than the presence of specific IgE antibodies:

        a. Radio-contrast dye. Probably related to activation of complement and direct release of mediators from mast cells by the dye itself. This reaction is not related to iodine allergy.

        b. Gamma globulin injection. May occur in patients receiving gamma globulin for hypogammaglobulinemia and is caused by aggregates of gamma globulin reaching the bloodstream and initiating complement activation. Products of complement activation can directly release mediators from basophils and mast cells.

c. **Some drugs** exert their effects directly on mast cells and basophils or by some other unclear mechanisms. These drugs include dextran preparations, narcotics (morphine, codeine), polymyxin B, curare, aspirin and other nonsteroidal anti-inflammatory drugs (in sensitive patients), metabisulfites and other preservatives in sensitive patients.

C. **Treatment** Any symptom of a systemic reaction may precede the development of life-threatening manifestations such as laryngeal edema or shock and should be treated aggressively and rapidly. The patient should be observed for several hours following resolution of a systemic symptom and admitted for observation if life-threatening symptoms have developed. **For specific treatment, see Table 1.**

D. **Prevention** The prevention of future reactions depends on identifying the causative factor through the following **diagnostic measures:**

1. **History.** A complete history of what the patient ate or was exposed to is the best diagnostic tool.

2. **Specific IgE determinations.** Allergy skin testing to foods or some drugs

TABLE 1. *Treatment of anaphylaxis*

General Measures

Inhibit antigen absorption: proximal tourniquet; local cooling (ice)
Maintain respiration: endotracheal intubation, tracheostomy for laryngeal edema; oxygen
Maintain circulation: monitor arrythmias; intravenous fluids: normal saline, albumin

Pharmacology

Class/name of drug	Dosage and administration	Side effects	Comments
Sympathomimetics			
Epinephrine	0.5 cc 1/1,000 s.c., q 15 min × 3 If patient in shock: 0.5 cc 1/10,000 i.v., q 15 min × 3	Tachycardia, arrythmias, headache	Decrease dose and monitor in patients older than 55 years or with cardiac history if shock is present
Terbutaline	2.5 mg s.c., q 15 min × 2	Tachycardia, arrythmias	Decrease dose if patient older than 55 years or has cardiac history
Antihistamines			
H₁: Diphenhydramine (Benadryl®)	50–100 mg i.m. (i.v. for shock)	Sleepiness	—
H₂: Cimetidine	300 mg i.m. (i.v. for shock)		
Methylxanthines			
Aminophylline	Load 0.9 mg/kg, then 0.1 mg/kg/hr i.v.	Nausea, vomiting, seizure	For wheezing
Corticosteroids			
Methylprednisolone	100–250 mg i.v., q 4–6 hr		Onset of action 4–9 hr

(penicillin, insulin, local anesthetics; see section V.) or the measurement of specific IgE in the circulation by radioallergosorbant test (RAST).

Once the causative factor is identified, the following **preventive measures** can be taken:

1. **Avoidance**—the most reliable and cost-effective modality.
2. **Immunotherapy** is useful only in a few instances, such as stinging insect hypersensitivity, and should be administered by a trained allergist.
3. **Desensitization** for drugs that are absolutely necessary, such as penicillin or insulin. See section V.

II. RHINITIS

A. Differential Diagnosis

1. **Allergic rhinitis** is due to the presence of specific IgE to **inhaled antigens**, including pollens, molds, animal danders, and dust. Pollen allergies are usually seasonal (spring—trees; summer—grasses; fall—weeds and some molds). Perennial symptoms may be due to indoor molds, house dust, or pets such as dogs, cats, or gerbils. **Symptoms** include paroxysms of sneezing (greater than three); clear nasal discharge; nasal stuffiness; itchy and watery eyes; itchy ears, nose, and palate; and other miscellaneous symptoms such as irritability, headaches, thin watery discharge, and conjunctival injection.

2. **Nasal structural abnormalities.** Nasal obstruction can occur from the presence of polyps, enlarged tonsils and adenoids, septal deviation, tumors, and foreign bodies. **Symptoms** include persistent bilateral or unilateral nasal stuffiness, anosmia, and, occasionally, purulent discharge. Physical signs include the direct visualization of a tumor, foreign body, or polyp "peeled grape" appearance.

3. **Rhinitis medicamentosa** is caused by **overuse** of topical decongestant, nose drops, or nasal sprays (Neo-Synephrine®, Afrin®, etc.). **Symptoms** are most frequently related to perennial nasal stuffiness which is relieved for a short time by the use of nasal spray. **Physical examination** reveals edematous, erythematous, and sometimes blue discoloration of nasal mucous membranes.

4. **Drug side effects.** Certain drugs will induce nasal stuffiness, e.g., reserpine, phenothiazines, other antihypertensive agents, and oral contraceptives. **Symptoms** are predominantly perennial nasal stuffiness. Physical examination is often nondiagnostic.

5. **Endocrine effects.** Rhinitis is most frequently associated with **hypothyroidism** or **pregnancy**. **Symptoms** are predominantly nasal stuffiness, especially during pregnancy. Signs are nondiagnostic.

6. **Infection.** Acute viral upper respiratory tract infection or chronic atrophic rhinitis are the most common causes. **Symptoms** include nasal stuffiness, rhinorrhea, and purulent discharge. Anosmia is frequently present. Signs include nasal mucosal inflammation with crusting and purulent discharge. This disease is usually self-limited.

7. **Vasomotor rhinitis.** This variety of rhinitis is frequently idiopathic and **diagnosed by exclusion** of other causes. Some patients have significant nasal eosinophilia and may have a variant of aspirin idiosyncracy syndrome. Symp-

toms include perennial rhinorrhea with a thin watery discharge, especially on exposure to cold air or associated with alcohol consumption or anxiety. Signs include minimal mucosal edema and watery nasal discharge.

B. Evaluation

1. **History** is a most useful diagnostic modality.

2. **Nasal smear for cytology.** The presence of eosinophils during symptomatic times suggests allergic rhinitis, although eosinophils may be present in patients with asthma or vasomotor rhinitis.

3. **Allergy skin test.** Done to inhalants and read as wheal and flare size in 15 to 20 min. It is useful to confirm history and as a potential guide for immunotherapy.

C. Treatment

1. **Avoidance.** For allergic rhinitis, avoidance of the offending antigen such as animals, molds, or dust is helpful, but total avoidance is frequently difficult. Discontinuation of nasal spray and changing medications that cause nasal stuffiness is essential. Thyroid replacement for patients with hypothyroidism frequently reverses nasal stuffiness. Nasal stuffiness related to pregnancy abates after delivery, but may recur if patient is placed on oral contraceptives.

2. Medications (See **Table 2** for antihistamine and decongestant administration.)

   a. **Antihistamines and decongestants** are useful in patients with most forms of rhinitis. Patients with rhinitis medicamentosa and vasomotor rhinitis may benefit from decongestants alone.

   b. **Nasal disodium cromoglycate** (cromolyn) is useful for patients with allergic rhinitis, since almost no side effects have been reported.

   c. Nasal **moisturization** with saline washes, water pick irrigation, and facial sauna may be useful for some patients with vasomotor rhinitis, especially in dry climates.

   d. **Corticosteroid** nasal sprays are useful in some patients with allergic rhinitis, vasomotor rhinitis with eosinophilia, rhinitis in pregnancy, and rhinitis medicamentosa when withdrawing from nose drops.

III. URTICARIA AND ANGIOEDEMA Acute urticaria is one or a few episodes lasting less than 6 weeks; chronic urticaria is recurrent or persistent urticaria of greater than 6 weeks' duration.

A. Causes Causes are found in less than 20% of patients.

1. **Drugs.** The most common causes of urticaria are drugs. Any drug, **especially antibiotics** such as penicillin and sulfonamide, can produce and IgE-mediated allergic reaction. Other drugs, such as **narcotics**, which are direct-mediator releasors, and **aspirin**, which can non-specifically exacerbate urticaria, are important to consider.

2. **Foods and additives.** Most common IgE-mediated reactions occur to seafood, peanuts, and other nuts. Dyes and additives such as yeast and preservatives may cause or precipitate urticaria by mechanisms that are not well defined.

3. **Infections.** Any chronic infection may be associated with urticaria, including

TABLE 2. Treatment of rhinitis

Generic name	Trade name	Dose and administration	Side effects	Comments
H₁ antihistamines (group)				
I: Ethanolamines				
Diphenhydramine HCl	Benadryl®	25–50 mg p.o. q.i.d.	Drowsiness	—
Carbinoxamine maleate	Clistin®	4 mg p.o. q.i.d.		
II: Ethylenediamine				
Tripelennamine	Pyribenzamine®	25–50 mg p.o. q.i.d.	Sedation	—
Methapyrilene HCl	Histadyl®	25–50 mg p.o. q.i.d.	GI upset	
III: Alkylamines				
Chlorpheniramine	Chlortrimeton®, Teldrin®, Histadur®	4 mg p.o. q.i.d. 8–12 mg p.o. b.i.d. (sustained release)	Less sedation	—
Brompheniramine maleate	Dimetane®, Dimetane® Extentabs®	4 mg p.o. q.i.d. 12 mg p.o. q.i.d.		
IV: Miscellaneous				
Hydroxazine	Atarax® Vistaril®	10–25 mg p.o. t.i.d.–q.i.d.	Anticholinergic effect, also good antipruritic agent	—
Promethiazine HCl	Phenergan®	12.5–25 mg p.o. t.i.d.	Sedation, antipyramidal effects	Antipruritic, antisertonin
Cyproheptadine	Periactin®	4 mg p.o. q.i.d.	Weight gain, sedation	—
Azatadine maleate	Optimine®	1–2 mg b.i.d.	Less sedation	—
Clemastine fumarate	Tavist®	2.60 mg t.i.d.	—	—
Decongestants				
Oral: Phenylpropanolamine HCl	Propadrine®	50–75 mg b.i.d.	Hypertension, insomnia	—
Pseudoephedrine HCl	Sudafed® Sudafed S.A.®	60 mg q.i.d. 120 mg b.i.d.		

Drug	Brand	Dosage	Comments	
Topical: Phenylephrine HCl	Neo-Synephrine®	2 sprays q 4–6 hr	Rebound nasal stuffiness if used more than 3 days	—
Oxymetazoline	Afrin®	2 sprays q 8 hr to q 12 hr		
Xylometazoline	Otrivin®	2 sprays q 12 hr		—
Antihistamines/decongestant combination				—
Triprolidine and pseudoephedrine	Actifed®	1 tab. p.o., t.i.d.–q.i.d.	Drowsiness, insomnia, hypertension	
Brompheniramine and pseudoephedrine and phenylpropanolamine	Dimetapp®	1 tab. p.o., b.i.d.	Drowsiness, less adrenergic stimulation	
Brompheniramine and pseudoephedrine	Drixoral®	1 tab. p.o., b.i.d.	Drowsiness, less adrenergic stimulation	More potent
Chlorpheniramine and phenylpropanolamine	Ornade®	1 tab. p.o., b.i.d.	Drowsiness, less adrenergic stimulation	—
Carbinoxamine and pseudoephedrine	Rondec®	1 tab. p.o., q.i.d.	Less drowsiness	—
	Rondec SR®	1 tab. p.o., b.i.d.	Less drowsiness	
Topical treatment Cromolyn Na	Rhinochrome 4%®	2 sprays, q.i.d.	Expensive, inconsistent response	—
Topical corticosteroids Dexamethasone	Decadron Turbinaire®	2 sprays, t.i.d.–q.i.d., each nostril	No adrenal suppression with recommended dose, nasal irritation	—
Flunisolide	Nasalide®	2 sprays, b.i.d.—t.i.d., each nostril	No adrenal suppression with recommended dose, nasal irritation	—
Beclomethasone	Beconase®	2 sprays, t.i.d.–q.i.d.	No adrenal suppression with recommended dose, nasal irritation	—
	Vacenase®	b.i.d.–t.i.d., each nostril		

helminthic, parasitic, fungal (dermatophytes), bacterial (dental abscesses, other occult sites), and viral (hepatitis B, infectious mononucleosis) infections.

4. **Insect stings.** Acute reactions with generalized urticaria can be seen following stings by bees, wasps, hornets, and yellow jackets. This may be part of an anaphylactic reaction.

5. **Contact urticaria** is most frequently seen with cosmetics or antigens such as grass or animal dander to which the patient is extremely sensitive.

6. **Systemic disease** may also be associated with urticaria, including:

   a. **Endocrine.** Hyperthyroidism, hyperparathyroidism.

   b. **Neoplastic** diseases. Carcinoma, lymphoreticular malignancy, polycythemia rubra vera, and mastocytosis.

   c. **Connective tissue** disease. Systemic lupus erythematosus, rheumatoid arthritis, and vasculitis.

7. **Physical urticaria.** A urticarial reaction may result from **physical stimuli** such as cold, pressure, sun exposure, exercise (cholinergic urticaria), or scratching (dermographism). The reaction usually comes on within minutes of exposure and rarely lasts more than an hour, except in patients with delayed pressure urticaria where onset is 4 to 6 hr.

B. Diagnosis

1. **History.** This is the most important part of the evaluation. In addition to a drug history, ingestion of proprietary medications, vitamins, and laxatives must be discussed.

2. **Skin tests** are important for evaluation of drug allergies, but only a few tests are available (see V.). Skin tests to food and insects are useful and appropriately done to confirm the history.

3. **Elimination diet.** This approach   for patients who have urticaria more than two or three times per week. Food diaries should be kept for patients who have infrequent urticarial episodes. Everything ingested in the 24 hr prior to the episode should be recorded and saved. These should be evaluated to identify common exposures.

C. Management

1. **Avoidance.** This is useful if the cause is identified by the above evaluations. Unfortunately, identification occurs in less than 20% of cases.

2. Treat underlying systemic disease. Suppressive therapy for hyperthyroidism, surgical removal of a parathyroid adenoma, or immunosuppressive therapy for systemic lupus erythematosus (SLE) will often result in resolution of associated urticaria.

3. Drug therapy. See Table 3.

D. Hereditary Angioneurotic Edema This is a rare disease transmitted as an autosomal dominant with onset in youth or early adulthood. A family history is not always present. Urticaria is not seen in this disease. It is due to the absence of an inhibitor (C1 INH) that blocks activation of the first component of complement. **Clinically,** patients develop cutaneous swellings in areas of trauma; laryn-

TABLE 3. *Pharmacological therapy of urticaria*

Class/name of drug	Dose administration	Side effects	Comments
Antihistamines			
H₁: Diphenhydramine (Benadryl®)	50 mg p.o., q.i.d.	Sleepiness	
Chlorpheniramine (CMT)	4 mg p.o., q.i.d.		
Cyproheptadine (Periactin®)	4 mg p.o., q.i.d.	Increased appetite	
Hydroxazine (Atarax®, Vistaril®)	25 mg p.o., t.i.d.		
H₂: Cimetidine	300 mg p.o., q.i.d.	Gynecomastia, rash	Interacts with multiple drugs
Sympathomimetics			
Ephedrine	25 mg p.o., q.i.d.	Tachycardia, insomnia	
Terbutaline	5 mg p.o., q.i.d.		
Corticosteroids			
Prednisone	Minimal daily dose	Pituitary-adrenal suppression, osteoporosis, hypertension, diabetes mellitus	Use only as last resort or for delayed pressure urticaria

geal edema, which is the most common cause of death; and abdominal pain, which may result in unecessary exploratory laparotomy. All patients have low C4 levels at all times and may have decreased CH50 and C2 levels during attacks. Approximately 85% of patients have low C1 INH levels and 15% may have normal immunologic measurements, but low functional activity.

Treatment

1. Emergency treatment is symptomatic, and laryngeal edema may require endotracheal intubation or tracheostomy.

2. Prophylactic treatment for elective or emergency surgery includes the administration of two units of fresh frozen plasma prior to surgery. **Long-term prophylactic treatment** with attenuated androgens, specifically **danazol** or **stanozolol**, have been effective in preventing attacks. **Side effects**, especially from stanozolol, include menstrual abnormalities and virilization in women, and elevated creatinine phosphokinase in men.

IV. ASTHMA

A. Definition Asthma is characterized by reversible obstructive airway disease. Obstruction may be initially reversed with bronchodilators or require more prolonged and progressive therapy with methylxanthines, bronchodilators, and even corticosteroids to observe reversibility.

B. Diagnosis Objective **pulmonary function testing** is necessary to confirm the presence of obstruction and, as noted above, bronchodilators to find reversibility.

1. Baseline pulmonary function testing without bronchodilators demonstrate FEV₁ less than 80% predicted with a normal or increased forced vital capacity (FVC), decreased peak expiratory flow rates, and increased airway resistance.

2. Bronchoconstrictive response occurs to low levels of histamine and methacholine administered by inhalation. Bronchoconstriction can be induced by graded exercise or isocapneic hyperventilation.

3. Precipitating factors to asthma attacks. All patients with asthma are not the same and have different factors that induce attacks. These should be identified (see Table 4) to provide better therapeutic control and patient awareness of disease.

C. Treatment   See Chapter IX.

V. DRUG ALLERGIES AND REACTIONS

A. Penicillins   This is the most common drug allergy. At present, diagnosis is difficult, since history is relatively unreliable (accurate in less than 20% of patients). Immediate hypersensitivity skin tests are more than 90% useful in excluding an allergic reaction, but are not yet commercially available. At present, if the history is positive and skin tests are unavailable, an alternative antibiotic should be used. Cephalosporins and their derivatives have the potential of cross-reacting with penicillin in a penicillin-allergic patient, but this is not well documented. If a penicillin or a semisynthetic penicillin is required for therapy, desensitization should be undertaken **(See Table 5 for desensitization protocol).**

B. Insulin

1. Clinical presentations

a. Urticaria, angioedema, and anaphylaxis are manifestations of IgE-mediated allergic hypersensitivity and may occur within minutes after injection.

TABLE 4. *Precipitating factors in asthma*

Factor	Type	Evaluation	Comments/treatment
Infection	Viral	Sputum examination	Vaccination
	Bacterial (sinus)	Sinus X-rays	Decongestants, humidification, nasal corticosteroids, antibiotics, surgery
Exercise	Cold dry environment, i.e., running	History; challenge	Pretreat with bronchodilator inhaler (Bronkosol®, Alupent®, Salbutamol®) Swimming
Irritants	Perfumes, smoke, cold air	History	
Drugs	Aspirin and nonsteroidal anti-inflammatory drugs Tartrazine	Nasal polyps; challenge carefully	Avoidance
	Beta-adrenergic blockers	History	Avoidance
Allergy	Inhalant: trees, grass, weeds, dust, molds, animals	History; season; exposure Skin testing, RAST Inhalation challenge (rarely necessary)	Avoidance, antihistamines, immunotherapy

TABLE 5. *Penicillin desensitization*

1. Crash cart with endotracheal tube available, i.v. running. Preferably performed in the intensive care unit.
2. Administer increasing doses every 15 to 30 min until reaction occurs or maximum level reached (pretreatment with antihistamines not helpful).

Dose	Intravenous method units	Oral method[a] units
1	10	100
2	20	200
3	40	400
4	80	800
5	160	1,600
6	320	3,200
7	640	6,400
8	1,280	12,800
9	2,500	25,000
10	5,000	50,000
11	10,000	100,000
12	20,000	200,000
13	40,000	400,000
14	80,000	200,000 s.c.
15	160,000	400,000 s.c.
16	300,000	800,000 s.c.
17	640,000	1,000,000 i.m.
18	1,250,000	Continue full
	Continue therapy	therapeutic dose

[a]Oral method is recommended unless other route is indicated.

h. Late reactions (delayed) are present as local indurated, erythematous, and pruritic areas at the injection site. These are usually self-limited and disappear after several days of continued insulin therapy.

2. Management

a. Skin testing for allergic reactivity can be done with kits commercially available from Eli Lilly.

b. Change Preparation. Change to skin test negative preparation (i.e., pork to beef, protamine to lente, single peak to single component) or try human insulin.

c. If allergic to all preparations, desensitization using regular human insulin administered subcutaneously may be helpful (see Table 6). Slow desensitization, administering a dose every 60 min until complete, may be used. If a severe reaction occurs, move back one step and resume schedule. Equipment for treatment of anaphylaxis should be at the bedside.

C. Local Anesthetics True allergies to local anesthetics are relatively rare. More commonly, **syncopal episodes** related to vasovagal reactions or toxic side effects from overdose or intravenous injection are seen. Allergic reactions to group I drugs are seen most commonly and true allergies to members of group II are extremely rare (Table 7).

TABLE 6. *Insulin desensitization schedule*

Dose	Concentration (units/ml)	Volume injected (ml)	Dose (units)
1	0.01	0.1	1/1,000
2	0.01	0.2	1/500
3	0.01	0.4	1/250
4	0.1	0.1	1/100
5	0.1	0.2	1/50
6	0.1	0.4	1/25
7	1.0	0.1	1/10
8	1.0	0.2	1/5
9	1.0	0.4	1/2
10	10.0	0.1	1
11	10.0	0.2	2
12	10.0	0.4	5

1. **Evaluation.** See Table 7.

2. **Management.** If a patient is allergic to any member of group I, then a preparation from group II may be used. No cross-reactivity exists among drugs in group II. For local reactions diphenhydramine hydrochloride (Benadryl®) 25 to 50 mg may be added to the preparation, or other preparations with local anesthetic activities such as promethazine hydrochloride (Phenergan®) may be used in severely sensitive patients.

D. **Radio-Contrast Dye**   Patients who have had previous reactions, such as shock, diffuse urticaria, wheezing, or other systemic anaphylactoid symptoms, are at a greater risk for reaction on reexposure to radio-contrast dye. This reaction is not mediated by specific IgE antibodies or related to iodine allergy. Although the mechanism is not totally well defined, it is likely related to direct mediator release and complement activation induced by parenteral injection of the highly concentrated radio-contrast dyes.

TABLE 7. *Local anesthetics: classification and evaluation*

Group I	Group II
(Para-aminophenyl group)	(Miscellaneous)
Procaine (Novocain®)	Xylocaine (Lidocaine)
Pontocaine	Carbocaine (Mepivacaine)
Benzocaine	Cocaine
Tetracaine	

Test for allergic sensitivity

Dose	Dilution	Route	(+) Reaction
1 drop	Undiluted	Prick or scratch	Wheal and flare in 15 min
0.02 cc	Undiluted	Intradermal injection	Wheal and flare in 15 min
0.1 cc	1:100 dilution	s.c. injection	Swelling
0.1 cc	1:10 dilution	s.c. injection	Swelling
0.1 cc	Undiluted	s.c. injection	Swelling
0.5 cc	Undiluted	s.c. injection	Swelling
1.0 cc	Undiluted	s.c. injection	Swelling

Group I all cross-react.
Group II do not cross-react.
Group III do not cross-react with group II.

1. **Diagnosis.** There is no reliable method for identifying patients who will develop systemic reactions to dye injections. Test doses are not helpful and may induce severe reactions. Skin tests are of no value.

2. **Management** of patients with previous reactions:

    a. Establish the necessity for the study and avoid unnecessary dye administration. Crash cart and equipment for treatment of anaphylactic reactions should be readily available.

    b. Intravenous access should be established.

    c. The following pretreatment may prevent reaction or decrease the severity:

    (1) Prednisone 50 mg by mouth (p.o.), q 6 hr × 3, starting 19 hr prior to procedure.

    (2) Diphenhydramine 50 to 100 mg intramuscularly, 1 hr prior to procedure.

    (3) Cimetidine 300 mg i.m., 1 hr prior to procedure.

VI. IMMUNODEFICIENCY DISEASES

A. **Evaluation**   The most frequent situation in which immunodeficiency diseases are suspected are those related to **infections**, either with unusual opportunistic organisms or with more common organisms such as the pyogenic bacteria, which are poorly responsive to antimicrobial therapy. An algorithm approach to evaluating patients with these types of infections is provided in Fig. 1. Some of the **laboratory evaluations**, such as sophisticated lymphocyte stimulation testing and subset evaluation, are available only in specialized laboratories, and consultation with an immunologist or pathologist should be sought.

B. **Acquired Immunodeficiency Syndrome (AIDS)**   This is a recently described syndrome initially seen in promiscuous homosexual males, but now appearing in Haitians, in drug abusers, and in patients receiving intravenous blood products such as multiple transfusions (e.g., hemophiliacs) and exchange transfusions. The disease manifests by **multiple opportunisitic infections** including candidiasis, pneumocystis pneumonia, cytomegalovirus infections, hepatitis B infections, and atypical mycobacterium infections. Patients have also been noted to develop rampant Kaposi's sarcoma. Mortality is extremely high, approaching 80% to 90% in 5 years. Diagnosis can be confirmed by presence of a lymphopenia, anergy, absent in vitro lymphocyte responsiveness, and an elevated T suppressor-to-helper cell ratio. To date, no treatment of the basic immunologic deficiency has been established. The hospitalized patient should be treated as a hepatitis B carrier and placed on stool and needle precautions, since transmission is probably through parenteral and possibly sexual exposure.

C. **Treatment**   Treatment of diseases of **cell-mediated immunity** is predominantly in the experimental category and an immunologist should be consulted.

Treatment of **deficiencies in humoral immunity**:

1. **IgA deficiency.** Gamma globulin should be avoided, and blood products should be used with extreme caution since some patients have antibodies to exogenous IgA. Washed red cells should be used for transfusion. Chronic antibiotic therapy is often useful for chronic sinus and pulmonary infections.

2. **Hypogammaglobulinemia.** Either acquired or hereditary hypogammaglobu-

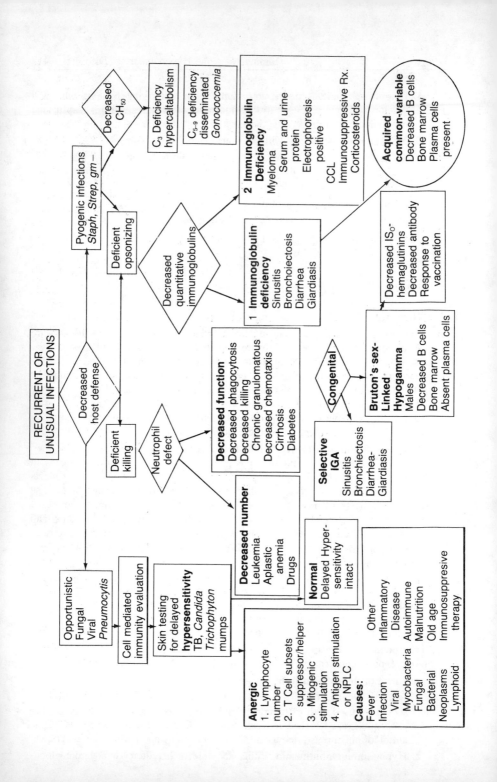

RECURRENT OR UNUSUAL INFECTIONS

Pyogenic infections *Staph, Strep, gm –*

Decreased host defense

Decreased CH$_{50}$

C$_3$ Deficiency hypercaltabolism

C$_{5-9}$ deficiency disseminated *Gonococcemia*

Deficient opsonizing

Deficient killing

Decreased quantitative immunoglobulins

2 Immunoglobulin Deficiency
Myeloma
Serum and urine protein
Electrophoresis positive
CCL
Immunosuppressive Rx.
Corticosteroids

Acquired common-variable
Decreased B cells
Bone marrow
Plasma cells present

1 Immunoglobulin deficiency
Sinusitis
Bronchoiectasis
Diarrhea
Giardiasis

Decreased IS$_0$-hemaglutinins
Decreased antibody
Response to vaccination

Neutrophil defect

Decreased function
Decreased phagocytosis
Decreased killing
Chronic granulomatous
Decreased chemotaxis
Cirrhosis
Diabetes

Congenital

Bruton's sex-Linked Hypogamma
Males
Decreased B cells
Bone marrow
Absent plasma cells

Selective IGA
Sinusitis
Bronchiectosis
Diarrhea-Giardiasis

Decreased number
Leukemia
Aplastic anemia
Drugs

Normal
Delayed Hyper-sensitivity intact

Opportunistic
Fungal
Viral
Pneumocytis

Cell mediated immunity evaluation

Skin testing for delayed **hypersensitivity**
TB, *Candida*
Trichophyton
mumps

Anergic
1. Lymphocyte number
2. T Cell subsets suppressor/helper
3. Mitogenic stimulation
4. Antigen stimulation or NPLC

Causes:
Fever
Infection
Viral
Mycobacteria
Fungal
Bacterial
Neoplasms
Lymphoid

Other
Inflammatory Disease
Autoimmune
Malnutrition
Old age
Immunosuppresive therapy

linemia can be treated with replacement therapy to attempt to maintain IgG levels above 200 μg/dl. Patients with low levels of gamma globulin, but normal levels of isohemagglutinins and normal antibody response to immunization should not be treated with gamma globulin. Replacement therapy can be administered by i.m. injection of standard gamma globulin preparations or i.v. administration of a purified gamma globulin preparation (Gamimune®, Cutter Biological). Anaphylactoid reactions can occur if aggregates are injected intravenously. Chronic suppressive therapy with **antibiotics**, including ampicillin and sulfonamides, has proved extremely useful in preventing chronic sinus and pulmonary infections.

VII. IMMUNE COMPLEX DISEASE

A. Clinical Presentation   Many clinical diseases in the category of connective tissue disease are characterized by the presence of **circulating immune complexes**. Such diseases include systemic lupus erythematosus (SLE), rheumatoid arthritis, and vasculitis. The presence and levels of circulating complexes frequently correlate with the presence and activity of vasculitic lesions and glomerulonephritis. Levels of total hemolytic complement and DNA binding correlate with the activity of the glomerulonephritis in some patients with SLE. Levels of cryoglobulins correlate with activity of vasculitis in some patient with rheumatoid arthritis.

1. **Clinical manifestations** of circulating immune complexes:

   a. Nephritis.

   b. Vasculitis. Leucocytoclastic venulitis and polyarteritis nodosa as diagnosed on skin or muscle biopsy.

   c. Bowel involvement is seen in SLE and vasculitis.

   d. Arthritis.

   e. Skin rashes: palpable purpura, urticaria, and maculopapular rashes.

   f. Fever.

   g. Cardiac involvement is rare.

   h. Neurologic. Peripheral neuropathies (rheumatoid vasculitis); CNS involvement is rare.

B. Evaluation   Many tests required to evaluate the presence of immune complex disease are not available in a routine pathology laboratory and necessitate sending serum to other laboratories or obtaining immunology consultation (see Table 8).

C. Management   The **goals** of treatment for immune complex disease include decreasing antigen load, decreasing antibody production, and suppressing the inflammatory response generated by the deposition of immune complexes in target organs. Modalities available include:

1. **Corticosteroids.** Decrease inflammatory response and may decrease antigen load by suppressing underlying disease activity.

2. Immunosuppressive drugs: Azathioprine (Imuran®), cyclophosphamide (Cy-

FIG. 1.   Evaluation of immunodeficiency.

TABLE 8. *Laboratory evaluation of immune complex disease*

Test	Result (normals)	Interpretation
Indirect tests		
Total hemolytic complement (CH_{50})	Varies per laboratory	Decreased levels indicate complement activation or congenital deficiency. May correlate with disease activity (SLE)
Complement components:		
C_3	Varies per laboratory	Decrease in any complement activation—both classical and alternative pathways—anything that activates complement
C_4	Varies per laboratory	Decrease in classical pathway activation (by immune complexes)
Direct quantitative measurements		
Cryoglobulins (mixed)	Normals per laboratory	Increase correlates with presence of circulating immune complexes and activity of disease (nephritis, vasculitis)
^{125}I C1q binding Raji cell binding Others: rheumatoid factor, bovine conglutinin, etc.	Predominantly research, tools available in specialized laboratories	Increased levels indicate increased levels of circulating complement binding substances—probable immune complexes
Measures of specific circulating antigens		
DNA binding	Dependent on laboratory	Increased levels seen in SLE may be useful to follow activity of renal disease
Hepatitis B antigens	Abnormal if present	Found in some patients with polyarteritis nodosa
Indication of tissue deposition		
Tissue staining with labeled antibodies (fluorescent, peroxidase, etc.) to immunoglobulins and complement components	Present if abnormal	Deposits seen in: Kidney in immune complex nephritis, Goodpasture's syndrome, IgA nephropathy In vessel walls in vasculitis Dermal/epidermal junction in SLE

toxan®), methotrexate, which function by decreasing both inflammatory response and immunologic reaction, ultimately decreasing antibody production.

3. Other modalities of direct immunosuppression or immune complex removal, including plasmapheresis, irradiation, thoracic duct drainage, leucopheresis. All of these are experimental procedures and should be used in institutions where protocols are available.

BIBLIOGRAPHY

Middleton, E. Jr., Reed, C. E., and Ellis, E. S. (1978): *Allergy Principles and Practice.* C. V. Mosby, St. Louis.

19.

Diabetes Mellitus and Hyperlipidemia

Craig N. Sadur

19.

Diabetes Mellitus and Hyperlipidemia

I. **DEFINITION AND CLASSIFICATION OF DIABETES MELLITUS** Primary **diabetes mellitus (DM)** is a disorder of carbohydrate (CHO), lipid, and protein metabolism characterized by absolute or relative insulin deficiency and associated with various complications and genetic predispositions. **Secondary DM** occurs as a result of another insult, e.g., pancreatic destruction or excess counterregulatory hormones (glucocorticoids, growth hormone, catecholamines, glucagon).

The National Diabetes Data Group diagnoses DM in men and nonpregnant women by one of three criteria. First is the combination of polyuria, polydipsia, and weight loss with "unequivocal elevation of plasma glucose." Second is the presence of repeated elevations of fasting plasma glucose (FPG) $\geqslant 140$ mg/dl. Third, on rare occasions a strictly executed oral glucose tolerance test (OGTT) is needed to prove the diagnosis with a 2-hr and 30-, 60-, or 90-min plasma glucose level of $\geqslant 200$ mg/dl. Plasma or serum glucose levels are approximately 15% greater than blood glucose values.

Primary DM can be divided into two major types. **Type 1 DM**, or insulin-dependent DM, tends to occur in nonobese children and in young adults and is associated with ketosis. These patients are insulinopenic and require insulin to sustain life. **Type 2 DM**, or noninsulin-dependent DM, usually afflicts adults, a larger percentage of whom are obese, and is not associated with ketosis. Whereas these patients demonstrate normal or even high serum insulin levels, DM develops because of an insulin-resistant state. Because of relative insulin deficiency, these patients often benefit from insulin therapy.

Impaired glucose tolerance (IGT) in men and nonpregnant women is diagnosed by an OGTT with an FPG < 140 mg/dl, pre-2-hr plasma glucose values of $\geqslant 200$ mg/dl, and a 2-hr level of 140 to 200 mg/dl. Patients with IGT are not considered to be diabetic and should not be labeled as such.

II. **DIET** The American Diabetes Association (ADA) offers some dietary guidelines. Prescribing a diet with the aid of a nutritionist/dietician may help with patient compliance.

   A. **Calories** Type 1 DM patients are rarely overweight and, therefore, do not require caloric restriction. Often these patients experience significant weight loss and will gain weight with institution of therapy. A general guideline is 35 kcal/kg body weight/day to reach or maintain ideal body weight. Individual caloric requirements, which depend on the age of the patient, general state of health, and energy expenditure, can determine adjusted caloric intake. Of **type 2 DM** patients, 80% are obese, a condition that contributes to the insulin-resistant state. In these patients a caloric restriction of 25 kcal/kg body weight/day should result in weight loss.

   B. **Carbohydrates** The trend has been to increase the percentage of CHO, now recommended as 50% to 55% of the total calories, in the diabetic diet. CHO is best provided in the complex form, e.g., potatoes, rather than simple or refined forms, e.g., "sweets."

C. **Proteins**   Proteins should compose 20% of the diet. Because of the lower fat content, fish and fowl are better meat protein sources than beef. Examples of vegetarian protein sources low in fat are soybeans and lentils.

D. **Fat**   A moderate fat restriction diet would include a lipid content of 25% to 30% of the total calories. Cholesterol content ideally should be less than 300 mg/day in conjunction with a polyunsaturated:saturated fat ratio of 1:0.

E. **Alcohol**   In small amounts (e.g., one glass of wine) alcohol may be allowed within the caloric recommendations. Of note, alcohol should be discouraged for DM patients with liver disease, hyperlipidemia, peripheral neuropathy, or hypoglycemia.

F. **Timing**   For DM patients who are receiving hypoglycemic therapy, particularly insulin, it is important to stress adherence to a schedule for meals. Calories should be divided into at least three meals a day. For patients on multiple insulin injections, an evening snack and sometimes midmorning and midafternoon snacks can prevent hypoglycemia. Extra calories, primarily in the form of CHO, may be ingested before a vigorous athletic event.

III. ORAL AGENTS

A. **Indications and Guidelines**   The "first generation" of **sulfonylureas** is listed in Table 1. These agents have **no role in type 1 DM** and are effective only with type 2 DM patients. Not all patients respond adequately to the drug despite the absence of aggravating factors, e.g., infection, dietary indiscretion. Many who respond initially will eventually fail to remain adequately controlled. Patients who fail one drug may respond to another. With the long half-lives of the drugs, changes in dosage should be delayed at least 3 days for tolazamide, tolbutamide, or acetohexamide and 1 week for chlorpropamide.

B. **Side Effects**   Sulfonylureas should be avoided in patients with significant renal or hepatic failure, pregnant women, or nursing mothers. Potential side effects include hypoglycemia, which can be particularly prolonged with chlorpropamide; potential hyponatremia with chlorpropamide and rarely tolbutamide; mild diuresis with tolazamide and acetohexamide; pancytopenia; and hepatocellular dysfunction. First-generation sulfonylureas, particularly chlorpropamide, have been associated with an "Antabuse syndrome," characterized by attacks of facial flushing following alcohol ingestion. Much controversy exists regarding the validity of the UGDP study that states that tolbutamide is associated with increased coronary artery disease.

TABLE 1. *Oral agents*

Name	Dosage range (mg)	Tablet size (mg)	Dose frequency
Tolazamide	100–750	100,250,500	q.d. or b.i.d.
Chlorpropamide	100–500	100,250	q.d.
Tolbutamide	500–3,000	250,500	b.i.d. or t.i.d.
Acetohexamide	500–1,500	250,500	q.d. or b.i.d.

IV. INSULIN

A. Type   Insulins vary in schedule of action, source, and degree of purity. The number and kinds of insulin have increased over the past few years (Table 2). Most of the insulin manufactured is a mixture of beef and pork, which has been adequate for the majority of patients. Purified preparations of pork insulin can help in the treatment of severe insulin allergy or insulin resistance and are theoretically advantageous in patients who will likely need insulin for only a temporary period, such as diet-controlled type 2 diabetics who require insulin during some acute illness or stress, gestational diabetes, and patients receiving insulin in hyperalimentation solutions. New lines of synthetic human insulin may also prove helpful with these patients.

The only concentration of insulin that should be used for routine use is **U-100**. Rare cases of severe insulin resistance in which large doses of insulin must be administered may require the more concentrated U-500 form.

Insulins also vary in duration of action. The three main types are short-, intermediate-, and long-acting. **Short-acting** insulin has an onset, peak, and duration of approximately 1, 2, and 6 hr; **intermediate-acting**, 3, 8, and 18 to 24 hr; and **long-acting**, 12, 18 to 24, and 36 hr. Some patients who have significant insulin antibodies and insulin resistance may experience an even longer duration of action for these agents.

B. Dosage Schedule   Whereas a type 1 patient almost always presents with diabetic ketoacidosis (DKA) requiring hospitalization, a type 2 patient frequently is an outpatient. If the latter patient's illness does not require hospitalization and insulin is to be instituted as an outpatient, then a conservative starting dose would be 15 U subcutaneous (s.c.) of intermediate-acting insulin, with adequate monitoring of blood glucose levels for subsequent readjustments.

Only a minority of diabetics, usually type 2 patients, demonstrate good 24-hr glycemic control with only one injection of intermediate-acting with or without short-acting insulin a day. **For most patients two injections a day are optimal.**

TABLE 2. *Insulin types*

Type	Species	Product
Short-acting	Beef-pork combination	Regular
		Semilente
	Pure pork	Regular
		Semilente
	Pure beef	Regular
Intermediate-acting	Beef-pork combination	NPH
		Lente
	Pure pork	NPH
		Lente
	Pure beef	NPH
		Lente
Long-acting	Beef-pork combination	PZI
		Ultralente
	Pure pork	PZI
	Pure beef	PZI
		Ultralente

The doses are best given one-half hour before breakfast and before the evening meal. Commonly, the morning dose consists of two-thirds of the total daily amount and includes a ratio of intermediate-to-short-acting insulin of 2:1 or 3:1, with the evening dose composed of a 1:1 ratio. Individual needs, however, may dictate a change in timing, ratio, and amount of insulin, depending on eating patterns, sleep schedules, and exercise routines. Bedtime snacks to prevent nocturnal hypoglycemia are very important for anyone taking an evening dose of insulin. Intermediate-acting insulin should not be changed more rapidly than every 2 days unless there is frank hypoglycemia or a blood glucose ⩾350 mg/dl. With a b.i.d. combination of intermediate- and short-acting insulins, specific changes in therapy can improve glucose levels at different times of the day (Table 3).

C. Technique For any patient starting to self-administer (or a family member who administers it to the patient) insulin, special attention to the technique of drawing insulin into the syringe, the method of s.c. injection, and injection sites are all important. Absorption of insulin is more rapid from an exercising limb, potentially leading to hypoglycemia. For example, a runner may want to inject his or her arm rather than leg (and take in more calories) before a run. Visually-impaired patients may have a particularly difficult time drawing up the insulin from the bottle. Syringes with magnifying lenses may help, or another person can draw up the dose and refrigerate the labeled syringe for a storage period of a few days.

D. Side Effects The main side effect of insulin is, of course, **hypoglycemia**, which can be greatly minimized by careful monitoring of blood glucose (see below). Hypoglycemia is more likely to occur with the development of renal failure; recovery from another illness without accompanying decreases in insulin dosage; onset of a disease, e.g., hypothyroidism, Addison's disease, hypopituitarism, that will lower insulin requirements; weight loss; decreased caloric intake; increased exercise; increased alcohol ingestion, especially when accompanied by starvation; and the onset of pregnancy.

Commonly, with the onset of therapy, **insulin allergy** can lead to local skin reactions (erythema, edema, mild pain), occurring 30 min to a few hours after injections, which are usually self-limited and require no specific therapy. In some cases, a switch to a purified pork preparation will help symptoms. With **severe cases**, coinjection of a small dose of glucocorticoid can help. If patients are expected to need insulin therapy for only a finite period, e.g., gestational diabetes, then either purified pork or human insulin should be prescribed. In rare patients, often who have previously taken insulin intermittently, **systemic insulin allergy**, characterized by urticaria, angioneurotic edema, and even anaphylaxis, can occur. Treatment consists of desensitizing doses of purified pork insulin with the first

TABLE 3. *Optimum b.i.d. combination insulin therapy*

Time of desired glucose change	Insulin to be changed	Time of desired glucose change	Insulin to be changed
Prebreakfast	Evening intermediate-acting dose	Predinner	Morning intermediate-acting dose
Prelunch	Morning short-acting dose	Prebedtime	Evening short-acting dose

dose of 0.001 U. Rare cases of severe **insulin resistance**, requiring hundreds of units of insulin for control, can often be improved by a switch to a purer insulin form. If the purified pork preparation fails to improve the resistant state adequately, then large doses of glucocorticoids, e.g., 60 mg/day of prednisone, may help.

Lipodystrophy is a benign s.c. condition associated with insulin injections and includes both hypertrophy and atrophy of the local adipose stores. Lipohypertrophy tends to occur at sites of repeated injection and may improve with avoidance of those locations. Lipoatrophy may improve with a switch to purified pork insulin. Severe lipodystrophy is associated with insulin resistance and hyperlipidemia.

E. **Goals of Insulin Therapy**   As with other regimens of DM care, the goal of insulin therapy needs to be individualized. An example would be the obese, type 2 diabetic who complies poorly with caloric restriction but who needs some glycemic control to reverse the symptoms of hyperglycemia. Similarly, for patients with chronic severe mental and/or physical debilities, "tight" control of glucose may be impractical or even harmful. For patients who are willing and able to monitor blood glucose carefully and frequently as needed, reasonable control throughout the 24-hr period is indeed achievable. Evidence exists that peripheral neuropathy and microvascular complications of the eye and kidney may be aided by improved glycemic control.

V. **PATIENT EDUCATION**   Patient, and often family, education is extremely important in DM care. Reading materials, classes, and other educational devices can supplement information given by the practitioner. Resources such as the ADA can aid in instruction. The patient-doctor-relationship is a key in signaling to the patient that a physician is available to help with acute and chronic aspects of diabetes care.

Psychological aspects of DM play major roles in how patients will respond to treatment. Patients view their own diseases quite differently and will have varying personal goals.

Patients with DM should be provided with "sick day rules," which, among other recommendations, should advise patients to continue administering insulin during any illness while trying to take in some calories and notifying medical help if problems persist. Every patient with DM should wear an **"alert" bracelet.**

VI. **GLUCOSE MONITORING**

A. **Urine Glucose**   Adequate glycemic control requires some monitoring of glucose levels. Urine glucose determinations, by the double-voided method (fresh urine sample approximately 15 min following previous urination) and measured by **Diastix®**, **Tes-Tape®**, or **Clinitest®** tablets, the first two being the most convenient, provide some indication of control and blood glucose levels above the usual threshold, 180 mg/dl, of glycosuria. However, measurements can be altered by medications. **Diastix® and Tes-Tape®** are subject to false negatives by ascorbic acid, levodopa, and salicylates whereas phenazopyridine can lead to false positives. False positives occur with **Clinitest® tablets**, with patients ingesting the following medications: ascorbic acid, chloramphenicol, levodopa, methyldopa, nalidixic acid, probenecid, salicylates, sulfonamides, and tetracyclines. In many patients, with or without neuropathy and nephropathy, the determinations can be quite misleading. For all patients a "negative" urine glucose does not distinguish between frank

hypoglycemia and normal blood glucose levels. Of note, swallowing Clinitest®
tablets can cause severe esophageal damage.

B. Urine Ketones   Although patients with type 1 DM should check urine ketones
during times of illness, routine testing is unnecessary. The simplest aid is the
Keto-Diastix®.

C. Blood Glucose   Self-monitoring of blood glucose is a convenient and relatively
inexpensive way to control glucose levels. Automated lancets provide simple and
relatively painless methods to obtain a blood sample by fingerstick. Finger infections are quite rare. Strips of paper with reagent (**Chemstrip bG™, Visadex®**)
or automated, portable glucose-determining meters (a number of products) allow
for accurate determinations of blood glucose.

VII. VACCINATION   Vaccination should be a routine part of diabetes care. Currently,
yearly influenza vaccines should be administered upon availability. One-time pneumococcal vaccinations are also recommended.

VIII. EXERCISE   Exercise should be encouraged in DM patients. Glucose levels, in
patients who are already reasonably controlled, can be lowered further with exercise.
For patients undergoing nonroutine extensive physical exertion, a supplement of calories, preferably in the form of carbohydrate, before the event can help prevent
hypoglycemia. The risk of developing hypoglycemia with exercise will also be diminished if the insulin injection is at a site other than that of an exercising limb. For
those who begin routine heavy physical activity, specific diabetic therapy may need
to be altered.

Patients who are in poor glycemic control often exacerbate hyperglycemia with
exercise. Thus, an exercise program should follow institution of adequate therapy in
the resting state.

IX. DIABETIC KETOACIDOSIS

A. Causes   DKA represents the state of severe metabolic derangement that can occur
in **type 1** patients. The most common etiologies for DKA are infections and/or
inflammation, poor compliance with medications, trauma, surgery, and other forms
of stress.

B. Diagnosis   The hallmark laboratory findings of DKA are hyperglycemia/glyco-
suria, ketonemia/ketonuria, and an anion gap metabolic acidosis.

C. Treatment   For each patient the physician should devise a **flow sheet** documenting frequent serial changes in glucose, electrolytes, pH, urine output, and
urine ketones as well as the administration of fluids, electrolytes, and insulin.

   1. Hypovolemia. Essentially all patients in DKA suffer from significant volume
   losses, the exception being the patient with severe renal failure who may show
   signs of volume overload. **Resuscitation** begins with aggressive replacement
   with intravenous (i.v.) normal saline (NS). For patients with frank hypotension, large bore i.v. lines should be placed for rapid saline infusion until the
   patient is normotensive. For patients with only orthostatic hypotension, at least
   1 liter of i.v. NS should be administered during the first hour, followed by at
   least 300 ml/hr. With that initial therapy, volume status should be carefully
   monitored. Total volume deficits average between 6 to 10 liters. Once marked
   improvement occurs, the patient, usually with hypernatremia (considering the

correction for hyperglycemia and hyperlipidemia), can be switched to i.v. 1/ 2 NS. After the patient is no longer orthostatic, i.v. maintenance fluids can be given.

2. **Hypokalemia.** Nearly all DKA patients develop significant total body potassium depletion and need potassium replacement. Because of the acidotic state, a higher proportion of the total body potassium will be extracellular, giving the serum potassium measurement a falsely elevated value. Thus, "normal" serum levels in an acidotic patient represent potassium depletion, mandating potassium therapy. If the DKA patient has hypokalemia, then the potassium depletion is likely to be even more severe. In most DKA patients oral potassium therapy is poorly tolerated initially, requiring i.v. administration (see XIV. C.). Ideally, all DKA patients should have continuous ECG monitoring, especially while receiving vigorous potassium replacement therapy.

3. **Acidosis.** Accompanying the anion gap acidosis are low serum bicarbonate levels. Overly aggressive administration with bicarbonate therapy during resuscitation of DKA can lead to potential problems, such as metabolic alkalosis, pulmonary edema, and perhaps cerebral edema. Thus, with an arterial pH of <7.1 it is reasonable to bolus 2 i.v. ampules (88 mEq) of sodium bicarbonate. In some instances repeat administration of bicarbonate therapy is needed to maintain an adequate pH of at least 7.1, after which replacement therapy should be discontinued.

4. **Hyperglycemia.** Most patients with DKA have significant hyperglycemia, which, in addition to the acidotic state, requires vigorous insulin therapy. For the past number of years more physicians are going to the "low-dose" regimen. Commonly, a **loading dose of 20 U of regular insulin i.v.** is followed by either **0.1 U/kg/hr continuous i.v. regular insulin drip** by "piggyback" solution with an infusion pump or **0.1 U/kg hourly intramuscular (i.m.) injections of regular insulin.** Although both are often equally effective, the i.m. injections may not be absorbed as efficiently in the patient with severe volume depletion. The key to insulin therapy with DKA is to monitor the blood glucose hourly, especially in the early course of therapy, with bedside checks via reagent strips or reflectance meters (see VI. C.). With this regimen, blood glucose levels should fall by an average of 75 to 100 mg/dl/hr. A rare patient with significant insulin resistance will not respond to the "low-dose" regimen with a fall in blood glucose. In that case, the dose of insulin must be doubled every 2 hr if there is no decrease. For most patients blood glucose should fall rapidly on the "low-dose" therapy. Once levels reach 300 mg/dl, 5% glucose should be added to the i.v. solutions to avoid hypoglycemia. After a level of 250 mg/dl is achieved, it is wise to begin to lower levels slowly by decreasing the insulin infusion rate to avoid hypoglycemia and possibly the rare occurrence of cerebral edema. An occasional patient with good renal glucose clearance presents with severe acidosis but only minimal hyperglycemia. In that instance, glucose should be administered intravenously from the outset of insulin therapy.

How long patients should remain on i.v. insulin is often unclear. Frequently, insulin is prematurely switched to the s.c. route, and the patient worsens metabolically and clinically. To avoid this situation, i.v. insulin can be tapered, but continued under careful blood glucose monitoring until ketonuria and acidosis are resolved (i.e., normalization of the anion gap) in a patient who is eating normally. Then a similar 24-hr dose of s.c. short-acting insulin can be substituted in q 6 hr doses, following q 6 hr checks of blood glucose for a brief period of time, usually 1 to 2 days before administering s.c. intermediate-acting insulin.

5. **Hypophosphatemia.** Phosphate stores are commonly depleted in DKA. Serum phosphorous levels are likely to fall significantly with standard therapy for DKA. The importance of this worsening remains unclear; but in the patient who is hypophosphatemic and normocalcemic, and for normal renal function, approximately one-half of the potassium in the form of i.v. potassium phosphate can be administered until phosphorous levels are normal. With replacement therapy, it is important to follow serum calcium levels to avoid a calcium–phosphorous product of more than 60 to 70.

6. **Cerebral edema.** Rarely, DKA patients, most often children and adolescents, develop cerebral edema while undergoing appropriate resuscitative therapy. This phenomenon may occur more often if there is a very rapid fall in blood glucose levels. Treatment should include glucocorticoids, mannitol, hyperventilation, and neurologic consultation.

7. **General supportive care.** DKA patients commonly have altered mental status requiring supportive care for obtunded or comatose patients, such as nasogastric intubation to prevent aspiration. If severe volume depletion exists, adequate monitoring of urine output is essential, including bladder catheterization if necessary.

8. **Underlying disease.** DKA may persist or relapse despite optimal supportive therapy unless any precipitating disease is adequately managed.

X. **HYPEROSMOLAR/NONKETOTIC COMA**   Hyperosmolar/nonketotic coma (HO/NK) represents the state of severe derangement for patients with type 2 DM.

A. **Diagnosis**   Typical laboratory values reveal severe hyperglycemia with mild, if any, serum and urine ketosis. Metabolic acidosis is usually from other causes, e.g., renal failure, lactic acidosis.

B. **Etiology**   Causes leading to HO/NK resemble those of DKA with an increased incidence of drugs, e.g., glucocorticoids, precipitating the disease state. Because the patient population with type 2 DM is older, there is a higher proportion suffering ischemic or thrombotic events.

C. **Treatment**   Guidelines for treatment of hypovolemia, hyperglycemia, hypokalemia, and hypophosphatemia are similar to those for DKA. Because of the increased incidence of underlying cardiac and/or pulmonary disease in these patients, monitoring may include a central venous pressure or a Swan-Ganz catheter. Bicarbonate therapy depends on the type and degree of the metabolic acidosis (see IV. C.).

XI. **HYPOGLYCEMIA IN DM**

A. **Etiology**   Various causes can lead to hypoglycemia in the DM patient. Commonly, skipped meals or unusual physical exertion result in hypoglycemia. Errors in administration of insulin therapy, such as mismatching of insulin concentration with syringes, failure to shake the vial adequately, i.m. injections, and previous injections into a vigorously exercising limb can all render low blood glucose levels. Patients who are recovering from some other intercurrent illness, such as myocardial infarction, will often experience hypoglycemia unless the dose of therapy is appropriately lowered. Any DM patient who continues to lower therapy requirements with repeated hypoglycemia should be evaluated for worsening renal function. The Somogyi effect must be considered in a patient who suggests symptoms of nocturnal or early morning hypoglycemia with periods of hyperglycemia or glycosuria while gaining weight. Factitious insulinization or overdose with oral agent therapy will occur with episodes of hypoglycemia. Other less common causes of diminishing hypoglycemic therapy requirements are hypothyroidism, hypopituitarism, or Addison's disease. Drugs that can exacerbate hypoglycemia are salicylates, alcohol, and (in type 2) sulfonylureas.

Not all patients with DKA, particularly those with severe autonomic dysfunction or receiving beta-blocking agents, may have adrenergic symptoms, e.g., tremor, palpitations, diaphoresis. Instead, they may experience only neuroglycopenic symptoms, e.g., decreased memory, light-headedness, syncope.

B. Treatment   For patients in a medical setting with severe hypoglycemia, an **i.v. ampule (50 ml) of D50W** can be followed with either a second ampule or continuous i.v. glucose, usually D5W, depending on the response. For patients out of the hospital, oral glucose in the form of candy, orange juice, or nondietetic soft drinks, the latter two working faster than the former, can improve the hypoglycemic state. Patients who suffer from severe autonomic dysfunction and who are more prone to severe hypoglycemic attacks may benefit by carrying a 1-mg ampule of glucagon for a quick s.c. or i.m. injection, followed by oral glucose administration. Failure to raise glucose levels appropriately calls for immediate medical assistance.

The mainstay of therapy remains prevention. Adequate insulin or oral agent therapy will diminish the likelihood and severity of hypoglycemia. Once hypoglycemia occurs without an obvious nonmedication etiology, hypoglycemic therapy should be reduced in dosage to prevent recurrence.

XII. PREGNANCY

A. Glycemic Control Before Conception   Pregnancy is a time when good glycemic control is of utmost importance. Because problems such as congenital anomalies developing in the first trimester are increased with suboptimal diabetic control, well-controlled glucose levels (i.e., essentially normal pre- and postprandial levels) should be maintained by diet or drug therapy before the time of conception in a patient considering pregnancy.

B. Diagnosis   In a patient with known pregestational DM, no special diagnostic tests are warranted. Because FPG levels fall during the first half of pregnancy, a repeated level of >105 mg/dl indicates gestational DM. With a normal FPG the National Diabetes Data Group suggests the following pregnant patients undergo an OGTT: first-degree relative with DM; previous history of stillborn or spontaneous abortion; previous history of a child heavy for delivery dates and/or with congenital malformations; maternal obesity; high maternal age; parity of 5 or more; and, repeated glycosuria. Normal gestational plasma glucose values following ingestion of a 100-g oral glucose load are <190 mg/dl at 1 hr, <165 mg/dl at 2 hr, and

<145 mg/dl at 3 hr. If two or more of these are reached or surpassed, the diagnosis is gestational diabetes. Due to the reduced threshold for glycosuria in pregnancy, **urine glucose studies should never be used alone to make the diagnosis.**

C. **Glycemic Control During Pregnancy**   Good control of blood glucose is mandatory during pregnancy to improve the course of gestation and outcome of the newborn. Early in the pregnancy the predominant effect is toward lower FPG levels because of the fuel demands of the fetus. The last half of gestation is characterized by more insulin resistance and, hence, a tendency toward higher glucose values stemming from such factors as increases in various diabetogenic hormones of pregnancy. Because of their high-risk state, pregnant diabetics should be evaluated frequently by an obstetrician and internist/endocrinologist.

Goals for blood glucose are to obtain fasting levels ≤ 100 mg/dl and 2-hr postprandial values ≤ 150 mg/dl. Care must be taken in avoiding maternal hypoglycemia (<60 mg/dl). As noted above, urine glucose determinations are notoriously misleading in pregnancy, mandating frequent monitoring of blood glucose.

D. **Type 1 DM**   Nearly all type 1 patients are best managed by multiple injections of s.c. insulin. Most commonly, this regimen includes a morning and evening combination of intermediate- and short-acting insulins. Adjustments in doses should follow the principles outlined in section IV. B. **Type 1 patients**, who by definition are insulinopenic, **must be prevented from becoming ketotic, which is severely detrimental to the pregnancy and fetus. Any ketosis or inability to keep adequate calories down are indications for immediate hospitalization** and vigorous resuscitation with fluids, electrolytes, and insulin. If DKA occurs, treatment is the same as outlined in section IX. C.

E. **Type 2 DM**   Type 2 DM patients, who are by definition insulin-resistant, are even more resistant during much of the gestation. Thus, adequate glycemic control often requires much higher doses of insulin in the final half of pregnancy than in the nonpregnant state.

As with any pregnant patient who is obese, pregnancy is not the time for weight reduction and should not be part of the therapeutic regimen until the postpartum state. The recommended gain in weight during gestation is 25 lb. The diet should be designed to include 30 to 35 kcal/kg/day and be composed of 45% CHO, 25% protein, and 30% fat. If diet alone can maintain normal pregnancy glucose levels, no other therapy is needed. If not, insulin therapy rather than oral agents should be used. Patients can start with 15 U single dose of intermediate-acting insulin in the morning and add short-acting insulin in the morning and then intermediate-acting insulin with or without short-acting insulin in the evening, adjusting according to the schedule of section IV. B., to reach good control.

F. **Gestational DM**   As with type 2 patients, diet therapy may suffice in producing good glycemic control in gestational DM patients. If not, then the same plan of instituting insulin therapy in type 2 patients should be used.

G. **Labor/Delivery**   Maternal, as well as neonatal, hypoglycemia often occurs postpartum. To avoid this occurrence, a continuous infusion of i.v. insulin by a physician experienced with this administration and delivery can control glycemia throughout labor. With the onset of labor or cesarean section, the patient can begin with the infusion rather than the usual s.c. doses of insulin. D5NS i.v. can be infused at a rate of at least 100 ml/hr while a "piggyback" solution of short-acting insulin (25 U in 500 ml of NS, concentration of 0.05 U/ml) is infused intravenously by infusion pump at a rate of 0.25 to 5 U/hr. Initial blood glucose levels need to be determined every 1 to 2 hr, while the insulin rate is adjusted, until a plateau is reached. Once a steady state is achieved, glucose levels can be checked every 4 hr. After delivery, the insulin infusion should be stopped with the glucose infusion maintained and s.c. short-acting insulin administered q 6 hr, following blood glucose determinations, until the patient is eating normally, at which time intermediate-acting insulin can be given.

If i.v. insulin therapy is not feasible, then a less optimal alternative is possible. On the day of delivery one-third to one-half the usual morning dose of intermediate-acting insulin is injected s.c., and a D5 i.v. solution is infused at a rate of at least 200 ml/hr, with close monitoring of blood glucose throughout the day.

H. Newborn   For any pregnant diabetic patient the pediatrician should be alerted to monitor the newborn carefully. Various potential complications can occur such as respiratory distress, hyperbilirubinemia, hypoglycemia, hypocalcemia, and sequelae of macrosomia.

XIII. SURGERY   During the stress of surgery, glucose tolerance often worsens. The choice of therapy needs to be individualized according to the patient's disease and extent of surgery performed.

Ideally, the blood glucose levels should remain between 150 and 200 mg/dl to prevent hypoglycemia and severe hyperglycemia. In addition, there is some evidence that the immune system functions best with a blood glucose below 200 mg/dl.

DM, as with any chronic disease, should be controlled before elective surgery is performed. Also, the surgery should be performed in the morning to minimize the time during which the patient must fast.

For procedures of less than 2 hr durations, less interventional therapy is required. Patients controlled on diet alone will not need therapy unless blood glucose levels exceed 250 mg/dl, at which time s.c. boluses of short-acting insulin can be given as needed. Likewise, type 2 patients on diet or oral agent therapy may not need insulin during short procedures. If they are on sulfonylurea therapy, the drug should be held the morning of surgery. If blood glucose exceeds 250 mg/dl, s.c. short-acting insulin should be administered. Type 1 patients who eat postoperatively can receive two-thirds of their usual morning insulin dose following surgery while a simultaneous i.v. 5% glucose solution is infused.

Longer operations often require more intensive insulin therapy. Because of the stress of surgery with increases in counter-regulatory hormones, plus the fasting state and various fluid and electrolyte demands, a continuous infusion of i.v. insulin, regulated by someone experienced in the technique, will result in the best glycemic control. Similar to the plan outlined in section XII. G. for the patient during labor and delivery, previous hypoglycemic therapy is held the morning of surgery. Starting the evening before surgery, 50 U of short-acting insulin is added to 500 ml (0.1 U/ml concentration) of a 5% glucose solution and administered as a "piggyback" via infusion pump. Depending on the patient's previous requirements, the starting dose can be ½ to 1 U/hr and adjusted as in section XII. G. Blood glucose levels need to be monitored in both the operating and recovery rooms. Following surgery the insulin, but not glucose, infusion can be discontinued with careful monitoring of blood glucose levels. Until normal eating has resumed, it is best to treat with q 6 hr s.c. short-acting insulin.

An alternative insulin therapy that will result in wider fluctuations of glucose is to administer two-thirds of the usual morning dose of intermediate-acting insulin, while infusing glucose, before surgery and supplement with s.c. short-acting insulin intra- and postoperatively as needed. Care must be taken to avoid hypoglycemia due to the different insulins "peaking" at the same time.

XIV. COMPLICATIONS

A. General   Much about the cause of complications from DM remains unknown. There is some evidence that good glycemic control lessens the risk of developing various complications.

B. Eyes   Diabetics suffer impairment of visual acuity for a variety of reasons, including refractive changes with fluctuations of blood glucose, cataracts, glaucoma, and diabetic retinopathy. All patients with DM should have a complete evaluation by an ophthalmologist at least yearly, depending on the severity of the eye disease. Whereas "tight" control of blood glucose levels is controversial in its role in the pathogenesis of the disease, optimal control of blood pressure helps impede the progression of retinopathy. Proliferative retinopathy and at times background retinopathy are best treated with laser photocoagulation therapy. Once a major vitreous hemorrhage has occurred, vitrectomy can often restore vision.

C. Kidneys   Patients should be monitored closely with 24-hr urinary creatinine clearance and protein at least yearly, again depending on the severity of the disease. All reversible causes of renal dysfunction, e.g., hypertension or urinary tract infection, should be evaluated and treated. Patients with significant renal disease should be followed by a physician familiar with diabetic nephropathy. When a creatinine reaches a chronic level of 2 mg/dl, the patient should be referred to a nephrologist. End-stage renal disease can be treated with hemodialysis, chronic peritoneal dialysis, or renal transplantation.

In addition to antihypertensive therapy, supportive care in the patient with nephropathy includes control of existing volume overload and adjustments of insulin therapy to correspond with changing requirements with advancing renal failure. Dietary plans should include restrictions in sodium, potassium, and protein. Some patients develop hyperkalemia (>5.5 mEq/liter) out of proportion to their degree of renal failure, presumably from a state of hyporenin-hypoaldosteronism. In addition to potassium restriction, fludrocortisone 0.05 to 0.2 mg by mouth q.d. (higher doses may benefit from b.i.d. therapy) will lower serum potassium levels. Potential complications of this therapy, however, include hypertension and volume expansion.

Absorbable or i.v. contrast solutions used for a variety of radiographic procedures, including oral cholecystography, should be avoided in all diabetic patients when possible, particularly in patients with renal dysfunction (serum creatinine >2.0 mg/dl). When administered, the patient should maintain an adequate volume throughout the procedure and should be followed for a few days for subsequent worsening of renal function. A 200-ml infusion of 20% mannitol before or with the contrast solution has also been proposed as a prophylactic measure.

D. Cardiovascular Hypertension is a common and often difficult problem in DM patients. Beta blockade is potentially dangerous in patients who become hypoglycemic because of the blunted recovery. Potassium-wasting diuretics can also worsen glycemic control in type 2 patients by impairing insulin release. Medications such as α-methyldopa may exacerbate or worsen the already impaired sexual function of many diabetic men. Also, various sympatholytic drugs worsen preexisting orthostatic hypotension.

Because the incidence and severity of ischemic heart disease is increased in DM, special attention to the reversible risk factors, hypertension, smoking, and hyperlipidemia, is warranted.

Peripheral vascular disease is also increased in DM. The mainstay of therapy is prevention of severe foot complications as outlined in the next section. In addition, because of frequent coexisting neuropathy, **use of heating devices on the lower extremities is to be discouraged. If ulceration occurs, meticulous local care is important.** Excessive pressure on the area, sometimes relieved with a specially fitted orthotic device but often requiring bedrest, also should be avoided. Often surgical consultation is helpful. If infection develops, broad-spectrum antibiotics as well as bedrest are needed. If gas-producing microorganisms are present, appropriate culture studies should identify them. In some cases, e.g., clostridia, surgical intervention is necessary.

E. Foot Care Daily foot care is an essential component of the management of the diabetic patient. Regular inspection, well-fitted shoes, avoidance of bare feet and of extremes in temperature, daily lubrication to reduce callouses, and special care in nail-cutting compose much of the plan required to prevent future complications. Frequently, patients, particularly those who are visually impaired, should be cared for by a podiatrist.

F. Neuropathy

1. **Peripheral neuropathy and mononeuropathy.** Diabetic neuropathy classically involves a stocking-glove distribution, but may present as a variety of mononeuropathies. If motor and/or sensory disturbances persist following adequate glycemic control, then a number of medications can be tried. A combination of fluphenazine (Prolixin®), 1 mg p.o. b.i.d.–t.i.d., and amitriptyline, starting dose 50 mg p.o. q.h.s. increasing by 25 mg every 3 to 4 days until an adequate response or a maximum dose of 200 mg/day is reached, phenytoin, 200 to 400 mg p.o. q.d., or carbamazepine, starting at 200 mg p.o. q.d., increasing by 200 mg every 2 days until a response is reached with 200 mg p.o. b.i.d.–t.i.d., have been used with varying success. Side effects are listed in chapter 23. If these medications fail to provide adequate relief, analgesia may be used. Symptoms may worsen while nerve conduction studies improve.

2. **Gastrointestinal neuropathy.** Gastroparesis, a diagnosis often made by exclusion of other upper gastrointestinal pathology, can be treated by smaller, more frequent meals and, if necessary, metoclopramide, 10 mg p.o. q.i.d. before meals. Potential side effects include drowsiness, fatigue, restlessness, and extrapyramidal changes.

Cholelithiasis and complications from cholecystitis are more common in type 2 patients. Cholecystectomy is, therefore, often indicated.

Diarrhea can be a severe problem in diabetics. After other causes, e.g., malabsorption, are excluded, the main treatment is symptomatic. Bulk-forming laxatives, such as psyllium (Metamucil®), 1 tsp in water or juice p.o. t.i.d., can improve the diarrhea. Other therapies are diphenoxylate hydrochloride, opiates, and cholestyramine (see Hyperlipidemia).

Diabetics, in suboptimal control, especially obese type 2 patients, often have fatty infiltration of the liver. At times, this disorder may cause abnormalities in the liver panel such as a rise in the alkaline phosphatase. No specific therapy is indicated, but other pathologic processes need to be considered and excluded.

3. **Flaccid bladder.** Neurogenic changes in the lower urinary tract often lead to impairment in bladder emptying, urinary stasis, and a propensity for infections. Frequent voiding, sometimes with suprapubic pressure applied, or, if necessary, q 4 hr bladder catheterization, can diminish the likelihood of large residual volumes. Occasionally, bethanecol, 20 to 50 mg p.o. q.i.d., will improve bladder emptying but should be avoided in patients with heart disease. Blood pressure should also be monitored for alterations.

4. **Orthostatic hypotension.** Postural blood pressure changes can be devastating for some patients with autonomic neuropathy. Aggravating medications, such as sympatholytic agents, must be reevaluated. Symptomatic measures include specially prescribed elastic hose, which can improve venous return to the heart, and elevation of the head of the bed with 8- to 10-in blocks. If necessary, fludrocortisone, 0.05 to 0.6 mg/day p.o. in q.d., b.i.d., or t.i.d. doses, depending on the total daily requirement, may be helpful. **Side effects** of fludrocortisone include volume expansion and supine hypertension, the latter which may be treated with a single dose of hydralazine or prazosin before bedtime. Occasionally, ephedrine 25 mg p.o. q.i.d. will improve blood pressure in the upright position for patients with autonomic insufficiency.

G. **Infections**   Certain infections, such as monilial vaginitis, otitis externa, and mucormycosis, are associated with increased frequency in DM. Any infectious process can worsen diabetic control. Conversely, there is evidence that suboptimal glycemic control can impair the body's immune systems. Thus, ideally, blood glucose levels should be maintained throughout the 24-hr period below 200 mg/dl during a patient's infectious state.

H. **Gonadal/Sexual**   Impotence is increased in incidence among diabetic men, presumably because of the neuropathic and vascular processes; nevertheless, reversible organic causes should be sought. Devices such as penile prostheses have aided in this problem.

In women with type 1 diabetes a higher incidence of premature ovarian failure occurs, a disorder that should be considered in the evaluation of menstrual disorders. If ovarian failure is documented, estrogen and progestin therapy should be instituted (in the absence of contraindications).

I. **Other Endocrinopathies**   Type 1 DM is associated with other endocrinopathies that are thought to have an autoimmune pathogenesis. Included in this group of endocrine disorders are Hashimoto's thyroiditis, Graves' disease, Addison's disease, and idiopathic hypoparathyroidism as well as pernicious anemia, myasthenia gravis, and vitiligo. Any clinical suspicion of these conditions in a patient with type 1 DM warrants appropriate evaluation and treatment.

XV. **DEFINITION OF HYPERLIPIDEMIA** Lipoproteins are structures composed of triglycerides (TG), cholesterol (CHOL), apoprotein, and phospholipid which allow the solubilization and transport of lipids to various tissues for cellular function or excretion. Patients with hyperlipidemia by definition have hyperlipoproteinemia. **Chylomicrons** are TG-rich lipoproteins that carry TG absorbed postprandially from the gut. **Very low density lipoproteins** (VLDL) are the transport forms of endogenously produced TG. Both chylomicrons and VLDL metabolize to form remnant particles which consist of a higher percentage of CHOL. Increased concentrations of **low density lipoprotein** (LDL), a CHOL-rich particle that is metabolized from VLDL remnants, are associated with an increased risk of atherogenesis. **High density lipoprotein** (HDL), produced independently from the VLDL-remnant-LDL cascade, is also CHOL-rich; but high levels of HDL in conjunction with normal total cholesterol levels are associated with a decreased risk of atherogenesis.

XVI. **DIAGNOSIS** Determinations for TG, total cholesterol, and HDL levels should follow a 12-hr fast and a 3-day abstinence from alcohol and ideally, should be measured while the patient is free of acute medical illness and off lipid-modulating drugs. Values of TG greater than 800 mg/dl, often associated with a creamy surface layer of refrigerated serum, indicate persistent chylomicronemia. Total CHOL consists of the CHOL found in VLDL, LDL (LDL CHOL), and HDL (HDL CHOL) particles. Of the TG-rich VLDL particle, 20% is CHOL. If the TG level is ≤ 400 mg/dl, LDL CHOL can be accurately estimated by the following equation:

$$LDL\ CHOL = Total\ CHOL - (\frac{TG}{5} + HDL\ CHOL)$$

to determine if the elevation of total CHOL is present only because of the elevation of TG. An increase in the amount of remnants should be suspected with a somewhat parallel increase in both TG and total CHOL and confirmed with the presence of a broad beta pattern in a lipoprotein electrophoresis. This test aids in the **diagnosis of broad beta disease** but in no other hyperlipoproteinemia.

When diagnosing hyperlipidemia, two principles should be remembered. One, lipid levels rise with age; and **two**, the higher the LDL CHOL level, even within the normal range, the greater the risk of developing atherosclerosis. Many "normal" values listed by laboratories tend to underdiagnose hyperlipidemia. A stricter criteria include the following upper limits of normal values:

TG = 100 + Age
Total CHOL = 200 + Age
LDL CHOL = 125 + Age

Once the diagnosis of hyperlipidemia has been established, acquired and familial causes should be considered. **Aggravating factors** include poorly controlled diabetes mellitus, obesity, alcohol, uremia, nephrotic syndrome, hypothyroidism, liver disease, dysglobulinemia, anorexia nervosa, pregnancy, Cushing's, and acromegaly. Drugs that commonly raise TG levels are estrogens and glucocorticoids. Obviously, treatment should be directed at reversing any underlying causes and/or discontinuing offending agents when possible. In all cases of hyperlipidemia immediate family members should be screened to detect familial hypercholesterolemia (the presence of only elevated CHOL levels in family members), familial hypertriglyceridemia (only elevated TG), and familial combined hyperlipidemia (elevations of both TG and total CHOL).

XVII. THERAPY

A. **Goals of Therapy**   It remains controversial whether or not hypertriglyceridemia, sporadic or familial, is an independent risk factor for atherosclerosis. The primary reasons for treating hypertriglyceridemia are to reverse the associated skin lesions and/or prevent the TG levels from exceeding 800 mg/dl in the postprandial state when chylomicronemia can possibly course to acute pancreatitis.

Elevated levels of LDL CHOL may occur sporadically, familially, as a part of broad beta disease, or in familial combined hyperlipidemia. All have an increased incidence of associated atherosclerosis, providing a rationale for lowering CHOL, particularly LDL CHOL, toward normal.

Because HDL CHOL appears to have some antiatherogenic properties, it is desirable to strive for higher levels in comparison to total CHOL. Regular exercise, which has been associated with higher HDL CHOL levels, can be a beneficial component of any therapeutic program.

B. **Diet**   Dietary education remains a cornerstone of the management of the hyperlipidemic patient. The physician should outline a diet to a nutritionist who can individualize a plan for the patient. Although a maximum decrease in TG and/or CHOL of only 25% may occur, this fall may be all that is needed in some patients. For overweight patients a weight-reducing diet should be prescribed. A model diet includes a limit of 100 mg/day of cholesterol with 15% of the calories as protein; 65% as carbohydrates, preferably in the complex form (e.g., potatoes, rice); and 20% as fat, which should have a polyunsaturated:saturated ratio of one (Table 4). Many patients will be unable to adhere to these guidelines, and a compromise diet should be substituted. For hypertriglyceridemic patients abstinence from alcohol is advisable.

C. **Drugs**   For most patients with hyperlipidemia, some form of medication is needed to lower lipid levels adequately. Table 5 summarizes the lipoprotein changes that occur with the different treatments. With any pharmacologic therapy, it is advisable to monitor serum lipids to determine changes in dosage.

1. **Triglycerides**

   a. **Gemfibrozil and clofibrate.** Triglycerides are best lowered by either gemfibrozil or clofibrate. **Gemfibrozil** is given in gradually increasing p.o. b.i.d. doses to 1,200 to 1,500 mg/day. Possible **side effects** include abdominal pain, nausea, vomiting, asymptomatic cholelithiasis, glucose intolerance, hyperuricemia, liver toxicity, hyperpigmentation, and rash. **Clofibrate**, 1 g p.o. b.i.d., has **similar side effects in addition to** rare associations with myalgias, arthralgias, impotence, and decreased libido. With hypertriglyceridemia, gemfibrozil or clofibrate may raise LDL CHOL levels in some patients, theoretically increasing the risk for atherogenesis. There has also been a questionable association between clofibrate and cancer.

   b. **Nicotinic acid,** which can also lower TG levels, should be started at 100

TABLE 4. *Cholesterol, fat, and fatty acid content of various foodstuffs*

	Cholesterol (mg/100 g food)	Fat (g/100 g food)	Saturated fat (g/100 g food)
Fish			
White fish, clams, scallops, oysters, and water-packed tuna	66	0.9	0.2
Shrimp, crab, lobster	112	1.7	0.2
Salmon	75	6.9	1.7
Poultry			
Chicken and turkey, no skin	87	4.9	1.3
Duck and goose, skin	91	33.4	8.0
Veal			
10% fat-trimmed roasts and chops, veal cutlets	99	11.1	4.7
15% fat-untrimmed loin roasts and chops	99	16.9	7.1
Beef, pork, and lamb			
10% fat-ground sirloin, trimmed lean beef and lamb	90	10.0	3.7
15% fat-ground round, untrimmed lean beef, trimmed lean pork	90	14.8	5.5
20% fat-ground chuck, untrimmed beef and lamb roasts, trimmed fatter beef and lamb	90	19.1	8.3
30% fat-ground beef and pork, shortribs, untrimmed, well-marbled steaks, chops (T-bone, etc.), ham	90	30.7	12.9
40% fat-spareribs, country-style ribs	90	38.9	10.5
Organ meats	300–2,000	4.8	1.6
Eggs			
White	0	0	0
Egg substitutes	0	4.2	1.2
Whole	504	11.5	3.4
Visible fats			
Most vegetable oils	0	100.0	13.0
Soft vegetable margarines	0	81.0	16.0
Soft shortenings	0	100.0	25.8
Butter	227	81.0	49.8
Coconut oil, palm oil, cocoa butter (chocolate)	0	100.0	74.6
Cheeses			
Count-down, dry-curd cottage cheese, tofu (bean curd), pot cheese, low-fat cottage cheese, St. Otho	6	2.1	0.9
Cottage cheese, Lite-Line, Chef's Delight, Breeze, Lite 'n Lively, part-skim ricotta	29	7.5	4.6
Cheezola, Scandic or Min Chol Hickory Farm Lyte, Pizza Pal, Saffola American[a]	12	24.5	4.7
Green River (lower fat cheddar), part-skim mozzarella, Neufchatel (lower fat cream cheese), Keil Kase, skim American	58	18.2	10.2
Cheddar, roquefort, Swiss, brie, jack, American, cream cheese, Velveeta, cheese spreads (jars)	106	35.0	20.6
Frozen desserts			
Water ices	0	0	0
Sherbet or frozen yogurt	4	1.2	0.8
Ice milk	14	5.1	3.2
Ice cream, 10% fat	40	10.6	6.6
Milk			
Skim milk (0.1% fat) or buttermilk	2	0.1	<0.1
1% milk	3	1.0	0.6
2% milk	6	2.0	1.2
Whole milk (3.5% fat)	14	3.5	2.2
Liquid nondairy creamers: store brands, Cereal Blend, Coffee Rich	0	11.0	8.5
Liquid nondairy creamers: Mocha Mix, Poly Rich, Mello	0	9.8	2.7

From Conner, W. E., Connor, S. L. (1982): *Med. Clin. North Am.*, 66:506–607, with permission.
[a]Cheeses made with skim milk and vegetable oils.

TABLE 5. *Drugs for treatment of hyperlipidemia*

Drug	Lipoprotein alteration	Drug	Lipoprotein alteration
Gemfibrozil	↓ VLDL, ↓ LDL, ↑ HDL	Colestipol	↑ VLDL,[b] ↓ LDL
Clofibrate	↓ VLDL, ↑ LDL,[a] ↓ LDL, ↑ HDL, ↓ remnants	Probucol	↓ LDL, ↓ HDL
Nicotinic acid	↓ VLDL, ↓ LDL, ↑ HDL	Neomycin	↓ LDL
Cholestyramine	↑ VLDL,[b] ↓ LDL	D-thyroxine	↓ LDL

[a]In occasional patients.
[b]In occasional patients with hypertriglyceridemia.

mg p.o. t.i.d. and gradually increased over a 3-month period to 2 to 4 g p.o b.i.d. before meals. The main **side effects** are flushing and pruritus, which can sometimes be prevented by pretreating with a prostaglandin inhibitor, e.g., aspirin 300 mg p.o., one-half hour before each dose. Other associated side effects are epigastric distress, hepatic dysfunction, glucose intolerance, hyperuricemia, and acanthosis nigricans.

2. Cholesterol

a. Cholestyramine and colestipol. The mainstays of lowering CHOL are the bile acid binding resins, **cholestyramine** and **colestipol.** Some patients, particularly those with concomitant hypertriglyceridemia, will increase their TG levels while taking these medications. If so, one of the TG-lowering drugs can be administered simultaneously. Both **cholestyramine and colestipol can lead to** constipation, rectal irritation, diarrhea, increased stool volume, heartburn, and a sensation of satiation. Moreover, cholestyramine can interfere with the absorption of thiazide, digoxin, thyroxine, and warfarin. Colestipol may be preferred by patients and physicians because of its flavorless quality, because of its need for a smaller volume of diluent and its antacid properties, and because it is less likely to interfere with other drugs. To improve compliance these drugs can be started at a low dose, one packet of cholestyramine (4 g) or colestipol (5 g) p.o. b.i.d., for several weeks. Then, either drug can be increased slowly to a maximum of 24 g/day of cholestyramine or 30 g/day of colestipol in b.i.d., t.i.d., or q.i.d. doses. To improve their taste and texture, the drugs can be taken in a variety of liquids, including juice, soft drinks, instant breakfast packets, and clear soups, or applesauce. Blenderizing the medicines in their vehicles may also improve the consistency. Side effects are often transient and can be reduced by temporarily decreasing the dose and increasing fluids. Frequently, simultaneous administration of a bulk-forming laxative-like psyllium taken 1 tsp in a glass of water b.i.d. can improve the most commonly encountered problems.

b. Miscellaneous. Second-line drugs are **gemfibrozil** and **nicotinic acid**, both of which can lower total CHOL while raising HDL CHOL. Both **probucol** and **neomycin** have CHOL-lowering properties. Probucol, which is well-tolerated, is given 500 mg p.o. b.i.d. Because it lowers HDL CHOL as well as LDL CHOL, it has some theoretical disadvantage. Neomycin is a poorly absorbed antibiotic given in a range of 0.5 to 2 g/day p.o. in a b.i.d. dose. **Toxicity** includes ototoxicity and renal damage, especially in patients with preexisting renal dysfunction. **Dextrothyroxine** lowers LDL CHOL similarly to L-thyroxine. Because the major side effect of this drug is hyperthyroidism, dextrothyroxine should be avoided.

BIBLIOGRAPHY

Diabetes

Alberti, K. G. M. M., and Thomas, D. J. B. (1979): The management of diabetes during surgery. *Br. J. Anaesth.*, 51:693–710.

Amico, J. A., and Klein, I. (1981): Diabetic management in patients with renal failure. *Diabetes Care*, 4:430–434.

Bradley, W. E. (editor) (1980): Aspects of diabetic autonomic neuropathy. *Ann. Intern. Med.*, 92:289–342.

Caplan, R. H., Pagliara, A. S., Beguin, E. A., et al. (1982): Constant intravenous insulin infusion during labor and delivery in diabetes mellitus. *Diabetes Care*, 5:6–10.

Christlieb, A. R. (1980): The hypertensions of diabetes. *Diabetes Care*, 5:50–58.

Coustan, D. R., Berkowitz, R. L., and Hobbins, J. C. (1980): Tight metabolic control of diabetes in pregnancy. *Am. J Med.*, 68:845–852.

Feinglos, M. N., and Lebevitz, H. E. (1980): Sulfonylurea treatment of insulin-independent diabetes mellitus. *Metabolism*, 29:488–494.

Fisher, J. N., Shahshahani, M. N., and Kitabchi, A. E. (1977): Diabetic ketoacidosis: low-dose insulin therapy by various routes. *N. Engl. J. Med.*, 297:238–241.

Galloway, J. A., and Bressler, R. (1978): Insulin treatment in diabetics. *Med. Clin. North Am.*, 62:663–680.

Karlsson, K., and Kjellmer, I. (1972): The outcome of diabetic pregnancies in relation to the mother's blood sugar level. *Am. J. Obstet. Gynecol.*, 112:213–220.

Knowler, W. C., Bennett, P. H., and Ballintine, E. J. (1980): Increased incidence of retinopathy in diabetics with elevated blood pressure. *N. Engl. J. Med.*, 302:645–650.

Kriesberg, R. A. (1978): Diabetic ketoacidosis: new concepts and trends in pathogenesis and treatment. *Ann. Intern. Med.*, 88:681–695.

Morris, L. R., McGee, J. A., and Kitabchi, A. E. (1981): Correlation between plasma and urine glucose in diabetes. *Am. Int. Med.*, 94(1):469–471.

National Diabetes Data Group (1979): Classification and diagnosis of diabetes mellitus and other categories of glucose intolerance. *Diabetes*, 28:1039–1057.

Rayfield, E. J., Ault, M. J., and Keusch, G. T., et al. (1982): Infection and diabetes: the case for glucose control. *Am. J. Med.*, 72:439–450.

Skyler, J. S. (1980): A plethora of insulins. *Diabetes Care*, 3:638–639.

Skyler, J. S., Skyler, D. L., Seigler, D. E., et al. (1981): Algorithms for adjustment of insulin dosage by patients who monitor blood glucose. *Diabetes Care*, 4:311–318.

Taub, S., Mariana, A., Barkin, J. S. (1979): Gastrointestinal manifestations of diabetes mellitus. *Diabetes Care*, 2:437–447.

Hyperlipidemia

Brunzell, J. D., Chait, A., and Bierman, E. L. (1978): Pathophysiology of lipoprotein transport. *Metabolism*, 27:1109–1127.

Conner, W. E., and Connor, S. L. (1982): The dietary treatment of hyperlipidemia. *Med. Clin. North. Am.*, 66:506–607.

Havel, R. J. (ed) (1982): Symposium on lipid disorders. *Med. Clin. North Am.*, 66:317–553.

Levy, R. I. (guest ed) (1983): Hyperlipoproteinemia: dietary and pharmacologic intervention (symposium). *Am. J. Med.*, 74(5A):1–36.

20.

Thyroid, Parathyroid, Adrenal, Genital, and Hypothalamopituitary Disorders

Richard Robbins

20.

Thyroid, Parathyroid, Adrenal, Genital, and Hypothalamopituitary Disorders

I. THYROID DISEASES

A. Hyperthyroidism Thyrotoxicosis describes a syndrome that is due to excess bioavailable thyroid hormone. The most frequent signs and symptoms in **thyrotoxicosis** are:

Signs	Symptoms
Tremor	Nervousness
Lid lag	Weight loss
Stare	Hyperdefecation
Tachycardia	Heat intolerance
Goiter	Palpitations
Hyperactive reflexes	Insomnia
Fever	Weakness

Graves' disease is a systemic autoimmune process that, in addition to the above syndrome, may cause proptosis, cheimosis, pretibial myxedema, hepatosplenomegaly, vitiligo, onycholysis, and lymphadenopathy.

Once the clinical diagnosis is suspected, the laboratory confirmation of thyrotoxicosis requires one of the following: an increased free T4 level, an increased free thyroxine index, an increased free T3, or a suppressed thyroid-stimulating hormone (TSH) response to thyrotropin-releasing hormone (TRH). A diagnostic schema is shown in Fig. 1.

Therapy. Recommendations are summarized in Table 1.

1. **Medical therapy.** Medical control of the thyrotoxic state should be attempted in the majority of patients. Of those individuals with mild Graves' disease, 20% to 30% may experience a long-term remission after a 6-month trial of thiourea drugs. In most patients with Graves' disease, however, medical therapy is designed to render the individual euthyroid prior to definitive therapy (surgery or ^{131}I). Beta blockade will very often be sufficient by itself to relieve the majority of symptoms. Oral contrast agents (ipodate, etc.), steroids, and iodine should be reserved for thyroid storm or cardiac decompensation in severe thyrotoxicosis. Lithium is indicated for mild to moderate thyrotoxicosis in individuals with a previous history of serious reactions to thiourea. Table 2 lists antithyroid drugs, their dosages and potential adverse reactions.

2. **Surgical therapy.** Goals of surgery in thyrotoxicosis are to **remove as much thyroid gland as possible** without damaging the parathyroid glands or their blood supply. Identification and preservation of the recurrent laryngeal nerves

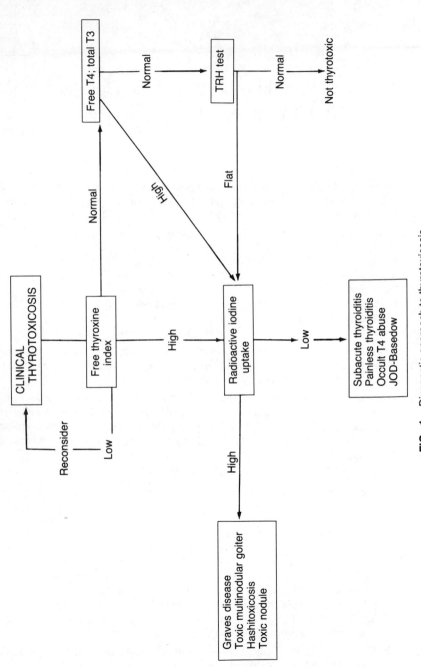

FIG. 1. Diagnostic approach to thyrotoxicosis.

TABLE 1. *Therapy of thyrotoxicosis*

Diagnosis	Recommended initial therapy	Persistence or recurrence
Graves' disease:		
Mild; small goiter	PTU 300–600 mg/day for 6 months then stop and observe	[131]I
Moderate	PTU 300–600 mg/day and β-blocker until euthyroid then [131]I	[131]I
Large goiter	Surgery	[131]I
Unreliable patient	Surgery	
Young patients	Surgery	
Toxic multinodular goiter	Surgery or [131]I (large dose)	[131]I
Toxic adenoma "hot nodule"	[131]I (large dose)	[131]I
Subacute thyroiditis	Aspirin (2-wk trial)	Steroids (2–3 months)
Painless/lymphocytic thyroiditis	β-Blocker (3 months)	Add steroids (2–3 months); watch for hypothyroidism
Hashitoxicosis	β-Blocker (3 months)	Steroids (2–3 months)

is also important. Thyroidectomy should be used initially only in patients with very large goiters or in recurrent thyrotoxicosis, especially in individuals with poor medication compliance.

3. **Radioactive iodine.** [131]I is indicated as the **definitive treatment** in mild to moderate thyrotoxicosis for most **adults.** Its use in thyrotoxic children and teenagers is still controversial and not recommended by many experienced thyroidologists. There is no firm evidence, however, that ^{131}I damages gonadal tissue or that individuals who have received doses under 20 mCi have any increased risk of developing thyroid cancer or leukemia.

[131]I is best administered 3 to 4 days after antithyroid medications [propyl-thiouracil (PTU), methimazole] have been withdrawn to allow adequate uptake by the thyroid. These drugs can be reinitiated 4 to 5 days after the [131]I. Full effects of ^{131}I may be seen as early as 6 weeks, but can take 6 months. Transient exacerbation of symptoms may occur days to weeks after the ^{131}I therapy because of increased release of preformed T4 and T3 from damaged cells (radiation thyroiditis). It is, therefore, prudent to continually maintain patients on drugs that interfere with the peripheral action of thyroid hormone (e.g., propranolol) throughout the course of ^{131}I therapy. PTU can be tapered and stopped as soon as signs or symptoms of hypothyroidism occur or between 8 to 12 weeks after ^{131}I if there are no clinical changes.

B. **Thyroid Storm** Thyroid storm is an **intense state of hyperthyroidism** seen only in patients with underlying thyrotoxicosis who develop another acute stress, usually a severe infection. Fever (greater than 40° C), tachycardia (more than 130 beats/min; often atrial fibrillation), dehydration, hypertension, and decreased mental acuity are the hallmarks of the disease. A decrease in **hypertension** before therapy indicates incipient shock. Therapy must be multivalent and includes:

1. **Iodine.** Initially 1 to 1.5 g of sodium iodine i.v. every 8 hr, which then can be changed to potassium iodide solution (SSKI) or Lugol's solution, 30 drops a day orally in divided doses. The major effect of iodine is to acutely decrease release of thyroidal T4 and T3.

TABLE 2. *Antithyroid drugs*

Generic name	Daily oral dosage	Side effects	Mechanism of action	Preparation
Propylthiouracil (PTU)	Initial: 300–600 mg in 3 or 4 divided doses; maintenance: 100–300 mg	Rash, leukopenia, pruritus, arthralgias, agranulocytosis 0.1%	Inhibits organification and coupling; decreases T4 → T3	PTU, tablets: 50 mg (preferred therapy in pregnancy)
Methimazole	Initial: 30–60 mg in 3 divided doses; maintenance: 5–20 mg	Rash, nausea, headache, leukopenia, agranulocytosis 0.01%	Inhibits organification and coupling	Tapazole® (Lilly), tablets: 5, 10 mg
Propanolol	40–200 mg in divided doses	Bradycardia, CHF, fatigue, impotence, fever	β-Blocker; inhibits T4 → T3	Inderal® (Ayerst), tablets: 10, 20, 40, 80 mg
Ipodate (iopanoic acid)	1 g single dose	Nausea, headache, urticaria, oliguria	Blocks T4 release; inhibits T4 → T3	Oragrafin sodium® (Squibb), capsules: 500 mg; Telepaque® (Winthrop), tablets: 500 mg
Glucocorticoids	Equivalent to 300 mg hydrocortisone	Hypertension, gastritis, edema, CNS effects, glaucoma, infections	Inhibits T4 → T3	Decadron® (Merck), tablets: 0.5, 1.5, 4 mg; Solu-Cortef® (Upjohn) for parenteral therapy
Lithium	600–1,200 mg in divided doses	Fatigue, rash, polyuria, increased WBC, nausea, tremor	Decreases T4 release; competes with iodine in T4 synthesis	Eskalith® (SK&F) capsules and scored tablets: 300 mg; Lithotabs® (Rowell), 300 mg
Iodine	5 drops 3 times a day	Metallic taste, excess salivation, rash, cough	Inhibits T4 release; initially inhibits T4 synthesis	SSKI (Upsher-Smith), 1 g/ml; Lugol's solution (Purepac); sodium iodide for i.v. use

2. **PTU.** To prevent intrathyroidal synthesis of thyroid hormones, this drug should be given as a **loading dose** of 1,000 mg followed by 450 to 600 mg daily in divided doses. Because of an increased number of side effects, methimazole is a second choice. Intravenous preparations of these drugs are not routinely available.

3. **Steroids.** Since **glucocorticoids** decrease T4 to T3 conversion and possibly decrease T4 release, the initial 3 to 4 days of therapy should include i.v. dexamethasone (8–12 mg/day in divided doses) or hydrocortisone (300 mg/ day in divided doses). This therapy also protects against the occasional co-existence of 1° adrenal insufficiency.

4. **Propranolol.** Beta blockers reduce the excess adrenergic tone and inhibit the conversion of T4 to T3. Propranolol can be used to treat the congestive heart failure (CHF) of thyroid storm, which it does primarily by decreasing heart rate.

5. **General support measures.** Mild reduction of central body temperature with a cooling blanket, conventional treatment of dehydration, CHF and any underlying infections are indicated. Aspirin should **not** be used as an antipyretic because it may displace T4 from binding globulins and lead to increased free T4 levels.

C. **Hypothyroidism** This very common condition (Fig. 2) is most often due to previous thyroid surgery or radioactive iodine. Spontaneously occurring hypothyroidism in the United States is most commonly due to autoimmune destruction (Hashimoto's disease). The **symptoms** of cold intolerance, tiredness, weight gain, hypersomnia, and constipation are so insidious that often they are not well-defined complaints. The **most common signs** include a "puffy" edema of the face and distal extremities; a dry, yellowish skin; hoarse voice, brittle hair and nails; and a slowing of muscle relaxation. Bradycardia and small pericardial effusions are common. Thyroid examination may reveal:

1. No palpable thyroid, suggesting agenesis in a child or hypothalamopituitary dysfunction in an adult.

2. A small, firm, micronodular goiter suggestive of Hashimoto's disease.

3. A moderate sized, smooth, diffuse goiter suggestive of dyshormonogenesis or prior Graves' disease.

4. A multinodular goiter consistent with dyshormonogenesis, iodine deficiency, or goitrogen ingestion.

Therapy. See Table 3 for preparations. Achieving the euthyroid state should be gradual and progressive. Elderly individuals or patients with underlying cardiopulmonary disease should be started on low doses (25–50 µg) of levothyroxine and slowly advanced until they are clinically and biochemically euthyroid. The **drug of choice is levothyroxine.** Using this drug allows replacement monitoring by measuring serum T4 levels. Individuals can control conversion of T3 or reverse T3 based on their own needs when replaced with levothyroxine. Use of preparations such as thyroglobulin, mixtures of T3 and T4, and T3 alone should not be routine.

Dessicated thyroid tablets may be less expensive than levothyroxine but variable bioavailability and difficulty in monitoring replacement levels by serum T4 deter-

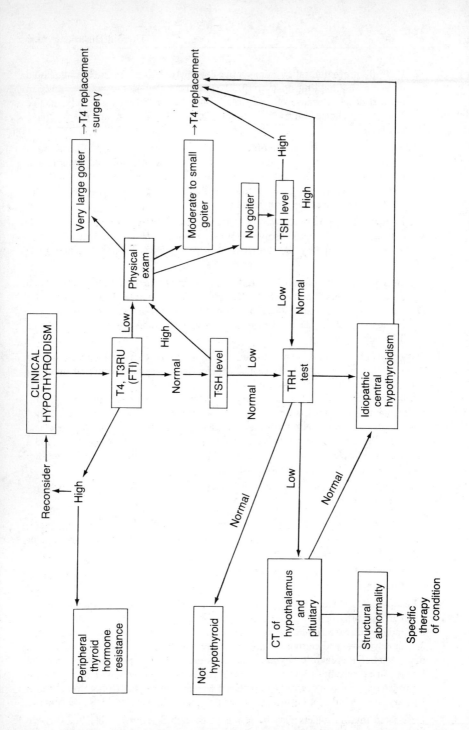

TABLE 3. *Thyroid preparation*

Generic name	Daily dose*a*	Dose equivalent to 0.1 mg L-thyroxine	Trade name
Levothyroxine (T4)	0.05 to 0.2 mg	0.1 mg	Synthroid® (Flint) Levothroid® (Armour)
Thyroid extract	60–180 mg	100 mg	Pork thyroid tablets (Armour) Beef thyroid tablets (Armour)
Liothyronine (T3)	15–75 μg	38 μg	Cytomel® (Smith, Kline & French)
Thyroglobulin	60–180 mg	100 mg	Proloid® (Parke-Davis)

*a*Varies with age.

minations has made this choice a distant second to L-thyroxine (Synthroid® or Levothroid®).

If the biochemical data and clinical estimates of the achievement of the euthyroid state are not in agreement, trials of minor adjustments in thyroid replacement are appropriate.

D. Myxedema Coma   This severe and often life-threatening condition usually arises slowly and gradually in the winter months in older women who have undiagnosed hypothyroidism or inadequate thyroid replacement. The precipitating cause is often a superimposed illness, most often a respiratory infection. In addition to classic signs of hypothyroidism, these individuals also manifest:

1. **Hypothermia**—which should be corrected gradually. Hypothermia causes apparent changes in arterial blood gas measurements. For each 1°C fall below 37°C the following corrections need to be made in order to calculate the true values:

   a. Subtract 0.015 units from measured pH.

   b. Add 4.4% to the measured P_{CO_2}.

   c. Add 7.2% to the measured P_{O_2}.

2. **Hypoventilation**—arterial blood gases must be analyzed by the formulas given above. Intubation and mechanical ventilation are often indicated to clear the mental depression of elevated P_{CO_2}.

3. **Hypotension**—the fall in blood pressure is exacerbated by bradycardia and often by pericardial effusion. This may also reflect coincident adrenal insufficiency. **Hydrocortisone** (100 mg i.v. every 8 hr) should be given for the first few days. **Intravascular dehydration** may also be present owing to fluids moving into third spaces, and repletion with normal saline is indicated. A central catheter to measure central venous pressure (CVP) is often very helpful, as many of the clinical estimates of CVP are unreliable in severe hypothyroidism. A number of **other sequelae** of hypothermia including paralytic ileus, decreased glomerular filtration rate, increased blood viscosity, thromboembolic events, a left shift of the O_2-hemoglobin dissociation curve,

FIG. 2.   Diagnostic and therapeutic protocol in hypothyroidism. FTI, free thyroxine index.

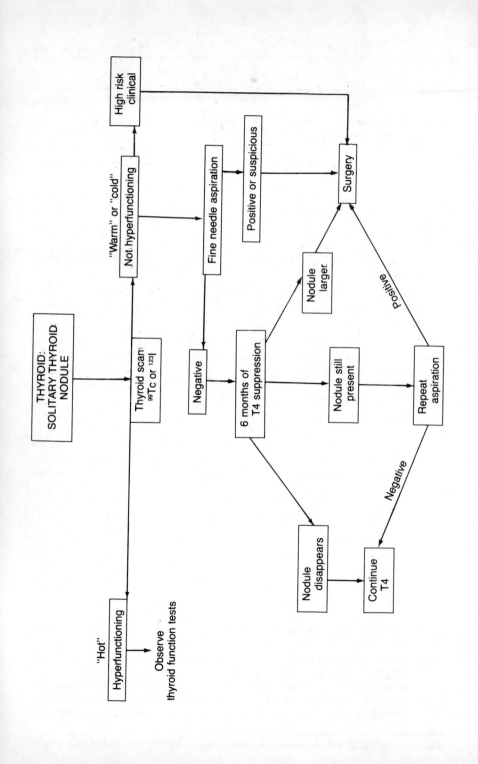

and hyperglycemia may occur. The presence of hypoglycemia in myxedema coma raises the likelihood of associated adrenal insufficiency. **Replacement Therapy.** Many specific regimens have been suggested for **replacement therapy** with the common goal of rapidly saturating all thyroid hormone receptors. The following regimen is suggested:

a. Intravenous administration of 300 to 500 μg of L-thyroxine initially.

b. Daily i.v. injection of 50 μg of L-thyroxine until medications by mouth (p.o.) can be given. Poor absorption by an edematous bowel precludes initiation of p.o. therapy or nasogastric tube. Since T4 and T3 conversion is often very low in hypothyroid coma, it may be useful to add 30 μg T3 i.v. initially and 25 μg i.v. daily with the 50 μg of T4.

All CNS depressants should be vigorously avoided in these patients during the initial recovery. The occurrence of myocardial infarction, hypophosphatemia, and hypokalemia should be anticipated during therapy.

E. **Thyroid Nodules**   Solitary nodules of the thyroid are very common, with an overall prevalence of 4% to 6% of the American population. Nodularity of the thyroid increases with age. The central diagnostic theme is to identify the subgroup (5% to 20%) in which the nodules are malignant. Nodules are at **higher risk of being malignant** when they are associated with a history of head and/or neck irradiation, rapid enlargement, vocal cord paralysis, fixation of the gland in the neck, "rock hard" texture, cervical lymphadenopathy, or in patients under 25 years of age. The sensitivity and specificity of any single test are low enough that multiple diagnostic criteria must be used (Fig. 3). As experience with fine needle aspiration increases, this procedure may become the diagnostic test of choice, but for now, the diagnostic protocol in Fig. 3 should be applied.

Current therapy (Fig. 4) for a malignant nodule in one lobe is controversial; however, since recurrence in the contralateral lobe may be as high as 20%, near total **thyroidectomy** followed by ^{131}I ablation of any remaining neck uptake 1 month later is recommended. Thyroid suppression with L-**thyroxine** (no TSH response to TRH) should be instituted and maintained for life only to be stopped for periodic ^{131}I total body scans.

Surgery for **locally invasive disease** in the neck should almost never exceed local neck dissection of lymph nodes. Radical neck dissections do not decrease recurrence rates and are associated with more morbidity and deformity than local dissection.

II. **DISORDERS OF MINERAL METABOLISM**

A. **Hypercalcemia**   The most common causes of hypercalcemia in medical patients are malignancy and hyperparathyroidism. Cancer may cause elevated serum calcium levels by metastatic bone destruction, by providing calcium-binding proteins (such as in myeloma), or by synthesizing factors that deplete the skeleton of calcium (e.g., osteoclast-activating factor, parathyroid hormone-like substances). Parathyroid hormone (PTH) hypersecretion may be primary from hyperplastic or adenomatous parathyroid glands, or it may be secondary to metabolic imbalances such

FIG. 3.   Diagnostic evaluation of the thyroid nodule.

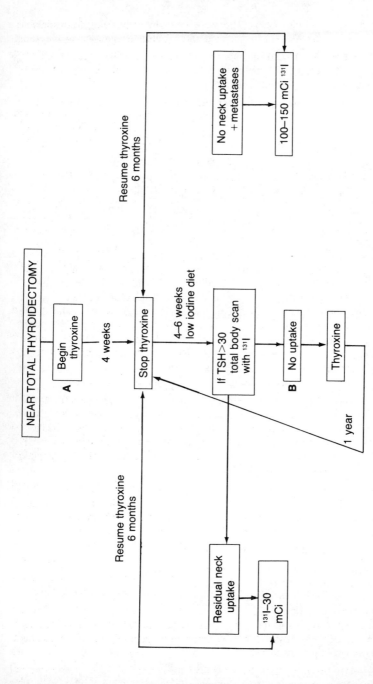

FIG. 4. Therapeutic options in thyroid malignancies. **A.** Thyroxine therapy in the setting of thyroid cancer postthyroidectomy is designed to replace thyroid hormone but must be given in doses high enough to suppress the TSH response to TRH. **B.** Two consecutive negative total body scans at 1-yr intervals can be taken to indicate a cure and further follow-up should consist of yearly clinical evaluations with lifelong thyroxine therapy.

as hyperphosphatemia and hypocalcemia (e.g., in renal failure). Thyrotoxicosis and vitamin D also stimulate excess calcium mobilization from gastrointestinal (GI) and bone sources. Hypercalcemia from inadequate renal calcium disposal is seen in familial hypocalciuric hypercalcemia and in individuals on thiazide diuretics.

Hypercalcemia causes a renal resistance to vasopressin and therefore is associated with polyuria. The **polyuria**, if not compensated, may lead to dehydration and further elevations of calcium, resulting in a dangerous cycle. Nephrocalcinosis and stone formation may ensue. Hypercalcemia and hypercalciuria may be associated with renal tubular acidosis and sodium and potassium wasting.

Common **complaints** of hypercalcemia patients include weakness, lethargy, constipation, anorexia, dyspepsia, and nausea. **Overt symptoms** usually indicate a serum calcium of greater than 12 mg/dl. Care must be taken in the diagnosis of hypercalcemia in individuals with elevated albumin levels. Total serum calcium increases 0.8 mg/dl for each gram of albumin above 4 mg/dl, whereas ionized calcium remains normal.

1. **Hydration therapy.** The great majority of hypercalcemia patients have volume depletion that should be corrected with normal saline at 100 to 200 ml/hr or half normal saline in patients with decreased cardiac reserve.

2. **Sodium diuresis therapy.** Achieving euvolemia may be associated with a decline in serum calcium. Persistent hypercalcemia can be treated by continued saline infusion in excess of urinary loss induced by furosemide (40–80 mg i.v. every 2–3 hr). Furosemide inhibits distal calcium reabsorption and increases calcium excretion.

3. **Calcitonin therapy.** Parenteral injections of this hormone may lower serum calcium rapidly but the effect is transient. Twenty to 25% of patients may not respond to calcitonin, which should be reserved for acute hypercalcemia emergencies. Calcitonin (Calcimar®) should be given i.m. in a dose of 4 Medical Research Council (MRC) units per kg and can be repeated every 6 to 12 hr if effective. If serum calcium does not fall by more than 1 mg% after two doses, other therapies should be attempted.

4. **Glucocorticoid therapy.** Corticosteroids lower serum calcium by interfering with vitamin D-dependent intestinal absorption of calcium as well as by decreasing bone turnover and possibly by increasing urinary calcium excretion. Steroids have proved **most useful in** hypercalcemia due to sarcoidosis, vitamin D intoxication, leukemia, lymphoma, myeloma, and breast cancer. The onset of the effect is gradual and may not be maximal until 36 to 48 hr of therapy.

Prednisone, dexamethasone, cortisone acetate, or similar drugs are recommended in doses equivalent to 300 mg of hydrocortisone daily followed by maintenance in the 50 to 100 mg/day range.

Occurrence of **side effects** including gastric ulcer formation, fluid and electrolyte abnormalities, hypertension, and Cushing's syndrome are not uncommon and should be anticipated.

5. **Phosphate therapy.** Phosphate supplements are useful in reducing intestinal calcium absorption and by decreasing the 1α hydroxylation of vitamin D. This

therapy should be **used only** in individuals with low serum phosphate levels, such as in maintenance therapy of primary hyperparathyroidism when surgical intervention is precluded.

Oral preparations such as Fleet Phospho®-Soda (10 ml t.i.d. starting dose) or Neutro-Phos® (750 mg t.i.d. starting dose) can be used, but elevated serum phosphorus or diarrhea may necessitate decreasing the dose. Intravenous phosphates should, in general, **not be used** because of tissue $Ca-PO_4$ deposition and occasional hypotension. However, in extreme hypercalcemic emergencies this form of therapy may rapidly lower serum calcium levels. Inorganic phosphate 1 to 1.5 g (as the potassium or sodium salt) should be infused i.v. over 6 to 8 hr, with careful monitoring.

   6. Dialysis. In patients resistant to initial conventional therapy, hemodialysis using a calcium-free dialysate may be the only means of treating severe hypercalcemia.

B. Hypocalcemia   Hypocalcemia is most commonly encountered after thyroid or parathyroid surgery. Other settings include hypomagnesemia, vitamin D deficiency, and acute pancreatitis. Serum calcium may be low in hypoalbuminemic states but ionized calcium remains normal. Hereditary causes such as pseudohypoparathyroidism and vitamin D-dependent rickets are uncommon. **Tetany** is the clinical hallmark of hypocalcemia. Subclinical tetany can be elicited by percussing the facial nerve (Chvostek's sign) or by Trousseau's maneuver with a blood pressure cuff. Depressed sensorium, dermatitis, brittle hair, and cataracts are often seen in chronic hypocalcemia.

Acute therapy requires judicious use of i.v. calcium, with 10% calcium gluconate being the most acceptable form. Calcium chloride 10% is very irritating to veins, but is equally effective in restoring calcium. An i.v. infusion of 200 mg of calcium (20 ml) can be given slowly over 20 min initially. Thereafter a constant infusion starting at 50 mg/hr can be instituted. The rate of calcium infused can be doubled every 4 to 6 hr until serum calcium reaches the 8 mg/dl range.

Chronic replacement therapy in surgically induced hypoparathyroidism is provided by oral calcium supplements (1–2 g/day; see Table 4) and by vitamin D (see Table 4). Replacement doses of both drugs may need to be slowly increased in certain "resistant" individuals, with careful monitoring of serum and urinary calcium. Urinary calcium should never exceed 300 mg in 24 hr.

C. Hypomagnesemia   This condition, which is surprisingly common in the hospital population, can be **a result of** excessive renal loss (e.g., diuretic use), poor intake (e.g., alcoholics), chronic diarrhea, high aldosterone states, and the use of certain aminoglycosides. The **clinical manifestations** include muscular irritability, mental status changes and arrythmias. **Laboratory studies** often reveal coincidence of hypokalemia and hypocalcemia. The hypokalemia may be protective of muscle spasms, which may be manifested when i.v. potassium is given to restore serum potassium levels. Calcium supplements will be relatively ineffective in correcting the hypocalcemia until Mg^{2+} stores are replete.

Oral Mg^{2+} supplements can be given, and doses of 500 mg magnesium orally (as Milk of Magnesia) three times a day (approximately 75 mEq) is a standard **starting dose.** Only approximately 50% of oral magnesium is absorbed. For more rapid

TABLE 4. *Oral therapy for hypoparathyroid states*

Calcium supplements	Starting daily replacement	Elemental calcium	Trade name
Calcium carbonate	2.5–3.75 g	1,000–1,500 mg	Os-Cal 500® (Marion)
Calcium gluconate	15–20 g	1,350–1,800 mg	Calcium gluconate USP
Calcium lactate	10–15 g	1,300–1,950 mg	Calcium lactate USP
Vitamin D supplements	Initial daily dose	Relative bioactivity[a]	Trade name
Ergocalciferol (D₂)	50,000 units	1	Deltalin® (Lilly)
Cholecalciferol (D₃)	50,000 units	1	Cholecalciferol USP
Dihydrotachysterol (DHT)	0.5–2.5 mg	3	Hytakerol® (Winthrop)
25 Hydroxycholecalciferol	25–200 µg	10	Calderol® (Upjohn)
Calcitriol [1,25(OH)₂D₃]	0.5–2 µg	1,000	Rocaltrol® (Roche)

[a]As compared with D₃.

correction, 10% magnesium sulfate may be given i.m. or i.v. An initial dose of 20 mEq can be repeated every 4 hr until there is clinical improvement.

III. ADRENAL DISEASES

A. **Adrenal Insufficiency**   This condition may arise from autoimmune destruction of the adrenal cortex (Addison's disease), hypothalamo-pituitary disorders, invasion of the glands by neoplastic or granulomatous processes, and in patients who have been on chronic steroid therapy. Clinical features of glucocorticoid and mineralocorticoid deficiency include:

Symptoms
nausea
vomiting
orthostatic dizziness
weakness
weight loss
hyperpigmentation
anorexia

Laboratory Studies
hyperkalemia
hyponatremia
hypoglycemia
eosinophilia
lymphocytosis
low urinary 17-hydroxycorticosteroid

1. **Diagnosis.** The diagnosis of primary adrenal insufficiency rests on demonstrating the inability of the adrenal to respond to adrenocorticotrophic hormone (ACTH). Two tests are available to assess this responsiveness:

a. **Cosyntropin (Cortrosyn)® test.** The patient receives an i.v. infusion of 25 units of ACTH or 250 µg of an ACTH analog (cosyntropin; 1-24 ACTH), which is given as an i.v. bolus. Serum cortisol is drawn at the beginning of the test (time 0) and 30 and 60 min after injection. The normal response would be an increase in serum cortisol of 15 µg/dl, with a minimum 60-min level of 25 µg/dl.

b. **Insulin-induced hypoglycemia test.** This procedure tests not only the response of the adrenal gland to ACTH but also the response of the pituitary to a metabolic stress. The test is performed by rapid i.v. injection of 0.10 units per kg of regular insulin to induce hypoglycemia. Peak ACTH levels are seen between 30 to 60 min after injection of insulin, and peak cortisol levels are seen 60 to 90 min after insulin injection. Again, a normal response of serum cortisol is an absolute value of at least 20 μg/dl and an increase of at least 10 μg/dl.

2. **Therapy.** Therapy for primary adrenal insufficiency includes physiologic replacement of both glucocorticoid and mineralocorticoid hormones. The relative potencies of various commercial products are shown in Table 5. Therapy for acute primary adrenal insufficiency requires an initial expansion of intravascular volume by normal saline and replacement stress doses of i.v. hydrocortisone as an **initial dose** of 100 to 150 mg i.v. bolus followed by 100 mg i.v. every 6 to 8 hr thereafter. A tapering schedule can then be used down to a maintenance dose of 30 mg/day. Hydocortisone will provide sufficient mineralocorticoid activity during the initial acute phase whereas chronic replacement therapy is best provided by fludrocortisone in a dose of 0.05 to 0.1 mg/24 hr. Secondary adrenal insufficiency, due to defects at the hypothalamic-pituitary level, do not require mineralocorticoid replacement because the renin-angiotensin-aldosterone pathway is intact; thus, in this situation hydrocortisone or cortisone acetate alone is usually sufficient to restore adrenal function.

B. **Cushing's Syndrome (Glucocorticoid Excess)** This condition is most often iatrogenic in individuals on steroid hormone therapy. Spontaneous Cushing's syndrome is due to ACTH producing pituitary tumors in 80% of cases; adrenal cortical adenomas account for 15% of cases, and the remainder are due to adrenal carcinomas or ectopic ACTH syndromes.

The most **common symptoms** are weakness, depression, weight gain, amenorrhea, frequent infections, hirsutism, and bone pain. Physical examination often reveals excess facial and supraclavicular fat, thin skin, ecchymoses, purple striae, centripetal obesity, muscle wasting, downy hirsutism, fungal skin infections, and hypertension.

Appropriate **screening tests** include an overnight dexamethasone suppression test (1 mg given p.o. at midnight; 8 hr later the fasting serum cortisol should be <5 μg/dl in normals) or preferably a 24° urinary free cortisol (UFC). If screening tests are positive they should be confirmed with a low-dose dexamethasone suppression test (0.5 mg p.o. q.i.d. for 48 hr with baseline and daily 24-hr UFC levels). If there is no suppression (less than a 50% fall in baseline UFC), a high-dose dexamethasone suppression test (consisting of 2 mg every 6 hr for 2 days) should

TABLE 5. *Oral replacement therapy for adrenal insufficiency*

Drug	Daily replacement dose (mg)	Duration of effects (hr)	Glucocorticoid potency[a]	Mineralocorticoid potency[a]
Hydrocortisone	30	6–8	1	1
Cortisone acetate	37.5	6–8	0.7	0.7
Prednisone	7.5	8–12	4	0.7
Dexamethasone	0.75	24–26	30	2
Fludrocortisone acetate	0.1	8–12	0.1	400
Triamcinolone	6	12–24	3	0

[a]Compared with hydrocortisone.

be performed. A decline in 24-hr UFC of greater than 50% indicates a **pituitary source** of the syndrome (Cushing's disease).

Serum ACTH levels less than 20 pg/ml indicate an **adrenal source**, whereas levels greater than 500 pg/ml suggest an **ectopic source**. ACTH levels in pituitary-dependent Cushing's syndrome are normal to slightly elevated (usually < 200 pg/ ml).

X-ray studies in Cushing's disease are notoriously misleading since many pituitary adenomas are below the resolution of average computed tomography (CT) scanners, and bony erosion of the sella occurs in less than 50% of patients. CT scans of the adrenals may show asymmetrical nodular changes even in pituitary Cushing's disease.

In patients with a pituitary adenoma **transsphenoidal surgery** is currently more efficacious than radiation therapy (4,500–5,000 rads).

Medical **management** of surgical or radiation failures includes the drugs listed in Table 6.

Bilateral adrenalectomy may be necessary in Cushing's disease resistant to conventional therapy directed at the pituitary level. **A suggested therapeutic approach is outlined in Fig. 5.**

C. **Endocrine Hypertension**

1. **Primary hyperaldosteronism.** Primary aldosteronism is due to either an adenoma or a hyperplasia of the adrenal cortex. **Hypokalemia**, which is present in virtually all patients on a normal sodium diet, is the cause of most of the symptoms, including weakness, tiredness, polyuria, polydipsia, headache, and paresthesias. There are no specific physical findings (i.e., no edema). Confirming **laboratory studies** include hypokalemia, hypernatremia (greater than 145 mEq/liter) in face of a low hematocrit, metabolic alkalosis, inappropriately high urinary K^+ (>20 mEq/liter) suppressed plasma renin activity, and elevated plasma aldosterone (PA).

The distinction between an adrenal adenoma and hyperplasia can be determined by measuring the response of PA to 2 to 4 hr of upright posture after 5 days of low-sodium diet. Patients with an adenoma will have no change or a fall in PA levels, whereas patients with adrenal hyperplasia frequently have an increase in PA after 4 hr of upright posture.

TABLE 6. *Drugs for the treatment of Cushing's syndrome*

Drug	Site of action	Dose and administration	Side effects
Aminoglutethimide	Adrenal	Orally 1–2 g/day	Lethargy, goiter, rash
Mitotane (*o,p'* DDD)	Adrenal	Orally 6–12 g/day	Anorexia, lethargy, elevated cholesterol, elevated serum alkaline phosphatase, nausea, diarrhea
Metyrapone	Adrenal	Orally 1–2 g/day	Nausea, diarrhea, hirsutism
Cyproheptadine	Pituitary	Orally 12–24 mg/day	Somnolence, weight gain, acne

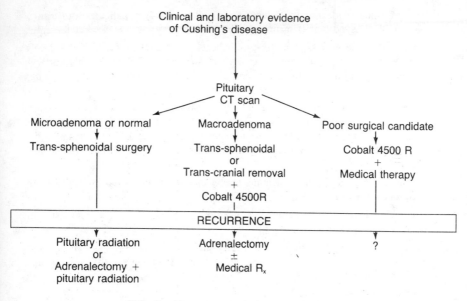

FIG. 5.   Management of Cushing's disease.

Localizing an adrenal adenoma is most effectively accomplished with an abdominal CT scan. If the results are equivocal, selective adrenal vein catheterization for measurement of PA levels is indicated.

Adenomas generally respond well to surgery whereas adrenal hyperplasia is best treated with spironolactone (200–400 mg/day).

2. **Pheochromocytoma.** A pheochromocytoma is a tumor arising in chromaffin cells, usually in adrenal medulla, which produces large amounts of norepinephrine (NE), epinephrine (E), and occasionally dopamine (DA). Intermittent release of large quantities of NE and E is associated with paroxysms of hypertension, headache, sweating, and papitations. Most patients still have baseline hypertension even between paroxysms.

Although less than 0.2% of all hypertension patients have a pheochromocytoma, its surgical curability and potentially fatal outcome require considering this diagnosis in all hypertensive patients.

In the appropriate clinical setting, the **screening test** should be a 24-hr urine collection for vanillylmandelic acid (VMA), metanephrine, and normetanephrine. These three screening tests taken together will detect more than 95% of patients with the disease.

Although a number of provocative tests have been developed to induce a release of catecholamines, the high degree of false positive and false negative tests, as well as the potential risk of sudden rises in blood pressure, makes these tests virtually obsolete. If overwhelming clinical criteria are not substantiated by elevated urinary catecholamine metabolites, a **phentolamine test** may be considered. This test is performed by pretesting a hypertensive patient with 1 mg of phentolamine i.v. If there is no response, the formal test of a 5 mg i.v. bolus will result in a blood pressure drop of >35 mm Hg systolic and >20 mm Hg diastolic if the hypertension is due to a pheochromocytoma. False positive tests are not unusual.

Localizing the tumor is best achieved by an abdominal CT scan. Selective adrenal vein catheterization studies should be reserved for CT scan negative patients with positive biochemical diagnosis and should be performed carefully because of occasional induction of a hypertensive paroxysm. In addition, a high degree of variability of adrenal vein cathecholamine gradients exists even in normal subjects.

Surgery is the treatment of choice for a pheochromocytoma. Alpha blockade with phenoxybenzamine (20–80 mg daily), and in those patients with persistent tachycardia beta blockade with propranolol (80–200 mg/day), should be accomplished preoperatively. Phentolamine and nitroprusside should be readily available intraoperatively. Preoperative hydration with saline may prevent sudden falls in blood pressure after the tumor is removed. **Careful attention to the type of anesthesia used is also important**, as ether and cyclopropane may increase sympathetic activity. Safe anesthetic agents include enflurane, ethrane, methoxyflurane, and sodium pentothal.

IV. **REPRODUCTIVE DISORDERS**

A. **Amenorrhea** Amenorrhea is diagnosed in any 16-year-old female who has never menstruated (primary) or in a woman who has had menses in the past but then experiences a 6-month interval with no vaginal bleeding. The diagnostic approach as shown in Fig. 6 is useful in most patients with amenorrhea.

Structural abnormalities of the outflow tract require formal gynecologic evaluation and chromosomal studies.

Individuals with idiopathic ovarian failure require estrogen replacement and progestin withdrawal every other month. Patients with chronic anovulation, most often due to the polycystic ovary syndrome (PCO), can also be cycled with progestin withdrawal every other month. Chances of fertility in the PCO group can be enhanced with the use of clomiphene citrate (50–150 mg p.o. daily for 5 days), which will induce ovulation in more than 60% of these patients. Tumors of the hypothalamo-pituitary region require specific endocrine-neurosurgical evaluation. **In all cases estrogen deficiency should not be allowed to continue as atrophy of estrogen-dependent tissue (breast, uterus, vagina), osteoporosis, and loss of libido are significant sequelae.**

B. **Hirsutism** The definition of this condition is highly variable as many women feel that they have excess facial hair. Racial and familial tendencies have a major influence on the amount of body hair, which is high in individuals of Mediterranean heritage but low in Orientals.

Most clinically abnormal hirsutism is felt to be due to excess androgen production or, less often, to increased sensitivity to normal female androgen levels. Hirsutism is not usually associated with overt estrogen deficiency but is associated with chronic anovulation and obesity.

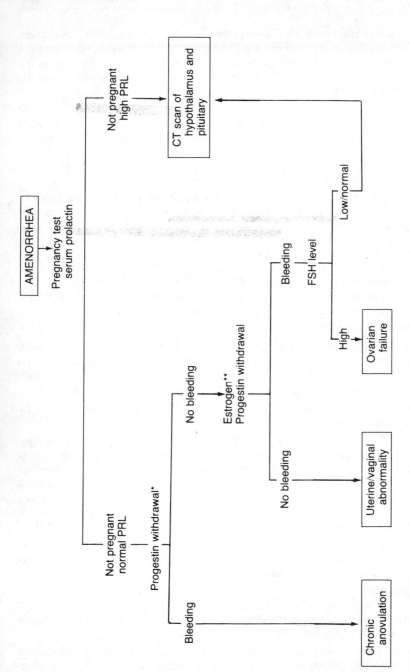

FIG. 6. Diagnostic approach to amenorrhea. *Progestin withdrawal may be done with either Provera® 10 mg p.o. for 5 days or progesterone in oil 200 mg i.m. **Estrogen priming may be accomplished with either Premarin® (2.5 mg) or estradiol (50 μg) p.o. daily for 21 days.

Signs of virilization suggest a much higher level of androgen production and an androgen-secreting tumor should be excluded.

Therapy is based on the use of medications that will inhibit either adrenal or ovarian androgen production. Glucocorticoids with low salt-retaining properties such as dexamethasone can be administered at bedtime (0.5–1 mg) to prevent the nighttime ACTH rise, a major stimulant to adrenal androgen production.

Estrogens, usually in the form of combination oral contraceptives, have also been used. Results are usually very gradual, and it may take 6 months before a clear response is evident. Some objective measurement of hair growth should be monitored.

Local therapy, including electrolysis and depilatories, may be preferable to years of medical treatment for hirsutism.

C. **Gynecomastia** Gynecomastia is defined as enlargement of the male breast. This is almost always due to growth of **glandular tissue.** The most common type of gynecomastia is that seen in pubertal boys which lasts for 3 to 4 yr. The necessary hormonal imbalance required for gynecomastia is an increase in the estradiol-testosterone ratio. A moderate decline in testosterone alone will usually not lead to gynecomastia. **Pathological gynecomastia** is seen in association with estrogen-producing tumors, thyrotoxicosis, Klinefelter's syndrome, hepatic failure, and with certain drugs. The following drugs may cause gynecomastia: spironolactone, digitoxin, cimetidine, and mitotane (o,p'-DDD). The common denominator in disease states that lead to gynecomastia (cirrhosis, Leydig cell tumors, adrenal carcinomas) is excess production of estradiol. No therapy is indicated for mild cases. Surgery, irradiation, and antiestrogens (e.g., tamoxifen) have been used, but **treatment of the underlying disease or elimination of the causative drug should be the initial approach.**

V. **NEUROENDOCRINOLOGY**

A. **Acromegaly** Acromegaly is a condition associated with growth hormone (GH) producing pituitary tumors, causing **soft-tissue enlargement** of the hands, feet, and face. Excessive sweating, glucose intolerance, osteoarthritis, peripheral neuropathies, and congestive heart failure occur in acromegaly.

Diagnosis in individuals with high clinical indices requires either failure of GH levels to suppress during a glucose tolerance test or fasting GH levels greater than 10 mg/ml in the absence of hyperglycemia.

Treatment with transsphenoidal surgery is slightly more effective than conventional radiotherapy (4,500–5,000 rads). Medical therapy with dopamine agonists (bromocriptine 20–30 mg/day) may be effective in certain individuals.

B. **Prolactinomas** Prolactinomas, which often present as amenorrhea-galactorrhea in women and as impotence with decreased libido in men, are the most common type of pituitary tumor. The **diagnosis** depends on demonstrating an elevated serum prolactin level in the appropriate clinical setting. A CT scan of the pituitary is the radiologic procedure of choice. Debate still persists, however, as to the initial treatment of choice. The initial high cure rates reported with transsphenoidal surgery are declining as recurrences are appearing years later. **Medical therapy** with bromocriptine is virtually always effective in lowering prolactin levels and may even shrink tumors in two-thirds of patients. Regrowth of tumors and elevation of prolactin levels are very common once the bromocriptine therapy is stopped, however. Radiation therapy is not indicated as a primary treatment modality.

C. Pituitary Reserve Testing   Testing the reserve of other pituitary hormones can be performed as follows:

1. **TRH test.** An i.v. bolus of 400 μg of TRH will test the responsiveness of TSH and prolactin. Serum samples should be drawn at 0, 30, and 60 min. Although age and sex determine responses to TRH, TSH levels should increase by 10 μU/ml by 60 min, and prolactin (PRL) levels should show at least a threefold increase.

2. **Gonadotropin-releasing hormone (GnRH) test.** GnRH luteinizing hormone-releasing factor (LRF) 200 μg is given as an i.v. bolus. Luteinizing hormone (LH) and/or follicle-stimulating hormone (FSH) levels are drawn 0, 60, and 90 min after injection. LH usually responds more than FSH, and females tend to be more responsive than males. Responses in women vary with the phase of the menstrual cycle. The lowest response in females is usually seen in the early follicular phase. LH should increase by at least 3 mIU/ml in males and at least 5 mIU/ml in females.

3. **Insulin tolerance test (ITT).** Hypoglycemia after an i.v. bolus of insulin (0.10 U/kg) stimulates the release of GH and ACTH. Hyperadrenergic symptoms should be allowed to proceed for at least 5 min before glucose is given. Blood sugar levels below 40 mg/dl are necessary for a valid test. GH should rise by at least 8 ng/ml or by threefold. (**Failure of GH to rise by ITT alone is not sufficient to diagnose GH deficiency.** Another provocative test such as L-DOPA, arginine, or exercise must also be blunted.) ACTH reserve is monitored by changes in serum cortisol levels. Serum cortisol levels must be drawn at 0, 30, and 60 min. Serum cortisol should increase by 10 μg/dl or to an absolute value over 20 μg/dl.

These three tests can be done simultaneously by injecting the TRH, GnRH, and insulin and drawing blood samples at the appropriate time. There exist many other tests for the reserve of each individual pituitary hormone. These can be found described in more detail in standard endocrinology texts.

BIBLIOGRAPHY

Adrenal

Aron, D. C., Findling, J. W., Fitzgerald, P. A., Fosham, P. H., Wilson, C. B., and Tyrell, J. R. (1982): Cushings' Syndrome: Problems in management. *Endocr. Rev.*, 3:229–244.
Krieger, D. T. (1983): Pathophysiology of Cushing's Disease. *Endocr. Rev.*, 4:12–43.
Nerup, J. (1974): Addison's disease—clinical studies. A report of 108 cases. *Acta Endocrinol.*, 76:127–139.
Sever, P. S., Roberts, J. C., and Snell, M. E. (1980): Pheochromocytoma. *J. Clin. Endocrinol. Metab.*, 9:543–568.
Weinberger, M. H., Grim, C. E., et al. (1979): Primary aldosteronism. *Ann. Intern. Med.*, 90:386–397.

Calcium

Agus, Z. S., Wasserstein, A., and Goldfarb, S. (1982): Disorders of calcium and magnesium homeostasis. *Am. J. Med.*, 72:473–478.

Lafferty, F. W. (1981): Primary hyperparathyroidism. *Arch. Intern. Med.*, 141:1761–1766.

Pituitary

Lufkin, E. G., Kao, P-C., O'Fallon, W. M., and Magan, M. A. (1983): Combined testing of anterior pituitary gland with insulin, thyrotropin-releasing hormone, and lutenizing hormone-releasing hormone. *Am. J. Med.*, 75:471–475.

Melmed, S., Braunstein, G. C., Horvath, E., Erzin, C., and Kovacs, K. (1983): Pathophysiology of acromegaly. *Endocr. Rev.*, 4:271–290.

Robinson, A. G., and Nelson, P. B. (1983): Prolactinomas in women: Current therapies. *Ann. Int. Med.*, 99:115–118.

Reproduction

Carlson, H. E. (1980): Gynecomastia. *N. Engl. J. Med.*, 303:795–802.

Hatch, R., Rosenfield, R. L., Kim, M. H., and Tredway, D. (1981): Hirsutism: Implications, etiology and management. *Am. J. Obstet. Gynecol.*, 140:815–830.

Hsueh, W. A., Hsu, T. H., and Federman, D. D. (1978): Endocrine features of Klinefelters Syndrome. *Medicine*, 57:447–463.

McDonough, P. D. (1978): Amenorrhea—etiologic approach to diagnosis. *Fertil. Steril.*, 30:1–15.

Thyroid

Chopra, I. J., Hershman, J., Pardridge, W., and Nicoloff, J. (1983): Thyroid function in nonthyroidal illness. *Ann. Intern. Med.*, 98:946–957.

Mazzaferri, E. L. (1981): Papillary and follicular thyroid cancer: a selective approach to diagnosis and therapy. *Annu. Rev. Med.*, 32:73–91.

Surge, D., McEvoy, M., Feeley, J., and Drury, M. I. (1980): Hyperthyroidism in the land of Graves: Results of treatment by surgery, radioiodine and carbimazole in 837 cases. *Q. J. Med.*, 49:51–61.

Van Herle, A. (1982): The thyroid nodule. *Ann. Intern. Med.*, 91:221–232.

21.

Nutritional Therapy

Boris Draznin

21.

Nutritional Therapy

I. BASIC FACTS OF NUTRITION   All of an individual's energy is derived from plant and animal food. Food energy values are customarily given in kilocalories (kcal). Proteins, fats, and carbohydrates are the energy-yielding substances. The typical American diet consists of approximately 15% proteins, 35% to 45% fats, and 45% to 55% carbohydrates. An energy deficit leads to utilization of the body's own substances and weight loss, whereas an excess of energy intake leads to weight gain and obesity. A negative or positive balance of 3,500 kcal results in either the loss or gain of approximately 1 lb.

A. Basal Metabolic Rate   Basal metabolic rate (BMR) is the amount of energy required to maintain the involuntary work of the body. One-fifth of the BMR is needed to maintain the functional activities of brain and nervous tissues. The functional activities of the liver, kidney, lungs, and heart consume an additional three-fifths. In adults, BMR is approximately 1 kcal/kg body weight (BW)/hr for men and 0.9 kcal/kg BW/hr for women. The BMR is influenced by size, shape, and weight of the individual, sex, age, rate of growth, sleep, body temperature, and state of nutrition.

B. Energy Requirement   The energy requirement of an individual is best determined from a record of daily activity. For practical purposes an individual's activity is classified as sedentary, moderately active, and active. Sedentary activity requires 30 to 35 kcal/kg BW, moderate activity requires 35 to 40 kcal/kg BW, and an active individual would need 40 to 45 kcal/kg BW.

1. Example 1: A sedentary 50-year-old man, 69 in tall (175 cm), weighing 150 lb (68 kg) has a body surface area of 1.82 m². His BMR is 35.8 kcal/m²/hr (Table 1). Thus, his BMR over the 24-hr period is:

BMR = 35.8 kcal/m²/hr × 1.82 m² × 24 hr = 1,564 kcal.

For sedentary activity add 400 to 800 kcal/day; for moderately active work add 800 to 1,200 kcal/day; for active work add 1,200 to 1,800 kcal/day.

Total daily energy requirement is equal to:

1,564 kcal + 600 kcal = 2,164 kcal.

2. Example 2 (for practical purposes): A sedentary man (same man as above) requires 30 to 35 kcal/kg BW/day. His total daily energy expenditure is

30–35 kcal/kg BW/day × 68 kg = 2,040–2,380 kcal/day.

C. Proteins   Proteins are complex organic compounds made up of both essential and dispensable amino acids. Essential amino acids cannot be synthesized in the body from other compounds and therefore must be provided by food. They are

TABLE 1. *Normal basic metabolic rates*

Age (yr)	kcal/m²/hr Men	Women	Age (yr)	kcal/m²/hr Men	Women
16	41.4	36.9	45	36.2	34.5
17	40.8	36.3	50	35.8	33.9
18	40.0	35.9	55	35.4	33.3
19	39.2	35.5	60	34.9	32.7
20	38.6	35.3	65	34.4	32.2
25	37.5	35.2	70	33.8	31.7
30	36.8	35.1	75 and over	33.2	31.3
35	36.5	35.0			
40	36.3	34.9			

From Wilmore, D.W. (1977): *The Metabolic Management of the Critically Ill.* Plenum Medical Book Company, New York.

leucine, isoleucine, lysine, methionine, phenylalanine, threonine, tryptophan, and valine. One gram of protein provides 4 kcal. The recommended daily allowance (RDA) for protein intake is 0.8 gm/kg BW/day for adults.

Except for hepatic coma, massive hepatic necrosis, and acute or chronic renal failure, which require a **decreased** amount of protein in the diet, a variety of pathological conditions such as fever, trauma, fractures, burns, cancer, and gastrointestinal disorders require **increased** protein intake.

D. Fats   Fats are essential and the most concentrated source of energy. They provide 9 kcal/g. In addition, they serve as carriers of fat-soluble vitamins. There is no RDA for fats. As little as 15 to 25 g of food fats per day is required to absorb the fat-soluble vitamins (A, D, E, and K) and to meet the body's requirement in essential fatty acids (linoleic acid).

E. Carbohydrates   Carbohydrates are commonly subdivided into monosaccharides (simple sugars), disaccharides (double sugars), and polysaccharides (starch, dietary fiber, and other complex compounds). One gram of carbohydrates yields 4 kcal. There is no specific RDA for carbohydrates. However, undesirable metabolic responses can be observed when daily carbohydrate intake decreases to less than 50 to 100 g/day.

II. Nutritional Assessment   Malnutrition is commonly due to a disease process. It is not surprising, therefore, to encounter malnutrition among hospitalized patients. The prevalence of protein-calorie malnutrition is said to be as high as 50% among surgical and medical patients in an average municipal or referral teaching hospital. A minimum of 5% of the patients in any acute care hospital will meet established criteria for severe malnutrition and require intensive nutritional support.

Congestive heart failure, obstructive pulmonary disease, infections, gastrointestinal disorders causing anorexia or discomfort with eating, renal and hepatic insufficiency, malignant and psychiatric illnesses are almost invariably accompanied by protein-calorie malnutrition of various degree. Most patients with this disorder demonstrate obvious or subtle signs of vitamin and mineral depletion. Folic acid is most commonly depleted. Deficiency of vitamins A, B_1, B_6, C, and niacin is also very frequently observed.

In addition to patients with acute or chronic illnesses, the thorough **assessment of nutritional status is especially important in** adolescents, pregnant and lactating women, and in the elderly. For example, it is well recognized that people of 65 years of age and older are likely to be deficient in calcium, iron, and ascorbic acid.

Nutritional assessment consists of five major components:

1. Clinical assessment.
2. Anthropometric measurements.
3. Biochemical assessment.
4. Dietary methodologies.
5. Evaluation of social environment.

All five aspects of nutritional assessment are equally important in composing the right picture of nutritional status of a given patient and in arriving at the appropriate conclusions in order to formulate the best plan for nutritional support. Thus, **thorough nutritional assessment includes:**

Medical history and current state of health, including a list of medications used.

Physical examination and evaluation of nutritional status, including height, weight, other anthropometric measurements, and dental evaluations. Careful attention should be directed at the presence of edema, muscle wasting, cheilosis, changes in hair, eyes, and skin.

Family history, social history, and any community factors that might relate to problems.

Nutritional history, including the presence or absence of weight change, information of dietary intake, food acceptance, vomiting, diarrhea, food habits, meal patterns, methods of food preparation and preservation, and daily calorie count.

Laboratory studies, including electrolytes, plasma proteins, BUN, alkaline phosphatase, cholesterol, urinalysis, stools for ova and parasites, others as indicated by a history and physical, and approximate X-ray studies.

There are 14 **undesirable practices** that can affect the nutritional status of hospitalized patients (Butterworth, 1974).[1]

1. Failure to record weight and height.
2. Frequent rotation of staff.
3. Diffusion of responsibility for patient care.
4. Prolonged i.v. feedings of glucose or saline.
5. Failure to observe patient's food intake.
6. Meals withheld for diagnostic tests.
7. Tube feedings in inadequate amount.
8. Ignorance of composition of vitamin mixtures and other nutritional products.
9. Failure to recognize increased nutritional needs due to injury or illness.
10. Failure to assess patient's nutritional status before and after surgery.

---

[1]Butterworth, C. E., Jr. (1974): The skeleton in the hospital closet. *Nutr. Today,* 9(2):4–8.

11. Failure to appreciate the role of nutrition in prevention and recovery from infection.

12. Lack of communication between doctor and dietician.

13. Delay in initiating an appropriate nutritional support.

14. Limited availability of laboratory tests to assess nutritional status.

After nutritional assessment is completed, therapeutic goals are established, and all undesirable elements are analyzed, the type of nutritional therapy should be chosen.

III. **Types of Nutritional Therapy**

A. **Standard Hospital Diet**   Standard hospital diet is appropriate for the majority of patients. Special adjustments are required for the patients with diabetes mellitus [American Diabetes Association (ADA) diet], gluten enteropathy, and hyperlipoproteinemia. Most commonly used hospital diets are listed in Table 2.

Special dietary maneuvers may be needed in order to provide high-protein and high-calorie diets, frequent feedings, and special diets for individual tastes. Selecting the nutritional therapy route is shown in Fig. 1.

Several important factors should be kept in mind when selecting the type of nutritional support.

1. Total nitrogen content must be adequate to meet the daily need.

2. All eight essential amino acids should be present.

3. The ratio of essential to total amino acids (E/T) should be 40% (except for the patients with uremia or hepatic failure).

4. L-amino acids are better utilized than DL-forms.

One must also recognize that giving glucose as a source of calories without nitrogen results in marked negative nitrogen balance. Thus, nitrogen/calorie ratio must be taken into account in choosing an appropriate type of nutritional therapy. The most commonly used nitrogen/calorie ratios range from 1:120 to 1:200.

TABLE 2. *Hospital diets*

Diet	Indications
Regular	No dietary restrictions
Soft	Progression from liquid to regular diet
Clear liquid	Acute illness, progression from NPO to oral feedings
Liquid	Moderate reduction in GI function
Pureed	For patients unable to chew or swallow solid foods
Low residue	Colitis, ileitis, diarrhea
High fiber	Diverticular disease, irritable bowel syndrome, constipation
ADA diet	Diabetes mellitus
Reduction	Obesity
Low fat (50 g/day)	Diseases of gallbladder, liver, and pancreas
Protein-restricted diet (60 g/day)	Renal or hepatic failure
Sodium-restricted diet (22, 44, 88 mEq/day)	CHF, hypertension, fluid retention
Potassium-restricted diet (60 mEq/day)	Renal failure

NPO, nothing by mouth; CHF, congestive heart failure.

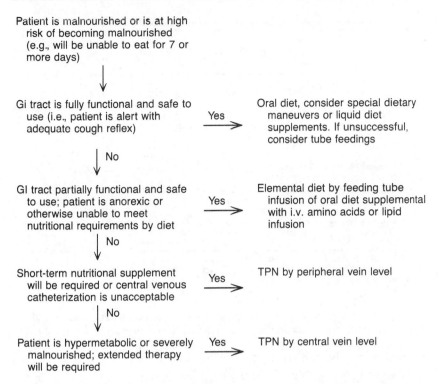

Patient is malnourished or is at high
risk of becoming malnourished
(e.g., will be unable to eat for 7 or
more days)

↓

Gi tract is fully functional and safe to
use (i.e., patient is alert with
adequate cough reflex)

Yes ⟶

Oral diet, consider special dietary
maneuvers or liquid diet
supplements. If unsuccessful,
consider tube feedings

↓ No

GI tract partially functional and safe
to use; patient is anorexic or
otherwise unable to meet
nutritional requirements by diet

Yes ⟶

Elemental diet by feeding tube
infusion of oral diet supplemental
with i.v. amino acids or lipid
infusion

↓ No

Short-term nutritional supplement
will be required or central venous
catheterization is unacceptable

Yes ⟶

TPN by peripheral vein level

↓ No

Patient is hypermetabolic or severely
malnourished; extended therapy
will be required

Yes ⟶

TPN by central vein level

FIG. 1.   Factors in the selection of nutritional therapy route. [From Willard, M.D. (1982): *Nutrition for the Practicing Physician*. Addison-Wesley Publishing Co., with permission.]

The requirement for electrolytes varies widely in individual patients and depends on volume and type of fluid loss, cardiovascular and renal status, type and amount of nutrients given. It is essential to monitor plasma electrolytes at frequent intervals, particularly when parenteral nutrition is administered.

B. **Multivitamin and Mineral Supplement**   Individuals who do not consume a basically adequate diet are advised to take a multiple vitamin-mineral supplement. This includes patients with protein calorie malnutrition, those on voluntarily restricted diets, pregnant and lactating women, elderly subjects, and patients who take mineral oil, stool softeners, cholestyramine resin, neomycin, methotrexate, oral contraceptives, phenytoin, penicillamine, diuretics, and alcohol.

C. **Liquid Diets**   Liquid diets require a **functioning digestive system** and are relatively complete foods. They are used as supplements or as substitutes for regular foods in patients with anorexia and depression and in those recovering from surgery, burns, or having difficulty with mastication. Most liquid diet supplements contain 1 kcal/ml. Individual tastes and factors such as tolerance to the protein and carbohydrate content in a supplement must be taken into account in prescribing a liquid diet supplement. Some commercially available liquid diet supplements are listed in Table 3.

TABLE 3. *Partial list of commercially available liquid diet supplements*

Product	Calories per serving	Protein in 1,800 calories (g)	Protein source	Comments
Free of milk protein and lactose:				
Precision LR	317	43	Egg white	Protein is of high biologic value
Precision HN[a]	300	75	Egg white	
Precision Isotonic	250	54	Egg white	300 mOsm/liter[a]
Lactose-free:				
Ensure®	240	63	Milk casein and soy protein	1 cal/ml
Ensure® Plus	250	66	Milk casein and soy protein	1.5 cal/ml
Isocal®	250	61	Milk casein and soy protein	350 mOsm/liter[a]
Containing milk protein and lactose:				
Meritene liquid	300	108	Milk casein	
Sustacal®	360	109	Milk solids and soy protein	

[a]Primarily for tube feedings; other products 435–625 mosm/liter
From Willard, M. D. (1982): *Nutrition for the Practicing Physician.* Addison-Wesley Publishing Co., with permission.

Hepatic acid, a formula containing increased branch-chain amino acids and decreased straight-chain amino acids, may be used in patients with hepatic encephalopathy. Amin-Aid, containing 6.35 g of essential amino acids and 0.25 g of histidine, may be used in patients with acute renal failure not undergoing dialysis.

D. Elemental Diets and Tube Feedings Elemental diets are composed of hydrolyzed protein or a mixture of chemically pure amino acids, a source of sugar, essential fatty acids, electrolytes, vitamins, and minerals. Table 4 provides the composition of selected commercially available elemental diets. Elemental diets are absorbed by **passive diffusion,** requiring minimal active digestion. Because they flow easily through small feeding tubes, they are commonly used for tube feedings. Indications for using elemental diets are outlined in Table 5. In Table 6 a sample administration schedule of an elemental diet is shown. **An infusion pump** is better than gravity and stop-cock arrangement in assuring a steady infusion rate.

TABLE 4. *Contents of elemental diets at full strength*

Product	Calorie /pkg	Calorie /pkg	Contents in 1,800 calories			
			Protein (g)	Na+ (mEq)	K+ (mEq)	Osmolality (mOsm/liter)
Standard Vivonex®	300	1	41	67	54	550
High Nitrogen Vivonex®	300	1	88	60	32	844
Vital®	300	1	75	31	54	450
Flexical®	250	1	41	27	58	723
Pregestimil®	a	0.67	59	49	65	496

[a]One-pound containers.
From Willard, M. D. (1982): *Nutrition for the Practicing Physician.* Addison-Wesley Publishing Co., with permission.

TABLE 5. *Indications for administration of elemental diets*

Persistent diarrhea
Fistulas of alimentary tract
Malabsorption
Acute pancreatitis
Short-bowel syndrome
Inflammatory bowel disease
Delayed postoperative intestinal function
Inability to eat
Inability to ingest adequate amounts of food
Food allergy (during elimination diet)

Fluid and electrolyte balance, liver, and renal function tests should be monitored. **Smaller feeding tubes made of soft plastic** are tolerated much better than traditionally used large vinyl or rubber feeding tubes.

Osmotic complications of tube feedings may result from the rate of administration, temperature and osmolality of feedings, presence of lactose, or bacterial contamination. A **tube feeding syndrome** consisting of hypernatremia and dehydration may be life-threatening if it is unrecognized. This syndrome is seen in patients who are comatose and cannot communicate their sense of thirst. Thus, **serum BUN and Na** levels must be monitored in these patients.

Nasogastric tubes, gastrostomy, and jejunostomy tubes are used for tube feedings. The first is seldom used in outpatient settings. A feeding **gastrostomy** provides a better tolerance to variations in infusion rates. Disadvantages of a feeding gastrostomy include regurgitation, belching, residual bad taste in the mouth, and increased risk of aspiration in patients with impaired cough reflects. Diluted pureed table foods or commercially blended pureed foods may be used for feedings. Both elemental and liquid diets may also be used.

E. **Peripheral Amino Acid Infusions** Peripheral amino acid infusions are used occasionally in hospitalized patients taking nothing by mouth in order to maintain their nitrogen balance. Travasol (3.5%) or aminosyn (3.5%) are most commonly used.

TABLE 6. *Sample administration schedule of slowly advanced elemental diet*

Day	Dilution of package concentration[a] (ml)	Continuous infusion rate (ml/hr)	Provides in 1 day	
			Calories	Volume (ml)
1	500	50	720	1,200
2	500	75	1,080	1,800
3	500	100	1,440	2,400
4	450	100	1,600	2,400
5	400	100	1,800	2,400
6	350	100	2,057	2,400
7	300[b]	100	2,400	2,400
8	300	125	3,000	3,000

[a]Using a 300-calorie package and continuous 24-hr infusion.
[b]Full strength, 1 cal/ml.
From Willard, M.D. (1982): *Nutrition for the Practicing Physician*. Addison-Wesley Publishing Co., with permission.

TABLE 7. *Indications for TPN*

Anorexia nervosa	Malignant diseases
Chronic vomiting and/or diarrhea	Renal failure
Malabsorption syndromes	Hepatic failure
Ileus or GI obstruction	Burns
Short-bowel syndrome	Trauma
Inflammatory bowel disease	Hypermetabolic states
Enterocutaneous fistulas	
Acute pancreatitis and	
pancreatic fistulas	

Although protein is spared during amino acid therapy, the fat stores are not. Enhanced utilization of fat stores results in mild **ketosis**. Ketosis in turn may cause electrolyte losses and hypovolemia. Amino acid therapy is contraindicated in the pregnant patient since ketosis may have an adverse effect on the outcome of the pregnancy.

F. **Total Parenteral Nutrition**   Indications for total parenteral nutrition (TPN) are outlined in Table 7. In general, parenteral nutrition is indicated when patients are unable to eat by mouth, and tube feeding is either contraindicated or has failed. Occasionally, TPN is used as an important supplement to oral feeding in patients with cancer, particularly those receiving chemotherapy or radiation therapy.

TPN should be instituted as early as possible to prevent further deterioration of nutritional status. Once started it should be pursued with vigor until patients are able to eat a reasonable amount of food by mouth.

The TPN is usually administered via the subclavian vein. A chest X-ray film must be obtained after catheterization and before the TPN solution is started.

Requirements for protein and calories are roughly proportional to the degree of injury, stress, or infection. Uncomplicated surgical procedures increase the BMR by 10%, major trauma by 10% to 25%, extensive infection by 20% to 50%, and burns by 50% to 125%. **The simplest practical formula** for calculating caloric requirements is as follows:

$$\text{Caloric requirement} = \text{BMR} + \text{stress factor} + 50\%$$

General guidelines for calculated i.v. nutrient requirements are presented in Table 8.

Examples of standard formulas for central TPN orders as administered at the University of Colorado Health Sciences Center are as follows:

1. Each 1,000 ml contains:
   aminosyn 8.5%—500 ml
   dextrose 50%—500 ml
   which is equal to:
   42.5 g of total protein
   6.7 g of nitrogen
   850 nonprotein calories
   127:1 ratio of nonprotein calories to 1 g of nitrogen.

TABLE 8. *Guidelines for calculating i.v. nutrient requirements*

1. 0.2–0.24 g nitrogen/kg BW
2. 40–45 kcal/kg BW
3. Nitrogen/calorie ratio ≈ 1:200
4. Energy derived on 50% basis each from glucose and fat
5. Optimum potassium/nitrogen ratio at least 5 mmol/l g
6. Optimum magnesium/nitrogen ratio 1 mmol/1 g
7. Optimum phosphorous intake 0.5–0.75 mmol/kg BW
8. Water-soluble vitamins
9. Essential elements: zinc, copper, manganese, iron

Modified from Dickerson, J. W. T., and Lee, H. A. (1978): *Nutrition in the Clinical Management of Disease.* Edward Arnold Publishers, Ltd.

a. Additives

Solution A	or	**Solution B**
(per 1,000 ml)		(per 1,000 ml)
potassium, 33 mEq		chloride, 17.5 mEq
sodium, 35 mEq		acetate, 45 mEq
magnesium, 5 mEq		MVI, 5 ml daily
acetate, 71 mEq		folic acid, 1 mg daily.
multivitamins (MVI), 5 ml daily		
phosphorus, 15 mM		
chloride, 49 mEq		
calcium (as gluceptate), 4.5 mEq		
folic acid, 1 mg daily.		

Order of solutions to be infused (e.g., ABAB, AABB, etc.).

b. Trace elements

(1) Standard mix/1,000 ml: Zinc 1 mg, chromium 4.0 mg, copper 0.4 mg, manganese 0.1 mg.

(2) Zinc only 1 mg/1,000 ml.

Do not give copper and manganese in biliary obstruction. Infuse TPN solution at **the rate** of 50 ml/hr initially, increase by 5 ml/hr as tolerated.

Infuse 10% **fat emulsion** (liposyn), 500 ml, once or twice a week over 6 hr.

2. Each 1,000 ml contains:
travasol 5.5%—500 ml
dextrose 50%—500 ml
total protein/liter = 27.5 g
nitrogen, 4.63 g
nonprotein calories, 850
nonprotein calories/g nitrogen, 184:1.

a. Additives

Solution A	or	**Solution B**

Solution A
potassium, 30 mEq
sodium, 35 mEq
magnesium, 5 mEq
MVI, 5 ml daily
phosphate, 30 mEq
chloride, 35 mEq
folic acid, 1 mg daily
calcium (as gluceptate), 4.5 mEq.

Solution B
chloride, 11 mEq
acetate, 17.5 mEq
folic acid, 1 mg daily
MVI, 5 ml daily.

Other orders as in the first example.

Solutions in schedule 1 contain less nonprotein calories per gram of nitrogen than solutions in schedule 2. Therefore, patients with severe negative nitrogen balance should be given TPN according to schedule 1.

Patients requiring a certain degree of protein restriction (e.g., renal failure) should receive solutions from the schedule 2.

The **order of solutions to be infused** (ABAB or AABB or AAAB, etc.) is dictated by the fluid and electrolyte status of the patient. Solution A is the major source of Na, K, PO_4, and Ca, and it should be infused in quantities sufficient to maintain normal fluid-electrolyte balance.

3. **Standing orders for TPN**

   a. Daily input and output, weight.

   b. Urine for glucose and acetone q 6 hr (blood glucose monitoring using readout or chemical strip material is preferable).

   c. Change in-line filter q 24 hr.

   d. Change CVP dressing q 2 days using sterile technique.

   e. SMA-6, BUN every Monday, Wednesday, and Friday.

   f. Complete blood count, prothrombin time, osmolality every Monday.

   g. Ca, Mg, P, total protein every Friday.

   h. LDH, SGOT, alkaline phosphatase q 2 weeks.

   i. **Do not** add anything to the TPN bottle once hung.

   j. **Do not** draw or infuse blood through CVP catheter.

   k. The catheter is to be used for **TPN only.**

   l. Vitamin K 10 mg i.m. every Monday and Thursday.

   m. Vitamin B_{12} 150 μg i.m. q 2 weeks.

4. **Intravenous lipid infusions** may be used to supplement caloric intake or to supply essential fatty acids in patients receiving TPN. Intralipid, 10% soybean oil emulsion with 1.2% egg yolk phospholipids and 2.25% glycerin (280 mosm/ liter), or liposyn, 10% safflower, is most commonly used. These emulsions contain 1.1 kcal/ml. Lipid emulsion should not be mixed with any other solutions and 500 ml is usually infused over 5 to 6 hr.

Because emulsified soybean oil is cleared from the bloodstream in a manner similar to that of chylomicrons, patients with hyperlipidemias may develop elevated serum lipids with i.v. lipid infusion. Lipid emulsion may also cause a transient decrease in pulmonary oxygen diffusion. Therefore, it may be contraindicated in patients with severe pulmonary disease. **Lipid emulsion should be used with caution in** severe liver disease, hyperlipidemic states, nephrotic syndrome, acute pancreatitis, allergies to eggs, and possibly diabetes.

5. In some patients, **extra insulin is added to the TPN solution** if blood glucose is not maintained below 150 mg/dl. Add 10 U of regular insulin to each 250 g of dextrose if blood glucose concentration is 150 to 200 mg/dl; add 15 to 20 U of insulin at the blood glucose concentration 200 to 250 mg/dl; add 25 or more units of insulin if blood glucose concentration exceeds 250 mg/dl.

6. **A chest X-ray film** must be obtained after catheterization and before the TPN solution is started. **Weight increases greater than 1.5 lb/day** are attributable to fluid retention rather than to weight gain. **At the conclusion of TPN therapy,** the solution is not shut off suddenly, because of the danger of hypoglycemia. When patients resume oral diet, TPN solution is decreased by 1,000 ml/day. TPN is continued, however, at 1,500 to 2,000 ml/day until the oral intake reaches 1,500 to 1,800 kcal/day. At this point, 5% or 10% dextrose is infused overnight at the rate of 100 ml/hr and the catheter is removed.

7. **Patients must be assessed** for effectiveness of i.v. nutrition during the course of therapy. Clinical well-being and maintenance of weight without edema are good signs. Improvement of wound healing, improved resistance to infections, positive nitrogen balance, increase in serum concentrations of transferrin and C_3 are all significant indicators of the effectiveness of the nutritional therapy.

8. Both **metabolic complications** and **complications resulting from subclavian vein catheterization** are listed in Table 9. Main complications of TPN are related to catheterization procedure, catheter sepsis, and, metabolic complications.

Metabolic complications are usually due to: inappropriate use of energy substrates; use of inappropriate energy substrates; poor monitoring; poor design

TABLE 9. *Complications of TPN*

Subclavian vein catheterization	Metabolic
Subclavian artery laceration	Hyperglycemia and glycosuria
Thoracic duct injury	Ketoacidosis
Pneumothorax	Osmotic diuresis and dehydration
Air embolism	Hyperchloremic acidosis
Brachial plexus injury	Prerenal azotemia
Catheter embolism	Hyperammonemia
Jugular thrombosis	Hypophosphatemia
Vena cava thrombosis	Liver enzyme abnormalities
Catheter fever and sepsis	Other mineral and electrolyte alterations
	Postinfusion hypoglycemia
	Headache
	Lethargy
	Tachycardia

of TPN regimen; failure to provide adequate amount of basic nutrients or other constituents (e.g., potassium or phosphate).

IV. **NUTRIENT-DRUG INTERACTION**   Drugs can affect taste, appetite, intestinal motility, absorption, and metabolism of nutrients. Conversely, changes in food intake, certain foods, or patterns of dietary consumption may alter drug absorption and response. For example, it is well known that **long-term anticonvulsant therapy** may lead to folate deficiency, osteomalacia, and rickets. **Cholestyramine** may cause loss of fat-soluble vitamins. **Long-term glucocorticoid therapy** results in an excessive loss of calcium and phosphorus, which may cause osteoporosis. **Mineral oil** reduces absorption of fat-soluble vitamins (A, D, E, and K). **Antacid therapy** causes alkaline destruction of thiamine within the bowel. **Antimicrobial** agents decrease utilization of folic acid, reduce absorption of vitamin B_{12} and calcium, and change intestinal flora, which may lead to malabsorption. **Cytotoxic drugs** inhibit and antagonize folic acid and interfere with vitamin B_{12} absorption. These are only a few examples of the effects of drugs on nutrition.

On the other hand, **energy and protein deficiency influence the metabolic pathways of drugs**. This is primarily related to the changes in the activity of microsomal drug-metabolizing enzymes in the liver. The effects of many minerals and vitamins on drugs' activity is well known to clinicians. Thus, a low potassium level increases the risk of digitalis-induced cardiac arrhythmias. Deficiency of ascorbic acid may enhance the toxicity of some muscle relaxants, thus increasing the risk of anesthesia.

Another important aspect of nutrient-drug interaction is the consumption of alcohol and/or caffeine. Both agents may alter significantly the rate of absorption and the clearance rate of many drugs, thus influencing the half-life of a variety of therapeutic agents. These and other nutrient-drug interactions mandate careful assessment and monitoring of the nutritional status of every patient on long-term drug therapy.

SUGGESTED LITERATURE

Elwyn, D. H. (1980): Nutritional requirements of adult surgical patient. *Critical Care Med.* 8:9–20.

Goodhart, R. S., and Shills, M. E.:*Modern Nutrition in Health and Disease.* Lea and Febiger, Philadelphia.

Grant, J. P. (1980): *Handbook of Total Parenteral Nutrition.* WB Saunders, Philadelphia.

Kinney, J. M. and Felig, P. (1979): The metabolic response to injury and infection. In: *Endocrinology, Volume 3,* edited by L. J. DeGroot. Grune and Stratton, New York.

Rudman, D., Millikan, W. J., Richardson, T. J., et al. (1975): Elemental balances during intravenous hyperalimentation. *J. Clin. Invest.* 55:94–104.

Silberman, H. and Eisenberg, D. (1982): *Parenteral and Enteral Nutrition for the Hospitalized Patient.* Appleton-Century-Croft, Norwalk, Connecticut.

Taylor, K. B. and Anthony, L. E. (1983): *Clinical Nutrition.* McGraw-Hill, New York.

Weinsier, R. L., Hunker, E. M., Krumdieck, C. L., and Butterworth, C. E. Jr (1979): Hospital malnutrition: A prospective evaluation of general medical patients during the course of hospitalization. *Am. J. Clin. Nutr.* 32:418–426.

22.

Skin Diseases

J. Clark Huff

22.

Skin Diseases

Optimum therapy for skin disease requires that a diagnosis be established by careful clinical assessment and diagnostic procedures such as examination of skin scrapings for fungus, a skin biopsy, or culture of skin lesions for microbial agents. However, even in instances in which a definitive diagnosis cannot be established immediately, nonspecific measures, such as symptomatic treatment for itching, may provide considerable benefit to patients.

I. NONSPECIFIC MEASURES FOR SKIN DISEASES

A. Symptomatic Treatment of Itching

1. **Oral antihistamines** may be valuable in suppressing the symptom of itching, but they are rarely totally effective. The side effects, such as sedation and anticholinergic effects, must be balanced against the therapeutic benefits. Use of oral antihistamines may be most appropriate prior to bedtime, a time when itching is often most severe and a time when a sedative dose of an antihistamine will not be as objectionable. The oral antihistamines most useful as antipruritic agents are the H_1 blockers, such as **diphenhydramine** or **hydroxyzine.** Dosages of 10 to 50 mg prior to bedtime may be given, and if sedation is not objectionable, 10 to 25 mg may be given every 4 to 6 hr during the day. Other antihistamines that may be used as antipruritic agents include **chlorpheniramine, tripelennamine, and cyproeptadine.**

2. **Topical measures for itching** are measures that provide a protective, soothing environment for pruritic skin or a cooling sensation on the skin surface.

    a. **Tub soaks** in a deep bathtub of lukewarm water for 10 to 15 min may provide relief from itching. Showers are not as helpful as soaking in a tub. Hot water should be avoided because of the rebound of itching that may occur afterward. Soaps, oils, and salts, such as sodium bicarbonate, are unnecessary additives to the tub.

    b. **Wet dressings,** soft absorbent cloth soaked in lukewarm tap water and applied to pruritic skin, may provide relief from itching. The excess water must be squeezed out of the cloth prior to application to the skin. A dry covering over the wet dressing will help secure the dressing in place, retard evaporation, maintain warmth, and protect bedding or furniture from the water. The evaporation of water from such dressings provides a cooling sensation that combats itching. If wet dressings are used over a large portion of the cutaneous surface, the cooling may induce shivering, and the patient may require a radiant heater.

    c. **Lubricating lotions** are liquid oil-in-water preparations that produce a cooling antipruritic sensation as the water evaporates from the skin surface.

Examples are Lubriderm® and Alpha Keri® lotions. Adding menthol 0.5% or camphor 0.5% to such lotions may provide an increased cooling sensation.

d. **Shake lotions,** such as calamine lotion, provide a cooling sensation and a protective covering on pruritic skin.

e. **Topical anesthetics** containing benzocaine or diphenyhydramine should **not** be used topically on the skin for itching because of the sensitizing potential of these medications.

B. **Therapy for Dry Skin and Chronic Dermatitis**   Dry skin is skin that does not contain an appropriate water content in the stratum corneum. Dry skin is manifested by scaling, fissuring, and sometimes itching and can be an important factor in the genesis of dermatitis. Elderly individuals and atopic individuals are particularly prone to dry skin difficulties. In arid climates and in unhumidified, heated, indoor environments, this problem may be accentuated. The measures appropriate for dry skin are generally applicable to any chronic dermatitis characterized by scaling and fissuring.

1. **Hydration of skin** is best achieved by tub soaks for 10 to 15 min prior to bedtime. **Use of soaps should be minimized** and limited primarily to intertriginous areas. Soaps such as Dove, Alpha Keri®, or Emulave® are less likely to irritate or further compromise the water-holding capacity of the stratum corneum.

2. **Lubrication of skin** with topical lubricating preparations is a means of sealing moisture into the stratum corneum to prevent its evaporation. The **greasier and more occlusive** the lubricant, **the more effective** it is in this regard. Cosmetic considerations and personal preferences are also important in the choice of a lubricant (Table 1). **Lubricants are best applied to moist skin immediately after hydration by tub soak.**

3. Infrequent bathing, along with the use of lubricants, may be necessary for a patient who cannot use the program of direct hydration followed by lubrication. The infrequent bathing approach is usually much slower and somewhat less effective than direct hydration.

C. **Therapy for Exudative Skin Diseases**   Blistering, oozing, or macerated skin is best treated topically by measures that are drying and debriding. In this instance, **wet dressings** are applied intermittently as needed, and the skin is allowed to dry after removal of the dressings. Such intermittent wet dressings (compresses) achieve drying, cleansing, and debridement. The same effects may be obtained by allowing dressings to dry next to the skin (wet to dry dressings), but the dry dressings may stick to the skin and removal may be uncomfortable. Soaking the dressing in aluminum acetate or aluminum chloride may provide the added drying, antibac-

TABLE 1. *Examples of lubricants*

Greases	Oils	Creams	Lotions
Petrolatum	Mineral oil	Eucerin	Lubriderm®
Aquaphor	Bath oils	Nivea	Alpha Keri®
Hydrophilic ointment		Aquacare®	

terial, and astringent benefits of these agents. An appropriate aluminum acetate solution may be obtained by diluting Burrow's solution 1:40 in water or by dissolving one Domeboro® or Bluboro® packet or tablet in a pint of water. One package of AluWets® in 12 to 16 oz of water provides an appropriate solution of aluminum chloride for wet dressings. If too concentrated, these aluminum salts may be quite irritating to inflamed skin.

D. Antiinflammatory Therapy with Glucocorticosteroid Drugs   Inflammatory dermatoses may respond nonspecifically to antiinflammatory therapy with glucocorticosteroid drugs. Care should be taken that these drugs are not inappropriately administered for skin diseases caused by infectious agents.

1. **Topical glucocorticosteroid therapy** is a convenient method of administering these drugs to the skin while avoiding many of the serious systemic side effects of these drugs. Even topical steroid therapy given for months to years may be attended by side effects, usually locally at the sites of application. Atrophy of the skin, telangiectasias, striae, and perioral dermatitis are such **local effects.** Although systemic absorption occurs, overt systemic side effects and clinically significant suppression of the hypothalamic-pituitary-adrenal axis are unusual. The nature of the skin disease being treated, the age of the patient, and the sites being treated are important considerations in the choice of a topical steroid (Table 2). Topical steroid treatment of infants' and children's skin, of intertriginous skin, of genital skin, or of facial skin should employ **lower potency preparations.** Therapy for inflammatory dermatoses characterized by thickening of the skin, scaling, and fissuring (chronic dermatitis) should employ primarily ointment **(grease)-based products,** whereas therapy for more exudative processes, with blistering and oozing, more often requires a **cream (oil in water) base. Gel or lotion bases** are most appropriate for hairy areas, such as the scalp. For an acute dermatosis, topical steroids may be applied every 2 to 4 hr, but for most chronic problems, careful application is rarely practical more than twice a day. **Because drugs are better absorbed if the stratum corneum is hydrated, optimal use of topical steroids may be achieved by combining their use with the topical measures that hydrate the skin.**

   a. **Tub soaks** combined with topical steroids are most appropriate for dermatoses characterized by thickening, scaling, and fissuring. After the tub

TABLE 2. *Examples of topical glucocorticosteroid preparations*

Lower potency	Medium potency	Higher potency
Hydrocortisone 0.25%–2.5%	Hydrocortisone valerate 0.2%	Betamethasone dipropionate
Prednisolone 0.5%	Desonide 0.05%	0.05%
Dexamethasone	Fluocinolone acetonide	Amcinonide 0.1%
0.04%–0.1%	0.01%–0.025%	Desoximetasone 0.25%
	Triamcinolone acetonide	Triamcinolone acetonide 0.5%
	0.025%–0.1%	Fluocinolone acetonide 0.2%
	Betamethasone valerate	Halcinonide 0.1%
	0.1%	Fluocinonide 0.5%
	Flurandrenolide 0.025%	Clobetasol 0.05%

soak, the topical steroid preparation in an ointment base is applied to the moist involved skin, and a bland lubricant is applied to the uninvolved skin.

  b. Wet dressings may be applied to the involved skin after application of a topical steroid cream for the treatment of inflammatory dermatoses. For dry, scaly, fissured dermatoses, the dressings are not allowed to dry, and the next application of the steroid is made to moist skin. For exudative dermatoses, the topical steroid cream is used under the intermittent wet compresses.

  2. Systemic glucocorticosteroid therapy should be used with **great caution for inflammatory dermatoses** and only after a diagnosis appropriate for such therapy has been established. Acute inflammatory dermatoses, which run a course of 1 to 4 weeks, are best treated with a tapering dose of oral prednisone, given as a single morning dose, beginning with 40 to 60 mg/day. Chronic inflammatory dermatoses are best controlled acutely with daily oral prednisone and chronically by careful tapering of daily dosages and conversion to alternate-day prednisone therapy.

II. TREATMENT OF SPECIFIC DISEASES

A. Dermatitis

  1. Atopic dermatitis is a chronic pruritic dermatosis of unknown etiology which may occur in certain predisposed individuals. The dermatitis usually displays the characteristics of a chronic dermatitis.

    a. Patient education is important so that the patient understands the chronic nature of the disease and the innate hyperreactivity of and tendency to pruritus in this special skin.

    b. Symptomatic treatment of itching with oral antihistamines, taken prior to bedtime, might be quite helpful.

    c. Dry skin therapy with hydration and lubrication once daily is appropriate in most cases.

    d. Avoidance of potential irritants, such as chemicals, alkali, and rough clothing, should be emphasized.

    e. Oral antibiotic therapy is needed if the dermatitis develops intense redness, tenderness, or oozing. Erythromycin, penicillin, or dicloxacillin at dosages of 250 mg q.i.d. for 7 to 10 days is usually effective.

    f. Topical antiinflammatory therapy with **steroid drugs** usually requires medium-potency products. Ointment bases, if tolerated by the patient, are most appropriate. Topical steroid application to areas of dermatitis after hydration by tub soak may be particularly effective. Atopic dermatitis on the face is best treated with 1% hydrocortisone cream.

    g. For extensive atopic dermatitis unresponsive to the above measures, tar and ultraviolet light therapy, as described for psoriasis (II.B.), may be helpful.

    h. Systemic glucocorticosteroid therapy should be **avoided** in atopic dermatitis.

  2. Nummular dermatitis is characterized by round pruritic areas of dermatitis, usually on the extensor skin of the extremities. The areas of dermatitis are usually chronic in nature, but in some instances may be more exudative, with oozing and crusting. The therapeutic measures for atopic dermatitis are also appropriate for nummular dermatitis.

3. **Allergic contact dermatitis** represents an acute dermatitis due to a delayed hypersensitivity reaction in the skin.

   a. **Removing the allergen** from the environment is critical to control of this problem. A thoughtful history and physical examination are invaluable in identifying possible causes. Patch testing is a helpful technique for demonstrating contact allergy.

   b. Symptomatic treatment of itching with **oral antihistamines** and topical measures may be of value.

   c. Therapy for exudative dermatitis with **wet compresses** is appropriate.

   d. Topical antiinflammatory therapy with glucocorticosteroid drugs is best combined with wet dressings. Medium- to high-potency preparations are usually necessary.

   e. Oral prednisone therapy, beginning with 40 to 60 mg/day and tapered over 2 to 3 weeks, is often needed for effective control of severe, widespread allergic contact dermatitis.

4. **Irritant contact dermatitis** due to contactants that alter the structural or functional integrity of the skin is best treated by removing the irritant and protecting the skin from the contactant. The therapeutic measures for atopic dermatitis may be worthwhile.

5. **Lichen simplex chronicus** is a thickened, pruritic, chronic dermatitis perpetuated by rubbing and scratching. Symptomatic treatment of itching and use of potent topical steroid ointments after hydration are worthwhile. Intralesional injection of thickened plaques with triamcinolone diacetate 5 to 10 mg/ml is frequently beneficial.

6. **Intertriginous dermatitis** (intertrigo) is a multifactorial dermatitis in occluded skin sites, such as under the breasts or in the creases of the groin. Therapy for exudative skin disease is helpful in cleansing, debriding, and drying the skin sites. Empirical topical therapy for candida along with a low-potency topical steroid twice a day may be quite effective.

7. **Seborrheic dermatitis** is defined by the presence of erythema and greasy scale around the brows, nasolabial folds, ears, scalp, or central chest.

   a. A shampoo containing 2.5% selenium sulfide (Exsel®, Iosel®, Selsun®) may be applied to the scalp for 10 min three times a week and washed out in order to suppress scaling in the scalp. Alternatively, shampoos containing salicylic acid (Sebulex®, Ionil, Vanseb®) are helpful in removal of scale.

   b. **Application of topical steroids** suppresses the inflammatory component of seborrheic dermatitis. Low-potency products, such as hydrocortisone, should be used for seborrheic dermatitis on the face and around the ears.

   c. Preparations containing sulfur and salicylic acid, and tar preparations (such as Pragmatar® cream), offer an alternative for topical therapy.

8. Stasis dermatitis is a dermatitis that occurs in an area of venous stasis, usually on the medial aspects of the lower legs near the ankles. Treatment of the venous stasis by elevation of the legs and support hose and treatment of the dermatitis by hydration and lubrication are essential elements for control of this problem. Use of topical steroid ointments may be combined with hydration. If stasis dermatitis becomes exudative, wet compresses and oral antibiotics are appropriate. Great care should be taken in the application of topical products to stasis dermatitis because of the high potential for the development of acute allergic contact dermatitis to ingredients in topical drugs.

B. Papulosquamous Eruptions

1. Psoriasis is a chronic skin disease with genetic and environmental determinants characterized by inflammation and hyperproliferation of the epidermis.

    a. Patient education should emphasize the chronic and variable course of the disease. The patient should understand that the disease is treatable but that the tendency of one's skin to develop psoriasis is not yet curable.

    b. Measures for symptomatic treatment of itching are appropriate in the unusual psoriatic patient with severe itching.

    c. Dry skin therapy, with hydration and lubrication, is helpful for removal of scale and softening of psoriatic plaques.

    d. Ultraviolet light, in particular the sunburn spectrum (UV-B), is quite effective in most psoriatics. Care should be taken not to burn the skin because the psoriasis may spread into damaged skin. When psoriasis responds favorably to ultraviolet light, the remission may be more long-lasting than with other forms of therapy. Both natural sunlight and artificial sun lamps are appropriate sources of UV-B.

    e. Topical steroids, usually medium- to high-potency products, used twice a day, produce clearing of many psoriatic lesions. They may be particularly helpful when applied to hydrated skin in an ointment form after a tub soak. Oftentimes a "rebound" flare of psoriasis is seen after topical steroids are discontinued.

    f. Topical tar preparations, in the form of coal tar derivatives (Estar®, T/Derm®), bath preparations (Balnetar®, Polytar®, Zetar®), or crude coal tar (1%–3% in petrolatum), may have a suppressive effect on psoriatic epidermis and sensitize the skin to long ultraviolet light (UV-A). The classical tar and light therapy for psoriasis (Goeckerman regimen) may be modified for outpatient use. Tar preparations are applied in the evening, left on the skin overnight, and wiped off in the morning with mineral oil. The skin is then exposed to an erythema dose of ultraviolet light, usually from an artificial light source. With this therapy, most psoriatics respond favorably, and clearing may persist for many months.

    g. Scalp therapy usually involves overnight application of a preparation to remove scale under a plastic shower cap. A phenol-saline solution (Baker's P&S®) may be quite helpful in this regard. Scale is mechanically removed with a comb in the morning, and a tar shampoo (Sebutone®, T-Gel®) is used to clean the scalp and hair. A topical steroid solution is then applied to the psoriatic lesions in the scalp. Tar shampoos and topical steroids may be sufficient for mild scalp psoriasis.

h. **Photochemotherapy,** the use of oral psoralen drugs along with long ultraviolet light (UV-A), may result in remarkable clearing of psoriasis. Special potent sources of UV-A are needed for this therapy, so the therapy is best performed in special photochemotherapy centers.

i. **Methotrexate,** given orally once a week, may be required for certain severe, disabling cases of psoriasis unresponsive to other therapy. Weekly dosages of 5 to 20 mg may be sufficient in many cases. Chronic low-dose methotrexate requires particular attention to potential liver damage and necessitates liver biopsies.

j. Systemic steroid therapy is contraindicated in psoriasis.

2. **Lichen planus** is an extremely pruritic skin disease with distinctive papules on the skin, oftentimes accompanied by oral or genital involvement. The disease may persist for months to years.

a. Symptomatic measures for itching should be employed.

b. Topical steroid therapy at least twice daily with medium- to high-potency creams or ointments may result in clearing and relief of symptoms.

c. Injection of triamcinolone diacetate 5 to 10 mg/ml into certain unresponsive lesions may also result in clearing.

d. Systemic glucocorticosteroid therapy with oral prednisone is justified in cases characterized by intractable, disabling itching. Most adults require 40 to 60 mg/day. If alternate-day therapy can be achieved with reasonable control, this dosage schedule is preferable. Unfortunately, the disease often flares as prednisone is withdrawn.

3. **Pityriasis rosea** is diagnosed by its characteristic clinical course and the morphology of the skin lesions. Serology to rule out secondary syphilis is often necessary. Symptomatic treatment for itching may be needed. Erythema doses of ultraviolet light may hasten the resolution of the eruption and assist in control of itching.

C. Inflammatory Follicular Diseases

1. **Acne vulgaris** requires use of multiple therapeutic modalities and individualization of therapy.

a. **Patient education** for acne requires explanation of the chronic nature of the disease, the need for 4 to 12 weeks for response to therapy, the necessity for long-term therapy, and the fact that **diet is rarely etiologically related.**

b. Elimination of irritants and trauma is also important. Modern acne therapy discourages the use of drying, irritating, or abrasive scrubs and topical products. Squeezing or excoriation of acne lesions may worsen the inflammation and subsequent scarring.

c. **Benzoyl peroxide** gels or lotions are applied once or twice daily in areas of skin prone to acne. The products must not be used simply on preexisting acne lesions. Both contact allergy and irritancy may be problems with benzoyl peroxide preparations. Products with 5% benzoyl peroxide are usually better tolerated than those with 10%.

d. **Topical antibiotics,** in particular those with erythromycin (Staticin®, A/T/S™, EryDerm®) or clindamycin (Cleocin-T™), may be quite effective. These must also be applied once or twice a day to the entire area where acne is occurring.

e. **Vitamin A acid or tretinoin** (Retin A®) used topically may be an effective means of preventing the formation of follicular keratin plugs. Cream (0.05%) or gel (0.025%) preparations are best tolerated. Topical therapy with vitamin A acid can induce irritation, and particularly sensitive areas of skin, e.g., eyelids, nasolabial folds, and perioral skin, should be avoided when using this product. Skin treated with vitamin A acid may be more sensitive to ultraviolet light, and protection from sunlight may be necessary.

f. **Oral antibiotics**—tetracycline 250 to 1,000 mg/day, erythromycin 250 to 1,000 mg/day, or minocycline 50 to 200 mg/day—may be invaluable in control of inflammatory acne. **Tetracycline is still the preferred drug.** Other antibiotics such as penicillin, semisynthetic penicillins, and cephalosporins are ineffective in acne therapy. The oral antibiotics may be divided into two doses a day rather than multiple doses. Instruction to patients must emphasize taking the oral antibiotics at times when absorption of the drugs is maximized. Once acne is controlled, dosages of oral antibiotics are slowly tapered.

g. Glucocorticosteroid drugs may play a role in control of **cystic acne.** Triamcinolone diacetate 5 mg/ml may be used for intralesional injection into acne cysts, and prednisone 40 to 60 mg/day for 3 to 4 weeks may assist in establishing initial control over severely inflammatory, scarring cystic acne.

h. Oral retinoid therapy with **13-cis retinoic acid** (Accutane®) is a valuable new tool for control of severe, scarring, cystic acne unresponsive to more conventional therapy. Because of the toxic nature of this drug and the important **side effects** (hypertriglyceridemia, myalgias, cheilitis, teratogenicity), use must be limited to appropriately selected patients, and patients must be followed closely through the 4 to 5 months of therapy by a physician experienced in the use of this drug. **Laboratory evaluation prior to therapy** should include pregnancy test, urinalysis, complete blood count with differential, BUN, liver function tests, and serum lipid levels. The cholesterol and triglyceride levels in the serum should be evaluated on a monthly basis. The daily dosage of this drug, 1 to 2 mg/kg, is divided into two doses and the drug is continued for 15 to 20 weeks. This drug is **absolutely contraindicated** during pregnancy and in nursing mothers.

2. **Acne rosacea** is treated with the same types of modalities as acne vulgaris. Oral tetracycline is often invaluable in control of rosacea.

3. **Perioral dermatitis** is an inflammatory process with both a dermatitis and an acneiform component. This problem is more common in women, and topical steroids used on the face are often important perpetuating factors. All topical steroids should be tapered or withdrawn while control is achieved with oral

antibiotics. Oral tetracycline 500 to 1,000 mg/day is usually the most effective drug. Subsequently, the tetracycline can be tapered slowly.

D. Cutaneous Infections

1. Bacterial infections are usually caused by pathogenic streptococci and staphylococci and respond to appropriate therapy for these organisms.

   a. Impetigo and secondarily infected dermatitis usually involve streptococci or a mixed flora and respond to 7 to 10 days of oral **erythromycin or penicillin** at 1 g/day. Therapy with topical antibacterial agents is less effective and usually inappropriate.

   b. Deeper infections (lymphangitis, erysipelas, cellulitis) may also respond to erythromycin or penicillin, but, because of the more serious nature of these infections, **hospitalization** for parenteral antibiotic therapy, blood cultures, and use of a drug that covers resistant staphylococci, such as dicloxacillin or oxacillin, are usually required.

   c. Infections more likely to be caused by staphylococci include bullous impetigo, furuncles, and carbuncles. In addition to appropriate incision and drainage for abscesses, drug therapy for resistant staphylococci is needed.

2. Viral infections

   a. Warts represent infection of keratinocytes with human Papillomavirus. Therapy involves destruction or removal of the infected epidermal cells that constitute the wart.

     (1) Paring of warts with a scalpel blade, freezing for 15 to 30 sec with liquid nitrogen in a swab or spray, or burning with an electric current (electrodessication) is a convenient mode of destructive therapy.

     (2) A blistering agent, cantharidin (Cantharone®), applied to a wart and occluded with tape for 24 hr may be invaluable for treating warts in children and for treating periungual warts.

     (3) Acids may be applied to warts to destroy and remove infected epidermis. Duofilm® (salicylic acid and lactic acid in flexible collodion) is a convenient product for patient use. Salicylic acid plaster (40%) along with paring is valuable for plantar wart therapy. The plaster is applied for 3 to 5 days at a time, and the site is pared before application of a fresh plaster.

     (4) Podophyllin 25% in tincture of benzoin is a particularly valuable treatment for warts in moist areas, such as on genital or perianal surfaces. The podophyllin is applied with a swab to the warts, and the area is washed in a tub in 3 to 4 hr. The therapy may be required every 1 to 2 weeks until control is achieved. The pain and irritation induced by podophyllin therapy may occasionally be severe.

   b. Molluscum contagiosum is an infection of keratinocytes with a pox virus. The destructive therapies described for warts may be helpful. The skin lesions of molluscum contagiosum may be scraped off with a sharp dermal currette. These lesions first may be frozen with liquid nitrogen or fluoroethyl spray and then scraped off with a currette while they are firm.

c. Herpes simplex infections are not easily treated. Severe primary infections or disseminated infections in compromised hosts may be shortened and the severity and symptoms lessened by proper treatment with acyclovir given intravenously. The severity of primary infections may be lessened somewhat by topical acyclovir (Zovirax®). No therapy has been shown to be clearly effective for recurrent herpes simplex. Protection from ultraviolet light may assist in preventing many episodes of recurrent herpes labialis. Symptomatic therapy for pain plus wet compresses may assist in management of certain severe cases.

d. Varicella and herpes zoster are caused by the same virus. Varicella is best treated with symptomatic measures for itching. Wet compresses and symptomatic treatment of pain are appropriate for herpes zoster. Studies have shown that systemic glucocorticosteroid therapy, given early in the illness, may diminish the occurrence of postherpetic neuralgia in older individuals. Prednisone is given in initial daily doses of 40 to 60 mg and is tapered over 3 weeks.

3. Fungal infections

a. Dermatophytes are fungal organisms with an affinity for keratinizing tissue such as the stratum corneum, hair, or nails.

(1) Stratum corneum infections, such as tinea corporis, tinea pedis, or tinea cruris, are best treated with topical antifungal agents. Effective products include tolnaftate (Tinactin®, Aftate®), haloprogin (Halotex®), miconazole (Monistat-Derm™), and clotrimazole (Lotrimin®). These products in a cream or liquid base should be applied two to three times a day to the affected area until the lesion has cleared. In chronic cases of tinea pedis, prolonged use of an ointment with salicylic acid (Whitfield's ointment) may be advisable.

(2) Hair infections (tinea capitis, tinea barbae) require systemic therapy with griseofulvin for 6 to 8 weeks. The microsize form in dosages of 500 to 1,000 mg/day is usually adequate. In highly inflammatory infections of hair with scarring alopecia, prednisone 1 mg/kg/day may be given concomittantly for the first 3 to 4 weeks to lessen the scarring. Because of the prolonged therapy needed and the rarity of tinea capitis in adults, great care should be taken to properly diagnose this problem in adults by fungal culture and microscopic examination of hair.

(3) Nail infections (onychomycosis) are extremely difficult to cure. Topical antifungal agents are rarely effective. Griseofulvin in the microsize form at a dosage of 500 to 1,000 mg/day may be necessary for 6 months for fingernails and 12 months or longer for toenails. Because of the relative unresponsiveness of nail infections, particularly those of toenails, proper trimming and filing of the infected nails may be more appropriate than specific antifungal therapy. Applying of 4% thymol in absolute alcohol to infected nails twice daily will have an antifungal effect and may be most appropriate for long-term therapy of onychomycosis.

b. **Tinea versicolor,** an overgrowth in the stratum corneum of an organism that may be a normal cutaneous resident, may respond to a number of therapies.

    (1) **Selenium sulfide suspension** (2.5%) (Selsun®, Exsel®, Iosel®) is applied to skin areas prone to develop this problem, usually the skin of the neck, trunk, and upper extremities, and is allowed to dry. The selenium sulfide is washed off in about 15 min. Daily treatments for 1 to 2 weeks may suffice, but intermittent, less frequent treatments may be needed in the future to prevent a relapse.

    (2) **Keratolytic agents** such as 3% salicylic acid in 70% alcohol, applied to the skin nightly for 1 to 3 weeks are often beneficial.

    (3) **Propylene glycol,** 50% in water applied to the skin one to two times a day, results in clearing over several weeks.

    (4) **Sodium thiosulfate,** 25% (Tinver® lotion) applied two times a day is also effective.

    (5) **Zinc pyrithione** shampoos (Head & Shoulders®, Zincon®, DHS Zinc®) may be used in the same fashion as the selenium sulfide suspension.

    (6) The topical antifungal agents effective for dermatophyte infections (clotrimazole, miconazole, tolnaftate, haloprogin) are also effective for tinea versicolor, but the expense of the quantity of medication needed to cover large areas of skin may be prohibitive.

c. **Candidiasis** represents a superficial overgrowth of *Candida albicans.* In treating this infection, consideration must be given to whether or not potentially correctable predisposing factors exist, such as antibiotic therapy, diabetes, glucocorticosteroid therapy, occlusion, or maceration.

    (1) **Intertriginous candidiasis** often occurs in the creases of the groin, under the breasts, or in other occluded or macerated skin, such as the corners of the mouth. Intermittent wet compresses and drying of the area are helpful measures. Topical medications effective against candida should be applied two to three times a day. Miconazole (Monistat-Derm™), clotrimazole (Lotrimin®, Mycelex®), nystatin cream (Mycostatin®), haloprogin (Halotex®), or amphotericin B (Fungizone®) used in a cream base are usually effective. Use of 1% hydrocortisone cream along with the topical antimicrobial agent will hasten healing.

    (2) **Thrush** is most easily treated with nystatin oral suspension, 1 teaspoon q.i.d. After being held in the mouth for 2 to 3 min, the suspension is swallowed. Clotrimazole troches held in the mouth are also effective.

    (3) **Vaginitis** caused by *Candida* is best treated once daily with miconazole cream (Monistat-Derm™) or clotrimazole cream or vaginal tablets (Gyne-Lotrimin®).

E. Infestations

  1. Pediculosis represents a transmissable infestation with lice adapted to living and feeding on human skin.

    a. **Pediculosis capitis** (head lice) is treated with 1% gamma-benzene hexachloride or lindane (Kwell®) shampoo, worked into the scalp, left on for 5 min, and then rinsed out. Treatment may be repeated in 7 days. After the first treatment, eggs (nits) must be mechanically removed from hair shafts with a fine-toothed comb. Soaking the hair in a warm, damp towel for 30 min prior to combing will help remove adherent nits.

  b. Pediculosis corporis (body lice) may be successfully treated by removing all clothing and a thorough bath or shower. Washing clothing in hot water destroys the lice. Dusting affected individuals with insecticides, such as 1% malathion powder, is also effective.

  c. Pediculosis pubis may be treated in a manner similar to pediculosis capitis.

 2. Scabies is usually caused by the human scabies mite, which burrows beneath the stratum corneum. The mite or the eggs can be demonstrated in scrapings of skin lesions.

  a. Symptomatic treatment for itching, which may be quite severe in scabies, is worthwhile.

  b. Lindane lotion (1% gamma benzene hexachloride) is applied to dry skin and is allowed to dry. All skin except for that of the head should be treated. One application to an adult requires about 60 ml. The skin is then washed in a tub or shower in 6 to 12 hr. Treatment may be repeated in 1 week. Close personal contacts, including family members and sexual partners, should also be treated once. Lindane is absorbed through the skin and may be neurotoxic. Alternative therapy should be considered in babies and in pregnant women.

  c. Crotamiton (Eurax®) cream, applied daily for 2 to 3 days, may also be effective.

  d. A traditional treatment for scabies is 5% sulfur in petrolatum applied nightly for three nights. The greasiness and odor may be objectionable.

  e. Clothes and bedding are washed in hot water after the first treatment for scabies. The employment of an exterminator is unnecessary.

F. Drug Rashes These rashes are usually widespread over the skin and maculopapular in character. Stopping potential causative drugs and symptomatic treatment for itching usually suffice.

G. Vesiculobullous Diseases These diseases are mediated by immunologic mechanisms and may require long-term and potentially dangerous drug therapy. Diagnosis should be confirmed by skin biopsy and immunofluorescence studies before treatment begins.

 1. Dermatitis herpetiformis is a chronic, pruritic papulovesicular eruption characterized by granular IgA deposits in the papillary dermis and along the basement membrane and by a bowel lesion similar to that of gluten sensitive enteropathy.

  a. Symptomatic measures for itching may be marginally beneficial.

  b. Dapsone at oral doses of 100 to 200 mg/day results in remarkable clearing and relief of itching. After the initial response, the dosage should be decreased to the smallest amount that maintains the disease under control.

Presumably, this drug works by affecting neutrophil function. The drug must be administered for years in order to maintain control.

Dapsone induces a chronic low-grade hemolysis of red blood cells and may induce serious **hemolysis** in patients with glucose-6-phosphate dehydrogenase (G-6-PD) deficiency. **Other adverse effects** include agranulocytosis, peripheral neuropathy, hepatitis, and allergic rashes. Prior to therapy, a complete blood count with differential, liver enzymes, and G-6-PD level should be evaluated. The blood count should be monitored weekly for the first month, monthly for the first 6 months, and biannually thereafter.

    c. Sulfapyridine given orally at dosages of 1 to 3 g/day may also be effective. Evaluation of blood counts and liver tests, in a manner similar to that recommended for dapsone, is advisable. Proper **hydration** is needed to minimize precipitation of the drug in the urinary tract.

    d. A strict **gluten-free diet,** followed for months to years, will lessen or obviate the requirement for dapsone or sulfapyridine therapy in dermatitis herpetiformis.

2. Bullous pemphigoid is a subepidermal bullous disease of elderly individuals, usually marked by the presence of antibodies that react with an antigen in the basement membrane zone of the skin.

    a. Symptomatic measures for itching may be needed.

    b. Oral prednisone at doses of 40 to 60 mg/day usually results in control of the disease after several weeks of therapy. The dosage may then be tapered and alternate-day therapy instituted.

    c. Oral azathioprine (Imuran®) at daily dosages of 1 to 2 mg/kg seems to have a steroid-sparing effect and facilitates control of the disease on lower prednisone dosages. Blood counts and liver tests should be followed during azathioprine therapy.

3. Pemphigus vulgaris is a mucocutaneous disease with intraepithelial blisters and nonhealing erosions. It is marked by antibodies that react with an antigen between epithelial cells.

    a. Oral prednisone at 60 to 120 mg/day may be needed for initial control. If blisters continue to arise after a week of therapy, even higher doses may be required. Once control is established and lesions healed, prednisone may be carefully tapered. If alternate-day prednisone administration can be achieved, side effects are minimized.

    b. Oral cyclophosphamide (Cytoxan®) or azathioprine at 1 to 2 mg/kg/day may be administered for its steroid-sparing effects.

    c. Intramuscular gold (Myochrysine® or Solganal®), used in a manner similar to its use in rheumatoid arthritis, may be effective in pemphigus. Because the response to gold may be slow (6 weeks or longer), its value is as a steroid-sparing agent or as therapy for mild cases.

H. Cutaneous Lupus Erythematosus   The skin lesions that may characterize lupus erythematosus (LE) include chronic (discoid), subacute, and acute lesions. Photosensitivity to ultraviolet light is evident in most cases of cutaneous LE. **Therapy** consists of photoprotection and antiinflammatory drugs.

1. **Protection from ultraviolet light** includes avoiding midday sunlight, protective with clothing, and wearing hats.

2. **Sunscreens** protecting against the sunburn spectrum of ultraviolet light (UV-B) are an essential part of therapy for cutaneous LE. Products containing para-aminobenzoic acid with high sun-protective factors (SPF-15) are most effective. Examples include Total Eclipse, PreSun® 15, and Super Shade 15. The sunscreen should be applied each morning to exposed skin.

3. **Medium- to high-potency topical steroids** applied to lesions two to three times daily may hasten resolution of inflammatory skin lesions.

4. Injecting chronic, scarring (discoid) skin lesions with triamcinolone diacetate 5 to 10 mg/ml may help control the inflammation and lessen scarring.

5. **Antimalarial drugs** may be quite valuable in treating cutaneous LE when the simpler measures described above are not effective. Chloroquin (250 mg/day), hydroxychloroquin (200–400 mg/day), or atabrine (100–200 mg/day) may be used. Improvement in the rash of LE is usually seen within 4 weeks. A number of **side effects** may be seen with antimalarial drugs, including skin pigmentation, drug rashes, myopathy, and gastrointestinal upset. Retinopathy, although unusual, can be a serious side effect. Patients taking chloroquin or hydroxychloroquin should have baseline eye examinations and reevaluations every 4 to 6 months while they are on these drugs.

I. **Urticaria** Urticaria represents a transient swelling in the skin that may have a variety of etiologies.

1. **Acute urticaria** often represents an immediate hypersensitivity reaction to some immunologic stimulus or a response to agents that degranulate mast cells.

   a. If a suspicious precipitating agent, e.g., food or drug, can be identified, it must be avoided.

   b. Oral antihistamine therapy with oral H_1 blockers should be given every 6 to 8 hr. These drugs are most helpful given prior to the onset of urticarial lesions and should be given according to a regular schedule. Hydroxyzine or diphenhydramine given at dosages of 10 to 25 mg are often beneficial.

   c. **Subcutaneous epinephrine** (0.3 ml of a 1:1,000 dilution) may be valuable in severe urticaria or urticaria with angioedema that may compromise airway patency. The injection may be repeated in 20 to 30 min.

2. **Chronic urticaria** is a pattern of recurring urticaria that persists for 2 months or longer. The etiology is often obscure.

   a. **Oral H_1 blockers** used prophylactically, as with acute urticaria, are usually beneficial.

   b. **Oral H_2 blockers** such as cimetidine (Tagamet®) at 1,200/mg/day, occasionally are useful adjuncts to the use of H_1 blockers.

   c. Attention to the avoidance of salicylate-containing medications and a salicylate-free diet is sometimes helpful in control of chronic urticaria.

3. **Physical urticaria** is a wheal-like reaction in the skin to physical provocation. Cholinergic urticaria and dermatographism are common examples of physical urticaria. Cholinergic urticaria is precipitated by heat, exercise, and sweating,

whereas dermatographism is caused by physical trauma, such as scratching or stroking the skin. These provoking stimuli should be avoided. Hydroxyzine, 10 to 25 mg, given regularly every 8 to 12 hr may minimize the reactivity of the skin.

J. Reactive Erythemas   Reactive erythemas are distinct erythematous eruptions that occur in the skin and are usually precipitated by an infection or drug.

1. **Erythema nodosum** is a sterile subcutaneous inflammatory process that most typically occurs on the pretibial skin of women.

   a. Bed rest and elevating the legs may be helpful.

   b. Nonsteroidal antiinflammatory drugs, such as aspirin or indomethacin, are valuable in control of the inflammation and pain.

   c. If a treatable or correctable precipitating factor can be identified, such as a streptococcal infection, fungal infection, oral contraceptives, or sarcoidosis, it should be treated or removed.

2. **Erythema multiforme** is an acute, self-limited cutaneous or mucocutaneous syndrome characterized by distinctive target lesions on the skin. Infections, in particular recurrent herpes simplex, and drugs are usually the precipitating stimuli.

   a. Symptomatic treatment for itching may be helpful.

   b. Oral antibiotics, such as erythromycin or penicillin at 1 g/day for 7 to 10 days, may be beneficial in treatment of purulent, secondarily infected oral lesions associated with cervical lymphadenopathy.

   c. Controlling the pain of oral erosions is facilitated by avoiding salty or spicy foods and drinks and maintaining a soft diet. Gentle debridement of purulent oral lesions with half-strength hydrogen peroxide (1½%) used as a mouthwash is often helpful. If a topical anesthetic is needed prior to meals, a convenient formula is equal parts of pectin-kaolin (Kaopectate®) and elixir of diphenhydramine, used as a mouthwash.

   d. Systemic glucocorticosteroid therapy is unnecessary for most cases of erythema multiforme, which are mild and self-limited. In severe cases with involvement of multiple mucosal surfaces, as may be seen in the Stevens-Johnson syndrome, systemic steroids given early may be helpful. Oral prednisone at 1 to 2 mg/kg/day may be given until spreading has ceased and then tapered over 2 to 3 weeks.

BIBLIOGRAPHY

Ahmed, A. R., Graham, J., Jordon, R. E., and Provost, T. T. (1980): Pemphigus: Current concepts. *Ann. Intern. Med.*, 92:396–405.

Ahmed, A. R., Maize, J. C., and Provost, T. T. (1977): Bullous pemphigoid. *Arch. Dermatol.*, 113:1043–1046.

Alexander, J. O. (1975): *Dermatitis herpetiformis.* W. B. Saunders Co., London.

Cram, D. L. (1981): Psoriasis: Current advances in etiology and treatment. *J. Am. Acad. Dermatol.*, 4:1–14.

Cunliffe, W. I., and Cotterill, J. A. (1978): *The Acnes.* W. B. Saunders Co., London.

Dubois, E. L. (1978):   Antimalarials in the management of discoid and systemic lupus erythematosus. *Semin. Arthritis Rheum.*, 8:33–51.

Epstein, J. H., and Farber, E. M. (1979): Current status of oral PUVA therapy for psoriasis. *J. Am. Dermatol.*, 1:106–117.

Fritz, K. A., and Weston, W. L. (1983): Topical glucocorticosteroids. *Ann. Allergy*, 50:68–76.

Goldstein, J. A., Socha-Szott, A., Thomsen, R. J., Pochi, P. E., Shalita, A. R., and Strauss, J. S. (1982): Comparative effect of isotretinoin and etretinate on acne and sebaceous gland secretion. *J. Am. Acad. Dermatol.*, 6:760–765.

Huff, J. C. (1984): Erythema multiforme. Current Issues in Dermatology. Vol. 1. G. K. Hall Medical Publishers, Boston. pp. 223–251.

Huff, J. C., and Weston, W. L. (1978): Eczematous dermatitis. In *Adolescent Dermatology*. W. B. Saunders Co., Philadelphia. pp. 86–122.

Katz, S. I., and Strober, W. (1978): The pathogenesis of dermatitis herpetiformis. *J. Invest. Dermatol.*, 70:63–75.

Lever, W. F. (1979): Pemphigus and pemphigoid. *J. Am. Acad. Dermatol.*, 1:2–31.

LeVine, M. J., White, H. A. D., and Parrish, J. A. (1979): Components of the Goekerman regimen. *J. Invest. Dermatol.*, 73:170–173.

Peck, G. L., Olsen, T. G., Yoder, E. W., et al. (1979): Prolonged remissions of cystic and conglobate acne with 13-Cis-retinoic acid. *N. Engl. J. Med.*, 300:329–333.

Penneys, N. S., and Eaglstein, W. H. (1976): Management of pemphigus with gold compounds. *Arch. Dermatol.*, 112:185–187.

Rajka, G. (1975): *Atopic Dermatitis*. W. B. Saunders, London.

Roenigk, H. H., Auerbach, R., Maibach, H. I., and Weinstein, G. D. (1982): Methotrexate guidelines revised. *J. Am. Acad. Dermatol.*, 6:145–155.

Storrs, E. J. (1979): Use and abuse of systemic corticosteroid therapy. *J. Am. Acad. Dermatol.*, 1:95–105.

Warin, R. P., and Champion, R. H. (1974): *Urticaria*. W. B. Saunders Co., London.

Weston, W. L. (1979): *Practical Pediatric Dermatology*. Little Brown & Co., Boston.

23.

Neurologic Diseases

Neil L. Rosenberg

23.

Neurologic Diseases

I. COMA

A. Definition and General Principles Coma is best defined as a state where there is complete loss of consciousness. State of consciousness is defined as one's level of arousal and interaction with the environment. Observers disagree about what lethargy, obtundation, stupor, and semicoma represent, so only coma is referred to when discussing alterations in consciousness. Since the same pathophysiologic processes that alter consciousness also produce coma, they can be considered varying degrees of the same phenomenon.

The presence of coma implies a disease process is affecting either **both cerebral hemispheres** or the **ascending reticular activating system** (ARAS) that runs from the pons to the diencephalon. Therefore, a process affecting one hemisphere, such as an infarction, should not produce coma unless there is secondary compression of the other hemisphere or brainstem.

B. Diagnosis

1. **History.** The importance of obtaining history rapidly when someone is brought to the emergency room in an unresponsive state is to assess whether a structural or nonstructural lesion is responsible for coma. Features in the history that suggest a **structural lesion** include trauma (suggesting subdural or epidural hematoma), prior history of stroke or tumor, chronic alcohol abuse (subdural hematoma), head and face infections (abscess, empyema, cerebritis), bleeding disorder (intracranial hemorrhage), and focal symptoms prior to onset of coma. In patients with **nonstructural or toxic/metabolic causes** of coma, frequently there is a history of prior medical illnesses such as liver, pulmonary, or renal disease or a prior history of drug abuse. A prior history of a psychiatric disorder is also important in relation to depression, drug overdose, and other attempts at suicide.

2. **General physical examination** may reveal the evidence of trauma even when there is no available history. **Battle's sign** is an ecchymosis of the mastoid process indicating fracture of mastoid, and **raccoon's eyes** in an ecchymosis in the periorbital region indicating orbital fracture. These signs may be the only evidence of basilar skull fracture. Examination for other evidence of bruises or hematomas, lacerations, and bleeding from nose or ears are also important signs. The **general appearance** of the patient may reveal evidence of either acute or chronic illness or even the presence of a particular systemic illness, such as the cherry-red color of the skin in carbon monoxide intoxication.

3. Neurologic examination. Although several aspects of the neurologic examination cannot be evaluated in a comatose patient, e.g., cerebellar function and coordination testing, the neurologic examination should be as complete as possible and emphasize the following:

a. **Observation.** In addition to the aspects of observation included in the general physical examination, the **position of the body and its parts** should be carefully observed. Is the patient lying in a natural position or is there flexor or extensor posturing? Are there any spontaneous movements and if so is there any asymmetry to these movements?

b. **Level of consciousness.** Observe and record the responses of patients to the following stimuli: normal verbal stimulus, loud auditory stimulus, mild physical stimulus (e.g., shaking), and noxious physical stimulus (e.g., pinching skin, pin prick, supraorbital notch or sternal pressure, or muscle or tendon pressure). Careful observation of the patient's responses will also provide information for sensory and motor examination and will be more informative than the use of such vague terms as lethargy or stupor.

c. **Respirations.** The depth and pattern of respirations may help in localizing and, occasionally, in determining the type of process. Respirations may be **depressed**, as commonly seen in drug overdose, or **stertorous**, as in postictal states. There are many irregular breathing patterns, the most common of which is the **Cheyne-Stokes** type of respiration. Cheyne-Stokes respiration occurs in many conditions (some without alteration in consciousness), and its presence implies bilateral deep hemisphere, diencephalon, or upper brainstem dysfunction. It is characterized by variable length periods of hyperventilation, which gradually taper off to apnea, also of variable duration; respirations resume slowly and gradually build up again to hyperventilation. Other respiratory patterns and their presumed locations of insult include **central neurogenic hyperventilation** (midbrain/upper pons), **apneustic** (lower pons), **irregular or ataxic** (medulla).

d. **Cranial nerves.** In a comatose patient, most cranial nerve functions cannot be evaluated fully and are generally limited to **observing motor responses:**

Nerve I: Olfaction cannot be tested.

Nerve II: Although the second cranial nerve is not usually helpful in evaluating a patient in coma, vision can be grossly tested when sudden movements are made toward the eyes with an object or with hands. If there is consistent blinking or closing of the eyes to visual threat, intact visual pathways can be assumed. A visual field defect, such as a homonymous hemianopsia, may also be found in this manner. **Too forceful a movement** toward the eyes may cause blinking by moving air into the eyes, testing the intactness of the fifth cranial nerve and not vision.

Funduscopy to look for **papilledema** and **hemorrhages** suggesting increased intracranial pressure should be performed in all comatose patients.

Nerves III, IV, and VI: Examining extraocular movements and pupils are perhaps the most important part of the cranial nerve examination in the patient in coma.

(1) Eye position. In a hemisphere lesion that destroys the **frontal eye fields**, eyes may be **conjugately deviated toward** the lesion (away from a hemiparesis). When a lesion affects the **pontine gaze center**, the eyes will be **conjugately deviated away** from the lesion (toward the hemiparesis). Dysconjugate gaze may suggest a specific cranial nerve palsy. Occasionally nystagmus may be seen at rest.

(2) Eye movements. If the patient is not responsive enough to follow commands and does not have spontaneous movements, eye movements can be evaluated by either **passive head turning** (doll's head maneuver or oculocephalic reflex) or **cold water calorics** (oculovestibular reflex). With passive and rapid head turning to one side, eye movements should **deviate to the opposite side in the normal state.** Absence or asymmetry of eye movements in response to head turning implies a destructive lesion at the pontine-midbrain level or deep metabolic/toxic coma of any cause.

Cold water calorics are also used to evaluate eye movements and are the response to irrigation of the intact tympanic membrane with cold water. After otoscopic examination reveals an intact tympanic membrane and a clear canal, the head is positioned at 30 degrees with respect to the horizontal, and between 20 and 30 ml of ice water is instilled into the canal and the eyes are observed. The normal response in a **conscious** patient consists of tonic deviation of the eyes toward the irrigated ear, followed by nystagmus. The **quick** component of the nystagmus is to the opposite side. The pneumonic **COWS** (cold-opposite, warm-same) can be used to remember this normal relationship. **In the comatose patient with an intact brainstem, only the deviation toward the irrigated ear is present and not full nystagmus.** Failure of conjugate deviation suggests a structural **ipsilateral** pontine-midbrain lesion. Dysconjugate gaze may indicate a third or sixth nerve lesion.

(3) Pupils. Size, shape, and reactivity (both direct and consensual responses) should be noted. **Bilateral midposition (3–5 mm) nonreactive pupils indicate midbrain lesion. Bilateral dilated and nonreactive pupils are seen in deep coma of any cause. Unilateral dilated and nonreactive pupil indicates third-nerve compression due to temporal lobe herniation.** Usually ptosis and abduction of the eye (due to unopposed lateral rectus muscle) are present in such cases. If not present, pharmacologic blockade (and psychogenic unresponsiveness) should be considered. **Small but reactive pupils are typically seen in metabolic causes of coma, pontine lesions, pilocarpine instillation, or narcotic overdose.** If pupils are pinpoint, making observation of reactivity difficult with the unaided eye, a magnifying glass can be useful.

Nerve V: An **open mouth** (decreased jaw tone) indicates severe unresponsiveness. Evaluation of corneal reflex bilaterally may indicate level of lesion. If the corneal reflex is absent unilaterally, an ipsilateral pontine lesion is present.

Nerve VII: Motor function can be evaluated by observation for increased width of palpebral fissure, drooping of angle of mouth, flattening of nasolabial fold, and drooling of saliva out of the angle of the mouth on the affected side. Response to noxious stimulus by facial grimacing may accentuate a facial paresis. **In facial weakness due to processes affecting the central nervous system above the seventh nerve nucleus, only the lower half of the face will be affected**, whereas involvement of the seventh cranial nerve nucleus or the nerve in its peripheral course causes paralysis of both upper and lower parts of the face.

Nerve VIII: Response to mild and loud auditory stimulus should be observed.

Nerves IX and X: Direct evaluation of palatal and pharyngeal function may not be possible, but presence or absence of the **gag** reflex should be tested bilaterally and any asymmetry noted.

Nerve XI: Head position at rest should be noted.

Nerve XII: Bulk and position of tongue and presence or absence of movements should be noted.

e. **Motor responses.** Much of this examination has already been performed when observing position, spontaneous movements, or postures and responses to noxious stimuli. Noxious stimuli may result in **decerebrate posturing** (extension, adduction, and internal rotation of arms and extension of legs), indicating a lesion of upper brainstem between red nucleus and vestibular nuclei or **decorticate posturing** (flexion and adduction of arms and extension of legs), indicating either a deep hemispheric lesion or a lesion just above the midbrain. Noxious stimulation may produce purposeful movement such as warding-off movements. Poorly organized or incomplete movements, especially when unilateral, suggest corticospinal tract dysfunction or damage.

C. **Etiologies** Etiologies of coma are many and beyond the discussion of this chapter. They can be categorized as traumatic, vascular, infectious, tumors, seizures, toxic/metabolic, or hypoxic etiologies.

D. **Laboratory Evaluation**

1. **Routine laboratory tests** should include a complete blood cell count (CBC) with differential leukocyte count, urinalysis, liver and renal function studies, electrolytes, blood glucose, calcium, EKG, chest X-ray, and toxic screen.

2. **Special studies**

   a. Computerized axial tomography (CAT) scan is the **best overall test** for evaluating a structural lesion and should be done in all patients in whom a **lumbar puncture** is contemplated for suspected meningitis or encephalitis.

   b. **Skull X-rays** have been replaced largely by the CAT scan and their routine use is controversial. However, they still are the best test to detect skull fractures when the CAT scan shows none.

c. Electroencephalograms (EEGs) are useful in cases where the CAT scan does not reveal the cause of coma. They may reveal evidence of seizure disorder or toxic/metabolic cause of coma.

d. Nuclear brain scan may be useful in selected cases where the CAT scan is normal (certain cases of cerebral infarction or cerebritis).

e. Angiography is used in selected cases where vascular etiology is suspected (e.g., vasculitis, basilar artery thrombosis).

f. Lumbar puncture.

E. Management and Treatment

1. Establish adequate **airway.** This may include intubation and mechanical ventilation.

2. Establish adequate circulation. Insert a large-bore intravenous (i.v.) catheter. Fluids may be necessary to maintain blood pressure and adequate perfusion of vital tissues.

3. Draw blood for studies mentioned above.

4. For possible **Wernicke's encephalopathy**, or if chronic alcohol abuse is known or suspected, give **thiamine** 100 mg i.v., then 100 mg intramuscularly (i.m.) daily for several days. Thiamine administration prophylactically **in all cases of coma** is a good practice, especially when no history is available, since Wernicke's encephalopathy may be precipitated in alcohol abusers by a large carbohydrate load.

5. Give **50 ml of 50% dextrose** solution i.v. to exclude hypoglycemia.

6. If there is some evidence that coma results from **narcotic overdose**, administer **naloxone**, 0.4 mg i.v. every 5 to 10 min as needed until consciousness returns. Response should occur within minutes in cases of narcotic overdose.

7. Manage cerebral edema and elevated intracranial pressure. The initial process in treating increased intracranial pressure (ICP) is to determine and treat the underlying cause if possible. Most **common causes** of increased ICP are trauma, large cerebral infarcts or hemorrhages, tumors, and subdural or epidural hematomas. The main **complications** of increased ICP are related to herniation of cerebral tissues through certain weak points and secondary brainstem hemorrhages. The **treatment** is as follows:

a. Monitor ICP with either surface or intraventricular monitors.

b. Fluid restriction.

c. Hyperventilation causes an immediate fall of ICP by reducing cerebral blood flow by causing hypocapnea. Pco_2 should be maintained between 20 and 30 mm Hg.

d. Administer **20% mannitol** solution at a dose of 1 gm/kg i.v. over 15 to 30 min. Maximum effects occur after 1 to 2 hr, and the original dose may be repeated every 4 to 12 hr. Since mannitol is an osmotic diuretic, **dehydration and acute renal failure** may occur unless fluid status and serum electrolytes, BUN, and osmolality are monitored closely. One problem with mannitol and glycerol (another osmotic diuretic) is that a **rebound increase**

in ICP can occur from retained mannitol in the brain, reversing the osmotic gradient with resultant increased brain water. When this happens, clinical deterioration of the patient's condition may occur.

e. **Steroids.** The glucocorticoid usually used to treat cerebral edema is **dexamethasone (Decadron®)**, although other similar parenteral glucocorticoid preparations can be used. Dexamethasone should be given initially at a loading dose of 10 mg i.v., followed by 4 to 6 mg i.v. or i.m. every 4 to 6 hr. The onset of the effect may take 6 to 12 hr and the effect peaks at 24 hr.

Note

8. **Manage specific processes.** See Section D.

9. **General care of the comatose patient** largely entails intensive nursing care which is crucial in overall management and prevention of complications.

   a. **Pressure sores** should be prevented by frequent turning, padding pressure points, and by using mattress pads (e.g., egg crate pads) or water mattress.

   b. **Joint contractures** should be prevented by early instituting passive range of motion exercises and foot boards. Contractures can occur in a few days if these measures are not used.

   c. **Corneal injuries** should be prevented by using methylcellulose eye drops and by taping eyelids closed.

   d. **Malnutrition** should be prevented by early institution of enteral or parenteral hyperalimentation. Nasogastric tube feedings in a patient with depressed level of consciousness may predispose to tracheal aspiration. If hyperalimentation is used, a small-diameter flexible tube should be used and the head elevated to help prevent tracheal aspiration.

   e. **Tracheal aspiration** should be prevented by frequent suctioning of mouth and nasopharynx and by placing the patient in the lateral decubitus position with neck extended and face turned toward mattress.

   f. Complications from poor **bladder** care should be avoided. Condom catheters should be used in male patients to prevent urinary tract infections from indwelling urinary catheters. Penile maceration, which may occur from condom catheters, can be avoided by frequent changes.

   g. Gastrointestinal bleeding may be prevented by use of antacids and/or cimetidine.

II. HEADACHE

A. **General Principles**   Headache is one of the most common complaints confronting both primary care physicians and neurologists. Although several hundred disorders can have headache as their chief complaint, most of these are related to acute infections or metabolic disorders and do not present a diagnostic problem. The most common headache problem facing the physician is that of the **chronic recurring headache.** Roughly 90% of chronic recurring headaches are caused by **benign** processes and are not related to an underlying structural, vascular or metabolic disorder. The majority of chronic recurring headaches are caused by vascular (migraine, cluster) or muscle contraction (tension) mechanisms, and although these are benign disorders, they are associated with substantial morbidity and missed work. The remaining 10% of chronic recurring headaches are related to underlying structural, vascular (subarachnoid hemorrhage, stroke), or other etiologies. One of the primary objectives, therefore, when first evaluating a patient with headache is to **screen for potentially life-threatening causes.** In addition to the chronic recurrent headache, one must decide when further evaluation and/or hospitalization is necessary when confronted with a patient with an **acute, severe headache** who has had no prior headache history. A simplified approach to evaluating the headache patient is shown in Fig. 1.

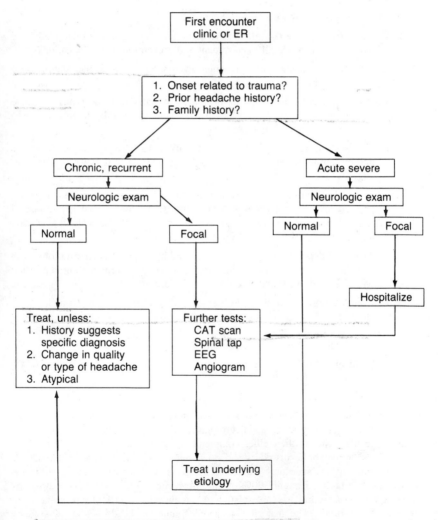

FIG. 1. Evaluation of the headache patient.

B. Etiologies of Chronic Recurrent Headaches

1. **Migraine** is a vascular headache characterized by recurrent, paroxysmal throbbing pain that is usually unilateral. In different attacks, opposite sides of the head may be affected or it may affect both sides simultaneously. Migraine may begin in childhood, but symptoms often include cyclical abdominal pain and vomiting, vertigo or motion sickness without accompanying headache. It is not until the teenage years when periodic headaches occur that the earlier symptoms are recognized as migraine equivalents. Age at onset of migraine headaches is usually between 20 and 35 years of age, but may occur at any age. Family history of migraine occurs in about 70% of patients.

   a. **Classic migraine** is preceded by a visual aura. This visual aura typically consists of scintillating scotomata that migrates in the visual field. This aura is believed to be due to ischemia of the occipital lobes and is followed in 5 to 15 min by a unilateral throbbing headache that gradually intensifies over several hours and may become bilateral. Other associated symptoms include visual blurriness, nausea, vomiting, photophobia, and irritability. Most headaches subside in 6 hr but may last up to 24 hr and occasionally longer.

   b. **Common migraine** is identical to the classic variety, except the visual prodromata do not occur. This variety is much more common than classic migraine, and the headaches last longer, often days at a time.

   c. **Complicated migraine** is the term used when the headache is accompanied by a persisting neurologic deficit. The neurologic deficit can precede, follow, or occur in the absence of headache. The persistent deficit implies that **cerebral infarction** has occurred.

      (1) **Hemiplegic migraine.** An attack of hemiparesis or hemiplegia, aphasia, confusion (depending on vascular territory affected) followed by contralateral throbbing headache is the typical course of this variety of migraine. The deficit may or may not resolve, and the diagnosis is made (after a negative workup) by a history of previous attacks and/or a family history of similar attacks.

      (2) **Ophthalmoplegic migraine.** This is a rare form of complicated migraine that usually starts in childhood. A headache history usually precedes development of ophthalmoplegia, which almost always affects the **oculomotor (third cranial) nerve.** After many years of this type of migraine, the ophthalmoplegia may become permanent.

   d. **Treatment**

      (1) **Preventive measures** include avoiding precipitating factors such as certain foods, especially chocolate, coffee, tyramine-containing cheeses, citrus fruits, alcohol, smoking, excessive fatigue, lack of sleep.

      (2) **Stress.** Though completely avoiding stress is not possible, counseling the patient in the recognition and management of stress is very important in the overall management of migraine headaches. Biofeedback may be of value in helping some patients with stress management.

(3) A patient's **anxiety** about the nature of headache needs to be addressed as many patients fear that their headaches are related to a brain tumor or stroke. **Depression** may also precipitate migraine headaches and needs to be treated appropriately.

(4) **Drug therapy.** Initiation of drug therapy involves the decision whether **abortive** or **prophylactic** therapy is indicated. In general, if a patient is having frequent (more than one per week) or severely disabling headaches, prophylactic treatment is indicated. Abortive therapy can be used simultaneously. Abortive and prophylactic drugs used in the therapy of migraine are listed in Tables 1A and 1B.

2. **Muscle contraction headache.** Also known as tension or psychogenic headaches, these headaches are very common in the general population. They usually come to the attention of a physician only when they become daily and refractory to the usual over-the-counter analgesics. Patients complain of an aching, pressure, or bandlike constriction that is typically bilateral and occipitonuchal in location. They tend to vary in intensity through the day and are present daily for weeks or years. They are associated with sustained contraction of the skeletal muscles of neck, head, and face in the absence of permanent structural change. They often occur or intensify in relation to emotional stress. In contrast to patients with migraine, patients with muscle contraction headaches tend to be in middle or older age groups at the time of the onset of their headaches. Treatment is difficult, especially when the headaches have been present for many years. To be successful, the treatment must be multifaceted.

a. **Physician attitude** is very important in influencing treatment outcome. Physicians who treat these patients as though they are "nervous," handle stress poorly, or are depressed will alienate the patient and fail in treating their condition. Simple reassurance that nothing is physically wrong inside their heads can help tremendously in the overall treatment program.

b. **Physical therapy.** Massage, particularly manual stretching of muscles of the neck, along with local heat to neck and shoulders, are important adjuncts in treating muscle contraction headaches.

c. **Relaxation techniques.** Relaxation may help lessen the severity of the headaches. Simple methods such as meditation, hypnosis, or yoga may help, but the most commonly used method is that of biofeedback. The value of these methods, though widely used, has not been established.

d. **Psychotherapy.** It is the rare patient who needs any more than a reassuring physician, who listens. Occasionally, however, **severe depression** with threats of suicide may require referral to a psychiatrist.

e. **Pharmacotherapy.** Drugs used in the treatment of muscle contraction headaches are listed in Table 2.

3. **Cluster headaches** are a variety of vasodilating headache and are of three major types. The typical variety is the **episodic** (periodic) variety where attacks occur daily for several weeks or months, stop abruptly, and are followed by a remission lasting months or even years. The other variants include **chronic** cluster, where no remissions occur, and the **atypical variants**, which include cluster-migraine and cluster-vertigo combinations. Cluster headaches are char-

acterized by excruciating, **always unilateral** (often orbital) pain that occurs in brief episodes lasting 20 min to 2 hr. The pain is maximal at its onset and has a sharp, boring quality. There is no associated prodrome as in migraine and nausea and vomiting are likewise absent. Headaches typically occur at the same time each night. Cluster is one of the few nonorganic headaches that will awaken a patient from sleep. Associated symptoms include tearing, nasal congestion and rhinorrhea, flushing of side of face and sweating. Signs present during an attack include ipsilateral bulging, pulsating temporal artery, conjunctival injection, and a Horner's syndrome. The typical cluster patient is an adult male (male:female ratio is 5–7:1) with facial features of ruddy complexion, "peau d'orange" skin, broad chin and skull, and telangiectasias. **Treatment** is pharmacologic and includes both abortive and prophylactic treatment. Drugs used in the treatment of cluster headache are listed in Table 3.

4. **Mixed muscle contraction–vascular headache.** With this headache, symptoms of both types, migraine and muscle contraction, exist during an attack. This type of headache typically occurs in a patient who has chronic muscle contraction headaches and who has unilateral or bilateral throbbing periodically when headache intensifies. **Treatment** usually consists of combination therapy or using medication that works in both types, such as amitriptyline.

5. **Trigeminal neuralgia** is the most common of the idiopathic cranial neuralgias and is characterized by severe paroxysmal pain in the distribution of one or more branches of the trigeminal nerve. The pain has a lightning-like quality and is brief in duration, usually lasting a fraction of a second to several minutes. Between attacks the patient is usually pain-free. The pain may be produced by stimulation of a trigger point on the face. These trigger points may be sensitive to cold or pressure or pain and may be triggered during swallowing, chewing, or toothbrushing. Trigeminal neuralgia usually occurs in adults over 40. Although most cases are idiopathic, further investigation is warranted if there are other associated neurologic signs or symptoms. Trigeminal neuralgia has been associated with dental or sinus disease, multiple sclerosis, and posterior fossa tumors.

Treatment is either medical or surgical. Medical treatment includes **phenytoin** (200–400 mg/day), **carbamazepine** [200–1,200 mg/day by mouth (p.o.)], **amitriptyline** (50 mg p.o. daily; increased by 25 mg/day every 2–3 weeks, up to 300 mg daily) and **baclofen** (10 mg p.o. t.i.d.). In patients who either relapse or fail to respond to medical therapy, neurosurgical referral should be sought. **Electrocoagulation of the gasserian ganglion** is the procedure of choice and affords relief to more than 90% of patients. The recurrence rate after surgery is very low.

C. **Other Disorders Commonly Associated with Headache**

1. **Temporal (giant cell) arteritis.** Temporal arteritis is an inflammatory arteritis of the elderly (usually over age 50) characterized by inflammatory infiltrates of lymphocytes and giant cells in the branches of the external carotid artery, most frequently the temporal arteries. The most dramatic complication is **visual loss** due to ischemic optic neuropathy, which can cause blindness in 12 to 24 hr. Most patients complain of headaches, but the location may be

TABLE 1A. *Abortive drugs used in the treatment of migraine*

Drug	Dosage	Side effects	Contraindications
Aspirin	600 mg p.o. q 4 hr as needed (prn)	GI bleeding, hypersensitivity	Hypersensitivity, active peptic ulcer disease
Acetaminophen	600 mg p.o. q 4 hr prn	Few short-term side effects	None
Ergotamine tartrate			
Oral	2 mg at onset and 1 mg every 30 min prn; maximum 6 mg/attack, 10 mg/wk	Nausea, vomiting, numbness, tingling, pain and cyanosis of limbs, chest pain, transient tachycardia, bradycardia, leg cramps	Occlusive vascular disease, sepsis, hepatitis, disease, renal disease, hypertension, pregnancy, hypersensitivity to ergot-containing medications, ergot-containing medications
Sublingual	2 mg at onset, and 1 mg every 30 min prn; maximum 6 mg/attack, 10 mg/wk		
Rectal	2 mg at onset; 2 mg after 1 hr if needed; maximum of 4 mg/attack, 10 mg/wk		
Intramuscular	0.5–1.5 mg; maximum 3 mg/wk		
Subcutaneous	0.5–1.5 mg; maximum 3 mg/wk		
Inhalation	1 inhalation at onset and 1 inhalation every 5 min prn; maximum 6 inhalations/day		
Isometheptene	130 mg p.o. at onset and 130 mg every hour prn; maximum 650 mg/day and 1,300 mg/wk	Drowsiness, nausea, and dizziness	Glaucoma, severe renal disease, hypertension, hepatic disease, organic heart, disease, concomitant use of monoamine oxidase inhibitors (MAOI)
Isometheptene (65 mg), acetaminophen (325 mg), dichloralphenazone (100 mg) (Midrin™) capsules	Same as isometheptene since that is limiting component	Same as isometheptene	Same as isometheptene
Steroids			
Dexamethasone	10–20 mg i.m. single dose	Fluid and electrolyte disturbance, hyperglycemia, increased susceptibility to infections, GI bleeding, osteoporosis, myopathy, cataracts, Cushingoid habitus	Systemic infections (especially fungal)
Prednisone	40 mg/day p.o. for 1 wk	Same as dexamethasone	Same as dexamethasone

TABLE 1B. *Prophylactic drugs used in the treatment of migraine*

Drug	Dosage	Side effects	Contraindications
Propranolol	10–140 mg b.i.d.–q.i.d.	Light-headedness, weakness, congestive heart failure, and bronchospasm in high-risk patients	Bronchial asthma, sinus bradycardia, greater than first degree AV block, congestive heart failure, cardiogenic shock, right ventricular failure secondary to pulmonary hypertension, allergic rhinitis during pollen season
Amitriptyline	50 mg p.o. at bedtime; increase by 25 mg every 3–4 wk until improvement or dose of 100–200 mg/day	Drowsiness, dry mouth, blurred vision, arrhythmias, urinary retention	Concomitant MAOI use; during acute recovery phase following myocardial infarction; hypersensitivity
Ergonovine maleate	0.2 mg p.o. t.i.d. for 3 months; stop for 1 month, then restart if needed	Same as ergotamine tartrate	Same as ergotamine tartrate
Methysergide	2 mg p.o. t.i.d. for as long as 3 months; stop for 1 month, then restart if needed	Fibrotic syndromes, nausea, vomiting, GI pain, diarrhea, drowsiness, dizziness, anxiety, hallucinations, psychotic reactions, muscle cramps, weight gain, hair loss	Existing fibrotic syndromes
Cyproheptadine	2–4 mg p.o. q.i.d.	Drowsiness, confusion, increased appetite, weight gain	Concomitant MAOI therapy; angle-closure glaucoma; prostatic hypertrophy; peptic ulcer disease; bladder neck obstruction; pyloroduodenal obstruction; elderly, debilitated patients
Phenytoin	200–400 mg p.o. daily	Dizziness, diplopia, ataxia	Hypersensitivity to phenytoin or other hydantoins
Clonidine	0.1 mg b.i.d.–t.i.d.	Orthostatic hypotension, impotence, depression, drowsiness, rebound hypertension (if withdrawn abruptly)	Hypersensitivity

MAOI, monoamine oxidase inhibitor.

TABLE 2. *Drugs used in the treatment of muscle contraction headaches*

Drug	Dose	Side effects	Contraindications
Analgesics			
Aspirin	Same as migraine	Same as migraine	Same as migraine
Acetaminophen	Same as migraine	Same as migraine	Same as migraine
Benzodiazepines			
Diazepam	5–30 mg/day	Sedation, dizziness, blurred vision, hypotension, depressed respiration	Hypersensitivity, acute narrow-angle glaucoma
Chlordiazepoxide	10–75 mg/day	Same as diazepam	Same as diazepam
Oxazepam	30–90 mg/day	Same as diazepam	Same as diazepam
Antidepressants			
Amitriptyline	Same as migraine	Same as migraine	Same as migraine
Imipramine	50 mg/day, adjusted upward to 300 mg/day	Same as amitriptyline	Same as amitriptyline

anywhere and not just in a temporal location. The erythrocyte sedimentation rate **(ESR) is elevated** in virtually all patients, usually to more than 50 mm/hr. Rigid, tender, nonpulsatile temporal arteries may be seen or felt. Diagnosis is confirmed by **temporal artery biopsy.** Even with serial sections through a large specimen, occasionally the biopsy will be normal. Under these circumstances, either biopsy of the opposite temporal artery should be undertaken or treatment initiated.

Treatment is with high-dose **corticosteroids** (prednisone 40–60 mg daily) and should be maintained for at least 6 months before tapering. Since temporal arteritis is a self-limited disorder, treatment can usually be discontinued after 6 to 18 months. Because of this high dose of daily corticosteroids, primarily to **prevent visual loss, complications** are common and include psychosis, myopathy, osteoporosis and vertebral body collapse, and gastrointestinal hemorrhage.

2. **Intracranial tumor.** Headache associated with intracranial tumor results either from traction on pain-sensitive intracranial structures or increased intracranial pressure. Although headache is a common symptom in patients with intracranial tumors, it is uncommon without other associated signs and symptoms. The "classic" tumor headache characterized by dull, nonthrobbing pain, which is worse upon arising in the morning, is uncommon. Headaches associated with intracranial tumors may be in any location, throbbing or nonthrobbing, mild or severe. It is the other associated localizing signs and symptoms, not the type or severity of headache, that should make one suspicious of an intracranial tumor.

3. **Subarachnoid hemorrhage** (see III. C.). An **acute, severe** headache (often described as explosive), with or without **alteration in consciousness,** low-grade **fever,** and with signs of **meningeal irritation** (nuchal rigidity, Kernig's or Brudzinski's signs) suggests subarachnoid hemorrhage. **Subhyaloid hemorrhages** are often seen on funduscopic examination. **Subarachnoid hemorrhage** is usually due to rupture of a saccular aneurysm, but can also be idiopathic, or secondary to arteriovenous malformations, trauma, or blood dyscrasias.

TABLE 3. *Drugs used in the treatment of cluster headaches*

Drug	Dosage	Side effects	Contraindications
Abortive			
Oxygen by mask	7–10 liters/min for 10 min	None	None
Ergotamine tartrate	Same as migraine	Same as migraine	Same as migraine
Prophylactic			
Methysergide	Same as migraine	Same as migraine	Same as migraine
Ergonovine maleate	Same as migraine	Same as migraine	Same as migraine
Prednisone	50 mg/day for 3 wk, then gradual taper	Same as migraine	Same as migraine
Indomethacin	25–50 mg p.o. t.i.d.	Gastric upset, GI bleeding	Allergy to indomethacin or have had bronchospastic reactions to other nonsteroidal antiinflammatory drugs
Lithium carbonate	300 mg p.o. b.i.d.– q.i.d. with blood level maintained between 0.5–1.5 mEq/liter	Tremor, other movement disorders, nausea, vomiting, diarrhea, weakness, ataxia, dizziness, seizures, arrhythmia, polyuria, goiter, hypothyroidism	Significant renal or cardiovascular disease, severe dehydration or sodium depletion, patients receiving diuretics

4. **Pseudotumor cerebri** (benign intracranial hypertension). Pseudotumor cerebri is a syndrome of diffuse increased intracranial pressure with headache as the most frequent presenting symptom. The headache is usually bilateral frontal and pressure-like in quality. **Papilledema** is always present. Transient (several seconds) obscurations of vision is another common complaint. Although sixth nerve palsies can occur as a nonlocalizing sign to increased intracranial pressure, other focal signs (hemiparesis, aphasia) do not occur. About **one-half of the cases** are idiopathic and occur in obese women with menstrual abnormalities. The **remaining cases** are due to one of several etiologies: hypervitaminosis A, tetracycline therapy, corticosteroids, chronic meningitis (infectious or neoplastic) and dural sinus thrombosis. It not uncommonly occurs during pregnancy. Workup includes a **CAT scan** to exclude a mass lesion and often suggests the diagnosis by the appearance of "slit-like" ventricles (small size). If the CAT scan is normal, lumbar puncture should be performed with careful attention to **opening pressure**. Pressure is usually increased to over 250 mm H₂O. Cerebral spinal fluid (CSF) is otherwise normal, except occasionally for decreased protein concentration. Since this condition is usually benign and many patients remit spontaneously after their diagnostic lumbar puncture, therapy is conservative. The one complication that arises from prolonged increased intracranial pressure is **visual loss**, therefore visual acuity and perimetry should be measured frequently until the intracranial pressure is lowered. Therapy consists of:

    a. Repeat lumbar punctures. Most patients can be successfully managed in this manner.

    b. Corticosteroids (prednisone 40–80 mg/day).

    c. Acetazolamide (250 mg p.o. t.i.d.).

    d. Surgery if visual loss is occurring; involves subtemporal decompression.

5. **Headache of nasal origin.** Some forms of vascular headache, especially cluster headaches, are frequently misdiagnosed as acute nasal sinusitis. The symptoms of acute nasal sinusitis, due to acute infection of the mucous membranes of the sinus, are referrable to the particular sinus involved (Table 4).

6. **Posttraumatic headache.** Along with a variety of other symptoms constituting the postconcussion syndrome, headache is a common complaint after head trauma. In most instances the pain disappears after several days to 3 months, but occasionally runs a protracted course over many years. In cases of prolonged headaches, they are often described as **vascular** in nature and may respond to migraine therapy. Less often they resemble muscle contraction or mixed muscle contraction-vascular headaches and should be treated as such.

7. **Postlumbar puncture headache.** The headache that occurs after a lumbar puncture is typically bilateral and throbbing, exacerbated by upright posture, and relieved by lying down. It is probably caused by a persistent leak of spinal fluid and may be prevented by use of a small (22 gauge) spinal needle. Conservative treatment with bedrest, hydration, and analgesics usually suffice, and the headache rarely lasts beyond one week. When these measures fail, an epidural blood patch over the puncture site using autologous blood usually gives immediate relief.

8. **Nonmigrainous vascular headaches.** A wide variety of disorders and headache syndromes have a vascular component. These include systemic infections, usually with fever (toxic headache), drugs causing vasodilatation (e.g., nitrates), postconvulsive states, "hangover" reactions, acute elevation of blood pressure (as in pheochromocytomas or in autonomic dysreflexia in paraplegics), hypoglycemia, hypercapnea, caffeine-withdrawal, and others. Treatment should be directed at the underlying etiology.

III. STROKE Stroke is the most common neurologic disease of adults and the third leading cause of death in the United States. Although several relatively rare diseases

TABLE 4. *Headache associated with acute nasal sinusitis*

Sinus	Location	Other signs/symptoms
Frontal	Frontal over sinus; may radiate to vertex or behind eyes	Tenderness in frontal area, fever
Maxillary	Over cheek; may radiate to upper teeth or forehead	Tenderness over cheek, postnasal drip, fever
Ethmoid	Between/behind eyes; may radiate to temporal region	Eyes tender, nasal obstruction, postnasal drip, fever
Sphenoid	Occipital, vertex, or frontal and eye regions	Postnasal drip, vertigo, forgetfulness, inability to concentrate, proptosis, diplopia, scotoma

are associated with cerebrovascular disease, many of which primarily cause strokes in young adults and children, strokes can generally be categorized as **ischemic** or **hemorrhagic**. Table 5 lists the major causes of stroke. Since there is no effective treatment yet to reverse the effects of stroke on the brain (pharmacologic protection), current efforts in stroke therapy are aimed at **preventing** worsening of an existing deficit or preventing additional deficits from occurring. Also identifying **risk factors** for stroke such as hypertension, cardiac arrhythmias, cardiac valvular disease, diabetes mellitus, polycythemia, oral contraceptives, and hyperlipidemia directs intervention to prevent stroke from occurring in these patients at risk.

A general outline for the approach to evaluation of the **acute stroke syndrome** is seen in Fig. 2. Guidelines for treatment of the acute stroke syndrome are presented in this section, but management will vary greatly from one center to another. A detailed description of these differences are controversial and beyond the scope of this text.

A. Ischemic Stroke   Although the treatment of ischemic cerebral infarction is controversial, there are several accepted treatment modalities depending on whether the infarction is caused by **extracranial occlusive vascular disease** due to atherosclerosis or primarily to **cardiac embolic** source.

    1. Transient ischemic attacks (TIA). TIAs are defined as episodes of transient and focal neurologic dysfunction of vascular origin which are rapid in onset

TABLE 5. *Major causes of stroke*

Ischemic
  Thrombotic occlusion of cerebral vessel or extracranial carotid
    artery
  Embolic
    Atheromatous plaque in vessel
    Cardiac source:
      Valvular (infectious or noninfectious endocarditis;
        rheumatic valvular disease)
      Mural thrombus (cardiomyopathy; hypokinetic segments
        secondary to myocardial infarction)
      Tumor (atrial myxoma)
  Vasculitis
    Primary CNS vasculitis (granulomatous angiitis of CNS)
    Systemic vasculitis (polyarteritis nodosa)
    Temporal arteritis
    Secondary to meningitis (tuberculous, cryptococcus,
      coccidioidomycosis)
    Meningovascular syphilis
    Drugs (amphetamines)
Hemorrhagic
  Intracerebral hemorrhage
    Hypertensive
    Cerebral amyloid angiopathy
    Anticoagulants
    Bleeding diatheses
    Hemorrhage into tumor
    Drugs (amphetamines)
  Subarachnoid hemorrhage
    Aneurysm
    Arteriovenous malformation
    Idiopathic

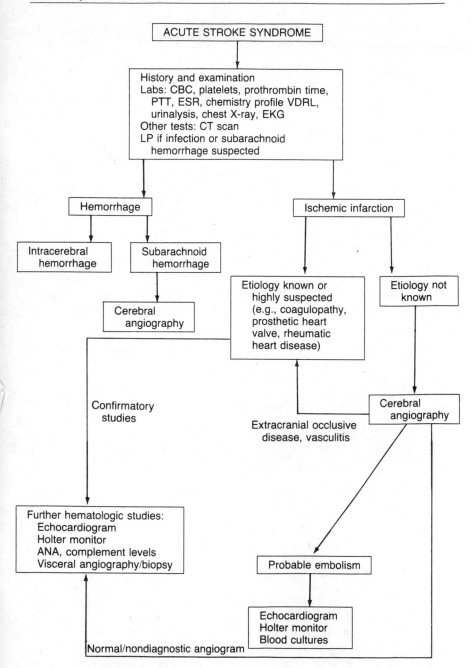

FIG. 2. Evaluation of the acute stroke syndrome.

and resolve within 24 hr. The 24-hr limit is artificial, and the majority of TIAs resolve within 60 min. TIAs are the most important warning of impending stroke and are seen in one-third to one-half of patients who develop completed strokes. They reflect dysfunction either in the carotid (anterior) circulation or in the vertebrobasilar (posterior) system. The pathologic processes that usually result in TIAs are **atherosclerotic stenosis, thrombosis, or embolism**, but other causes must be excluded. **Other causes** of transient neurologic deficits that resemble TIAs include subdural hematomas, tumors (especially meningiomas), hypoglycemia, hyperviscosity syndromes (polycythemia vera), complications of cardiac disease (arrhythmias, mitral valve prolapse), orthostatic hypotension, migraine, aneurysms, and arteriovenous malformations.

2. **Reversible ischemic neurologic deficit (RIND).** RINDs are prolonged reversible neurologic deficits that can last for days or even weeks. RINDs and TIAs are both caused by the same underlying pathologic processes.

3. **Stroke-in-evolution.** Stroke-in-evolution refers to the situation in which a neurologic deficit increases over a 24- to 48-hr period in the carotid artery distribution, or over a 72-hr period in the vertebrobasilar artery distribution. The increasing deficit may be due either to enlarging area of infarction or to cerebral edema. **Atherosclerosis** is the underlying pathologic process, but emboli can occasionally have a stuttering course.

4. **Completed stroke.** Completed stroke refers to the situation in which neurologic deficits of varying degrees of severity, as a result of cerebral infarction, remain stable for more than 24 hr in the carotid artery distribution and for more than 72 hr in the vertebrobasilar distribution. Completed stroke may be caused by **atherosclerotic extracranial vessel disease** or **cardiac embolic disease**. Therapy will vary, depending on the underlying cause.

5. **Lacunar infarction.** Lacunar infarctions, or lacunes, are small (0.2–1.5 mm), deep cerebral infarctions most commonly associated with a history of **hypertension**. They most commonly occur in the basal ganglia, internal capsule, thalamus, and pons. Because of their small size and typical locations they often produce **specific syndromes** that are not easily confused with syndromes of large-vessel occlusion. **Specific syndromes** include pure motor stroke, pure sensory stroke, sensorimotor stroke, hemiballismus, clumsy hand dysarthria syndrome, and homolateral ataxia and crural paresis.

B. **Treatment of Ischemic Stroke** Treatment modalities vary, depending on the type of ischemic stroke that has occurred and on whether one is addressing **acute** or **chronic** therapy. In Table 6 therapy for the different varieties of ischemic stroke, both medical and surgical is summarized. Drug dosages are summarized in Table 7.

C. **Hemorrhagic Stroke**

1. **Intracerebral (parenchymal) hemorrhage.** Intracerebral hemorrhage usually presents with the sudden onset of neurologic deficit often associated with headache and depressed level of consciousness or even coma. Small hemorrhages, however, are often impossible to distinguish clinically from ischemic strokes. The hemorrhage may stay confined to the parenchyma or may rupture into the ventricular system, subarachnoid space, or both. If such a rupture

TABLE 6. *Treatment of ischemic strokes*

Stroke type	Acute therapy		Chronic therapy	
	Medical	Surgical	Medical	Surgical
TIA	Antiplatelet aggregation drugs: Aspirin Dipyridamole (not proven) Anticoagulation—Heparin (controversial)	Carotid endarterectomy	Antiplatelet aggregation drugs (shown useful in males only) Anticoagulation—Coumadin® (controversial) Treat risk factors	Carotid endarterectomy
RIND Stroke-in-evolution	Same as TIA Anticoagulation—Heparin	Same as TIA Carotid endarterectomy (controversial)	Same as TIA Anticoagulation—Coumadin®	Same as TIA Carotid endarterectomy (if patient makes significant recovery)
Completed stroke Embolic (cardiac)	Anticoagulation—Heparin (to prevent reembolization, unless infarct hemorrhagic or severe)	None	Anticoagulation—Coumadin®	None
Thrombotic	None of proven value	None	No drugs of proven value; treat risk factors	Carotid endarterectomy (if patient makes significant recovery)
Lacunar stroke	None	None	Control hypertension	None

TABLE 7. *Drugs used in treatment of ischemic stroke*

Drug	Dosage	Side effects	Contraindications	Mechanism of action
Aspirin	325 mg p.o. b.i.d. or 650 mg p.o. b.i.d.	GI bleeding, hypersensitivity	Active peptic ulcer disease, hypersensitivity	Prevents platelet aggregation
Dipyridamole[a]	100 mg p.o. t.i.d.–q.i.d.	Nausea, vomiting, hypersensitivity, headache, dizziness, weakness	Hypersensitivity	Prevents platelet aggregation
Sulfinpyrazone[a]	200 mg p.o. t.i.d.	GI bleeding, urolithiasis, anemia, leukopenia, thrombocytopenia	Active peptic ulcer disease	Prevents platelet aggregation
Heparin	Initial i.v. bolus of 5,000–10,000 units followed either by continuous infusion of 1,000 units/hr or repeated boluses of 5,000 units every 4 hr (maintain PTT 2–3 times normal)	Bleeding problems	Active peptic ulcer disease, severe hypertension, patients at risk of falling, bleeding diatheses	Antiplatelet aggregation and reduced coagulation
Sodium warfarin (Coumadin®)	2–15 mg p.o. daily (maintain PT 1.5–2.5 times normal)	Bleeding problems	Same as Heparin	Reduces thrombus formation

[a]May be used alone or in combination with aspirin (not proven, under investigation).
PT, prothrombin time; PTT, partial thromboplastin time.

occurs, the prognosis is less favorable. The most frequent cause of intracerebral hemorrhage occurs from rupture of the small penetrating arterioles of the brain secondary to **hypertension**. The usual locations of hypertensive hemorrhages are putamen (60%), thalamus (15%), pons (5%), cerebellum (10%), and lobar (10%). When a hemorrhage occurs in a superficial lobar location, or the patient is not hypertensive, other etiologies of cerebral hemorrhage need to be considered. These include anticoagulants, bleeding diatheses, aneurysmal cerebral hemorrhage (often mycotic), cerebral amyloid angiopathy, tumor, and trauma.

a. Diagnosis. The diagnosis and location of a hypertensive hemorrhage can often be made on history and certain neurologic signs (Table 8). **The one instance where it is critically important for an early diagnosis to be made is that of a cerebellar hemorrhage, because surgical evacuation of the hematoma may result in complete recovery.**

A **CAT scan** is the next step and the most valuable test in the diagnosis of intracerebral hematoma. Virtually 100% of intracerebral hematomas will be seen on a CAT scan; however, small posterior fossa hemorrhages may be overlooked unless carefully sought on the CAT scan. Although almost all intracerebral hemorrhages will produce bloody spinal fluid, the advent of CAT scanning has obviated the need to perform lumbar punctures.

b. Treatment

(1) Lower blood pressure to near normal range.

(2) Treat cerebral edema or increased ICP (refer to I. E. 7.).

(3) Ventricular shunting for obstructive hydrocephalus may improve outcome, particularly in association with cerebellar hemorrhage. This procedure, however, by reducing pressure above, may cause upward herniation of the cerebellum and death.

(4) Surgical evacuation of a cerebellar hematoma as noted earlier can be lifesaving. A putaminal or thalamic hemorrhage in the nondominant hemisphere or a large lobar hematoma may be evacuated if indicated. Evacuation of a pontine hematoma has only rarely been attempted.

TABLE 8.   *Clinical features of hypertensive hemorrhages*

Location	Clinical signs
Putamen	Contralateral hemiparesis, hemisensory loss, homonymous hemianopsia, decreased level of consciousness. Other signs (aphasia, neglect), depending on whether dominant or nondominant hemisphere is affected
Thalamus	Contralateral hemiplegia, hemisensory loss, **downward deviation of eyes**, restricted upgaze, skew deviation, decreased level of consciousness
Pons	**Early coma, reactive pinpoint pupils**
Cerebellum	Occipital headache, dizziness or true vertigo, ipsilateral appendicular ataxia, truncal ataxia, signs of ipsilateral brainstem compression. Alert initially, can progress rapidly to coma and death

2. Subarachnoid hemorrhage. Spontaneous subarachnoid hemorrhage, a sudden bleeding into the subarachnoid space without associated head trauma (the most common cause of secondary subarachnoid hemorrhage), is usually the result of rupture of a **saccular aneurysm.** Saccular aneurysms are caused by congenital defects in the arterial wall and occur most commonly at sites of arterial branching of the middle cerebral artery. **Less frequent causes** of subarachnoid hemorrhages include other types of aneurysms, arteriovenous malformations, blood dyscrasias, and intracerebral hemorrhages that dissect into the subarachnoid space. In many instances, an etiology is not found, and cryptic arteriovenous malformations, which are too small to be seen with angiography, are presumed to be the cause. Clinical features of subarachnoid hemorrhage are discussed in section I. *page 510*

a. Diagnosis

(1) Lumbar puncture. Bloody cerebrospinal fluid is diagnostic of subarachnoid hemorrhage. Differentiation of "true" subarachnoid hemorrhage from a "traumatic" lumbar puncture can be accomplished by either the presence of **xanthochromia** after centrifuging the CSF sample (if xanthochromia is present, blood has been in the CSF for several hours, implying subarachnoid hemorrhage) or by checking the red blood cell count in first specimen tube and last specimen tube (if cell counts are the same, it implies that subarachnoid hemorrhage has occurred).

(2) A **CAT scan** will reveal evidence of subarachnoid blood in between 90% and 95% of cases. Therefore, all patients suspected of having subarachnoid hemorrhage should undergo spinal fluid examination even with a normal CAT scan. A CAT scan with contrast enhancement may reveal the etiology of subarachnoid hemorrhage (aneurysm, arteriovenous malformation) and should be performed in all cases of subarachnoid hemorrhage.

(3) Cerebral angiography should be performed on all four major vessels, since localization of an aneurysm is rarely possible on clinical grounds. Saccular aneurysms are also frequently multiple. In patients with normal angiograms, especially children, spinal angiography to look for spinal vascular malformations should be considered.

b. Treatment. Surgical repair of aneurysms is the treatment of choice but is dependent on many variables. First, and perhaps most important, is that a large percentage (some estimate up to 50%) of patients who have subarachnoid hemorrhage from a ruptured aneurysm will die before reaching a hospital. These patients are of course not available for surgical treatment. Of the patients who reach the hospital, surgical treatment is generally reserved for those without depressed level of consciousness, with mild neurologic deficit, and with aneurysms in a location that is surgically accessible. **Recurrent hemorrhage** and **vasospasm**, the two major causes of morbidity and mortality in the immediate posthemorrhage period, also need to be prevented or effectively managed if the patient is to be considered for surgery.

(1) Prevention of recurrent hemorrhage

    (a) Treat hypertension if present.

    (b) Avoid fluctuations in blood pressure by keeping the patient in a dark, quiet room and by using sedation with a benzodiazepine or barbiturate.

    (c) Administer prophylactic anticonvulsants to prevent seizures.

    (d) Prevent straining with bowel movements by using stool softeners such as dioctyl sodium sulfosuccinate (100 mg p.o. t.i.d.).

    (e) Epsilon-aminocaproic acid (Amicar®) is an antifibrinolytic agent that works by preventing lysis of the clot formed at the point of bleeding from an aneurysm, thus preventing rebleeding. Although most reports suggest that antifibrinolytic agents are beneficial in preventing rebleeding, the effectiveness of these drugs has not been definitively proven. If used, aminocaproic acid is generally given i.v. at the dose of 30 to 36 g/day via continuous infusion. **Side effects** include nausea, cramps, diarrhea, tinnitus, headache, skin rash, thrombophlebitis, and pulmonary embolism.

(2) Treatment of vasospasm. Vasospasm usually first occurs 2 to 3 days after subarachnoid hemorrhage, peaks in about 1 week, and resolves over the next 2 to 3 weeks. Vasospasm can cause focal neurologic signs or depressed level of consciousness. The cause of vasospasm is not known but is presumed to be due to the release of vasospastic substances from the subarachnoid blood. The degree of vasospasm is proportional to the amount of blood in the subarachnoid space, and a CAT scan may be useful in predicting which patients may develop problems from vasospasm and its severity.

Many approaches to preventing or treating vasospasm have been tried, including **vasodilating agents** (carbon dioxide, nitroprusside, nitroglycerine) and **pressors** (dopamine, isoproterenol). All have proved unrewarding. Initial clinical studies using one of the **calcium channel blockers, nifedipine**, has shown some promise in preventing and reversing vasospasm.

(3) Surgery. There are several procedures for surgical management of aneurysms (clipping neck of aneurysm, wrapping it with muscle, tying off internal carotid artery in neck). However, the major controversy in surgical treatment of aneurysms is deciding the **optimum time** for surgery. Generally, surgery has been performed 1 to 2 weeks following subarachnoid hemorrhage, when the patient's neurologic condition has stabilized. The recent trend has been to operate within the first several days of hemorrhage in an attempt to reduce complications of rebleeding and vasospasm.

IV. **SEIZURES**   Seizures are the clinical manifestations of a paroxysmal disorder of cerebral function occurring as the result of discharge of a group of neurons. The results of this paroxysmal discharge is transient impairment of consciousness, motor activity, sensation, or behavior. Epilepsy (seizure disorder) is a disorder characterized by **recurrent** seizures that are not due to a known process or to cerebral lesion. Although most commonly witnessed seizures are grand mal (generalized tonic-clonic), a seizure can present in many different ways. It is often difficult on first encounter with a patient who has had some type of "spell" (often not witnessed) to be able to differentiate seizure from other paroxysmal disorders such as syncope, narcolepsy, transient ischemic attacks, migraine, paroxysmal vertigo, and trigeminal neuralgia. Patients may also have an episodic disorder resembling seizures that are related to hysteria or malingering (pseudoseizures). A simplified classification of seizure types with clinical descriptions appear in Table 9.

TABLE 9. *Adult seizure classification based on clinical characteristics of seizure*

Major category	Clinical features	Drug of choice	Other drugs[a]
Partial			
Simple (elemental)	Generally no impairment of consciousness. Focal motor (Jackson's seizure) or sensory symptoms (or mixed), autonomic symptoms	Phenytoin	Carbamazepine Valproic acid Primidone Phenobarbital
Complex	Consciousness impaired, automatisms, cognitive or affective symptoms, aura	Phenytoin or carbamazepine	Primidone Phenobarbital Valproic acid
Secondarily generalized	Either simple partial or complex partial, which evolve into generalized tonic-clonic seizures (grand mal)	Phenytoin	Phenobarbital Carbamazepine Primidone Valproic acid
Generalized			
Absence (petit mal)	Staring, blinking, brief lapses of awareness, occasionally facial twitching, automatisms (rare), quickly returns to normal activity	Ethosuximide or valproic acid	Clonazepam Methsuximide
Tonic-clonic (grand mal)	Sudden loss of consciousness, major motor activity, postictal state (confusion, drowsiness, headache). May have purely tonic or purely clonic convulsions; no true aura	Phenytoin	Phenobarbital Carbamazepine Valproic acid Primidone
Myoclonic	Single or repetitive jerks of body part	Clonazepam	Valproic acid Phenobarbital Phenytoin
Atonic	Brief loss of postural tone and resulting fall (risk of serious head trauma). Brief loss of consciousness	Phenytoin	Clonazepam Phenobarbital Valproic acid Carbamazepine

[a]Drugs are listed in order of preference.

A. Evaluation

1. **History.** Diagnosis of a seizure disorder is primarily dependent on a careful **history-taking**. Although the patient may be unable to describe the event himself because of impairment of consciousness, the presence or absence of preictal phenomena (aura) is important in proper classification of the seizure type. A reliable witness can often clearly describe the event if closely questioned. A carefully obtained history will often reveal that a patient is having **recurrent attacks that are relatively stereotyped**, suggesting a seizure disorder. Further details of family history, past medical history, and birth history are also obtained. Birth history may reveal evidence of prenatal (intrauterine infections), natal (birth injuries), or postnatal (respiratory distress, metabolic insults, infections) complications that are associated with the appearance of epilepsy in later life. History of alcohol use or of other drugs or toxic exposures is important.

2. **General physical examination** may reveal evidence of a medical disorder associated with seizures. Particular attention should be made examining the **skin** and looking for facial or other skeletal **asymmetries**. Asymmetries of face and body may result from early injury to the contralateral hemisphere, and skin abnormalities may suggest one of the phakomatoses, which often have an accompanying seizure disorder.

3. **Neurologic examination** may reveal localizing signs suggesting an underlying cerebral lesion as possible etiology of seizures.

4. **CAT scan** is routinely done in patients with a new onset seizure disorder. A CAT scan may demonstrate a structural lesion (neoplasm, abscess, infarction, hemorrhage), evidence of old birth injury (porencephaly), congenital malformation, or familial disorder (tuberous sclerosis) associated with seizures.

5. **EEGs** are normal in up to 40% of patients with a known seizure disorder. When the EEGs show epileptiform activity, they can aid in the classification by **appearance** (generalized or focal), **rate of discharge** (e.g., 3 cps as seen in classic petit mal seizures), and whether the **background** (i.e., the average frequency and organization of activity of the EEG) is normal or abnormal (e.g., background activity is markedly disrupted in the Lennox-Gastaut syndrome but normal in idiopathic generalized tonic-clonic epilepsy). The EEG may need to be repeated several times and with sleep deprivation (which lowers seizure threshold) if it is initially normal before seizure activity is seen. Treatment should not be delayed, however, even with a normal EEG if a seizure disorder is strongly suspected. Patients who are in poor control and/ or the diagnosis of seizure disorder is in doubt may be candidates for EEG with sphenoidal or nasopharyngeal electrodes (for suspected complex partial seizures of temporal lobe origin) or intensive inpatient video monitoring with continuous EEG recording.

6. **Routine laboratory tests** should include CBC with differential leukocyte count, chemistry profile, ESR, and urinalysis. If infection is suspected, **lumbar puncture** for CSF evaluation is indicated.

B. Treatment   After the evaluation of the patient with a seizure disorder, either an etiology will be found (symptomatic seizure) or one is probably dealing with an idiopathic seizure disorder (epilepsy). In symptomatic seizures one treats the specific disease causing the seizures with or without antiepileptic drugs. Idiopathic seizures are treated by choosing the appropriate drug for the particular seizure type (Table 9). Common antiepileptic drugs (anticonvulsants) and their characteristics are listed in Table 10.

General guidelines for the use of anticonvulsants in the treatment of seizure disorders are outlined in Fig. 3.

C. **Status Epilepticus** In generalized tonic-clonic (grand mal) status epilepticus, seizures either follow one another so frequently that there are no intervening periods of consciousness (i.e., each additional seizure begins before the preceding postictal period ends) or there are continuous seizures. The most **common causes of status epilepticus** are noncompliance with anticonvulsant drug regimen in patients with known seizure disorder, alcohol withdrawal, strokes, idiopathic, head trauma, cerebral tumors, metabolic disorders, drug overdose, intracranial infections, or cardiac arrest (hypoxia). Prognosis for status epilepticus depends on the **underlying cause** and the **duration** of status. Patients who develop status secondary to head trauma, brain tumors, or encephalitis have a worse prognosis than patients who were noncompliant in taking anticonvulsants. The longer a patient remains in status the worse the prognosis primarily because of **hypoxia**. The emergency management of patients in generalized tonic-clonic status epilepticus is outlined in Table 11.

V. **DIZZINESS AND VERTIGO** "Dizziness" is a term often used by patients to describe symptoms including light-headedness, true vertigo, or unsteadiness of gait. Since the causes of dizziness are numerous (Table 12), a systematic approach to evaluating the dizzy patient is necessary. Because even the most intelligent, verbal patient may have difficulty defining whether he is experiencing dysequilibrium, vertigo, or even syncope, all must be thought of as synonymous and evaluated in the same systematic way.

A. **Evaluation**

1. **The history** should concentrate on the **characteristics of the symptom** (persistent or episodic, frequency, duration, severity), presence of any **associated symptoms** (difficulty hearing, tinnitus, ear discomfort, diplopia, blurred vision, loss of consciousness, paresthesias, weakness), and **exacerbating or remitting factors** (change in head or body position, fatigue, medications, sleep, eyes open or closed).

2. **Physical examination.** A complete general and neurologic examination should be performed in all patients but should concentrate on several specific aspects (Table 13). Some important differences between central and peripheral "dizziness" and nystagmus are listed in Table 14.

3. **Laboratory tests** should include CBC, ESR, 5-hr glucose tolerance test, thyroid function tests [including thyroid-stimulating hormone (TSH)], Venereal Disease Research Laboratory (VDRL) test for syphilis and fluorescent treponemal antibody absorption test (FTA-ABS) chemistry screen, urinalysis.

4. **Formal audiometric testing** should be performed if abnormalities are found on physical examination or if there is a history of hearing loss.

5. **Electronystagmography** (ENG) is indicated for quantitative recording of nystagmus. Direction, velocity, and duration can be quantitated for sponta-

TABLE 10. Characteristics of common anticonvulsant drugs

Drug	Dosage and administration (mg/kg/day)	Therapeutic plasma level (μg/ml)	Side effects	Laboratory parameters to follow	Plasma half-life (hr)
Carbamazepine	10–20 (p.o.) 2–3 divided doses	4–12	Skin rash, hypersensitivity, drowsiness, GI upset, cholestatic jaundice; aplastic anemia, pancytopenia; inappropriate antidiuretic hormone secretion	CBC, platelets, liver function tests (every 3 months)	8–30
Clonazepam	0.01–0.3 (p.o.) 3 divided doses	0.015–0.075	Sedation, ataxia	None	30
Ethosuximide	10–20 (p.o.) 2–3 divided doses	40–100	GI upset, sedation, ataxia, increased (or onset of) generalized tonic-clonic seizures, rare hematologic suppression, and abnormal liver function tests	CBC, liver function tests (every 3–6 months)	48–72
Methsuximide	5–20 (p.o.) 3 divided doses	40–100	GI upset, sedation, ataxia, hematologic suppression, abnormal liver function tests	Same as ethosuximide	
Phenobarbital	1–5 (p.o., i.m., i.v.), 1–3 divided doses	15–30	Sedation, ataxia, hyperactivity (children), osteomalacia	CBC and serum calcium (every 6 months)	48–96
Phenytoin	5–7 maintenance (p.o.), 1–3 divided doses, 18 loading dose (p.o., i.v.)	10–20	Ataxia, GI upset, gingival hyperplasia, hirsutism, osteomalacia, lupus-like syndrome, hematologic suppression, abnormal liver function tests, hypersensitivity, megaloblastic anemia	CBC, liver function tests, serum calcium (every 6 months)	18–24
Primidone	10–25 (p.o.) 2–3 divided doses	6–12	Sedation, ataxia, hyperactivity (children)	CBC (every 6 months)	6–12

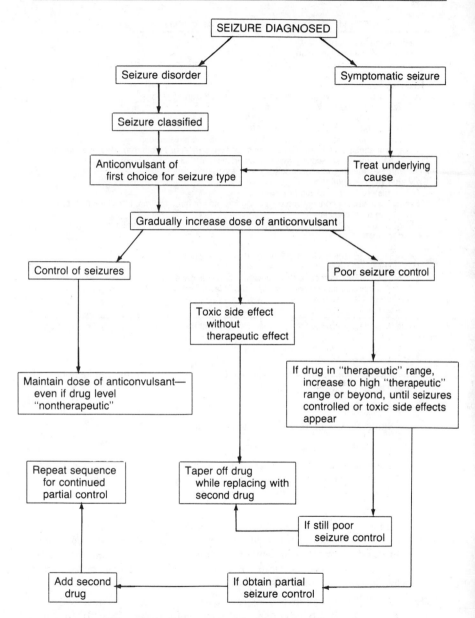

FIG. 3. General guidelines in the treatment of seizures.

TABLE 11. *Emergency management of patients in status epilepticus*

Immediate management
  Ensure adequate oxygenation
  Blood tests: CBC, serum glucose, chemistry profile, anticonvulsant levels, toxic screen
  Thiamine—100 mg i.v.
  Glucose—25–50 g i.v.
  Anticonvulsant therapy[a] (monitor blood pressure, EKG, respirations)
    Diazepam 5–10 mg i.v. (rate = 2 mg/min)
    Phenytoin 18 mg/kg i.v. (rate = 50 mg/min)
    Phenobarbital 20 mg/kg i.v. (rate = 100 mg/min)
    Paraldehyde solution (15 cc in mineral oil) rectally administered
    General anesthesia if seizures continue (sodium amytal or halothane). May need to use
      a neuromuscular blocking agent (pancuronium at 1–5 mg i.v.) to control motor
      manifestations and allow adequate ventilation
Early after seizure control or initiation of therapy
  Obtain history (from relatives or friends)
  Examination should concentrate on looking for signs of head trauma, CNS infection, or
  focal neurologic signs
  Check results of initial laboratory tests and either treat underlying condition or order
  further tests
Later evaluation
  EKG (difficult to obtain while patient is suffering a seizure)
  CAT scan
  Lumbar puncture if suspect CNS infection (virtually all patients in generalized tonic-clonic
  status will be febrile immediately afterward; if fever persists, CSF examination is
  indicated)
  Other tests if indicated

[a]Should be done in stepwise fashion, with additional anticonvulsants added only if seizures continue.

neous, positional, and caloric-induced nystagmus. Recording can be done with eyes open or closed.

6. Radiographic studies

  a. Skull films with Towne and Stenver's views.

  b. Cervical spine films.

  c. Cerebellopontine angle studies to evaluate for acoustic neuroma: internal auditory canal films; polycyclic tomography of petrous bone; and, CAT scan (higher yield with metrizamide or air contrast instilled via lumbar puncture).

  7. Brainstem auditory-evoked responses (BAER) is a very sensitive, noninvasive test to evaluate central auditory pathways. **Findings are most commonly abnormal when acoustic neuroma is present.** Because of the cost of radiologic tests as well as its sensitivity, BAERs should be the first test performed when acoustic neuroma is suspected.

B. Treatment The approach to the management of the dizzy patient will vary, depending on the underlying etiology and severity of symptoms. Specific treatment aimed at the underlying disorder is often available. However, often there is no effective specific therapy for the disorder, or the patient may need **symptomatic** relief from his dizziness or vertigo in addition to specific treatment of the disorder. Treatment is usually in the form of a **vestibular suppressant**, given either orally (for mild or recurrent dizziness or vertigo) or parenterally (for acute, severe

TABLE 12. *Major causes of "dizziness"*

A   Neurologic
    Vascular disease (vertebrobasilar insufficiency)
    Brainstem lesions
    Multiple sclerosis
    Acoustic neuroma
    Cerebellar disorders
    Vertiginous ("tornado") epilepsy
    "Multiple sensory" deprivation syndrome
    Drug-induced (e.g., anticonvulsants)
    Basal skull malformations
    "Cervical" vertigo
    Metabolic (e.g., hypothyroidism)
B   Otolaryngologic (peripheral labyrinthine)
    Labyrinthitis
    Vestibular neuronitis
    Ménière's disease
    Posttraumatic vertigo
    Benign positional vertigo
    Drug-induced (e.g., aminoglycoside antibiotics)
C   Cardiovascular
    Orthostatic hypotension
    Arrhythmias
    Hypersensitive carotid sinus
D   Psychiatric
    Hyperventilation syndrome
    Conversion reaction
    Affective disorders

vertigo). Use of these drugs in the treatment of dizziness or vertigo is outlined in Table 15. Other methods of treatment when a patient has acute, severe vertigo are use of **visual fixation,** which inhibits nystagmus and subsequently diminishes vertiginous sensation, and **mental relaxation.**

VI. **DEMENTIA AND DELIRIUM**   The syndromes of dementia and delirium are both characterized by **global deterioration of the intellectual function** caused by **organic factors.** However, where the etiologies of dementia are usually **chronic and irreversible,** delirium is generally **acute and reversible.** Other major differences between and common clinical features of dementia and delirium are listed in Table 16. Despite the differences in clinical features, the same underlying disorder can often present as either dementia or delirium. If a delirious patient has a markedly depressed level of consciousness, he or she will need to be evaluated as patients in coma. In this section only dementia is discussed unless otherwise stated. The causes of dementia are numerous (Table 17), and since most are irreversible, an avid **search for treatable causes** should be the primary concern of the clinician when confronted with a demented patient.

A. **Evaluation**

1. **History** should be obtained from relatives and friends, as well as from the patient, and should concentrate on premorbid personality and health, and onset (sudden or insidious) and progression of intellectual deterioration (stepwise or gradual).

TABLE 13. *Most important tests on physical examination in the dizzy patient*

Cardiovascular
  Blood pressure with postural determinations
  Valsalva maneuver
  Carotid sinus massage
Audiologic
  Otoscopy
  Weber[a]
  Rinne[b]
Neurootologic
  Spontaneous nystagmus
  Induced nystagmus
    Gaze-evoked
    Head in standard positions
    Nylen-Barany maneuver (checking for nystagmus
      with head tilted in various positions)
  Calorics (cold and/or warm water)
  Hyperventilation for 3 min

[a]Weber—performed by placing vibrating tuning fork over forehead. **Conductive hearing loss lateralizes to involved side,** whereas in **neurosensory hearing loss it is heard best in the uninvolved ear**.
[b]Rinne—performed with tuning fork over mastoid process (bone conduction) and then held directly in front of ear (air conduction). Normally, air conduction lasts longer than bone conduction. In **conductive hearing loss, air conduction is decreased and bone conduction is spared**.

2. **General medical** and **neurologic** examinations should be performed to evaluate for the presence of underlying medical illness and focal cerebral disease, respectively.

3. **Mental status examination** should be detailed and include appearance and behavior, mood, alertness, orientation, speech (content, comprehension, naming, repetition), memory (immediate recall, short-term, remote), calculations, and reading and writing.

4. **Neuropsychologic testing** may help elucidate difficulties on mental status examination regarding diffuse versus focal involvement or organic versus nonorganic causes of apparent dementia.

5. **Laboratory tests for all patients with dementia**

   a. **Blood tests:** CBC, ESR, VDRL, FTA-ABS, electrolytes (sodium, potassium, chloride, carbon dioxide), serum calcium and phosphorus, liver function tests, renal function tests (BUN, creatinine), serum vitamin B_{12} and folate, thyroid function tests [L-triiodothyronine (T3) uptake, thryoxine (T4), TSH].

   b. **Urinalysis** to look for evidence of renal or hepatic disease.

   c. **Chest X-ray.**

   d. **CAT scan** to look for presence or absence of focal or diffuse atrophy, hydrocephalus, or mass lesion.

   e. **EEG** for evaluation of cerebral physiology. Most patients with dementia

TABLE 14. *Characteristics of peripheral and central symptoms and nystagmus*

Characteristics	Peripheral	Central
Dizziness		
Onset	Sudden	Often insidious
Duration	Minutes to days	Weeks to months
Dysequilibrium	Severe	Usually mild
Worsening with motion	Marked	Mild
Associated auditory complaints	Common	Uncommon
Other neurologic signs	Absent	Present
Eye closure	Worse symptoms	Decrease in symptoms
Nystagmus		
Spontaneous	Horizontal or rotary; usually unidirectional	Any or all directions; usually multidirectional
Positional		
Latency	2–20 sec	None
Duration	Less than 30 sec	More than 60 sec
Fatigability	Disappears with repetition	Does not fatigue
Position	Present in only one position	Present in multiple positions
Direction	To one side only	May change direction with change of head position
Incidence of occurrence	90% of all cases of nystagmus	10% of all cases of nystagmus
Examples	Labyrinthitis	Multiple sclerosis

have some degree of diffuse slowing. Slowing, however, may be **focal** or there may be evidence of a **paroxysmal** disturbance of cerebral activity (e.g., Creutzfeldt-Jacob disease).

    f. Lumbar puncture with particular attention to **pressure** (normal or low in "normal pressure hydrocephalus"), **VDRL** (almost always positive in neurosyphilis), **cell count** (elevated in chronic infectious process), **Gram stain** (for acid-fast bacilli), and **cultures** (for fungus, tuberculosis, bacteria).

6. Additional laboratory tests if indicated:

    a. Toxic screen of urine and/or blood.

    b. Isotope cisternography if other studies (e.g., CAT scan and opening pressure during lumbar puncture) suggest normal pressure hydrocephalus.

    c. Cerebral angiography for suspected vascular disease.

    d. Nuclear brain scan if focal lesion is suspected and CT scan is normal.

    e. Brain biopsy is only rarely indicated if certain infectious (e.g., progressive multifocal leukoencephalopathy, herpes simplex encephalitis) or rare degenerative or storage disorders are suspected.

B. Treatment

    1. Specific treatment should be instituted if a definitive diagnosis of a reversible disorder is made (e.g., hypothyroidism).

TABLE 15. *Medical management of dizziness and vertigo*

Drug	Dosage and administration	Side effects
Antihistamines		
Meclizine	12.5–25 mg p.o. b.i.d.-t.i.d.	Sedation, dry mouth, blurred vision, nausea
Cyclizine	50 mg p.o. t.i.d. (can be given rectally or i.m. if vertigo is severe with nausea and vomiting)	Same as meclizine
Dimenhydrinate	25–50 mg p.o. t.i.d. (can be given rectally or i.m. if vertigo is severe with nausea and vomiting)	Same as meclizine
Diphenhydramine	50 mg p.o. t.i.d. (can be given i.m. or i.v. if vertigo is severe with nausea and vomiting)	Same as meclizine
Benzodiazepines		
Diazepam	5–10 mg p.o. t.i.d. or 5–10 mg i.v. if vertigo is severe with nausea and vomiting	Sedation, dizziness, blurred vision, hypotension, depressed respiration
Chlordiazepoxide	40 mg p.o. t.i.d.	Same as diazepam
Belladonna alkaloids		
Scopolamine	0.6 mg p.o. q. 6 hr (can be given s.c. or i.v. if vertigo is severe with nausea and vomiting)	Dry mouth, drowsiness, fatigue, restlessness, irritability, disorientation, delirium, coma
Atropine sulfate	0.4–0.8 mg i.m. or i.v. q. 4 hr if vertigo is severe with nausea and vomiting	Same as scopolamine
Phenothiazines		
Promethazine	25 mg p.o. q. 6 hr (can also be given rectally, i.m., or i.v. if vertigo is severe with nausea and vomiting)	Drowsiness

TABLE 16. *Characteristics of dementia and delirium*

Characteristics	Dementia	Delirium
Onset	Insidious	Sudden
Depressed level of consciousness	No	Yes
Reversibility	Uncommon	Common
Personality change	Yes	Yes
Recent memory impairment	Yes	Yes (related to clouded level of consciousness)
Disorientation	Later feature	Early feature
Performance of tasks	Does well on familiar ones, poorly on unfamiliar ones	Related to level of consciousness
Hallucinations	Uncommon	Common
Autonomic signs (rapid pulse, flushed skin, dilated pupils, intense emotional states, fever)	No	Yes

TABLE 17. *Diseases causing dementia*
Primary diffuse degenerative diseases of the central nervous system

Primary diffuse degenerative diseases of the central nervous system
  Alzheimer's disease ("presenile" and "senile" forms)
  Pick's disease
  Huntington's chorea
  Progressive supranuclear palsy
  Spinocerebellar degenerations
  Parkinson's disease
Metabolic and hematologic disorders
  Hypothyroidism
  Disorders of calcium metabolism
  Chronic liver disease
  Chronic renal disease (uremia and "dialysis encephalopathy")
  Recurrent hypoglycemia
  Vitamin deficiencies:
    Vitamin B_{12} (pernicious anemia)
    Folate
    Thiamine (Wernicke-Korsakoff syndrome)
    Niacin (pellagra)
  Hyponatremia
Vascular disorders
  Multiinfarct dementia
  Binswanger's disease
Infections
  Chronic meningitis:
    Fungal (especially cryptococcus)
    Bacterial (especially tuberculosis)
  Brain abcess
  Neurosyphilis
  Subacute sclerosis parencephalitis
  Creutzfeldt-Jakob disease
  Progressive multifocal leukoencephalopathy
Toxins and drugs
  Heavy metals
  Bromides
  Alcohol
  Chronic, multiple drug use
  Carbon monoxide
Brain tumors
Head trauma
  Chronic subdural hematoma
Normal pressure hydrocephalus
Psychiatric disorders
  Depression
  Schizophrenia

2. **Nonspecific treatment** is essential even if the disorder is irreversible.

a. Counseling to both patient and family.

b. **Maintaining familiar environment.** This aspect of care is very important, since any change of surroundings may prove to be very disruptive to a demented patient.

c. **Environmental manipulation** especially to lead to a more structured environment, can utilize a patient's residual functions to cope with his or her surroundings.

d. **Medications**

(1) Depression

(a) Amitriptyline 50 to 300 mg p.o. at bedtime.

(b) Nortriptyline 25 mg p.o. t.i.d. to q.i.d.

(c) Imipramine 50 to 300 mg p.o. at bedtime.

(d) Doxepin 75 to 150 mg p.o. at bedtime.

In addition to treating the depression that commonly occurs in patients with dementia, **all patients diagnosed as having dementia should be given a trial with antidepressant medications.** This statement reflects the high frequency (perhaps up to 25%) of patients with dementia who suffer from depressive psychosis ("pseudodementia") as well as the inability at times to clinically differentiate depressive psychosis from Alzheimer's disease.

(2) Mild anxiety

(a) Diazepam 2 mg p.o. t.i.d.

(b) Chlordiazepoxide 5 mg p.o. t.i.d.

(3) Extreme agitation and psychotic symptoms

(a) Haloperidol (Haldol®) 0.5 to 1 mg p.o. b.i.d. to t.i.d.

(b) Chlorpromazine (Thorazine®) 25 mg p.o. b.i.d. to t.i.d.

(c) Thioridazine (Mellaril®) 25 mg p.o. b.i.d. to t.i.d.

(4) Insomnia

(a) In acutely disturbed and agitated patients with insomnia, the following tranquilizers intramuscularly are the treatment of choice: **haloperidol** (2 mg i.m.), **chlorpromazine** and **thioridazine** (25 mg i.m.). Otherwise, the following drugs can be used.

(b) Chloral hydrate 500 mg p.o. at bedtime.

(c) Diphenhydramine (Benadryl®) 50 to 100 mg p.o. at bedtime.

(d) Promethazine hydrochloride (Phenergan®) 25 to 50 mg p.o. at bedtime.

VII. ACUTE NEUROMUSCULAR WEAKNESS   Few clinical problems are as alarming to both patient and clinician as that of the onset of rapidly progressive generalized weakness. The weakness may be due to a variety of etiologies and may result from dysfunction at any of the following levels of the motor system: upper motor neuron; lower motor neuron; peripheral nerve; neuromuscular junction; and, muscle. Disorders of the upper motor neuron causing weakness have been discussed in other sections of this chapter, and this section is devoted to discussion of the diagnosis and management of those neuromuscular disorders associated with rapidly progressive generalized weakness. The clinical and laboratory diagnoses of these disorders are summarized in Table 18. Specific management of several of the more common of these disorders is discussed below briefly. Initial management should aim at **preventing tracheal aspiration and/or pneumonia** due to bulbar dysfunction and **respiratory failure** (see I.).

A. Evaluation

   1. The **history** should concentrate on whether there is a prior diagnosis of a

TABLE 18. *Differential diagnosis of acute weakness*

Disorder	Clinical features	Laboratory
Lower motor neuron		
Poliomyelitis	Viral prodrome Asymmetric paralysis Meningeal signs Bulbar signs	CSF pleocytosis
Peripheral nerve		
Guillain-Barré syndrome	Recent viral illness, immunization or trauma Ascending paralysis and areflexia Sensory symptoms but not signs	CSF albuminocytologic dissociation Marked slow nerve conduction velocities
Tick paralysis	Typically in children Weakness, areflexia, bulbar symptoms, numbness	Find the tick and remove it
Diphtheria	Recent membraneous pharyngitis Palatal weakness Eye accommodation weakness (big pupils) Neuropathy late	Culture C diphtheriae organism
Porphyria	History of psychiatric, abdominal or cutaneous symptoms Guillain-Barré-like clinical picture	Excretion of excessive porphyrins in urine
Neuromuscular junction		
Myasthenia gravis	Fluctuating weakness Ptosis, diplopia, dysphagia, dysarthria	Positive Tensilon test Decrement with repetitive stimulation EMG Positive acetylcholine receptor antibody
Botulism	History of recent home canned food ingestion GI distress Rapid onset bulbar symptoms, paralysis, areflexia Dilated pupils (rare)	Increment with repetitive stimulation EMG Normal CSF Toxin in food, blood or stool
Organophosphate poisoning	History of insecticide exposure GI distress, sweating, agitation, twitching, small pupils Delayed neuropathy	Identification of organophosphate containing substance
Muscle		
Inflammatory myopathy (rapidly progressive)	Proximal weakness Dysphagia, but not other bulbar dysfunction Myalgia in 50%	Elevated CPK Myopathic EMG Inflammation on biopsy
Periodic paralyses	History of recurrent bouts of weakness Family history Speech, respiration spared	High or low serum K
Rhabdomyolysis	Recent strenuous overexertion Trauma or toxin (ETOH) exposure Swollen, tender extremities	Elevated CPK Myoglobinuria (positive benzidine test in urine without RBCs)

From Simon, D. B., Ringel, S. P., and Lacy, J. R. (1983): Neuromuscular emergencies. In: *Neurologic Emergencies*, edited by M. P. Earnest, pp. 219–258. Churchill Livingstone, New York, with permission.

neuromuscular disorder or recurrent episodes of weakness (periodic paralysis); history of recent viral illness (common in Guillain-Barré syndrome); home canned food ingestion (botulism); history of psychiatric, abdominal, or cutaneous symptoms (porphyria); sensory symptoms (peripheral neuropathy); myalgias (polymyositis; rhabdomyolysis); dysphagia (common in myasthenia gravis and polymyositis); diplopia (botulism, myasthenia gravis); gastrointestinal disturbance (toxins such as botulism or organophosphate poisoning); or acute cholinergic symptoms such as miosis, sweating, and muscle fasciculations (organophosphate poisoning).

2. The general **physical examination** is usually unrevealing although the **skin** manifestations of acute intermittent porphyria or dermatomyositis may be present.

3. The **neurologic examination** should concentrate on pattern of weakness, deep tendon reflexes, sensory loss, and muscle atrophy (Table 19).

4. **Laboratory tests**

   a. **Blood tests:** serum glucose and electrolytes (especially potassium); serum creatine phosphokinase (CPK); chemistry screen; urine for porphobilinogen, myoglobin, heavy metals; botulinum toxin assay; acetylcholine receptor antibody (if myasthenia gravis is suspected).

   b. **Electrophysiologic tests** (nerve conduction velocity, electromyography, and repetitive stimulation) are the most useful diagnostic tests for the evaluation of rapidly progressive generalized weakness and should be performed as soon as possible. If a neuropathy is present, differentiation into demyelinating (conductions slowed markedly) or axonal (mild slowing) variety can be done with nerve conduction velocities. Nerve conduction velocities are normal in all other disorders of the neuromuscular system. Repetitive stimulation studies produce a decremental response in myasthenia gravis and an incremental response in botulism and the myasthenic syndrome of Eaton-Lambert. Needle electromyography may reveal myopathic changes (polymyositis and rhabdomyolysis) or neuropathic changes (lower motor neuron and peripheral nerve disorders).

TABLE 19. *Clinical features associated with disorders of neuromuscular system*

Level of neuromuscular system affected	Pattern of weakness	Reflexes	Atrophy	Sensory loss
Lower motor neuron	Asymmetric; may have bulbar signs	Absent or diminished	Yes	No
Peripheral nerve	Symmetric, predominantly distal; may have bulbar signs	Absent or diminished	Yes	Yes (may be mild)
Neuromuscular junction	Bulbar signs common, diplopia, ptosis, fatigability	Preserved (absent in botulism)	No	No
Muscle	Proximal	Preserved	No	No

    c. Lumbar puncture will usually help in the diagnosis of Guillain-Barré syndrome where there is elevated protein and generally few white blood cells (albuminocytologic dissociation).

    d. Muscle and nerve biopsies may be valuable in certain situations, but are not done routinely.

B. Treatment

  1. Lower motor neuron—poliomyelitis—supportive.

  2. Peripheral nerve

    a. Guillain-Barré syndrome treatment is primarily **supportive.** The use of **corticosteroids** is generally not of value in this disorder, although a high percentage of patients (50%) who have a chronic form of this disease will respond. **Plasmapheresis** for treatment of Guillain-Barré syndrome is currently under investigation.

    b. Tick paralysis. Find and remove tick.

    c. Diphtheria. Supportive.

    d. Porphyria. Supportive plus removal of exacerbating factor (especially medications) if possible.

  3. Neuromuscular junction

    a. Myasthenia gravis

      (1) Prevention of tracheal aspiration and respiratory support.

      (2) Treatment of precipitating factors

        (a) Thyroid abnormalities.

        (b) Infections of the pulmonary and urinary tracts.

        (c) Drugs (usually prescribed medications).

      (3) Anticholinesterase agents

        (a) Pyridostigmine (Mestinon®) 60 mg p.o. t.i.d. This dosage can be increased or decreased, depending on symptomatic improvement or side effects, and can be given i.m. or i.v. at a dosage of 2 mg every 2 to 3 hr.

        (b) Neostigmine (Prostigmin®) 15 mg p.o. every 3 to 4 hr. This can be given i.m. or i.v. at a dose of 0.5 mg every 2 to 3 hr.

      (4) Corticosteroids (primarily in the form of prednisone) can be used in either high or low doses, daily or alternate-day regimens. No regimen is more efficacious than another, although a low-dose alternate-day regimen that gradually increases the dose may have fewer problems with **exacerbation of weakness** in myasthenia gravis. Such exacerbation of weakness is more associated with high-dose/daily program, especially during the first 5 days after initiating corticosteroids.

      (5) Immunosuppressive agents (usually azathioprine or cyclophosphamide) may be beneficial if the patient does not respond to corticosteroids.

      (6) Plasmapheresis may result in remarkable increase in strength rather quickly and is of most benefit during crisis until other therapy becomes effective or in **preparation for thymectomy.** Some physicians have used the combination of plasmapheresis/immunosuppressive agents as a primary therapy in myasthenia gravis, although, in general, this is impractical because of the need for repeated attempts at plasmapheresis.

(7) **Thymectomy** is standard therapy in the long-term management of myasthenia gravis in most centers. The indications for thymectomy, however, are not clear, except in cases of thymoma, and whether or not thymectomy is beneficial is not known.

b. **Botulism.** Treatment is primarily supportive, although **guanidine hydro-chloride** starting at 15 mg/kg/day, gradually increasing to 50 mg/kg/day given p.o. every 4 hr, may be beneficial for some aspects of the weakness (primarily extremity and extraocular muscle). The major short-term side effect of guanidine is gastrointestinal upset, and bone-marrow suppression has been reported with chronic use. Therapy against the toxin is started with the trivalent antitoxin (against botulinus toxin A, B, E) at 10,000 units i.v. given in single dose.

c. **Organophosphate poisoning** may be treated with the following drugs:

(1) Pralidoxime chloride 1 g i.v. May repeat dose after 20 min.

(2) Atropine 1 g i.v. or i.m. every 20 to 30 min as needed.

4. **Muscle**

a. **Inflammatory myopathies** are treated with corticosteroids and/or immunosuppressive drugs.

b. **Periodic paralyses** can be treated with **acetazolamide** (250 mg p.o. t.i.d.), which can dramatically reduce the number of paralytic attacks. Treatment of acute attacks will vary depending on the variety of periodic paralysis. Hypokalemic periodic paralysis is treated acutely with oral potassium chloride (2–10 g). Hyperkalemic periodic paralysis can be treated with oral glucose (2 g/kg) plus regular insulin (15–20 units subcutaneously). Dietary manipulation may also be beneficial in the prevention of further attacks.

c. **Rhabdomyolysis.** The treatment is supportive; this includes an increase in solute excretion (e.g., mannitol) to prevent acute renal failure.

VIII. **MULTIPLE SCLEROSIS** Multiple sclerosis (MS) is the most common demyelinating disease of the nervous system and one of the most common neurologic disorders in the United States. Since any area of the central nervous system may be affected, symptoms and signs vary widely among individual patients. The most common symptoms and their approximate frequency of occurrence both initially and later in the course of the disease appear in Table 20. Signs on the neurologic exam may reflect damage of virtually any area of the central nervous system.

A. **Diagnosis**

1. **History** may reveal evidence of neurologic dysfunction affecting several areas of the nervous system and may fit one of several clinical courses followed by patients with MS: **relapsing-remitting** (most common variety, usually with

TABLE 20. *Frequency of occurrence of symptoms in MS*

Symptom	Percent[a]	Symptom	Percent[a]
Visual (blurred vision)	35/66	Ataxia of gait	20/40
Diplopia	13/34	Sphincter/sexual	10/60
Weakness	43/88	impairment	
Paresthesias	13/87	Facial pain	5/20
Vertigo/dizziness	10/80	Cognitive impairment	2/40

[a]Initial symptom occurring eventually during course of disease.

onset between ages 20 and 40); **relapsing-remitting/progressive** (usually with progression after many years of a relapsing-remitting course); **progressive** (occurring in about 10% of patients who experience relatively steady worsening from onset without clear exacerbations and remissions); **benign** (occurring in up to 30% of patients, who usually have exacerbations with remissions and little or no disability many years after initial symptoms); and **malignant** (a rare form with rapid progression resulting in severe disability or death in several weeks to a few years after the onset). Prognosis depends on the course of the disease and cannot be defined with certainty early in the disease course.

2. **Neurologic examination** should be consistent with **multiple lesions** in the white matter of the central nervous system.

3. **Laboratory tests** are helpful in evaluating patients with suspected MS, but none are diagnostic. The various tests available and their degree of positivity in cases of definite MS are listed in Table 21. It should be emphasized that since no test listed is specific for MS, they must all be interpreted in light of the clinical manifestations. **The diagnosis of MS is largely based on clinical criteria and should not be made solely on an abnormality of a laboratory test.**

B. **Treatment** Treatment of MS is aimed at three general areas: **stopping progression, shortening acute exacerbations, and symptomatic treatment** of complications.

1. **Stopping progression.** Numerous types of therapeutic intervention have been

TABLE 21. *Ancillary tests used in evaluation of suspected cases of MS*

Test	% Positive in definite MS[a]
Cerebrospinal fluid	
Gamma globulin elevation (>12% total protein)	75
Mild (<100 mg%) protein elevation	25
Lymphocytic pleocytosis	25
IgG index [(CSF IgG/albumin)/(serum IgG/albumin)]	80–90
"Oligoclonal bands"	85–95
Evoked responses	
Visual	80–90
Brainstem	60–70
Somatosensory	70–80
All three combined	90–100
CAT scan	40–60

[a]Percent positivity in cases of probable and possible MS are successively lower.

tried to halt progression of MS. None has been proven to be of benefit; however, recent therapeutic attempts in treatment of chronic progressive MS may be of value. This has been primarily in the form of **immunosuppressive** therapy. Many agents are currently under study.

2. **Shortening acute exacerbations.** An **exacerbation** of MS is defined as the development of new signs or symptoms, or significant worsening of existing symptoms over a period of 1 to 2 days. Mild fluctuations in fixed symptoms are common in patients with MS and are usually due to physical or emotional stress and should not be confused with acute exacerbations.

Adrenocorticotrophic hormone (ACTH) is the only drug that has shown to be of benefit in shortening acute exacerbations of MS in a large cooperative study evaluating ACTH versus placebo. No study has compared various **steroid** preparations in the treatment of acute exacerbations, but these drugs may also be of value. An acceptable regimen for ACTH is:

Days	Units s.c. or i.m.
1–5	40 b.i.d.
6–8	30 b.i.d.
9–11	20 b.i.d.
12–14	10 b.i.d.
15–17	5 b.i.d.
18–20	5 daily
21,23,25	5 each day

Adverse reactions of ACTH therapy include **hypokalemia** (can be prophylactically treated with potassium chloride 20 to 40 mEq daily or follow potassium levels and replace as needed); **fluid retention** (can treat with low sodium diet or a diuretic, especially if associated with **hypertension**); **gastric irritation** (should prophylactically use nonconstipating antacids); **insomnia, mental alterations** (anxiety, restlessness, depression, euphoria, or even frank psychosis); **menstrual irregularities**; and **infection** and **sepsis.**

Oral corticosteroids can also be administered instead of ACTH for an acute exacerbation. They are more convenient than ACTH because of the oral route of administration plus there are fewer side effects. An acceptable regimen for oral prednisone is:

Days	mg/day
1–5	50
6–9	40
10–13	30
14–17	20
18–21	10
22–25	5

3. **Symptomatic therapy for complications of MS**

   a. **General therapeutic management** should consist of a **daily exercise program** (outlined by a physical therapist skilled in the management of MS patients), **well-balanced diet, adequate rest,** and **avoidance of physical** (e.g., fevers) and **emotional stress.**

b. **Spasticity**

(1) **General measures** should concentrate on preventing and treating infections (especially urinary tract infections) and other sources of noxious stimuli that can cause an increase in underlying spasticity.

(2) **Drugs** commonly used in the treatment of spasticity are:

(a) **Baclofen** (15–80 mg p.o. daily in three divided doses). Baclofen is the **drug of choice** in the treatment of spasticity from MS. Major side effects include light-headedness, nausea, drowsiness, and dry mouth.

(b) **Diazepam** (4–40 mg p.o. daily in divided doses). Major side effects include drowsiness, fatigue, ataxia, weakness, and physical dependence.

(c) **Dantrolene** (25–50 mg p.o. daily initially; may be gradually increased to a maximum of 400–500 mg/day). The major problem with dantrolene is that it always causes generalized weakness at therapeutic doses, which may make its use intolerable in many patients. Other side effects include hepatitis, diarrhea, light-headedness, and drowsiness.

(3) Treatment of severe spasticity when drug therapy fails consists of either **chemical** [**phenol** (5%–25% in oil or glycerin) intrathecally] or **surgical** destruction of reflex arch with either **anterior rhizotomy** or **peripheral nerve section.** Anterior rhizotomy is the surgical procedure of choice since remaining sensation is left intact. Spasticity may also be treated by sectioning the tendons and muscles involved in the spasms. This form of therapy is only temporary, however, since the muscle connections regenerate and spasticity reappears.

c. **Ataxia and tremor,** when present, are some of the most disabling features of MS. Medical therapy has been tried with various medications, but is usually unsuccessful. Extremity weight cuffs or a cervical collar may benefit some patients, and treatment of stress and anxiety may also be beneficial.

d. **Bowel and bladder dysfunction** are common in MS. When bladder dysfunction is present, evaluation should include urinalysis, urine culture and sensitivity, cystometrogram, cystoscopy and i.v. pyelogram (IVP) for further delineation of the problem so that proper therapy can be initiated. Bowel incontinence is an uncommon problem, although constipation is common. Constipation can usually be managed with bran or other bulking agents and with increased fluid intake.

e. **Sensory impairment** is resistant to treatment but when **pain** is a component (e.g., trigeminal neuralgia or other painful dysesthesia), treatment is with either **phenytoin** (300 mg daily), **carbamazepine** (400–1,200 mg daily), or amitriptyline (50 mg p.o. daily, increased by 25 mg/day every 2–3 weeks up to 300 mg daily).

f. **Psychologic impairment** may include depression, euphoria, psychosis, and dementia and needs to be treated individually.

IX. PARKINSON'S DISEASE Parkinson's disease is the most common movement disorder characterizing dysfunction of the basal ganglia and is a major cause of neurologic disability in the elderly.

A. Diagnosis   Since there are no biochemical markers or pathognomonic signs, the diagnosis of Parkinson's disease depends on clinical observation.

The major clinical features include:

1. **Tremor,** the most characteristic of the clinical features, is coarse (3–5 cps) and is most prominent in distal muscles. It is usually present at rest and decreases with movement.

2. **Bradykinesia** consists of decreased voluntary movements and loss of associated movements. Examples of bradykinesia are "masked" facies and difficulty initiating walking.

3. **Rigidity** is characterized by abnormally increased muscle tone with a "cogwheel" resistance to passive movement.

4. **Poor postural reflexes** result in difficulty maintaining body posture so that the patient assumes a flexed position when walking. Late in the disease course, postural reflexes may become so impaired that the patient is unable to sit unassisted.

5. **Less prominent clinical features** include increased sweating and salivation, thermal paresthesias (unpleasant burning sensation affecting an area of the body), painful cramps in the feet and legs, edema of one or both legs (probably due to stasis from decreased movement of the extremity), the "striatal toe" (tonically dorsiflexed great toe), and respiratory dyskinesia.

B. Differential Diagnosis   When several major clinical features are present, the diagnosis of Parkinson's disease is not difficult. Perhaps the most commonly misdiagnosed problem as Parkinson's disease is a **normal elderly person.** With aging many people develop some degree of stooped posture, bradykinesia, and/or tremor. These people do not have Parkinson's disease, although they have some parkinsonian features, and will not respond to medications used to treat Parkinson's disease. Disorders that are occasionally mistaken for Parkinson's disease include familial (benign essential) tremor, progressive supranuclear palsy, olivopontocerebellar atrophy, "arteriosclerotic" parkinsonism, Shy-Drager syndrome, and striatonigral degeneration.

C. Treatment   The basal ganglia have high concentrations of the neurotransmitters **dopamine** and **acetylcholine.** The normal balance of dopaminergic (inhibitory) and cholinergic (excitatory) allows for smooth control of voluntary movements. Since in Parkinson's disease there is an absolute deficiency in dopaminergic input, the goal of treatment is to balance the activity of the basal ganglia by either **enhancing dopaminergic** activity or by **reducing cholinergic** activity or **both.**

General guidelines in the use of antiparkinsonian **drugs** are as follows:

1. Select drugs with the fewest side effects for initial therapy (e.g., amantadine and/or anticholinergic agents).

2. Delay use of L-DOPA as long as possible. L-DOPA (or Sinemet®) are the most useful drugs used in the treatment of Parkinson's disease, but seem to have a limited period of usefulness after which they lose their effectiveness. In addition, L-DOPA has numerous acute and chronic complications.

TABLE 22. *Drug therapy of Parkinson's disease*

Drug	Major clinical indications	Dosage and administration	Side effects	Contraindications
Dopaminergic agents				
L-DOPA	Rarely used alone anymore without peripheral decarboxylase inhibitor (carbidopa) bradykinesia, rigidity	250 mg p.o. t.i.d. initially; gradually increase to 2–6 g p.o. daily	Nausea, vomiting, anorexia, cardiac arrhythmias, hypotension, abnormal involuntary movements, hallucinations, insomnia, nightmares, depression	Narrow-angle glaucoma, concurrent use of MAO inhibitors
L-DOPA/Carbidopa (Sinemet®)	Bradykinesia, rigidity	25 mg/100 mg (carbidopa/L-DOPA) p.o. t.i.d. initially; gradually increase to maximum of 2 g L-DOPA p.o. daily	Same as L-DOPA but with less nausea/vomiting, anorexia, cardiac arrhythmia	Same as L-DOPA
Amantadine (Symmetrel®)	Useful for short-term (6–8 wk) adjunct to L-DOPA therapy	100 mg p.o. daily or b.i.d.	Depression, congestive heart failure, urinary retention, livido reticularis in lower extremities, confusion, drowsiness	Severe congestive heart failure
Bromocriptine	Useful when L-DOPA causes severe wearing-off reactions (marked increase in symptoms prior to next dose) or dyskinesia allows reduction of L-DOPA dose	2.5 mg p.o. t.i.d. initially; gradually increase to 15–90 mg p.o. daily	Similar to L-DOPA, less dyskinesia, more confusion, hallucinations, delusions, pulmonary fibrosis	Psychosis, ischemic heart disease, active peptic ulcer disease, pulmonary fibrosis
Anticholinergic agents				
Benztropine (Cogentin®)	Tremor, bradykinesia, rigidity; alone or in combination with L-DOPA	0.5–2.0 mg p.o. b.i.d.–t.i.d.	Dry mouth, dizziness, blurred vision, confusion, agitation, urinary retention (esp. when prostatic hypertrophy in males)	Psychosis, prostatic hypertrophy
Trihexyphenidyl (Artane®)	Tremor, bradykinesia, rigidity; alone or in combination with L-DOPA	1.0–5.0 mg p.o. b.i.d.–t.i.d.	Same as benztropine	Same as benztropine
Biperiden (Akineton®)	Tremor, bradykinesia, rigidity; alone or in combination with L-DOPA	1.0–3.0 mg p.o. t.i.d.	Same as benztropine	Same as benztropine

3. If tremor is the major clinical feature, an anticholinergic agent is the drug of choice. Drugs useful in the treatment of Parkinson's disease are outlined in Table 22.

Surgical treatment in the form of **ventrolateral thalamotomy** is rarely performed anymore and is reserved for patients with incapacitating symptoms resistant to drug therapy.

BIBLIOGRAPHY

Acute Neuromuscular Weakness

Grob, D. (1981): Acute neuromuscular disorders. *Med. Clin. North Am.*, 65:189–207.
Ringel, S. P. (1979): Clinical presentations in neuromuscular disease. In: *Handbook of Clinical Neurology*, Vol. 40, edited by P. J. Vinken and G. W. Bruyn, pp. 295–348. North-Holland, Amsterdam.
Simon, D. B., Ringel, S. P., and Lacy, J. R. (1983): Neuromuscular emergencies. In: *Neurologic Emergencies*, edited by M. P. Earnest, pp. 219–258. Churchill Livingstone, New York.
Streib, E. W. (1983): Signs and symptoms of acute neuromuscular diseases seen in the emergency room. *Semin. Neurol.*, 3:58–67.

Coma

Fisher, C. M. (1969): The neurological evaluation of the comatose patient. *Acta. Neurol. Scand.*, 45 [Suppl.36]:1–56.
Levy, D. E., Bates, D., Caronna, J. J., Cartlidge, M. B., Knill-Jones, R. P., Lapinski, R. H., Singer, B. H., Shaw, D. A., and Plum, F. (1981): Prognosis in nontraumatic coma. *Ann. Intern. Med.*, 94:293–301.
Plum, F., and Posner, J. B. (1980): *Diagnosis of Stupor and Coma*, 3rd ed. F. A. Davis, Philadelphia.
Posner, J. B. (1975): The comatose patient. *JAMA*, 233:1313–1314.

Dementia and Delirium

Barnett, R. E. (1972): Dementia in adults. *Med. Clin. North Am.*, 56:1405–1418.
Katzman, R., and Terry, R., editors (1983): *The Neurology of Aging*. F. A. Davis, Philadelphia.
Task Force sponsored by the National Institute of Aging (1980): Senility reconsidered: treatment possibilities for mental impairment in the elderly. *JAMA*, 244:259–263.
Watson, R. T., and Heilman, K. M. (1974): The differential diagnosis of dementia. *Geriatrics*, 29:145–154.
Wells, C. E., editor (1977): *Dementia*, 2nd ed. F. A. Davis, Philadelphia.

Dizziness and Vertigo

Drachman, D. A., and Hart, C. W. (1972): An approach to the dizzy patient. *Neurology*, 22:323–328.
McCabe, B. F. (1973): Central aspects of drugs for motion sickness and vertigo. *Adv. Otorhinolaryngol.*, 20:458–469.
Symposium on Vertigo (1967): *Arch. Otolaryngol.*, 85:497–560.
Wolfson, R. J., editor (1973): Symposium on vertigo. *Otolaryngol. Clin. North Am.*, 6:1–320.

Headache

Dalessio, D. J. (1972): *Wolff's Headache and Other Head Pain*, 3rd ed. Oxford, New York.
Dalessio, D. J. (1978): Mechanisms of headache. *Med. Clin. North Am.*, 62:429–442.
Packard, R. C., editor (1983): Symposium on headache. *Neurol. Clin.*, 1:359–569.
Raskin, N. H., and Appenzeller, O. (1980): *Headache*. W. B. Saunders, Philadelphia.

Multiple Sclerosis

Antel, J. P., editor (1983): Symposium on multiple sclerosis. *Neurol. Clin.*, 1:571–785.
Bauer, H. J. (1978): Problems of symptomatic therapy in multiple sclerosis. *Neurology*, 28:8–20.

Hart, R. G., and Sherman, D. G. (1982): The diagnosis of multiple sclerosis. *JAMA*, 247:498–503.

McAlpine, D., Compston, N.DD., and Acheson, E. D., editors (1972): *Multiple Sclerosis: A Reappraisal*, 2nd ed. Churchill Livingstone, Edinburgh and London.

McFarlin, D. E., and McFarland, H. F. (1982): Multiple sclerosis. *N. Engl. J. Med.*, 307:1183–1188.

McFarlin, D. E., and McFarland, H. F. (1982): Multiple sclerosis. *N. Engl. J. Med.*, 307:1246–1251.

Rose, A. S., Kuzma, J. W., Kurtzer, J. F., Namerow, N. S., Sibley, W. A., and Tourtelotte, W. W. (1970): Cooperative study on the evaluation of therapy in multiple sclerosis: ACTH vs. placebo. Final report. *Neurology*, 20[suppl.]:1–59.

Parkinson's Disease

Boshes, B. (1981): Sinemet and the treatment of parkinsonism. *Ann. Intern. Med.*, 94:364–370.

Calne, D. B. (1977): Developments in the pharmacology and therapeutics of parkinsonism. *Ann. Neurol.*, 1:111–119.

Calne, D. B., Kebabian, J., Silbergeld, E., and Evarts, E. (1979): Advances in the neuropharmacology of parkinsonism. *Ann. Intern. Med.*, 90:219–229.

Fahn, S., Cote, L. J., Snider, S. R., Barrett, R. E., and Isgreen, W. P. (1979): The role of bromocriptine in the treatment of parkinsonism. *Neurology*, 29:1077–1083.

Kock-Weser, J. (1976): Drug therapy of parkinsonism. *N. Engl. J. Med.*, 295:814–818.

Seizures

Delgado-Escueta, A. V., Treiman, D. M., and Walsh, G. O. (1983): The treatable epilepsies. *N. Engl. J. Med.*, 308:1508–1514.

Delgado-Escueta, A. V., Treiman, D. M., and Walsh, G. O. (1983): The treatable epilepsies. *N. Engl. J. Med.*, 308:1576–1584.

Penry, J. K., and Newmark, M. E. (1979): The use of antiepileptic drugs. *Ann. Intern. Med.*, 90:207–218.

Roger, J., Lob, H., and Tassinari, C. A. (1974): Status epilepticus. In: *Handbook of Clinical Neurology*, Vol. 15, edited by P. J. Vinken and G. W. Bruyn, pp. 145–188. North-Holland, Amsterdam.

Schomer, D. L. (1983): Partial epilepsy. *N. Engl. J. Med.*, 309:536–539.

Woodbury, D. M., Penry, J. K., and Pippenger, C. E., editors (1982): *Antiepileptic Drugs*, 2nd ed. Raven Press, New York.

Stroke

Barnett, H. J. M., editor (1983): Symposium on cerebrovascular disease. *Neurol. Clin.*, 1:1–358.

Brust, J. C. M. (1977): Transient ischemic attacks: natural history and anticoagulation. *Neurology*, 27:701–707.

Buonanno, F., and Toole, J. F. (1981): Management of patients with established ("completed") cerebral infarction. *Stroke*, 12:7–16.

Easton, J. D., and Sherman, D. G. (1980): Management of cerebral embolism of cardiac origin. *Stroke*, 11:433–442.

Genton, E., Barnett, H. J. M., Fields, W. S., Gent, M., and Hoak, J. C. (1977): XIV. Cerebral ischemia: the role of thrombosis and of antithrombotic therapy. *Stroke*, 8:150–175.

Millikin, C. H., and McDowell, F. H. (1978): Treatment of transient ischemic attacks. *Stroke*, 9:299–308.

Yatsu, F. M. (1977): Pharmacologic basis of stroke therapy. In: *Clinical Neuropharmacology*, edited by H. Klawans, pp. 113–150. Raven Press, New York.

24.

Acute Poisoning and Drug Overdose

Allen J. Sedman

24.

Acute Poisoning and Drug Overdose

Toxic ingestions account for approximately 30,000 deaths per year in the United States and are responsible for 10% to 20% of adult medical service admissions. Although toxin ingestion is frequently a presenting complaint, the diagnosis of poisoning in suicidal or comatose patients, in children, and in the elderly is often difficult. Factors that should alert the clinician to possible toxin ingestion are given in Table 1.

I. **SUPPORTIVE CARE** Supportive care is the basis of therapy for most poisonings except those that are rapidly fatal, such as cyanide or insulin intoxication, and require the immediate use of a specific antidote.

   A. **Respiratory Evaluation**

   1. **Assessment of respiratory function** is achieved by noting the rate, depth, and pattern of respiration although arterial blood gases often are needed to determine adequacy of ventilation and oxygenation.

   2. **Airway management** is summarized in Fig. 1. Suction apparatus must be available should it be necessary to clear the airway.

   B. **Cardiac Stabilization**

   1. **Cardiopulmonary resuscitation** should be started for patients with absent pulse and blood pressure.

   2. **Intravenous access.** At least one large bore intravenous catheter should be placed in any patient with a significant drug intoxication. Venous blood may be collected at this time for future laboratory studies.

   3. **Hypotension.** Although many factors may contribute to the hypotension seen after drug ingestion, correction of volume depletion and of acid-base and electrolyte abnormalities usually results in normalization of blood pressure. **Rapid volume expansion** with **lactated Ringer's solution, normal saline, or 5% dextrose in normal saline** is recommended. Vasoactive agents such as norepinephrine or phenylephrine also may be required in unresponsive individuals. Central venous pressure or pulmonary capillary wedge pressure should be monitored in any patient with hypotension refractory to the above measures.

TABLE 1. *Factors that should alert the clinician to possible toxin ingestion*

History of previous drug ingestion, suicide attempt, depression, or other psychosocial problem
Age of less than 5 years
Rapid onset of unusual signs or symptoms
Symptom complex involving many organ systems not identifiable as a specific syndrome or disease entity

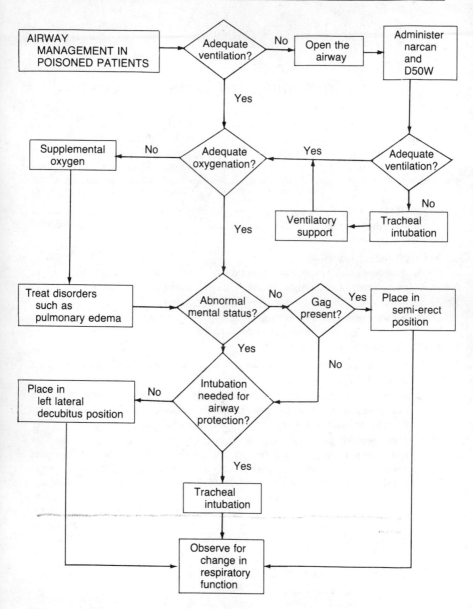

FIG. 1. Strategy for airway management. Comatose patients or those with rapidly decreasing mental status or status epilepticus should be intubated. Absent gag reflex is not an absolute indication for intubation.

4. Hypertension. Blood pressure elevations in poisoned patients usually are modest, short-lived, and require no therapy. However, ingestion of some drugs such as amphetamines or cocaine may result in profound increases in blood pressure that must be treated promptly as described in Chapter 4.

5. Cardiac rhythm should be monitored and symptomatic, life-threatening dysrhythmia treated. Intravenous **lidocaine** 1 mg/kg with a 1 to 4 mg/min infusion, followed in 20 min by a 0.5 mg/kg intravenous bolus, is the **antiarrhythmic of choice.** However, optimum management of arrhythmia often requires identifying the intoxicant. For example, when life-threatening arrhythmia resulting from digoxin intoxication is unresponsive to conventional therapy, it should be treated with digoxin antibody fragments.

C. Temperature Regulation **Hyperthermia** or **hypothermia** may occur following the ingestion of a wide variety of toxins, including salicylates, cocaine, phenothiazines, and anticholinergic drugs. Euthermia should be achieved by using antidotes, antipyretic agents, and a cooling or heating apparatus.

D. Empiric Therapy Empiric therapy with intravenous **thiamine** 100 mg, **50% dextrose in water** 100 ml, and **naloxone hydrochloride** 0.4 mg (2 ampules) should be given to patients with depressed mental status, hypotension, or hypoventilation. Propoxyphene hydrochloride (Darvon®) intoxication may require 2 mg (10 ampules) of naloxone hydrochloride for complete antagonism of central nervous system depression.

E. Seizure Therapy Repetitive seizures that compromise metabolic function or patient therapy require treatment. Although the type of ingestion may dictate a specific type of anticonvulsant therapy, for most poisonings, **diazepam** 2 mg/min (up to 20 mg) until seizures terminate, with an intravenous **phenytoin** loading dose of 18 mg/kg (maximum rate of infusion = 50 mg/min) is recommended.

F. Acid-Base and Electrolyte Disorders **Acid-base** and **electrolyte disorders** should be corrected rapidly to maximize cardiac and respiratory function and help prevent arrhythmia and seizures.

II. SPECIFIC THERAPY Indications for the use of specific therapeutic modalities are often controversial and depend on the type and size of ingestion, condition of the patient, and underlying pathophysiologic conditions such as renal insufficiency, congestive heart failure, or liver disease.

A. Identification of the Intoxicant Most specific therapy requires that the intoxicant be identified. Steps helpful in the identification of a specific poison include:

1. History and physical examination with attention to the amount, type, and time of ingestion, and examination of heart, lungs, abdomen, and nervous system.

2. Laboratory studies

a. Serum electrolytes, glucose, BUN, creatinine, and **osmoles.**

b. Arterial blood gas.

c. Complete urinalysis with attention to sediment.

d. Urine ferric chloride for salicylates.

e. Serum drug levels.

f. Urine, serum, and gastric lavage specimens for toxicological screening. A history of suspected intoxicants will facilitate drug screening by laboratory personnel, and consultation with the drug assay laboratory will ensure that appropriate "high-yield" samples are sent for analysis.

3. Contact a **regional poison control center** for help with difficult intoxications or for information regarding specific therapeutic measures once an intoxicant has been identified.

B. Antidotes   Antidotes are available for about 5% of all poisonings. They may prove to be life-saving and are summarized in Tables 2 and 3.

C. Prevention of Toxin Absorption

1. **Decontamination of skin** to prevent dermal injury or transdermal drug absorption should begin after the removal of all contaminated clothing. The

TABLE 2. *Emergency antidotes*

Poison	Antidote	Adult antidote dose	Clinical features of intoxication
Acetaminophen	Acetylcysteine	140 mg/kg p.o. followed by 70 mg/kg p.o. q 4 hr for 3 days	No unique signs or symptoms
Arsenic	British antilewisite or	5 mg/kg i.m. followed by 2.5 mg/kg q 8–12 hr for 7 days	Nausea, vomiting, diarrhea, neuropathy, encephalopathy, and Mees' lines
	Penicillamine	250 mg p.o. q 6 hr for 10 days	
Atropine	Physostigmine salicylate	0.5–2.0 mg i.v. over 3–5 min and repeated q.45–60 min as needed	Dry skin, fever, mydriasis, agitation, and hallucinations
Carbon monoxide	Oxygen	100% F_iO_2	Headache, depressed mental status, syncope, tachypnea, and convulsions
Cyanide	Amyl nitrite	2 pearls for 15–30 sec every min until sodium nitrite is administered	Ataxia, dyspnea, convulsions, mydriasis, and almond or silver polish breath
	Sodium nitrite	10 ml of 3% solution i.v. over 3–5 min	
	Sodium thiosulfate	50 ml of 25% solution i.v. over 10 min	
Digoxin	Digoxin antibody Fab fragments	As per experimental protocol	Nausea, vomiting, delirium, syncope, arrhythmia, and hyperkalemia
Ethylene glycol	Ethyl alcohol	600 mg/kg of 100% alcohol initially, followed by 75–250 mg/kg/hr of 100% alcohol to maintain blood alcohol level at 100 mg/dl. May be administered i.v. as a 10% solution in D5W or can be given p.o.	Drunkenness, seizures, osmolar-gap, anion-gap metabolic acidosis, and oxylate crystals in the urine

TABLE 3. *Emergency antidotes*

Poison	Antidote	Adult antidote dose	Clinical features of intoxication
Gold	British antilewisite or	5 mg/kg i.m. followed by 2.5 mg/kg q 8–12 hr for 7 days	Nausea, vomiting diarrhea, neuropathy, encephalopathy, and Mees' lines
	Penicillamine	250 mg p.o. q 6 hr for 10 days	
Iron	Deferoxamine mesylate	1 g i.m. q 4–8 hr	Nausea, vomiting, diarrhea, abdominal pain, convulsions, and anion-gap metabolic acidosis
Insulin	Glucose	50–100 ml of D50W i.v.	Hunger, anxiety, diaphoresis, weakness, nausea, vomiting, coma, and convulsions
Lead	Calcium disodium versenate	12.5 mg/kg i.v. q 6 hr given over 1 hr in D5W for up to 5 days	Nausea, vomiting diarrhea, neuropathy, depressed mental status, and microcytic anemia with basophilic stippling
	British antilewisite	See gold	
Mercury	See gold		
Methyl alcohol	See ethylene glycol		Blindness; oxylate crystals are not formed
Nitrites, nitrates	Methylene blue	1–2 mg/kg i.v. over 5 min	Depressed mental status, orthostatic hypotension, tachypnea, and cyanosis
	Oxygen	100% F_iO_2	
Opiates, pentazocine HCL; propoxyphene HCl	Naloxone HCl	0.4 mg i.v.; may repeat as necessary; 2.0 mg may be needed for pentazocine or propoxyphene	Depressed mental status, euphoria, respiratory depression, and miosis
Organophosphates	Atropine sulfate	0.5–2 mg i.v. and repeated as necessary	Salivation, larcrimation, defecation, urination, miosis, and pulmonary congestion
	Pralidoxine chloride	1–2 g i.v. over 15–20 min. An additional 0.5 g/hr may be required	

affected areas should be washed with copious amounts of soap and water and measures taken to protect hospital personnel from self-contamination.

2. Prevention of gastrointestinal absorption

a. Evacuation of gastric contents should begin as soon as possible following an acute toxin ingestion. However, since the absorption of large overdoses of drugs tends to be slower than the absorption of usual therapeutic doses, gastric emptying is indicated even several hours after acute toxin ingestion. Strategies for evacuation of gastric contents are outlined in Fig. 2. **Contraindications** to the use of forced emesis include the ingestion of petroleum distillates or caustic substances, i.e., acids and bases. Gastric lavage should not be used following the ingestion of these caustic materials. Hemorrhagic diatheses are a relative contraindication to both types of gastric evacuation.

b. **Chelation of gastric and bowel contents.** Chelation of unabsorbed toxins in the gastrointestinal tract, i.e., iron with deferoxamine, occasionally may be of value.

c. **Surgical removal of toxins from the gastrointestinal tract** has been life-

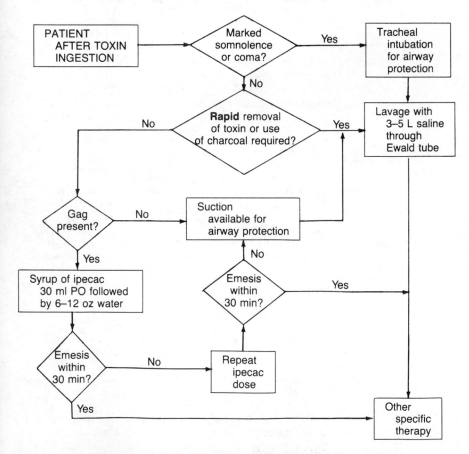

FIG. 2. Strategy for the evacuation of gastric contents. Syrup of ipecac may be administered through a nasogastric tube in uncooperative individuals.

saving following massive ingestions of iron and other heavy metals. Drug bezoars also can be effectively removed in this manner.

d. **Adsorption of drugs and chemicals to activated charcoal particles** effectively decreases their extent of absorption and thereby limits toxicity. Following gastric emptying, 50 to 100 g of **activated powdered charcoal** in 8 oz of water or 20% sorbitol should be given orally or by gastric tube. Although most toxins are adsorbed to activated charcoal, some small molecular weight toxins such as cyanide, lithium, and iron are not bound. On the other hand, acetylcysteine may be ineffective in the treatment of acetaminophen poisoning if given with activated charcoal, since it is readily adsorbed to this material. Therefore, the use of activated charcoal should be avoided in acetaminophen overdose, or previously administered charcoal should be removed by gastric lavage prior to the oral administration of acetylcysteine.

e. **Elimination of toxins in the stool.** Cathartics have traditionally been used to hasten the elimination of toxic substances in the stool despite lack of evidence that catharsis decreases total toxin absorption. However, since the administration of cathartics is relatively safe, this practice is still recommended. Following the instillation of activated charcoal, 30 g of **magnesium sulfate** or **sodium sulfate** in 300 ml of water should be given. **Contraindications** to the administration of cathartics include adynamic ileus, severe diarrhea, intestinal obstruction, abdominal trauma, renal failure (magnesium sulfate), and congestive heart failure (sodium sulfate).

D. **Enhancement of Toxin Elimination** Enhancement of toxin elimination is based on the premise that rapid removal of toxins from the bloodstream should result in improved patient survival. Unfortunately, many techniques used to accelerate toxin elimination such as emergent hemodialysis and/or hemoperfusion are associated with significant morbidity and rarely mortality. Therefore, the benefit of enhanced toxin elimination must be weighed against the risk of the removal technique.

1. **Forced diuresis** may enhance the elimination of certain drugs that are excreted in the urine and are not widely distributed in the body or highly plasma-protein bound. Increased urine flow may result in enhanced drug excretion, and alteration of urine pH can be used to decrease the reabsorption of ionizable toxins from urine to blood. Types of forced diureses are discussed below, and Table 4 indicates drugs amenable to each type of therapy. **Complications** of therapy include cerebral and pulmonary edema, congestive heart failure, and electrolyte (particularly hypokalemia) and acid-base abnormalities; thus, fluid

TABLE 4. *Elimination of drugs increased by forced diuresis*

Amphetamines (Ac)	Phenobarbital (Al)
Bromides (Sa)	Salicylates (Al)
Fenfluramine (Ac)	Strychnine (Ac)
Isoniazid (Al)	Quinidine (Ac)
Phencyclidine (Ac)	Quinine (Ac)

Ac, acid diuresis; Al, alkaline diuresis; Sa, saline diuresis.

status, serum electrolytes, arterial blood gases, and urine output should be monitored closely. Forced diuresis obviously cannot be used in patients with renal failure.

   a. **Forced saline diuresis** results in enhanced drug excretion solely through an increase in urine flow rate. Since passive reabsorption remains largely unaffected, only modest increases in toxin elimination are achieved. Initially, **5% dextrose in water** or **0.45% saline** at a rate of 500 ml/hr should be given to maintain a urine flow of 3 to 6 ml/kg/hr. A diuretic such as furosemide, 20 mg intravenously, may be needed to prevent volume overload. Addition of an osmotic agent, such as mannitol or urea, may prove more effective than forced saline diuresis alone because it also decreases the proximal tubular resorption of some drugs.

   b. **Forced alkaline diuresis** results in elevation of urinary pH above the pK_a of acidic compounds and thereby enhances their elimination by decreasing the amount of unionized drug available for reabsorption. Urinary pH should be maintained above 7.5 by the administration of 1 mEq/kg/hr of intravenous **sodium bicarbonate**; i.e., 3 ampules of sodium bicarbonate can be added to 1 liter of quarter normal saline administered at 500 ml/hr. Urine pH should be checked frequently to assure adequate alkalinization. The use of **acetazolamide** for alkalinization of urine is **not recommended** since systemic acidosis resulting from its use may lead to increased tissue permeability of acidic compounds and increased toxicity.

   c. **Forced acid diuresis** can effectively enhance the excretion of basic compounds in a manner analogous to that described above. **Ammonium chloride**, 20 mg/kg intravenously or orally every 6 hr, or **ascorbic acid** 0.5 to 2.0 g intravenously or orally every 4 hr, should provide an optimal urinary pH of 4.5 to 5.5. Urine flow rate should be 3 to 6 ml/kg/hr.

2. **Chelation** of iron and many heavy metals with deferoxamine, British antilewisite, or penicillamine, results in a markedly increased clearance of these compounds and helps minimize their toxicity. A regional poison control center should be contacted regarding the treatment of these intoxicants.

3. **Dialysis**

   a. **Gastrointestinal dialysis** is based on the finding that **repeated doses of activated charcoal** increase the clearances of drugs that have been absorbed into the systemic circulation. The treatment is devoid of significant adverse effects and appears most suited to toxins that are excreted partly in the bile and undergo enterohepatic recirculation. The clearances of phenobarbital, carbamazepine, phenylbutazone, digitoxin, and nadolol are markedly increased by repetitive doses of activated **charcoal 20 to 60 g orally** or by gastric tube **every 4 to 6 hr.**

   b. **Hemodialysis** is effective for the removal of small membrane-permeable, water-soluble toxins that are not highly bound to plasma proteins nor widely distributed throughout the body. Table 5 lists compounds that are not effectively removed by hemodialysis. Although hemodialysis can enhance the elimination of several hundred compounds, it is the mainstay of therapy only for intoxication with **ethylene glycol** and **methanol**. For other inges-

TABLE 5. *Drugs **not** effectively removed by hemodialysis*

Amitriptyline	Digitoxin	Opiates
Atropine	Digoxin	Pargyline
Chlordiazepoxide	Diphenhydramine	Phenelzine
Chloroquine	Doxepin	Promazine
Chlorpromazine	Ergotamine	Promethazine
Chlorpropamide	Imipramine	Protriptyline
Desipramine	Methaqualone	Secobarbital
Diazepam	Nortriptyline	Trifluoperazine

tions the risks of hemodialysis, which include infection, hemorrhage, extracorporeal clotting, hematomas, and hemodynamic instability, often outweigh the benefits of enhanced toxin removal. Hemodialysis is reserved for the therapy of life-threatening ingestion that has not responded to conventional measures or that cannot be managed conservatively because of the severity of the ingestion or because of the presence of hepatic or renal disease. Table 6 lists guidelines for the use of hemodialysis.

c. **Peritoneal dialysis** is used when hemodialysis or hemoperfusion is indicated but cannot be performed or in children who are too small for hemodialysis. Its major advantage is simplicity. **Disadvantages and potential complications** include lack of efficiency, peritoneal infection, intraabdominal trauma, and respiratory compromise.

d. **Charcoal or resin hemoperfusion** can enhance the elimination of a large number of poisons that are adsorbed to activated charcoal or polystyrene resin. They may be used for life-threatening intoxications (Table 6) involving hemoperfusable toxins. **Complications** include hemorrhage, thrombocytopenia, infection, and sorbent embolization.

4. The role of **plasmapheresis** and **exchange blood transfusion** in the treatment of poisoning remains unclear. However, they should be most applicable to the treatment of life-threatening intoxications by highly plasma protein-bound toxins that are not well removed by hemodialysis or hemoperfusion, i.e., chromate poisoning.

5. **Immunopharmacological therapy** utilizes antibody fragments to bind specific antigens (toxins) and thereby enhance their elimination from the circulation and minimize toxicity. Fab fragments directed toward digoxin molecules

TABLE 6. *Criteria for consideration of hemodialysis or hemoperfusion[a]*

Severe clinical intoxication with abnormal or widely fluctuating vital signs, including hypotension despite appropriate therapy, apnea, or severe hypothermia
Compromised function of an excretory or metabolic organ for the intoxicant
The presence of a material that is metabolized to a more toxic substance. Conversions of methanol to formaldehyde and ethylene glycol to oxalic acid are examples
Progressive clinical deterioration despite aggressive supportive care
Severe acid-base or electrolyte disturbances not responding to therapy
Ingestion and probable absorption of a potentially lethal dose of toxin
Potentially fatal toxin blood concentration
Prolonged coma

[a]A sufficient quantity of the toxin must be removed by hemodialysis or hemoperfusion.

have been successfully used to treat life-threatening digoxin intoxication unresponsive to conventional therapy.

E. **Psychiatric Consultation**   All patients presenting with intentional drug overdose should be seen by a psychiatrist.

III. **SPECIFIC TOXINS**   Fewer than 20 agents are responsible for 90% of intentional drug ingestions. The most frequently involved toxins are reviewed here.

A. **Acetaminophen**

1. **Toxicology.** Hepatic injury, cell death, and liver failure following acetaminophen poisoning result from the formation of a toxic metabolite and the inability of hepatic glutathione to detoxify this compound. **Hepatic toxicity** can be seen with acute acetaminophen ingestions as low as 7.5 g but is best **predicted by acetaminophen plasma concentrations** measured at least 4 hr after the time of ingestion (Fig. 3).

2. **Clinical manifestations.** Anorexia, nausea, vomiting, malaise, pallor, and diaphoresis occur during the first 24 hr but tend to resolve during the second day when hepatic necrosis becomes evident as transaminases and bilirubin rise and prothrombin time is prolonged. Hepatic failure, including jaundice, bleeding diathesis, hypoglycemia, and encephalopathy, presents at 3 to 5 days and often results in death.

3. **Management**

a. **Supportive care** is the cornerstone of management. However, **antidotal therapy must be used to treat significant intoxications** (Fig. 3).

b. **Acetylcysteine** (Mucomist®), the **preferred antidote**, is believed to prevent hepatotoxicity by providing sulfhydryl groups that bind the toxic metabolite. Acetylcysteine therapy should begin as soon as possible following large ingestions. The decision to continue therapy or institute acetylcysteine treatment should be based on a determination of acetaminophen plasma concentration at least 4 hr after drug ingestion. Therapy begun more than 24 hr after acute ingestion generally is ineffective. **Acetylcysteine therapy** consists of an oral loading dose of 140 mg/kg followed by oral doses of 70 mg/kg every 4 hr for 3 days. Activated charcoal should be avoided or removed by gastric lavage prior to the administration of acetylcysteine because charcoal effectively binds this antidote and may decrease its effectiveness. Acetylcysteine may be given intravenously (experimental protocol) to patients with persistent vomiting, intestinal ileus, or other contraindications to oral administration. However, intravenous use is associated with the potential risk of anaphylaxis.

B. **Alcohol (Ethanol)**

1. **Toxicology.** Central nervous system depression is the hallmark of alcohol intoxication. Blood levels of 300 to 400 mg/dl may result in respiratory depression, a major cause of death following alcohol ingestion.

2. **Clinical features** include nausea, vomiting, slurred speech, ataxia, and altered mental status. Hypothermia, cardiac arrhythmia, aspiration pneumonia, gastrointestinal hemorrhage, metabolic acidosis, acute hypoglycemia, pancreatitis, shock, or death can result from acute alcohol intoxication.

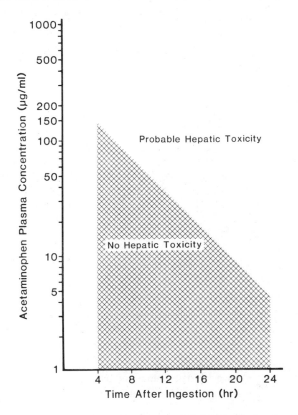

FIG. 3. Rumack–Matthew nomogram for acetaminophen poisoning. Reprinted from Rumack, B. H. (1975): *Pediatrics*, 55:873, with permission of the American Academy of Pediatrics.

    3. Management is supportive, with particular attention to respiratory status, serum glucose, electrolyte and acid-base abnormalities. **Thiamine** 100 mg should be given to all chronic alcohol abusers prior to the administration of glucose to avoid Wernicke-Korsakoff syndrome.

C. Aspirin

    1. Toxicology. The toxic properties of salicylates result primarily from their ability to stimulate respiration and disturb metabolic pathways. Ingestion of 10 g of aspirin usually results in toxicity and the degree of poisoning correlates well with serum salicylate levels obtained at least 6 hr after ingestion (Fig. 4).

    2. Clinical manifestations. Toxicity is manifested by nausea, flushing, vomiting, abdominal pain, tachypnea, **diaphoresis**, tinnitus, deafness, disorientation, irritability, lethargy, coma, and seizures. Following acute ingestions, hyperpnea and respiratory alkalosis precede the anion-gap metabolic acidosis that results from toxic effects on biochemical pathways. Hypovolemia, hypoglycemia or

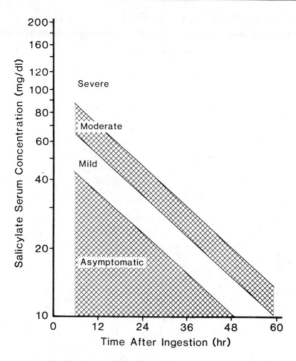

FIG. 4. Done nomogram for salicylate poisoning. Reprinted from Done, A. K. (1960): *Pediatrics*, 26:805, with permission of the American Academy of Pediatrics.

hyperglycemia, hypokalemia, pulmonary edema, hyperthermia, rhabdomyolysis, purpura, and gastrointestinal hemorrhage may also result from drug intoxication. Death usually results from cardiovascular collapse.

3. Management

    a. Supportive care is of paramount importance, with particular attention to correction of systemic acidosis, fluid, electrolyte, and glucose abnormalities, and control of body temperature.

    b. Specific therapy includes

        (1) Gastric emptying followed by administration of activated **charcoal** and a **cathartic** (II. C. 2. a., d. and e.).

        (2) Forced alkaline diuresis can be used to enhance the excretion of salicylates (II. D. 1. b.).

        (3) Hemodialysis effectively removes salicylates from the bloodstream but should be considered only for life-threatening intoxications (II. D. 3. b.).

D. Barbiturates

    1. Toxicology. Toxic effects of barbiturates are almost entirely due to progressive central nervous system depression. Respiratory depression is the usual cause of death, although cardiac depression and shock may contribute to mortality following large overdoses. Barbiturates are divided into two major groups: **long-acting**, less lipid-soluble compounds such as phenobarbital and barbital, and **short-acting**, highly lipid-soluble secobarbital, pentobarbital, and hexobarbital. Specific therapy is directed primarily at enhancing the elimination of the less well-sequestered, long-acting barbiturates.

2. **Clinical manifestations** include stupor, coma, areflexia, respiratory depression, adult respiratory distress syndrome, hypotension, shock, hypothermia, and bullous skin lesions. Patients may present with clinical brain death and a flat EEG yet recover fully following resolution of the acute intoxication.

3. **Management**

   a. **General supportive** care is the cornerstone of management. Attention should be directed to ventilatory support and protection of the airway, since aspiration pneumonia is the most common complication of coma accompanying barbiturate overdose.

   b. **Specific therapy**

   (1) **Gastric emptying** followed by the administration of **charcoal** and a **cathartic** should be performed as rapidly as possible (II. C. 2. a., d., and e.).

   (2) **Forced alkaline diuresis** will enhance the excretion of phenobarbital and barbital but has little effect on the short-acting barbiturates (II. D. 1. b.).

   (3) **Gastric dialysis** with repeated doses of **activated charcoal** is highly effective in the removal of long-acting barbiturates. Use of this technique may **triple the clearance** of phenobarbital and shorten the duration of coma (II. D. 3. a.).

   (4) **Hemodialysis and hemoperfusion** enhance the elimination of long-acting barbiturates but have no impact on the clearance of short-acting compounds. Because of its morbidity, hemodialysis is reserved for life-threatening intoxications unresponsive to the measures described above. The effectiveness of gastric dialysis may supplant the use of hemodialysis or hemoperfusion.

E. **Narcotics**   Narcotics are a diverse group of drugs including not only heroin, morphine, and codeine, but also synthetic compounds such as meperidine, butorphanol, propoxyphene, pentazocine, methadone, and nalbuphine.

   1. **Toxicology.** Toxicity is manifested primarily by central nervous system depression. Respiratory depression is the major cause of death although vascular collapse may occur following massive overdoses.

   2. **Clinical manifestations.** The hallmarks of narcotic overdose are **coma, respiratory depression,** and **miosis.** However, hypoxia and respiratory acidosis may result in mydriasis, shock, and cardiovascular collapse. Other complications include convulsions and narcotic-induced pulmonary edema.

3. Management

a. **Immediate** attention should be given to the **assessment and maintenance of ventilation and oxygenation.** Tracheal intubation and supplemental oxygen may be required. Supportive therapy should be given as necessary.

b. **Specific therapy**

(1) **Gastric emptying** and the administration of **activated charcoal** and a **cathartic** are indicated for the treatment of narcotic ingestions (II. C. 2. a., d., and e.).

(2) **Naloxone,** a pure narcotic antagonist, is capable of reversing the pharmacological effects of opioid agents. Initial naloxone dosage is 0.4 mg (2 ampules) intravenously but 2 mg (10 ampules) may be required to antagonize the effects of pentazocine or propoxyphene. Since the duration of naloxone action may be as short as 20 min and the effects of many narcotics, especially methadone, last much longer, repetitive doses of naloxone and careful patient observation often are required.

F. Phenothiazines

1. **Toxicology.** Toxicity is characterized by central nervous system depression, extrapyramidal reactions, central and peripheral anticholinergic manifestations, alpha-adrenergic blockade, and depressant effects on myocardial contractility, automaticity, and conduction.

2. **Clinical manifestations** are varied. Central nervous system findings include confusion, delirium, hallucinations, sedation, stupor, coma, respiratory depression, loss of thermoregulation, and seizures. Tachycardia, mydriasis, ileus, urinary retention, constipation, dry mucous membranes, and flushed, warm dry skin characterize anticholinergic signs and symptoms. Alpha-adrenergic blockade is manifested by hypotension, and cardiac toxicity, related to a direct, quinidine-like effect, results in decreased myocardial contractility, hypotension, and dysrhythmia. The most common arrhythmia is sinus tachycardia but supraventricular tachycardia, impaired conduction, and ventricular arrhythmia may occur. Extrapyramidal reactions include akathesia, akinesia, a Parkinson-like syndrome, and dystonic reactions.

3. **Management**

a. **General supportive care.** Electrocardiographic monitoring is required for all patients following significant phenothiazine ingestion. Lidocaine and phenytoin are the agents of choice for treating life-threatening ventricular arrhythmia, and since phenothiazines result in QT and QRS interval prolongation, the use of quinidine or procainamide is contraindicated. Although this arrhythmia rarely results in death, patients should be monitored until arrhythmia-free for at least 24 hr.

b. **Specific therapy**

(1) Since phenothiazines inhibit gastric motility, **gastric emptying** is **indicated regardless of the time of ingestion.** Activated charcoal and a cathartic also should be given (II. C. 2. a., d., and e.).

(2) **Diphenhydramine hydrochloride,** 25 to 50 mg orally or parenterally, or benztropine mesylate, 1 to 2 mg orally or parenterally, relieves

extrapyramidal symptoms. Following treatment of acute extrapyramidal reactions, diphenhydramine 25 to 50 mg orally t.i.d. should be continued for 1 to 3 days to prevent recurrence of symptoms.

(3) **Hemodialysis** is ineffective in the treatment of phenothiazine poisoning since these compounds are highly protein and tissue bound.

G. **Tricyclic Antidepressants**   Representative compounds include amitriptyline, nortriptyline, imipramine, desipramine, protriptyline, maprotiline, and doxepin.

1. **Toxicology** of these compounds is similar to that described for phenothiazines. Extrapyramidal reactions are not a prominent feature of tricyclic antidepressant overdose. **Cardiotoxicity** is the major source of mortality in these patients. A QRS interval duration of greater than 100 msec is a poor prognostic sign and indicates severe toxicity.

2. **Clinical manifestations** are similar to those presented for phenothiazine intoxication.

3. **Management**

a. **Supportive care**

(1) Aggressive supportive care should be instituted, including **continuous electrocardiographic monitoring.**

(2) **Sodium bicarbonate,** 0.5 to 2 mEq/kg by intravenous bolus, followed by an intravenous infusion of sodium bicarbonate, 3 ampules (132 mEq) in quarter normal saline, to maintain a blood pH of 7.5 is the agent of choice for treatment of tricyclic antidepressant-induced cardiac dysrhythmia. For an arrhythmia that does not respond to sodium bicarbonate, either **phenytoin,** 18 mg/kg intravenously (maximum rate of infusion = 50 mg/min), or **physostigmine salicylate,** 1 to 2 mg every 30 to 60 min by slow intravenous injection, is the next agent of choice. Lidocaine is of questionable efficacy and as for phenothiazines, the use of **quinidine or procainamide** is **contraindicated. Propranolol** is recommended for the treatment of supraventricular arrhythmia but should be used with caution if hypotension, conduction defects, reactive airway disease, or congestive heart failure are present. Severe bradyarrhythmia or heart block unresponsive to medical therapy is treated with pacemaker insertion. All patients should be monitored until arrhythmia-free for at least 24 hr.

(3) **Diazepam** is the drug of choice for the treatment of seizures. In individuals unresponsive to conventional therapy, physostigmine salicylate, 1 to 2 mg every 30 to 60 min by slow intravenous injection, may be used for seizure management.

(4) Since physostigmine salicylate has a **very narrow therapeutic index** and short-lived pharmacologic actions, its use to reverse coma or control agitated patients is **not** recommended.

b. **Specific therapy**

(1) **Gastric emptying** should be followed by administration of **activated charcoal** and a **cathartic** (II. C. 2. a., d., and e.).

(2) Gastric dialysis with repetitive doses of activated charcoal may enhance elimination because tricyclic antidepressants undergo extensive enterohepatic recirculation (II. D. 3. a.).

(3) Hemodialysis and hemoperfusion have no role in the treatment of tricyclic antidepressant intoxication because the extensive degree of protein- and tissue-binding severely limits the amount of drug that can be removed utilizing these techniques.

BIBLIOGRAPHY

Haddad, L. M., and Winchester, J. F. (1983): *Clinical Management of Poisoning and Drug Overdose*. W. B. Saunders Company, Philadelphia.

Levy, G. (1982): Gastrointestinal clearance of drugs with activated charcoal. *NEJM*, 307:676–678.

Neuvonen, P. J. (1982): Clinical pharmacokinetics of oral activated charcoal in acute intoxications. *Clin. Pharmacol.*, 7:465–489.

Rumack, B. H. (1977): *Management of Acute Poisoning and Overdose*. Rocky Mountain Poison Center, Denver.

Winchester, J. F., Gelfand, M. C., Knepshield, J. H., and Schreiner, G. E. (1977): Dialysis and hemoperfusion of poisons and drugs—update. *Trans. Am. Soc. Artif. Intern. Organs*, 23:762–842.

25.

Psychiatric and Sexual Disorders

Steven L. Dubovsky

25.

Psychiatric and Sexual Disorders

I. DEPRESSION

A. General Considerations Although 15% to 30% of the general population suffers from depression, and the same proportion holds true for all medical patients, lack of familiarity with diagnostic criteria and treatment methods results in only 10% of depressed patients receiving adequate treatment. Recent research suggesting that many depressions have a biological as well as a psychological component has led to increased use of medications and electroconvulsive therapy (ECT) in addition to psychotherapy. Of the prescriptions written for antidepressants, 60% are written by nonpsychiatric physicians.

B. Diagnosis

1. Depressed patients usually display a **disturbance of mood** (dysphoria) characterized by sadness, crying spells, discouragement, irritability, and hostility. Approximately 70% of depressed patients suffer anxiety as well. In **masked depression**, multiple somatic complaints or insomnia are more apparent than dysphoria.

2. A change in thinking in depressed patients is characterized by **negative views of the self, the environment**, and the future, as indicated by guilt; lowered self-esteem; self-hatred; loss of interest in occupational, social, and sexual activities; hopelessness; helplessness; difficulty concentrating; indecisiveness; and suicidal thoughts.

3. **Multiple somatic complaints,** particularly fatigue, insomnia, weakness, headaches, abdominal pain, chest pain, back pain, nausea, and vomiting, commonly are symptoms of depression.

4. **Vegetative signs,** which may indicate disordered hypothalamic function, include insomnia (especially early-morning awakening), diurnal variation of mood or other symptoms (worse in morning and better later in the day), decreased or increased appetite with corresponding weight change, psychomotor slowing, and constipation.

5. **Psychosocial disturbances** that may be due to covert depression include frequent job changes, disorganized behavior, disheveled or dirty demeanor, neurotic or compulsive thoughts, and unusual preoccupation with religion.

6. Many depressed patients have experienced a **recent loss** of an important person, of status, health, income, or an ideal.

7. **A past history of depression or of response to antidepressants or ECT** increases the suspicion that the current episode is due to depression.

TABLE 1. *Illnesses that may cause depression*

Organic brain syndrome	Multiple sclerosis
Viral infections (hepatitis,	Systemic lupus
infectious mononucleosis)	erythematosus
Pneumonia	Anemia
Pancreatic carcinoma	Hypokalemia
Endocrine disease (thyroid,	Rheumatoid arthritis
adrenal, parathyroid,	Congestive heart failure
pituitary)	

8. Depression and related disorders appear to have a genetic component, resulting in an increased **family history of depression, response to treatment for depression, mania, suicide, alcoholism, and antisocial behavior** in depressed patients.

9. **Laboratory tests.** For unknown reasons, depression may be associated with abnormalities on a number of tests of endocrine function.

   a. Although it is still controversial, the **dexamethasone suppression test** (DST) holds the most promise for clinical diagnosis. Dexamethasone 1 mg is given at 11:00 p.m., and serum cortisol is measured the next day at 4 p.m. for outpatients and at 4:00 and 11:00 p.m. for inpatients. When there is no physiologic explanation (e.g., Cushing's disease), patients who do not suppress serum cortisol below 5 μg/dl are likely to be depressed, regardless of their actual symptoms. A negative DST (i.e., serum cortisol values of 5 μg/dl or below) however, does not exclude the diagnosis of depression.

   b. Some authorities feel that a blunted elevation of thyroid-stimulating hormone (TSH) 30 min following an infusion of thyrotropin-releasing hormone (TRH) **(TRH stimulation test)** in the absence of thyroid disease is also correlated with a diagnosis of depression. However, if the suspicion of depression is great enough to warrant a TRH stimulation test, a trial of antidepressants is probably indicated, and the test may not be necessary.

C. **Treatment**

   1. **Physical illnesses** (Table 1), which may present with depression as the only obvious complaint, should be excluded before therapy for depression is instituted, and **medications** (Table 2) that may produce depression as a side effect should be discontinued or changed.

   2. Since many depressions arise in the context of an interpersonal stress (often

TABLE 2. *Medications that produce depression as a side effect*

Antihypertensives (reserpine,	Adrenal seroids and
methyldopa, clonidine,	ACTH[a]
spironolactone)	L-DOPA
Propranolol	Alcohol
Antianxiety drugs	Withdrawal from
Oral contraceptives	amphetamines and
	cocaine

[a]Adrenocorticotrophic hormone.

a loss), **psychotherapy** is an important component of any treatment approach. Useful techniques include:

a. Recognizing the importance of the physician to the patient and of the patient's sensitivity to rejection. Such recognition leads to **regular appointments**, maintenance of a **positive, hopeful attitude**, and **maximum physician availability** to the acutely depressed patient with a minimum of cross-coverage.

b. Setting realistic goals in medical and psychological therapy that the patient can accomplish.

c. Discussing emotions and thoughts that may be outside the patient's awareness, such as:

   (1) Unresolved grief.

   (2) Covert anger and **guilt** about feeling angry at loved ones.

   (3) Desire to **feel better without having to work at it.**

d. Helping the patient **confront unrealistic negative attitudes** and feelings of helplessness while demonstrating to the patient that he is not as powerless as he feels.

3. Antidepressants in common use are described in Table 3.

  a. The use of medications should be considered in the presence of:

   (1) Past history or family history of response to an antidepressant or ECT.

   (2) Family history of depression.

   (3) Significant vegetative signs.

   (4) Severe or psychotic symptoms.

   (5) Symptoms that do not appear in response to a psychosocial stress.

   (6) Failure to respond to psychotherapy.

   (7) Positive DST.

  b. Guidelines for selecting an antidepressant include the following:

   (1) Begin with a medication that the patient or a blood relative has responded to in the past and avoid medications to which there is a history of a negative response.

   (2) Sedating antidepressants such as amitriptyline, doxepin, and trazodone are useful for depression which is accompanied by anxiety, and insomnia, whereas less sedating medications such as desipramine, amoxapine, and maprotiline are used for retarded depressions.

   (3) Claims that doxepin and amoxapine are less cardiotoxic have recently been questioned.

   (4) Amoxapine has a more rapid onset of action but, as neuroleptics, tends to cause abnormal movements.

   (5) Maprotiline and amoxapine lower the seizure threshold and should not be given to epileptics.

   (6) Trazodone, amoxapine, maptrotiline and protriptyline are less anticholinergic.

TABLE 3. *First-line treatment of depression*

Drug	Usual daily dose (mg)	Interactions[a]	Side effects[a]	Management of overdose[a]
Tricyclic antidepressants:				
Amitriptyline (Elavil®)	150–300 (30–50)	Interferes with action of guanethidine, clonidine, and bethanedine	Anticholinergic (may precipitate glaucoma and urinary retention)	Death may occur at 1,200 mg of imipramine; not uncommon with 2,000 mg
Nortriptyline[e] (Aventyl®)	50–150 (25–50)	Decreased blood levels with barbiturates and alcohol	Postural hypotension	Physostigmine 0.5–2 mg i.v. for coma; repeat every 30–90 min
Protriptyline (Vivactil®)	10–60	Hypertension with amphetamines, norepinephrine, phenylephrine, MAOI	May precipitate heart block if preexisting BBB	Gastric lavage early plus activated charcoal
Imipramine[b,c] (Tofranil®)	150–300 (30–50)	Decreased effect of L-DOPA	Quinidine-like effect	Dialysis and diuresis of no va ue
Desipramine[e] (Pertofrane®)	150–250 (25–50)	Increased phenytoin toxicity	Weight gain, especially with amitriptyline	Phenytoin for cardiac toxicity and seizures
Trimipramine (Surmontil®)	50–300		Can cause impotence	Diazepam for seizures
Doxepin (Sinequan®)	75–150 (25–50)		? Sudden death	Alpha agonist action may be blocked
Amoxapine[c,d] (Ascendin®)	150–300 (25–75)		May be teratogenic (limb deformities)	
Tetracyclic antidepressant:			Excreted in breast milk	
Maprotiline[d] (Ludiomil®)	150–300 (25–50)			
Heterocyclic:				
Trazodone[c,d] (Desyrel®)	150–400 (50–150)			

( ) Indicates recommended geriatric dose range.
[a]These interactions, side effects, and management of overdose are similar for most antidepressants.
[b]Recommended pediatric dose = 2.5–4.5 mg/kg/day.
[c]Have been used for endogenous anxiety and phobias.
[d]Less postural hypotension.
[e]Appear to have a therapeutic window (less effective at blood levels below 50 mg/ml or above 150 mg/ml).
MAOI, monoamine oxidase inhibitor.
BBB, bundle branch block.
MHPG, 3-methoxy-4-hydroxyphenylglycol.

c. With the exception of trazodone, all antidepressants may be given in **one dose at bedtime** to make use of sedating side effects for sleep, to decrease daytime sedation and bothersome anticholinergic side effects, and to enhance patient compliance. However, this dosage regimen may cause nightmares in some patients.

(1) If the patient reports adverse effects after a test dose of 25 mg of amitriptyline or its equivalent, he is unlikely to continue taking the drug.

(2) If the patient tolerates the test dose, increase the dosage by 25 to 50 mg every other night until therapeutic levels are reached (Table 3). Blood levels should be obtained for nortriptyline and desipramine to monitor their therapeutic windows (decreased likelihood of response below 50 ng/ml or above 150 ng/ml), or to check for noncompliance or rapid metabolism in nonresponders.

(3) Antidepressants may take 3 to 4 weeks to take effect.

(4) If medications are effective, they should be continued for 9 to 12 months and then withdrawn at a rate of 25 mg/week. Reemergence of symptoms indicates the need for reinstitution of the drug at the previous dose. Rapid withdrawal may cause malaise or seizures.

(5) Patients with a past history of **mania** may require concomitant lithium therapy to prevent a manic response to the antidepressants. Uses, precautions, and interactions of lithium, which may also prevent recurrent attacks of depression and which may be effective for some acute depressions, are summarized in Table 4.

d. Failure to respond to an antidepressant is usually due to failure to prescribe an adequate dose, to noncompliance, to misdiagnosis, or to interaction with another drug that lowers blood levels. If these causes are excluded, an antidepressant effect may be achieved in a nonresponder by:

(1) Increasing the dose of the antidepressant.

(2) Changing to an antidepressant with a **different presumed mechanism of action** (imipramine, desipramine, doxepin, amoxapine, and maprotiline are thought to increase brain levels of norepinephrine, whereas amitriptyline and trazodone are serotoninergic).

(3) Administering a **second line treatment** (Table 5):

(a) Monoamine oxidase (MAO) inhibitors are especially useful when appetite and sleep are increased or psychomotor slowing, and self-pity are prominent.

(b) Neuroleptics may ameliorate depressions accompanied by agitation, delusions, hallucinations, or severe incapacitation.

(c) Low doses (25 μg) of **T3** added to standard therapy improves some treatment-resistant depressions, even if thyroid function is normal.

(d) Short-term administration of **methylphenidate** in low doses may improve depression that occurs in the context of a chronic medical

TABLE 4. *Use of lithium carbonate*

Drug	Usual daily dose (mg)	Special characteristics and indications	Interactions	Side effects	Management of overdose
Lithium carbonate	900–2,400 (therapeutic serum concentration = 0.5–1.5 mEq/l)	Proven effective for management and prophylaxis of mania Useful in prevention of recurrent depression with past history of mania (bipolar depression) and some recurrent unipolar depression May be useful in treatment of some depressions Useful for management of cluster headache and neutropenia	Diuretics increase blood levels High doses of neuroleptics with lithium may cause neurotoxicity, especially in hot weather ↑ lithium toxicity with antibiotics (esp. tetracycline) ↓ lithium levels with phenothiazines ↑ lithium levels with indomethacin and methyldopa Rapid cycling between mania and depression may occur when lithium and tricyclics are combined	GI: Nausea, vomiting, diarrhea, abdominal pain Dazed, tired feeling Fine tremor Thirst, polyuria nephrogenic diabetes insipidus Nontoxic goiter Irreversible renal carnage Hyperparathyroidism Leukocytosis Toxicity (>2 mEq/l) delirium, coma, muscle tone, fasciculations Highly teratogenic Excreted in breast milk	Osmotic diuresis to increase excretion: mannitol, diuretics, $NaHCO_3$ Intravenous saline may hasten urinary excretion of lithium Dialysis

TABLE 5. *Second-line antidepressant regimens*

Drug	Usual daily dose (mg)	Special characteristics and indications	Interactions	Side effects	Management of overdose
MAO inhibitors: Phenelzine (Nardil*)	60	Resistance to tricyclics Phobic-anxiety states Panic attacks Atypical depression[a] Tranylcypromine only for inpatients Phenelzine may also be an antihypertensive	Severe hypertension with sympathomimetics, methyldopa, tyramine-containing foods, meperidine, L-DOPA, antihistamines, tricyclics, many others Potentiation by thiazide diuretics	Anticholinergic Anorexic Irritability Impotence Postural hypotension Liver damage Infertility and fetal resorption in animals	Lethal dose = 6–10 times daily dose Treat hypertension with phentolamine 2–5 mg i.v. or chlorpromazine 50–100 mg i.m.
Tranylcypromine (Parnate*)	20				
Antipsychotics: Chlorpromazine	50–300[b]	Useful in agitated depression, depression with marked anxiety, or psychotic depression	May interfere with some antihypertensives Additive anticholinergic side effects Potentiation of CNS depressants by sedating antipsychotics Phenobarbital decreases blood levels	Anticholinergic Postural hypotension (less with haloperidol) Quinidine-like effect (esp. thioridazine) Parkinsonian side effects (thioridazine) Sudden death (thioridazine) Tardive dyskinesia (thioridazine) Impotence (thioridazine)	Fluids—but diuresis ineffective for removal Treat hypotension with **pure alpha agonist** (e.g., phenelphrine) Do **not** use α, β stimulators, as α action may be blocked, resulting in pure beta stimulation and hypotension Warm for hypothermia Seizures and arrhythmias rare Treat anticholinergic effect with physostigmine Dialysis ineffective
Thioridazine (**never** give >800 mg/day)	50–300				
Haloperidol	1–10				
Loxapine	10–50				
Stimulants: Methylphenidate	10–25	Useful in elderly and medically ill patients		Tolerance and addiction rare in depressed patients	
Other adjuncts: T_3 (Cytomel*)	25–50 μg	May enhance responsiveness to tricyclics, especially in women	May be safely combined with MAO inhibitors		
L-Tryptophane + pyridoxine (vitamin B_6)	4–15g/200/mg	Serotoninergic (B_6 is a necessary cofactor)			

[a] Increased sleep; worse at night; increased appetite; initial insomnia; anxiety; lethargy.
[b] Doses used to treat schizophrenia and mania are higher.

illness or an organic brain syndrome. Tolerance and addiction are rare in these circumstances.

(4) **ECT** is the most effective treatment for depression. It is indicated for severe, life-threatening, or treatment-resistant depression.

D. Suicide   Suicide results in a 5% to 15% mortality rate in depression. The majority of patients who kill themselves visit a primary care physician before their deaths, and up to 75% communicate their intent directly or indirectly before their deaths.

1. **Risk factors** indicating significant danger of suicide should be evaluated in **all** depressed or unhappy patients.

   a. **Diagnosis.** Most suicide victims are depressed and/or alcoholics. Patients with organic brain syndromes, patients with a history of narcotic abuse, and patients with schizophrenia also have higher suicide rates.

   b. **Present illness.** A recent loss or persistent complaints of insomnia are common in suicidal patients. Hopelessness is also a danger sign.

   c. **Past history.** The risk of successful suicide increases with the number of previous attempts, especially if they were carefully planned or dangerous or if three or more attempts were made, and with a past history of impulsive behavior.

   d. **Family history.** Patients who have lost a family member through suicide are at greater risk of killing themselves, as are those with family members who overtly or covertly want the patient to die.

   e. **Associated illnesses.** Chronically and terminally ill patients may be at greater risk of committing suicide.

   f. **Demographic factors.** The risk is highest in socially isolated, white, older, men.

   g. **Physician's reaction.** Patients may communicate suicidal intent **nonverbally** and make the doctor feel that they may be suicidal. **Such instinctive impressions should be taken seriously.**

2. Since suicidal patients often do not volunteer suicidal thoughts, **evaluation of immediate risk** must be by direct questioning about whether the patient:

   a. Ever feels so bad that life does not seem worth living.

   b. Has thoughts of committing suicide.

   c. Has a specific plan that can be carried out.

   d. Has rehearsed the plan (e.g., by placing an unloaded gun to his head).

   e. Sees no reason not to die.

3. **Treatment**

   a. High risk patients must be **hospitalized immediately** and placed under **constant observation.**

      (1) Most patients are relieved to have suicidal intent uncovered and consent to voluntary admission to a medical or psychiatric floor. In most states, a suicidal patient who refuses admission can be hospitalized involuntarily for 72 hr by any physician who can state that the patient is

dangerous to himself or to others because of a mental illness (e.g., depression).

(2) Patients who are extremely agitated or who threaten to leave can be restrained or sedated.

(3) Psychiatric evaluation of all suicidal patients should be requested as quickly as possible.

b. Immediate risk usually **decreases within a few days** if the patient can be kept from acting on self-destructive impulses.

c. Treatment for depression should be instituted rapidly.

d. Suicide risk, which may increase as depression subsides, should be monitored throughout treatment, and the patient encouraged to notify the physician or nursing staff immediately if suicidal feelings return.

E. **Prognosis**   Although it may remit spontaneously within 6 to 12 months, depression tends to become chronic in up to 40% of patients. The risk of chronicity is increased by lack of adequate treatment.

Depression has a strong tendency to recur, with symptoms reappearing within 2 years in up to 90% of patients in some studies. When symptoms recur, or the DST becomes positive, antidepressant therapy should be reinstituted promptly.

II. ANXIETY

A. **General Considerations**   Anxiety is a prominent complaint in 10% to 15% of medical outpatients, in 10% of inpatients, and in 2% to 5% of otherwise healthy individuals. Like depression, anxiety may represent an **exogenous** response to an external stress or a psychological conflict, or it may be **endogenous**, in which case it is presumably related to as yet unidentified biological factors. Examples of endogenous anxiety are **panic attacks** in which unpredictable episodes of intense dread, often accompanied by signs of autonomic arousal, occur spontaneously, and **phobias** that are not precipitated by exposure to a frightening situation. Endogenous forms of anxiety may lead to **anticipatory anxiety**, a form of exogenous anxiety in which the patient learns to fear spontaneous anxiety attacks.

B. **Diagnosis**   Even when an anxious mood is not apparent, signs of arousal such as tachycardia, palpitations, urinary frequency, diaphoresis, dry mouth, headache, or hyperventilation syndrome may be due to anxiety.

C. **Psychological Causes**   Hospitalized patients may be anxious about death, the mutilating effects of illness or surgery, losing control, or closeness to or dependency on others. Some inpatients, particularly those whose dependent status induces **regression** (psychological functioning appropriate to childhood and consisting of low frustration tolerance, frequent complaints, and difficulty tolerating being alone), develop **separation anxiety** (demands for attention whenever they are separated from important caretakers and family) and **stranger anxiety** (distress when confronted with new personnel, including new house officers). Anxiety that appears during hospitalization may also be due to an **organic brain syndrome** caused by the illness, to prescribed medications or to withdrawal from CNS depressants, or it may signal the emergence of a covert psychosis. 30% of apparent cases of anxiety are due to an underlying **depression.**

D. Treatment

1. **Illnesses** in which anxiety may be a presenting complaint because of stimulation of the sympathetic nervous system, increased heart rate or unknown mechanisms (Table 6) should be excluded before standard treatments for anxiety are applied. Some **drugs**, especially amphetamines, monosodium glutamate, and caffeine, may produce anxiety as a side effect, whereas neuroleptic-induced increased motor activity (akathisia) mimics anxiety and often makes the patient feel anxious because he cannot stop moving around. Abstinence from most centrally acting drugs is also commonly associated with anxiety.

2. **Psychological techniques** depend on first determining the cause of the patient's anxiety. For example, if the patient is anxious because he does not understand the illness or procedure, care should be taken to **explain** it to him in greater detail. Asking the patient to describe his understanding of his situation may reveal unrealistic fears that respond to reassurance. Patients who worry that they will be less attractive, powerful, or important and attempt to reassure themselves with excessive demonstrations of their beauty, strength, or importance—e.g., by exercising conspicuously shortly after a myocardial infarction—may be reassured that they still possess these attributes (e.g., "only a person of great strength would be able to lie still and cooperate with treatment even if he felt that he did not need to be in the hospital"). Patients who are afraid of loss of control should be permitted as much control as possible, for example, by tailoring medication schedules to their preference. Patients who become anxious when they are left alone should receive unlimited visiting by familiar people and frequent checks from the nursing staff. If they also seem to become upset when they are confronted with new faces, visits by unfamiliar people and changes of staff and physicians should be minimized whenever possible.

3. **Adjunctive measures** are particularly helpful to patients who are afraid of or cannot tolerate medications. Patients with acute anxiety or pain who are not threatened by relaxation are good candidates for **hypnosis**, whereas **biofeedback** is best applied to people who feel more comfortable with a machine or who have specific physiologic reactions to anxiety such as hypertension or migraine headache.

TABLE 6. *Illnesses that may produce anxiety*

Tumors
  Pheochromocytoma, carcinoid
Endocrine and metabolic
  Hypoglycemia, hyperthyroidism, hypocalcemia, Cushing's
    syndrome, porphyria
Cardiopulmonary
  Mitral valve prolapse, arteriosclerotic heart disease, paroxysmal
    tachycardias, COPD[a], pulmonary embolus, hypoxemia, asthma
Neurologic
  Temporal lobe epilepsy, organic brain disease, multiple sclerosis,
    cerebrovascular disease
Infections
  Tuberculosis, brucellosis

[a]Chronic obstructive pulmonary disease.

4. Antianxiety medications (Table 7).

a. Benzodiazepines are most likely to relieve exogenous anxiety (e.g., reactions to illness) when symptoms are **acute** and the patient is **motivated** to improve. Patients with limited psychological resources may need long-term benzodiazepine therapy, but patients who have not been receiving antianxiety drugs chronically should be told in advance that psychological and physical dependency can best be avoided if the drugs are only prescribed for 2 to 4 weeks.

(1) Benzodiazepines should be prescribed for no more than 1 to 2 weeks, if at all, for patients with a history of **drug or alcohol abuse.**

(2) To prevent the patient from becoming increasingly preoccupied with anxiety and medication because symptoms are not controlled, benzodiazepines should be prescribed in an **adequate dose.**

(3) Because of their long half-lives, most benzodiazepines can be prescribed in **one or two daily doses**, with the majority of the medication being administered at night to minimize daytime sedation and to enhance sleep.

TABLE 7. *Some antianxiety drugs*

Class	Examples	Usual daily dose (mg)	Comment
Benzodiazepines	Diazepam (Valium®)	4–20	Abstinence syndromes may be delayed; more common with more than 40–60 mg/day of diazepam or equivalent
	Chlordiazepoxide (Librium®)	20–100	
	Clorazepate (Tranxene®)	15–22.5	
	Oxazepam (Serax®)	30–45	
	Lorazepam (Ativan®)	1–10	Cimetidine increases blood levels of diazepam and chlordiazepoxide
	Alprazolam (Xanax®)	1.5–6	
	Flurazepam (Dalmane®)	15–30	
	Temazepam (Restoril®)	15–30	Alprazolam is the first benzodiazepine of choice for endogenous anxiety
	Triazolam (Halcion®)	0.25–0.75	
			Fatalities with overdose rare unless taken with alcohol or other drugs or with doses >700 mg/day
			Slow onset of action for temazepam makes it a poor choice for initial insomnia
			Rebound insomnia with triazolam
			Flurazepam can cause sedation short-term
Sedative autonomic antihistamines	Hydroxyzine (Atarax®)	100–200	No tolerance or dependence
	Diphenhydramine (Benadryl®)	100–200	Anxiety reduction less reliable than benzodiazapines
			May be useful as hypnotic in elderly
Beta-blocking agents	Propranolol (Inderal®)	40–120	Useful for anxiety with autonomic manifestations
			Also helpful for stage fright
			Effective in agitated, demented patients

(4) Lower doses and **shorter-acting preparations** (e.g., lorazepam) are preferable in **older** and **brain-injured patients** to prevent paradoxical excitement or oversedation.

(5) Patients who do not feel better after 2 weeks of treatment with benzodiazepine are unlikely to benefit later from that drug.

(6) Alprazolam may relieve anxiety mixed with depression.

(7) Although physical dependence is a definite concern in patients taking more than 40 to 60 mg of diazepam or its equivalent for more than a month, habituation and abstinence syndromes may occur at lower doses. Withdrawal symptoms, which consist of anxiety, agitation, delirium, and sometimes seizures, may not appear until 10 to 14 days after abrupt discontinuation of the drug. Despite these concerns, addiction to benzodiazepines that are prescribed appropriately in medical practice is extremely rare.

b. Although their antianxiety action is less predictable, **sedative-autonomic antihistamines** such as diphenhydramine (Benadryl®) and hydroxyzine (Atarax®) may be prescribed for patients in whom addiction is a concern and for older patients.

c. Beta-blocking agents may decrease stage fright and anxiety accompanied by tachycardia or other signs of autonomic arousal.

d. Neuroleptics (antipsychotic drugs) are indicated for acute mania and schizophrenia and for chronic schizophrenia. Short-term administration of nonsedating neuroleptics (e.g., trifluoperazine, thiothixene) may relieve anxiety without producing unwanted sedation, while anticholinergic side effects may decrease gastrointestinal manifestations of anxiety. However, longterm side effects, especially tardive dyskinesia, preclude prolonged administration unless a chronic or recurrent psychosis is ameliorated by a neuroleptic.

e. Because **barbiturates** and related compounds like **meprobamate, glutethimide**, and **etchlorvynol** produce tolerance, addiction and dangerous abstinence syndromes and are potentially lethal when taken in overdose, they should **never** be prescribed de novo for anxiety or insomnia. Patients taking these medications should be withdrawn gradually whenever possible.

f. Symptoms of **endogenous anxiety** (e.g., bouts of extreme anxiety or phobias unrelated to precipitating events) may respond well to medications that are not generally used for exogenous anxiety.

(1) The safest initial drug is **alprazolam**, up to 2 mg t.i.d. Alprazolam must be **discontinued gradually** to avoid withdrawal seizures.

(2) If symptoms are not substantially improved within 2 weeks of treatment with alprazolam, **impramine, amoxapine**, or **trazodone** should be administered for 1 month in standard antidepressant doses. Patients who do not respond to these antidepressants may improve with a **MAO inhibitor.**

E. Insomnia Insomnia, a common complaint in medical inpatients, is often a symptom of anxiety, pain, depression, or the discomfort of sleeping in a strange bed.

When physical disorders that disturb sleep, especially **organic brain syndromes, gastroesophageal reflux** and **sleep apnea**, are not present, benzodiazepine hypnotics (Table 7) should be offered as required (p.r.n.) to the patient rather than routinely administered.

1. **Flurazepam** has a long duration of action and may produce daytime sedation; however, insomnia on withdrawal is rare.

2. **Temazepam** has an intermediate duration of action and is more helpful to patients who have difficulty remaining asleep than to those who cannot fall asleep.

3. Because **triazolam** is short-acting, it is useful for patients with initial insomnia and does not cause a hangover; however, rebound insomnia may occur when the drug is withdrawn.

III. AGITATION

A. **General Considerations** Agitation, the **behavioral manifestation of anxiety**, may be encountered in the office, in the emergency room, or in the inpatient wards. The acutely agitated medical patient is likely to be suffering from an organic brain syndrome caused by illness, medications, or drug or alcohol withdrawal.

B. **The Assaultive Patient** If the patient is assaultive, diagnostic efforts may have to be deferred until the **safety of physician and patient** can be guaranteed.

1. All agitated or frightening patients should be asked if they are **armed**. If the patient is armed a security guard or the police should disarm the patient if he does not surrender the weapon immediately. The physician should **never** participate directly in efforts to subdue or disarm a patient.

2. A **calm, reassuring approach** may decrease anxiety and with it, agitation.

3. If the patient does not relax, **restraint** may be necessary. One person should be assigned to each limb while a fifth coordinates the activity. Restrained patients must be under **constant** observation to prevent escape, strangulation, or myoglobinuria caused by prolonged struggling.

4. If the patient retains some control, **medication** may be offered orally. If not, drugs may be administered parenterally.

   a. If an organic brain syndrome may be present, administration of **haloperidol, paraldehyde, or hydroxyzine** is the safest.

   b. When the diagnosis is uncertain, a **benzodiazepine** or **haloperidol** may be effective. The onset of action of intramuscular benzodiazepines is too slow to be useful in emergency situations.

   c. Severely agitated patients with a well-defined **acute functional psychosis** (schizophrenia or mania) should be given a **sedating antipsychotic drug** (e.g., chlorpromazine) or should be rapidly tranquilized with 1 mg of haloperidol every one-half to 1 hr.

C. **Mental Status Examination** When the patient is calmer, a **mental status examination** must be performed to exclude organic brain disease.

1. Acute organic brain syndromes are characterized by a fluctuating level of

consciousness, disturbed attention and concentration, disorientation to time and place but not to person, and loss of short-term memory and abstracting ability.

a. Agitation in patients with organic brain syndromes often decreases with orienting the patient, reminding the patient of his location, of the reason for his hospitalization, of the names of physicians and nurses, and with keeping the lights on at night, minimizing visits by unfamiliar people, and providing a clock and calendar.

b. Agitation or organic brain syndromes caused by abstinence from tranquilizers, sleeping pills, or alcohol is treated with decreasing doses of phenobarbital or pentobarbital.

c. Demented patients with unpredictable assaultiveness may respond to propranolol, 80 to 320 mg/day.

IV. MULTIPLE PHYSICAL AND PSYCHIATRIC SYMPTOMS

A. **Multiple Somatic Complaints** When an occult physical illness is not present, **multiple somatic complaints** without an obvious etiology may be due to a psychiatric disorder, especially if factors listed in Table 8 are present.

Psychiatric conditions that may be associated with multiple physical complaints include grief, depression, anxiety, conversion hysteria, hypochondriasis, psychoses, organic brain syndrome malingering, and factitious disorder (Munchausen's syndrome).

Management of the patient with chronic complaints in excess of demonstrable pathology depends on the etiology. Mourning should be encouraged when physical complaints mimic the symptoms of a loved one who has died, whereas patients who consciously simulate disease for an obvious gain (malingering) or for the sole purpose of becoming a patient (factitious disorder) should be confronted. Anxiety, depression, and psychosis should be treated vigorously, whereas conversion symptoms usually resolve spontaneously.

Hypochrondriasis and related "somatization disorders" are characterized by behavior that is oriented toward demonstrating how sick the patients are. The symptoms intensify when the patients are told that they are not too ill and decrease in intensity when they are informed that they are sick and will receive regular ongoing follow-up. Although these patients complain that medications and other treatments are ineffective, they are unwilling to relinquish any drug to which they have become attached. Since physical symptoms are used to express emotions, excuse failures

---

TABLE 8. *Factors suggesting that unexplained physical complaints may be psychogenic*

Onset of symptoms in association with an obvious stress
Idiosyncratic or overly dramatic description of symptoms in great detail
Refusal to consider possible influence of psychological issues
New symptoms appear when the patient is otherwise improving
Pain experienced with equal intensity in two different locations at the same time
Multiple complaints present since adolescence

in life, and ensure ongoing contact with a physician, the goal of management is to accept the patient's psychological need for his symptoms while minimizing, but not abolishing, the amount of dysfunction the patient must demonstrate.

1. Although **the patient's claim to having a "bona fide" illness should not be challenged**, and his **suffering should be acknowledged without a promise of relief**, endless tests that may reveal minor abnormalities must be avoided. The patient may be told that although not all illnesses can be measured by currently available methods, **the physician believes that the patient's symptoms are real.**

2. **Ongoing follow-up by the same physician** is essential. Without regular contact with a doctor, the patient is likely to continue to demonstrate his illness in an attempt to prove that he needs continued care. Return appointments should be scheduled in advance **whether or not the patient feels ill** so that he may learn that ongoing care-taking is not dependent on feeling sick.

3. **Periodic rehospitalization** may be necessary at times of increased stress or when the patient is unsure of the physician's interest. A **discharge date should be agreed upon in advance** and should not be contingent on the patient's feeling entirely well.

4. The patient should be told that since the illness is a chronic one, too many emergency calls will discourage long-term care. Numerous calls between scheduled visits, regardless of their content, indicate that appointments should be scheduled more frequently.

5. Because the suggestion that their symptoms are psychogenic implies that the illness is not "real," most hypochondriacal patients are threatened by attempts to explore emotional conflicts and refuse to consider psychiatric consultation. It is best **not to insist on psychological insight** and to allow the patient, over time, to wonder whether stress plays a role in the worsening of symptoms.

6. While it is impossible to avoid prescribing medications, drugs should, whenever possible, be **mild and nonaddicting** (e.g., vitamins, antihistamines, and nonsteroidal anti-inflammatory drugs). **Analgesics should be prescribed regularly** rather than on a p.r.n. basis, which encourages preoccupation with pain and its relief. **Narcotics should be avoided.**

7. Care must be taken **not to dismiss manifestations of an intercurrent illness** that the patient exaggerates as he does all distress.

B. Drug Effects   Psychiatric medications may produce a number of side effects (Table 9) that **mimic physical or psychiatric disorders**. Most hypnotics, tranquilizers, and neuroleptics, and many antidepressants, can produce **CNS depression and paradoxical excitement** in elderly patients and in brain-injured patients, and many antidepressants and antipsychotic drugs produce anticholinergic and antiadrenergic side effects. Acute and chronic neurologic syndromes are common with neuroleptic therapy.

C. Psychiatric Symptoms   Psychiatric symptoms may also appear in response to many **medications or to nonprescription drugs used in medical practice.** Although virtually any medication can produce an acute organic brain syndrome, some preparations cause specific psychiatric disturbances (Table 10) unaccompan-

TABLE 9. *Some side effects of psychiatric drugs*

Syndrome	Manifestations
CNS depression	Lethargy, drowsiness, depression, decreased activity
Paradoxical reactions to tranquilizers and sedating drugs	Agitation, restlessness, excitement, insomnia, psychosis
Anticholinergic symptoms	Fever, tachycardia, blurred vision, dry mouth, constipation, urinary retention
Alpha adrenergic blockade	Orthostatic hypotension; interference with alpha adrenergic drugs
Retinitis pigmentosa	Pigmentary retinopathy with thioridazine >800 mg/day
Peripheral neuropathy	Caused by tricyclics, disulfiram, carbamazepine, or depression (due to prolonged sitting)
Extrapyramidal syndromes	
Parkinsonism	Rigidity, tremor, mask-like facies, hypersalivation, shuffling gate, appearing within a month, abating within 6 months
Acute dystonia	Torticollis, oculogyric crisis, opisthotonus, dystonic movements
Akathisia	Inner restlessness, inability to sit still, leg movements, fidgeting, agitation
Tardive dyskinesia	Involuntary abnormal movements of face and tongue; choreoathetoid movements of limbs and trunk appearing months to years after initiation of neuroleptic therapy
Catatonia	Waxy flexibility, negativism, withdrawal, parkinsonism. May be caused by antipsychotics, amphetamines, aspirin, ACTH, porphyria, diabetic ketoacidosis, hypercalcemia, hepatic encephalopathy, pellagra, glomerulonephritis
Neuroleptic malignant syndrome	Muscular rigidity, hyperthermia, stupor, coma, tachycardia, labile blood pressure, respiratory distress, diaphoresis, incontinence. Develops over 1–3 days, hours to months after starting haloperidol or thioridazine, or after withdrawal of sedative hypnotics. 20%–30% fatality. Treat with dantrolene
Irreversible mixed neurological syndrome	Fever, ataxia, lethargy, weakness, confusion, extrapyramidal syndromes, paralysis with lithium + haloperidol and thioridazine
Heat stroke	May occur in hot weather in patients taking anticholinergic drugs (decrease sweating) and neuroleptics (decrease thirst)
Lenticular opacities and pigmentation of skin, lens, and cornea	Seen in patients on long-term and/or high-dose neuroleptic therapy, especially chlorpromazine and thioridazine

ied by an alteration in cognition or consciousness. Whenever unexplained physical or mental changes occur, medications that may be responsible should be discontinued or changed if possible.

V. SEXUAL DISORDERS

A. General Considerations Sexual dysfunctions are common in medical patients, who seldom volunteer the problem unless they are asked directly. A survey of marital and sexual functioning should therefore be routine in all patients.

B. Treatment Techniques used to **treat** sexual dysfunctions include **reassurance** that the problem can be treated and **education** about sexual anatomy, physiology,

TABLE 10. Partial list of commonly used drugs that may produce psychiatric symptoms

Medication	Side effects
Corticosteroids and ACTH[a]	Depression, anxiety, mania hallucinations, paranoia
Cimetidine	Hallucinations
Anticonvulsants	Hallucinations, depression
Digitalis	Nightmares, paranoia, aggressiveness
L-DOPA	Depression, hallucinations, mania, nightmares, paranoia, aggressiveness
Amantadine	Nightmares, neurological symptoms
Indomethacin	Depression, hallucinations, paranoia
Propranolol	Depression, hallucinations, nightmares, paranoia
Ketamine	Nightmares, hallucinations, crying, changes in body image
Sulindac	Paranoia, aggressiveness

[a]Adrenocorticotrophic hormone.

and technique. With few exceptions, **both partners** must be involved in treatment, and **communication of sexual likes and dislikes** should be encouraged while **marital problems** that may be contributing to the problem are evaluated. During treatment a **ban** is placed on **intercourse** to relieve **performance anxiety**, and **physical pleasuring sessions** are prescribed in which the couple is instructed to take turns applying massage and other **nongenital forms of contact.** The couple then proceeds to **genital contact** and eventually to **intercourse.** Specific techniques are added for particular dysfunctions.

C. **Organic Causes**   Organic causes of sexual dysfunction (Tables 11 and 12) are not uncommon. For example, 40% to 45% of cases of impotence are caused by physical factors.

D. **Premature Ejaculation**   This is treated if the couple defines it as a problem. Recent onset of premature ejaculation suggests marital discord or disease of the

TABLE 11. Medications that may produce sexual dysfunctions

Sexual dysfunction	Medication
Loss of libido	Sedative-hypnotics, alcohol, narcotics, adrenal steroids, antiandrogens, chronic use of amphetamines and cocaine
Increased libido	L-DOPA, androgens, acute use of amphetamines, cocaine, and hallucinogens
Impotence	Anticholinergics, antiandrogens, reserpine, guanethidine, methyldopa, thioridazine, haloperidol
Retrograde ejaculation	Thioridazine
Retarded ejaculation	Haloperidol

TABLE 12. Some illnesses that may produce sexual dysfunctions

Any debilitating or painful illness	Multiple sclerosis
Genital and rectal disease	CNS disease
Alcohol and drug abuse	Peripheral neuropathy
Venereal disease	Liver disease or other cause of increased
Thyroid disease	estrogen or decreased androgen
Diabetes mellitus	

urethra, prostate, or CNS. Specific techniques, added to general approaches, must be practiced for a year in order to retrain the sexual response.

1. In the **start-stop technique**, the patient masturbates to the point of ejaculatory inevitability and then ceases all stimulation until his erection has receded halfway. The procedure is repeated four to five times, first by the patient alone and then by the couple during physical pleasuring sessions. When the couple has learned the technique, it is then practiced during intercourse in the female superior position.

2. The **squeeze technique** follows the same sequence but adds strong pressure on the penis by the partner, whose thumb is placed on the ventral surface of the frenulum and first and second fingers on the dorsal surface.

E. **Impotence**   Impotence is treated by focusing attention on pleasurable aspects of lovemaking, allowing erections that occur during physical pleasuring sessions to recede repeatedly until the patient and partner no longer worry about losing them. If erections are lost at any point in therapy, pleasuring sessions without genital contact are reinstituted.

F. **Inability to Reach Orgasm**   Inability to reach orgasm through intercourse may not be a dysfunction, since 60% to 70% of all women cannot reach an orgasm without manual or oral clitoral stimulation.

1. The simplest approach is to teach the partner to provide clitoral stimulation during intercourse.

2. If lax pubococcygeal muscles are present, exercises to strengthen them by repeatedly closing the rectal or urethral sphincter may be helpful.

3. Women who have never been orgasmic through any means should be taught to stimulate themselves to orgasm in order to learn approaches that may be helpful during intercourse.

G. **Difficulty with Lubrication**   Lubrication difficulty in women is analogous to impotence in men and is treated in a similar manner. **Sensory awareness exercises** during pleasuring sessions help the patient to focus her attention onto the pleasures of physical contact and away from worries about whether she will be able to lubricate. Older women who do not respond to reassurance that arousal takes longer with age may benefit from vaginal estrogen creams.

BIBLIOGRAPHY

Dubovsky, S. L., and Weissberg, M. P. (1982): *Clinical Psychiatry in Primary Care* (2nd Ed). Williams and Wilkins, Baltimore.
Hackett, T. P., and Cassem, N. H., editors (1978): *Handbook of General Hospital Psychiatry.* Mosby, St. Louis.
Mechanic, D. (1962): The concept of illness behavior. *J. Chronic Dis.*, 15:189–194.
Medical Letter (1981): Drugs that cause psychiatric symptoms. *Med. Lett.*, 23:9–12.
Murphy, G. L. (1975): The physician's responsibility for suicide. *Ann. Intern. Med.*, 82:301–309.
Strain, J. J., and Grassman, S., editors (1976): *Psychological Care of the Medically Ill.* Appleton, New York.

Subject Index